NURSE'S REFERENCE LIBRARY ®

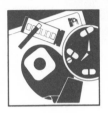

Patient Teaching

Nursing87 Books ™
Springhouse Corporation
Springhouse, Pennsylvania

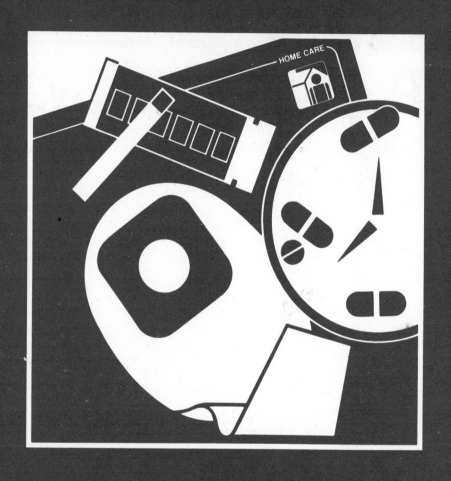

NURSE'S REFERENCE LIBRARY ®

Patient Teaching

Nursing87 Books ™
Springhouse Corporation
Springhouse, Pennsylvania

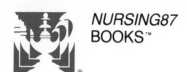

NURSING87
BOOKS™

Springhouse Corporation Book Division

CHAIRMAN
Eugene W. Jackson

VICE-CHAIRMAN
Daniel L. Cheney

PRESIDENT
Warren R. Erhardt

VICE-PRESIDENT AND DIRECTOR
Timothy B. King

VICE-PRESIDENT, BOOK OPERATIONS
Thomas A. Temple

VICE-PRESIDENT, CORPORATE OPERATIONS
Bacil Guiley

PROGRAM DIRECTOR, REFERENCE BOOKS
Stanley E. Loeb

Home care aids in this book, indicated by the graphic symbol shown here, may be reproduced by office copier for distribution to patients or their caregivers. Written permission is required for any other use or to copy any other material in this book.

Printed in the United States of America.

NRL10-011286

Library of Congress Cataloging-in-Publication Data
Patient teaching.

    (Nurse's reference library)
    "Nursing87 books."
    Bibliography: p.
    Includes index.
    1. Patient education.   2. Nurse and patient.
I. Springhouse Corporation.   II. Series.
[DNLM: 1. Patient Education—nurses' instruction. W 85 P298]
RT90.P3743   1987   610'.7'1   86-23001
ISBN 0-87434-086-1

NURSE'S REFERENCE LIBRARY®

Staff for this volume

EXECUTIVE EDITOR
Matthew Cahill

CLINICAL DIRECTOR
Barbara McVan, RN

ART DIRECTOR
Sonja E. Douglas

Clinical Editor: Joanne Patzek DaCunha, RN, BS

Contributing Clinical Editors: Margaret L. Belcher, RN, BSN; Kathleen Hannon, RN, BSN; Donna L. Hilton, RN, CCRN, CEN; Julie Tackenberg, RN, MA, CNRN

Text Editors: H. Nancy Holmes, Patricia Minard Shinehouse

Associate Editors: Elizabeth L. Mauro, June Norris

Contributing Editors: Martin DiCarlantonio, Barbara Hodgson, Roberta Kangilaski, Kevin J. Law, Alan Linn, Virginia Peck, Evelyn S. Ringold, Marylou Webster

Drug Information Manager: Larry Neil Gever, RPh, PharmD

Editorial Services Manager: David R. Moreau

Copy Editors: Diane M. Labus, Doris Weinstock, Debra Young

Contributing Copy Editors: Jaclyn A. Bootel, Sandra Buckley, Mary Durkin, Traci Ginnona, Wendy Walker

Production Coordinator: Sally Johnson

Senior Designer: Matie Anne Patterson

Designers: Linda Franklin, Antonia Gealt, Christopher Laird, Mary Wise

Illustrators: Maryanne Buschini, Steve Cusano, Design Management, Steve Early, Peter Gerritsen, John Gist, Linda Gist, Robert Jackson, Polly Krumbhaar-Lewis, Mark Mancini, Frank Margasak, Robert Neumann, Taylor Oughton, Patricia Perelburg, George Retseck, Eileen Rudnick, Dennis Schofield, Lauren Simeone, Joan Walsh

Art Production Manager: Robert Perry

Art Assistants: Loretta Caruso, Donald Knauss, Mark Marcin, Robert Wieder

Director of Composition/Editorial Services: David C. Kosten

Typographers: Elizabeth DiCicco, Diane Paluba, Nancy Wirs

Senior Production Manager: Deborah C. Meiris

Assistant Production Manager: Timothy A. Landis

Assistants: Maree E. DeRosa, Marlene C. Rosensweig

Special thanks to Ethel Halle, Carlos Lummus, and Minnie Bowen Rose, RN, BSN, MEd, who assisted in the preparation of this volume.

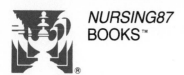

NURSING87
BOOKS™

NURSE'S REFERENCE LIBRARY®

This volume is part of a series conceived by the publishers of *Nursing87®* magazine and written by hundreds of nursing and medical specialists. This series, the NURSE'S REFERENCE LIBRARY, is the most comprehensive reference set ever created exclusively for the nursing profession. Each volume brings together the most up-to-date clinical information and related nursing practice. Each volume informs, explains, alerts, guides, educates. Taken together, the NURSE'S REFERENCE LIBRARY provides today's nurse with the knowledge and the skills that she needs to be effective in her daily practice and to advance in her career.

Other volumes in the series:

Diseases	Assessment	Practices
Diagnostics	Procedures	Emergencies
Drugs	Definitions	Signs & Symptoms

Other publications:

NEW NURSING SKILLBOOK™ SERIES

Giving Emergency Care Competently
Monitoring Fluid and Electrolytes Precisely
Assessing Vital Functions Accurately
Coping with Neurologic Problems Proficiently
Combatting Cardiovascular Diseases Skillfully

Nursing Critically Ill Patients Confidently
Dealing with Death and Dying
Managing Diabetes Properly
Giving Cardiovascular Drugs Safely

NURSING PHOTOBOOK™ SERIES

Providing Respiratory Care
Managing I.V. Therapy
Dealing with Emergencies
Giving Medications
Assessing Your Patients
Using Monitors
Providing Early Mobility
Giving Cardiac Care
Performing GI Procedures

Implementing Urologic Procedures
Controlling Infection
Ensuring Intensive Care
Coping with Neurologic Disorders
Caring for Surgical Patients
Working with Orthopedic Patients
Nursing Pediatric Patients
Helping Geriatric Patients
Carrying Out Special Procedures

NURSING NOW™ SERIES

Shock	Drug Interactions	Respiratory Emergencies
Hypertension	Cardiac Crises	Pain

NURSE'S CLINICAL LIBRARY®

Cardiovascular Disorders
Respiratory Disorders
Endocrine Disorders
Neurologic Disorders

Renal and Urologic Disorders
Gastrointestinal Disorders
Neoplastic Disorders
Immune Disorders

Nursing87 DRUG HANDBOOK™

NURSING YEARBOOK87

CLINICAL POCKET MANUAL™ SERIES

Diagnostic Tests	Cardiovascular Care	Surgical Care
Emergency Care	Respiratory Care	Medications and I.V.s
Fluids and Electrolytes	Critical Care	Ob/Gyn Care
Signs and Symptoms	Neurologic Care	Pediatric Care

NURSE REVIEW™

Contents

HOW TO TEACH PATIENTS

1 Understanding Basic Concepts

2 Assessing Learning Needs

3 Planning and Teaching

4 Evaluating Your Teaching

WHAT TO TEACH PATIENTS

5 Core Teaching Topics

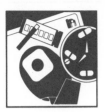

Advisory Board

At the time of publication, the advisors, clinical consultants, and contributors held the following positions.

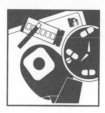

Clinical Consultants

Cheryl Conatser, RN, MS, Clinical Nurse Specialist, Children's Medical Center of Dallas

Sandra J. Cornett, RN, PhD, Patient Education Coordinator, Ohio State University Hospitals, Columbus

Ruth A. Crabbe, RN, MS, CNRN, CRRN, Assistant Professor of Clinical Nursing, University of Southern California, Los Angeles

Carolyn Garson, RN, MSN, University of Pennsylvania School of Nursing, Philadelphia

Sheila A. Glennon, RN, BSN, MA, CCRN, Critical Care Consultant, New York

Christine Grady, RN, MSN, CS, Clinical Nurse Specialist—Allergy, Immunology, Infectious Diseases, National Institutes of Health, Bethesda, Md.

Kathleen Whittaker Groves, RN, MS, Nursing Instructor, Department of Surgical Nursing, The Johns Hopkins Hospital, Baltimore

Marcia J. Hill, RN, MS, Manager, Dermatology, Methodist Hospital, Houston; Assistant Clinical Professor, Baylor College of Medicine, Houston

Jeanette D. Hines, RN, MA, Associate Professor, School of Nursing, San Diego State University

Leah S. Kinnaird, RN, MS, Director of Health Promotion, Baptist Hospital of Miami

Pamela Peters Long, RN, BSN, Director, Institute for Cancer Control, Northside Hospital, Atlanta

Mary Ann Marks, RN, MS, ACCE, Family Life Education Coordinator, Department of Health Promotion, Baptist Hospital of Miami

Ann R. Miller, RN, MS, Ambulatory Nurse Specialist, Beth Israel Hospital, Boston

Nina Olesinski, RN, MSN, Clinical Nurse Consultant, Ophthalmology and Otolaryngology, Eye and Ear Infirmary, University of Illinois, Chicago

Jo-Ellen Quinlan, RN, MSN, Gastrointestinal Nurse Clinician, Division of Gastroenterology, Children's Hospital, Boston

Dorothy A. Ruzicki, RN, PhD, Patient Education/Research Coordinator, Sacred Heart Medical Center, Spokane, Wash.

Kay Freeman Sauers, RN, BSN, MS, Clinical Nurse Specialist in Orthopedics, Trauma Rehabilitation Unit, Montebello Hospital Center, Baltimore

Janice Selekman, RN, DNSc, Associate Professor, Thomas Jefferson University, Philadelphia

Arlene B. Strong, RN, MN, ANP, Adult Nurse Practitioner, Anticoagulation Clinic and Cardiology, Veterans Administration Medical Center, Portland, Ore.

Gail Thatcher, RN, MSN, Patient Education Coordinator, Albert Einstein Medical Center–Northern Division, Philadelphia

Contributors

Arlene L. Androkites, RN, BSN, CNP, Nurse Practitioner in Oncology, Dana Farber Cancer Institute, Boston

Regina Blumenstein Butler, RN, Hemophilia Coordinator/Hematology Nurse Specialist, The Children's Hospital of Philadelphia

Marlene M. Ciranowicz, RN, MSN, Independent Nurse Consultant, Dresher, Pa.

Maribel J. Clements, RN, MA, Clinical Associate, Puget Sound Blood Center, Seattle

Charmaine Cummings, RN, MSN, Clinical Nurse Educator, Neurology, Eye and Aging Research Nursing Service, National Institutes of Health, Bethesda, Md.

Betty Dale, RN, BSN, Head Nurse, Operating Room, Abbott-Northwestern Hospital, Minneapolis

Rosemary Drigan, RN, MEd, CRNP, Nurse Practitioner in Oncology, Dana Farber Cancer Institute, Boston

Catherine Kelley Foran, RN, MSN, Independent Nurse/Consultant, Cherry Hill, N.J.

Gerri George, RN, MSN, President and Cofounder, SBI/Some Body Maternity Fitness Program, Bala Cynwyd, Pa.

Richard K. Gibson, RN, MN, JD, Critical Care Nurse, Kaiser Foundation Hospital, San Diego

Sandra K. Crabtree Goodnough, RN, MSN, Director, Research Support Services, Hermann Hospital, Houston

Janice F. Hansen, RN, CMA, Patient and Community Health Education Coordinator, Rutland (Vt.) Regional Medical Center

Miriam R. Horwitz, RN, MS, President, Executive Search Consultants, Inc., Boston

Lynn Kreutzer-Baraglia, RN, MS, Assistant Professor, West Suburban College of Nursing, Oak Park, Ill.

Deborah J. LaCamera, RN, BSN, CIC, Nurse Epidemiologist, Clinical Center, National Institutes of Health, Bethesda, Md.

Patricia W. McAlary, RN, MS, Clinical Assistant to the Director, Boston Pain Center, Spaulding Rehabilitation Hospital

Marianne K. Ostrow, RN, BSN, Clinical Nurse III, Thomas Jefferson University Hospital, Philadelphia

Beverly A. Post, RN, MS, Infection Control Coordinator, Louis A. Weiss Memorial Hospital, Chicago

Madeline T. Pozzi, RN, MSN, Clinical Nurse IV, Clinical Nurse Specialist, Orthopedics, Thomas Jefferson University Hospital, Philadelphia

Pamela Rowe, RN, BSN, MEd, Assistant Director for Nursing Education, Mary Hitchcock Memorial Hospital, Hanover, N.H.

Dorothy A. Ruzicki, RN, PhD, Patient Education/Research Coordinator, Sacred Heart Medical Center, Spokane, Wash.

Mary Jo Sagaties, RN, MSN, FNP-C, Nurse Practitioner/Ophthalmic Photographer, Leahey Eye Clinic, Lowell, Mass.

Ellen Shipes, RN, MN, ET(C), MEd, Clinical Nurse Specialist, Enterostomal Therapy, Vanderbilt University Hospital, Nashville, Tenn.

Frances J. Storlie, RN, PhD, CANP, Director, Personal Health Services, Southwest Washington Health District, Vancouver

Joan E. Watson, RN, PhD, Assistant Professor, Graduate Program in Nursing Education, School of Nursing, University of Pittsburgh

Janette R. Yanko, RN, MN, CNRN, Neuro Clinical Nurse Specialist, Nursing Department, Research and Development, Allegheny General Hospital, Pittsburgh

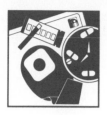

Foreword

Today, your nursing responsibilities are more likely than ever before to involve decisive patient teaching—especially in light of growing professional, fiscal, and legal demands for better patient education.

But how confident do you feel in your role as a teacher? Do you sometimes worry that you won't have enough time to teach your patients all they need to know before they're discharged? Are you sometimes uncertain about the best way to present information? Do you have trouble obtaining teaching materials that your patients can understand?

Patient Teaching, the latest volume in the Nurse's Reference Library, provides the resources and the guidelines you need to teach patients confidently and competently. For easy reference, this book is divided into two major sections: how to teach patients and what to teach them. The first section is designed to help you improve your teaching skills and avoid common pitfalls. The second section covers the teaching content for various disorders, tests, treatments, and home care procedures.

The initial four chapters of the book constitute the first section. Chapter 1 presents basic principles of teaching and learning: How people learn best and differences in learning styles. It also discusses the legal implications of patient teaching for nurses. Chapters 2 through 4 parallel the nursing process: Chapter 2 covers assessment of learning needs, then Chapter 3 explains how to plan and effectively implement your teaching. Chapter 4 tells you how to evaluate what the patient has learned and how well you've taught.

The next 16 chapters cover what to teach the patient. Chapter 5 covers the core information you'll have to teach each patient, such as hospital routines, facts about the disorder, and an explanation of treatments.

Chapters 6 through 16 deal with different body systems and include the disorders that involve significant patient teaching. Each disorder is covered in a standard format, beginning with an introduction that identifies the major teaching topics for that disorder and singles out any difficulties to anticipate in teaching. After this introduction is a section called *Describe the disorder*, which serves as a synopsis of the type, causes, and pathophysiology of the disorder.

The next section, *Point out possible complications*, underscores the importance of effective teaching by describing the complications that may occur if the patient doesn't comply with the prescribed medical regimen. The following section, *Teach about tests*, discusses the diagnostic tests for which you may have to prepare a patient. The final section, *Teach about treatments*, reviews the types and rationales of treatments that may be done in the hospital or in the patient's home. It emphasizes the teaching points that will help the patient prevent recurrence or aggravation of the disorder.

Special chapters on infection and cancer address the unique teaching challenges of these disorders. A chapter on comfort and support covers such teaching topics as pain control and care of the dying patient and his family. And a chapter on health promotion gives advice on diet, exercise, accident prevention, and other considerations for maintaining lifelong health.

Throughout the book, you'll find numerous charts, illustrations, and special features that will make your teaching easier and more effective. For example, you'll discover more than 80 *home care aids* that you can photocopy and give to patients. Clearly written and illustrated, these invaluable aids offer step-by-step instructions, guidelines, and tips for a wide range of home health care topics—from taking medications to caring for a tracheostomy tube.

Another feature of this book that you'll find useful are the diagnostic test charts in each body-system chapter. These charts summarize the purpose and teaching points for hundreds of tests. Equally useful drug charts outline the adverse reactions, interactions, and major teaching points for commonly prescribed drugs. And special *Surgery* sections discuss selected procedures.

What's more, a special graphic symbol, *Checklist*, identifies the major topics to cover when you teach about a given disorder. Another graphic symbol, *Inquiry*, alerts you to question-and-answer guides that prepare you for questions that patients are likely to ask about their disorder or treatment.

The book closes with an appendix that summarizes your teaching responsibilities in more than 50 selected health problems. And a directory of health organizations tells you where to obtain additional information.

In short, *Patient Teaching* is a comprehensive, easy-to-use reference that helps you teach patients effectively and efficiently. Now more than ever, when you have only limited time to spend with each patient, you need to make every teaching moment count. *Patient Teaching* can help you achieve this goal by improving your teaching skills and by outlining your teaching responsibilities.

Dorothy A. Ruzicki, RN, PhD

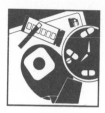

Overview

As nurses, we've always taught our patients. But never before has there been so great a need for us to be truly expert teachers, learning and practicing the most effective techniques. The social, technologic, and economic changes currently rocking the health care industry demand more masterful patient education. And it's up to us to meet this demand.

The trend toward health promotion

Social changes account for some of the most profound trends in health care today. For example, over the past decade, more and more people have become interested in personal health and fitness. What's more, as research has linked certain cardiovascular diseases and other health problems to life-style practices, more and more people have taken steps to correct unhealthful habits.

Today, nurses are in the forefront of health promotion. Day in and day out, we teach patients how to prevent illness, achieve wellness, and ultimately maintain health. And increasingly, we're doing our teaching in alternative health care settings, such as community nursing centers, urgent care centers, and ambulatory care units.

This trend toward health promotion has also gained momentum because people are living longer than ever before, thanks to continued medical advances. That makes teaching patients how to maintain good health even more crucial. But what happens when chronic illness threatens to diminish the advantage of a longer lifespan? Then, your teaching must emphasize the importance of compliance to achieve the best quality of life possible. To help persuade chronically ill patients that good health care can make a difference, you'll need to encourage them to become active partners in planning and providing their own care.

Getting patients to comply with prescribed treatment has always been a primary goal of patient teaching. But today, we're educating patients so they can make better decisions about their health care and assume greater responsibility for it. To help patients become well-informed health care consumers, we must be prepared to teach them and their families on a more sophisticated level. For example, when discussing treatment choices, we must present thorough, unbiased information about each option—its advantages and disadvantages, plus its possible side effects or complications.

The technology explosion

Technologic changes—in the form of new and better tests, treatments, and medical equipment—are being introduced into many hospitals at such a rapid rate that "accepted" knowledge and techniques are constantly becoming obsolete. This influx of new technology makes it crucial for us to remain up to date and well informed, so we can provide our patients with the latest information. Consider, for example, the proliferation of self-testing equipment, such as computerized blood pressure monitors and blood glucose meters. As this type of "high-tech" equipment becomes available for home use, our teaching responsibilities will increase to smooth the patient's transition from hospital to home.

Soaring health care costs

Economic changes, designed to control costs, are behind some of the most far-reaching trends affecting the health care industry. In particular, the revised system of federal reimbursement for Medicare—from a retrospective to a prospective payment system based on Diagnosis-Related Groups (DRGs)—has shortened the average hospital stay. As a result, patients are more likely to be discharged while still needing complex equipment, such as mechanical ventilators, or skilled care, such as postoperative wound care. And you'll have only limited time in which to prepare them and their families for such home care.

Fortunately, patient teaching has two big payoffs when it comes to controlling costs: It makes the patient more self-sufficient by bolstering his confidence in caring for himself, and it teaches him to anticipate postdischarge complications and seek medical attention early—at times, preventing rehospitalization.

Preparing for the future

If we're to meet the demand for more masterful patient education, we must prepare today. After all, teaching—like nursing—is a skill that must be practiced to be mastered. And *Patient Teaching* is the guide we need to practice that skill efficiently and effectively. In particular, I found the book's discussion on documentation and the legal implications of patient teaching for nurses especially informative. After all, if a patient incurs harm because he lacked information about his condition or care, he may sue his nurse for negligence.

I urge every nurse—from the staff nurse in a large hospital to the home care nurse in a small community—to invest in a copy of *Patient Teaching*.

Frances J. Storlie, RN, PhD, CANP

1

Understanding Basic Concepts

Understanding Basic Concepts

Introduction

In the past, we've taught patients because they've needed to know about their illnesses, their tests and treatments, and their home care regimens. Today, we still teach for the same reasons. But we do so with a new outlook on teaching brought about by growing professional, fiscal, and legislative demands for more efficient patient education. More than ever before, we need to be masterful teachers, learning and practicing the most effective techniques.

What is patient teaching?

First of all, it's something we do formally, with planning and deliberation. We also do it informally, whenever we take time to answer a patient's spontaneous question. We do it through explanation, demonstration, role playing, and teamwork.

Teaching, in effect, is an active process that aims to produce an observable change in the patient's behavior or attitude. The key words here are *active*, *process*, and *change*.

Active reflects the need for the patient's involvement. *Process* signals an ongoing series of actions or events that aim to help the patient learn how to maintain or improve his current health status. And *change* refers to acquiring new knowledge, new skills, or new values or beliefs.

How to teach effectively

To be effective teachers, we must do our own homework. We must control the learning environment, establish priorities for what our patients need to learn, supply instructional materials, and enlist the help of other staff members. We must also use appropriate teaching techniques and evaluate their outcome. More often than not, we do prepare for teaching, perhaps unconsciously. For example, by providing privacy while teaching, we control the learning environment and help reduce the patient's anxiety. By deciding that a newly diagnosed diabetic needs to learn injection technique and site rotation before leg and foot care, we establish priorities for learning. By supplying him with pictures and pamphlets, we reinforce or supplement our oral teaching.

Besides doing our homework, we need to look at our "classroom" to be effective teachers. A hospital or clinic, after all, isn't usually an inviting place for learning. Its staff, rules, and rituals are typically unfamiliar to the patient. As a result, the patient often feels especially vulnerable, creating a barrier to learning that we must overcome to teach effectively.

In contrast to the emotional distance a hospital or clinic setting invites, the relationship between ourselves and patients is likely to be closer than that between most teachers and learners. As nurses, we provide both physical and emotional care, allowing an intimacy rarely found in other teaching situations.

Who benefits from effective teaching?

The patient, of course. He benefits by learning how to maintain or improve his current condition. However, because the patient is the targeted beneficiary of this process, we typically evaluate teaching solely on the change produced in his attitude or behavior. Teaching, though, is a reciprocal activity: you may change your teaching methods as a result of the patient's feedback.

You and your patient aren't the only ones who benefit. Effective teaching also benefits the entire health care system. Research is beginning to show that the patient who has been taught about his condition and treatment seems to be leaving the hospital earlier. And the patient who's better able to understand and implement his home care plan has allowed more efficient use of personnel and equipment.

Thus, the hospital, clinic, and community as a whole can benefit from effective patient teaching.

THE CLIMATE FOR TEACHING

The Changing Direction of Patient Teaching

Within the past decade, various socioeconomic factors, role redefinitions, and revised professional standards have combined to change the direction of our teaching efforts. Perhaps the two areas of greatest change involve the patient's role as an active participant in health care and our role in assessing learning needs and planning to meet them.

The patient as participant

In the past, our teaching efforts usually focused on gaining the patient's passive compliance with the prescribed medical regimen. Today, the thrust of our efforts has shifted toward promoting the patient's active involvement in his care plan.

What brought about this shift in emphasis? One factor is the growing consumer awareness of health care issues and services. For example, today's patient is more likely to seek a second opinion before surgery or to ask for explanations of drug effects. The mother of a child with chronic otitis media may tell the doctor, "Don't start Billy on that antibiotic—he's never responded to it in the past and we'll just waste time." Before, she probably would have automatically followed the doctor's orders rather than pose objections.

Of course, not all of your patients will be as assertive as Billy's mother. Rather, most patients you encounter will probably fall somewhere in the middle—between a passive learner and an active one. This middle group of patients, though, can be favorably influenced by teaching that's well planned and well carried out.

Patient's bill of rights

In 1972, the American Hospital Association gave formal support to this new participatory outlook by publishing "A Patient's Bill of Rights." While not a legal document, this bill attempts to set a standard for state-of-the-art health care and to ensure quality care and greater satisfaction for both patient and health care provider. Seven statements in the "Bill of Rights" deal with information the patient receives and accord him the right to know about his health problem, health status, treatments, alternative care measures, and continuing care requirements, and about hospital regulations. This recognition of the patient's right to information promotes his participation in his health care. It also challenges nurses to assess the patient's readiness to learn and to incorporate the patient's goals into the care plan.

Changes in the health care payment system

Another major influence on your teaching role has come from the legislative response to soaring health care costs. These escalating costs, especially Medicare costs, have resulted from a *retrospective* payment system—a system that paid for care after it was provided and failed to discourage inefficient use of personnel, time, and equipment. In 1983, the U.S. government's Health Care Financing Administration responded by developing a *prospective* payment system—a system that pays a fixed fee, established in advance, for a specific illness, or diagnosis-related group (DRG). This system has dramatically affected medical and nursing practice and has shortened the average hospital stay.

Under this new system, patients may be discharged from the hospital even though they require continued care at home, which, of course, increases the demand for timely and effective teaching. Patients may undergo batteries of diagnostic tests and procedures as outpatients, which naturally doesn't reduce, and in fact often increases, their teaching needs. Patients may also undergo same-day surgery, but they and their families now need to know about postoperative care measures imperative to safety and comfort—such as positioning after a tonsillectomy and administration of analgesics.

Shortened hospital stays require intensive patient teaching, as well as planning for follow-up care and teaching by someone other than the care

planner, such as a home health nurse. Because of decreased time with the patient and his family in the hospital, we nurses need to teach "survival skills" first—those skills that the patient must have to care for himself safely and effectively upon discharge. As a result, we need to set priorities in our teaching plan.

Growing numbers of acutely ill patients

Under DRGs, the hospitalized patient today is usually more acutely ill than in the past. This means that his physiologic needs are necessarily more complex, which puts an even greater burden on your time. Understandably, you may find it difficult to monitor one patient with renal failure, provide wound care for another, balance fluids and electrolytes in a third, and still teach a fourth about respiratory distress syndrome. Setting priorities in situations like these isn't easy, but it's necessary.

Even given enough time and your commitment to teach, you may still be faced with a patient so ill that you question his ability and readiness to learn.

Increased longevity

Medical advances have helped significantly extend life expectancy and, as a result, have increased the number of chronically ill patients. And because many of these patients live independently and assume responsibility for their own care, they need to become willing partners in planning it. Our responsibility is increasingly to teach these patients self-care in a way that encourages collaboration and mutual problem solving. For example, in teaching an elderly diabetic about proper nutrition and exercise, you'll need to recognize the patient's preferences and test the feasibility of your instructions. In teaching a Parkinson's patient about safety, you'll need to know about his willingness and ability to modify his home environment to facilitate daily activities.

THE CHALLENGE OF TEACHING ACUTELY ILL PATIENTS

Because the typical hospitalized patient today is more acutely ill than in the past, you're facing a challenge in providing appropriate teaching. The patient's physical care alone can demand such large blocks of your time and can involve such complex equipment and procedures that teaching often is incomplete or, worse yet, not done at all.

The illustration here shows the range of demands acute illness places on the patient and you. These demands underscore the need for planning your teaching carefully to make learning effective.

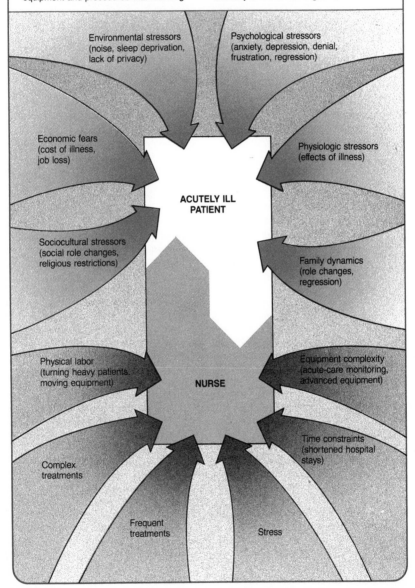

Environmental stressors (noise, sleep deprivation, lack of privacy)

Psychological stressors (anxiety, depression, denial, frustration, regression)

Economic fears (cost of illness, job loss)

Physiologic stressors (effects of illness)

ACUTELY ILL PATIENT

Sociocultural stressors (social role changes, religious restrictions)

Family dynamics (role changes, regression)

Physical labor (turning heavy patients, moving equipment)

Equipment complexity (acute-care monitoring, advanced equipment)

NURSE

Complex treatments

Time constraints (shortened hospital stays)

Frequent treatments

Stress

Legal Implications for Nurses

Greater patient participation in health care has led to an informed-consent philosophy, which promotes educated decision making by patients. In the past, for example, an epileptic patient was told when to take his medication; if he failed to take it as directed, he was considered noncompliant. Today, an epileptic patient can help plan medication regimens around his own lifestyle needs and identified trigger factors. Similarly, an epileptic patient who decides to stop her anticonvulsant medication while pregnant, if adequately informed, is no longer considered noncompliant but to be making a personal health decision.

In effect, we're now educating patients so they can make better decisions about their health care and assume greater responsibility for it. However, we still bear the responsibility for providing appropriate teaching.

Nurse practice act
The legal basis for our patient-teaching responsibilities rests in the nurse practice act. Although somewhat different from state to state, this act establishes licensing procedures and defines the practice of nursing within each state's jurisdiction. These guidelines for practice describe the nurse's participation in health education and are regarded as a professional standard.

Using the nurse practice act and the patient's bill of rights, the courts have placed responsibility on the nurse for timely and appropriate teaching. Several cases clearly illustrate this point. For example, in the 1944 case *Bernard v. Gravois*, a family alleged that a nurse failed to teach them how to use an electric heating pad correctly and that because of her oversight the patient burned himself. However, the court decided that the nurse had indeed given proper instruction and that the patient's injury occurred when a family member negligently carried out the instructions.

A Louisiana court ruled on a similar issue in 1983 (*Crawford v. Earl K. Long Hospital et al.*). The case involved a young boy who had been struck in the head with a baseball bat. The boy was examined by a doctor in the emergency department and found asymptomatic. The doctor then told a nurse to telephone the boy's mother and ask her to have someone take the boy home. The mother came to the hospital and took her son home. The next morning, she found him dead. In court, the mother alleged that she was given no instructions by the nurse or doctor to wake her son at regular intervals to check for arousability and coherence. But the nurse testified that she had indeed instructed the patient's mother. In fact, she pointed out that she had insisted for instructional purposes that the mother come to the hospital to pick up her son instead of letting the boy return home in a taxi, as the mother had requested.

In both of these cases, the court absolved the nurse of liability for the patient's poor outcome, with the verdict hinging on her implementation of teaching responsibilities.

A safeguard
Clear, complete documentation provides your legal protection if a patient claims he was harmed by improper teaching. In fact, failure to properly document your teaching can be interpreted in a court of law to suggest that you provided substandard nursing care even if you taught the patient thoroughly and felt confident about his response. So, complete documentation of your teaching and the patient's response to it represents your best defense against malpractice claims. An old saying can be applied to patient teaching: if you didn't document it, you didn't teach it.

TEACHING AND LEARNING

How Nurses Teach

Learning takes place through a planned sequence of activities. These activities can be formal—such as structured individual or group teaching sessions—or informal—such as conversations and the incidental instructions that are given during routine patient care. Whether carried out formally or informally, the teaching process goes through four steps familiar to every nurse: assessing, planning, implementing, and evaluating. But accomplishing these tasks involves more than just providing the patient with information.

Assessing

A careful assessment of your patient's learning ability and his learning needs related to his health problem forms the cornerstone of effective patient education and must precede any teaching. Your assessment must also address the patient's emotional readiness to learn. Trying to teach a patient about ostomy pouch application without recognizing that he's still unwilling to look at his stoma can only frustrate both you and the patient. This patient isn't emotionally prepared to learn the procedure even if it *is* on the teaching plan.

Assessment necessarily includes interviewing the patient's family members. This is most important when the patient is a young child or is mentally incapacitated, since you'll be directing most of your teaching to the family. In general, however, viewing the patient as a member of his family is vital to the teaching process, since the family network has the potential to facilitate or hinder your teaching efforts.

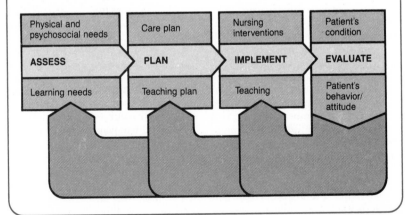

HOW THE TEACHING PROCESS PARALLELS THE NURSING PROCESS

The steps of the teaching process parallel those of the nursing process, but they take a different slant. The nursing process emphasizes planning and implementing care based on assessing the patient's physical and psychosocial needs. The teaching process identifies teaching content and methods based on assessing the patient's learning needs. Both processes are circular, with ongoing assessment and evaluation constantly redirecting your planning and teaching.

Physical and psychosocial needs	Care plan	Nursing interventions	Patient's condition
ASSESS	**PLAN**	**IMPLEMENT**	**EVALUATE**
Learning needs	Teaching plan	Teaching	Patient's behavior/ attitude

Assessing family dynamics—the way family members relate to the patient and to each other—will also help you tailor your teaching plan to the patient's learning needs. The wife who says, "Let me tell him what the tests show," or the husband who says, "I don't want my daughter to know her mother has cancer just yet," is regulating the flow of information among family members. Such regulation affects the way the patient and family adapt to a crisis.

Of course, the family is a dynamic unit. Its function and reliability as a unit will change as each member reacts to various stressors throughout the patient's hospitalization. Not all families have the ability to maintain cohesion and the growth of their members, and these families especially can present a formidable teaching problem. For example, attempting to teach a behavior modification program to the divorced parents of a head-injured child can be difficult if poor communication exists between the parents. Continuity of care may be affected when each parent interprets the program according to a personal perception of the child.

A family's learning readiness and needs require ongoing assessment. That's because the family's willingness and ability to learn will affect the patient's learning progress. So, when dealing with the patient's family, be sure to observe both verbal and nonverbal communication. Doing this will help you identify family members who can hinder the patient's learning and thus require you to modify your teaching plan. It will also help you identify family members who can provide you with accurate information about the patient and can support him when you're implementing the teaching plan. Often a family member can persuade a patient to follow instructions or to attempt procedures he refused to try for you.

Planning
As a teacher, one of your roles is to design a plan that enhances patient learning. To do this effectively, you'll need to clarify objectives, set priorities, and organize information. In addition, you'll need to choose appropriate teaching methods and select supporting material.

Your teaching plan should include specific learning goals that you and your patient have agreed upon and the teaching strategies that will best help him meet these goals. For an ostomy patient, you're responsible for deciding which tasks he's ready to learn now and which need to be postponed until he's emotionally ready. For a same-day surgery patient, you're responsible for ensuring continuity of care by providing a mechanism for follow-up teaching.

Implementing
Actually carrying out your teaching plan necessarily involves all the other steps in the teaching process. As you interact with the patient, you're constantly reassessing how well he's learning and then planning again to make your teaching more effective.

Evaluating
The final step in the teaching process leads you to examine how well the patient has learned the necessary material—and, by extension, how well you've taught it. Often, evaluation restarts the teaching process, because it provides direction for changes in the other three steps that can help your patient meet his established learning goals. It also enables you to refine your skills as a teacher and to develop more effective methods.

Documenting
One goal of your teaching plan is to provide continuity of care for your patient. And one way to accomplish this is through careful documentation.

Your documentation should reveal what teaching you've planned and accomplished, and what the patient has learned. This information saves time and prevents duplication of patient-

DOCUMENTING YOUR TEACHING

Accurate and detailed documentation helps assure continuity in teaching. It tells other members of the health care team what has been planned for the patient, what has already been carried out, and what remains to be done. It ensures that no one duplicates teaching efforts.

Careful documentation also protects you legally. If the patient claims he was harmed because you supplied inadequate instructions or provided none at all, your legal protection rests on documentation of your teaching and the patient's response. Documentation can support your judgment in setting priorities for learner needs, selecting teaching methods, and evaluating

---

Westphal, Joseph ①
SS 860-46-3954

Date ② Time
1-14-87 0900

③
64 y.o. man c̄ newly diagnosed Parkinson's requiring flexibility exercises for mobility. Pt + health care team have agreed
on exercise program. Pt has agreed to perform exercises ④
b.i.d. to his level of tolerance. Pt exhibits positive coping
mechanisms + personal relations, which should aid learning.
⑤   Maggi Breezler, RN

1100 ⑥
Flexibility exercises initiated c̄ ⑦ explanation + demonstration
of upper extremity activities. Explanation presented separately from questions, as pt prefers to "understand what ⑧
to do c̄ doing the activity. Pt return demonstrated ⑨
exercises under supervision + then independently 3 error ⑩
Pt states he knows how to do the exercises. Illustrated ⑫
examples left c̄ pt for his review. ⑪ Maggi Breezler, RN

1500
Pt needs assistance c̄ transfer to chair. On-off syndrome
being considered by M.D. Lower extremity exercises discussed
+ demonstrated. Pt unable to perform exercises. Pt correctly ⑬
indicates yes-no regarding execution of these exercises. Will
evaluate actual performance of exercises at another time.
                                        Maggi Breezler, RN

1-19-87
1400
Pt states, "Exercises are no use. This disease will stop me
whenever it wants." Pt anger at disease presenting a barrier ⑭
to discharge teaching. Discharge planning + teaching being
done c̄ wife until pt willing to participate. Discharge instructions given to wife, who demonstrates knowledge of inform- ⑮
ation by correctly responding to questions. Arrangements
made c̄ community nurse for home safety
evaluation. ⑯   Maggi Breezler, RN
⑰

learned tasks. For instance, statements of your patient's willingness and ability to learn can support your suggestion that certain teaching be done at a later date or even after discharge.

The following example—for a patient with Parkinson's disease—shows the kind of information you should document.

1. Patient's name and social security number on every record page

2. Date and time of each teaching session

3. Patient's health status and corresponding learning needs

4. Precise learning goal(s) agreed on by health care team and patient

5. Identified learning enhancements

6. Actual teaching you carry out

7. Specific teaching methods you use

8. Patient's characteristics as a learner

9. Precise description of exactly what occured, avoiding broad terms such as "learned well" and "seems to understand"

10. Your evaluation of patient's change or learning

11. Patient's response to teaching/learning experience, using his own words and behaviors

12. Specific teaching materials you use

13. Indications that patient or family member understands instructions

14. Identified learning barriers

15. Final progress notes with discharge teaching about diet, medications, physical activity, and follow-up care

16. Legible writing

17. Your signature

teaching activities. It allows other members of the health care team to begin instruction where you've left off—something that's especially important in units with floating staff and frequent reassignments.

• *What to include.* Since 1976, the Joint Commission for the Accreditation of Hospitals (JCAH) has mandated that medical records show evidence of informed consent and final progress notes. These notes should include specific instructions to the patient and/or his family about physical activity, medication, diet, and follow-up care.

The JCAH requires documentation that the patient not only received instruction in these areas but also understood it. This documentation must include the patient's response to teaching and an assessment of his progress toward learning goals.

With this information, it's possible for you and others to evaluate teaching effectiveness. (See *Documenting Your Teaching.*)

How Your Teaching Approach Affects Learning

So much of the teaching process rests on accurate assessment of the patient's learning readiness and ability. Thus, understanding the developmental stages of personality can aid your assessment: you can assess the patient against models of psychosocial and intellectual (cognitive) development.

All aspects of development are continuous, concurrent, and interrelated. Just as a person follows a pattern of physical growth and development, he also follows patterns of emotional, psychological, and cognitive development. These patterns conform to stages, and the characteristics of growth (developmental tasks) within the stages have been described by Erikson, Piaget, and others. The patient's level of physical, emotional, and psychological development directly influences his readiness and willingness to learn.

Erikson's developmental stages

Psychoanalyst Erik Erikson describes the physical, emotional, and psychological stages of development and relates specific issues, or developmental work or *tasks*, to each stage. For example, if an infant's physical and emotional needs are met sufficiently, he completes his task—developing the ability to trust others. However, a person who's stymied in an attempt at task mastery may go on to the next stage but continue to carry with him the remnants of the unfinished task. For example, if a toddler isn't allowed to learn by doing, he develops a sense of shame and doubt in his abilities, which may complicate later attempts at independence. Similarly, a preschooler who's made to feel that the activities he initiates are bad may develop a sense of guilt that hinders his taking the initiative later in life. (See *Erikson's Stages of Development*, page 11.)

Piaget and cognition

Much of your teaching involves cognitive abilities: sharing information with the patient and looking for signs that he understands it. As a result, it's important to understand cognitive stages.

Child psychologist Jean Piaget describes the mechanism (cognition) by which the mind processes new information. Piaget says a person assimilates, or understands, whatever information fits into his established view of the world. When information doesn't fit, the person must reexamine and adjust his thinking to accommodate the new information. Piaget describes four stages of cognitive development and relates them to a person's ability to accommodate and assimilate new information.

The *sensorimotor* stage lasts from birth to 2 years. In it, the child learns about himself and his environment through motor and reflex actions. Thought derives from sensation and movement. The child learns that he's separate from his environment and that aspects of his environment—such as his parents or favorite toys—continue to exist even though they may be outside the reach of his senses. Your teaching, then, for a child in this stage should be geared to the sensorimotor system. You can modify behavior by using the senses: a frown, a stern or soothing voice—all serve as appropriate techniques to elicit desired behavior.

The *preoperational* stage begins about the time the child starts to talk and continues to about age 7. Using his new knowledge of language, the child begins to use symbols to represent objects, and early in this stage he also personifies objects. He's now better able to think about things and events that aren't immediately present. But he's unable to think through a series of actions; he still must perform them. Oriented to the present, the child has difficulty conceptualizing time. His thinking is influenced by fantasy—the way he'd like things to be—and he assumes that others see situations from his point of view. He assimilates information and then changes it in his mind to fit his ideas.

Because of the child's undeveloped sense of time and vivid fantasies, you'll be challenged to present information in a time frame that allows for questions and learning without fostering rumination. Using neutral words, body outlines, and equipment a child can touch gives him an active role in learning.

The *concrete* stage begins to appear at the time the child enters first grade and lasts into early adolescence. During this stage, accommodation increases. The child develops an ability to think abstractly and to make rational judgments about concrete or observable phenomena, which in the past he needed to physically manipulate to understand. Concrete objects must be within sight, however, for these thought

ERIKSON'S STAGES OF DEVELOPMENT

Infant
Trust vs. mistrust
Needs maximum comfort with minimal
uncertainty in order to trust himself,
others, and environment

Toddler
Autonomy vs. shame and doubt
Works to master physical environment
while maintaining self-esteem

Preschooler
Initiative vs. guilt
Begins to initiate, not imitate, activities;
develops conscience and sexual identity

School-age child
Industry vs. inferiority
Tries to develop a sense of self-worth
by refining skills

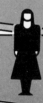

Adolescent
Identity vs. role confusion
Tries integrating many roles (child, sibling,
student, athlete, worker) into a self-image
under role model and peer pressure

Young adult
Intimacy vs. isolation
Learns to make personal commitment to
another as spouse, parent, partner

Middle-aged adult
Generativity vs. stagnation
Seeks satisfaction through productivity
in career, family, civic interests

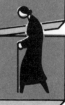

Older adult
Integrity vs. despair
Reviews life accomplishments, deals with
loss and preparation for death

processes to occur. In teaching this child, giving him the opportunity to ask questions and to explain things back to you allows him to mentally manipulate information.

The *formal operations* stage brings cognition to its final form during adolescence. A person reaches this stage when he no longer requires the physical presence of concrete objects to make rational judgments. At this point, he's capable of hypothetical and deductive reasoning. Teaching for the adolescent may be wide-ranging, since this problem solver usually considers many possibilities, leading him to deal with a problem from many perspectives.

Knowles and adult development

Using Piaget's and Erikson's work as a foundation, educator Malcolm Knowles has studied the adult learner. Not surprisingly, he feels that the adult learner has many of the cognitive abilities of Piaget's adolescent. However, Knowles considers an adult's life experiences as a crucial additional factor. He thinks that as the individual matures:

• his self-concept moves from dependency to self-direction.

• he accumulates a growing reservoir of experience that becomes a resource for learning.

• his readiness to learn becomes increasingly oriented to the developmental tasks of his various social roles.

• his time perspective changes from one of postponed application of knowledge to immediate application.

• his orientation to learning shifts from subject-centered to problem-centered.

If you examine personal and cognitive development and compare teaching approaches, you can see that children tend to be dependent as learners, while adults need to be independent and exercise control. For example, you'll usually teach an adult patient with migraine headaches some method of relaxation. Since an adult has more control over his time than a child does, you can logically allow him to decide which method fits his life-style and self-

image. Of the possible methods, progressive muscle relaxation, which usually requires 10 to 20 minutes at a time to perform, may not appeal to a busy executive. Visualization may be more effective because it conforms to his time constraints.

Implications for assessment

Inaccurate assessment of a patient's developmental stage can misdirect your planning and hamper your teaching. For instance, not recognizing a 15-year-old's concern about his appearance and his standing among his peers may damage your rapport with him and create a learning barrier.

A complicating factor in your assessment is that chronologic age and developmental stage aren't always related. Throughout life, people move sequentially through developmental stages, but most also fluctuate somewhat among stages, often in response to outside stressors. These stressors, which include illness and hospitalization, can cause a person to temporarily regress to an earlier stage. Sometimes a person may not achieve the task expected of his chronologic age. So, you'll need to address your patient at his current developmental stage, not at the stage you'd expect him to be because of his chronologic age.

How to Maximize Your Teaching Effectiveness

In some situations, you'll have the time to sit down and develop a formal teaching plan. But in others, you'll be confronted with a "teachable moment" when the patient is ready to learn and is asking pointed questions. Invariably, these moments seem to come while you're in the midst of a dressing change or a catheterization. At times like these, you face a dilemma: to teach or not to teach. Having a knowledge of basic learning principles will help you take best advantage of these moments. Here are some principles proven to enhance teaching and learning.

Seize the moment

Teaching is most effective when it occurs in quick response to a need the learner feels. So, even though you're elbow deep in decubitus care, you should make every effort to teach the patient

SAVING TIME FOR TEACHING

Sometimes, teaching patients what they need to know seems impractical—there's too much to cover and not enough time to do it. If you find yourself hard-pressed for time to teach, try using this method:
• List the patient's learning needs.
• Rank these needs: most important first, next most important second, and so on.
• Write your "teaching-to-be-done" list based on this ranking.

This method helps you distinguish the patient's *learning* needs from his *nursing care* needs. It also helps you organize your time and can quickly redirect your actions after an interruption.

Of course, the hardest part is ranking the patient's learning needs. To simplify this task, classify each learning need as:

• *immediate* (one that must be met promptly, such as teaching the patient who's being discharged in 2 hours) or *long range*
• *survival* (life-dependent, such as teaching the warning signs of adrenal crisis) or *related to well-being* (nice to know but not essential, such as describing the effects of stress in cardiovascular disease)
• *specific* (related to the patient's disorder or treatment, such as preparing him for upcoming cholecystectomy) or *general* (teaching that's done for every patient, such as explaining hospital visiting hours).

After you've classified the patient's learning needs, establish priorities. An immediate survival need, for example, would take top priority.

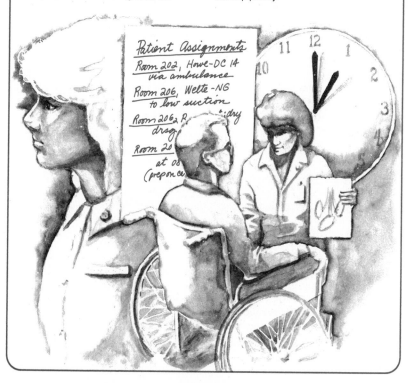

when he asks, "What can I do to stop getting so many open sores?" Your formal teaching plan may be in the patient's chart or in your desk and the slides may be in the head nurse's office, but the patient is ready to learn. So satisfy his immediate need for information now, and augment your teaching with more information later.

Involve the patient in goal setting

Merely presenting information to the patient doesn't ensure learning or change. For learning to occur, you'll need to get the patient actively involved in identifying his learning needs and goals. As the teaching process continues, you can further involve him by selecting teaching strategies and materials that require his direct activity, such as role playing and return demonstration (see *Promoting Your Patient's Involvement in Learning*, page 15). Regardless of the teaching strategy used, giving the patient the chance to test his ideas, to take risks, and to be creative will promote learning.

Begin with what the patient knows

You'll find that learning moves faster when it builds on what the patient already knows. A patient who's been on peritoneal dialysis and now must undergo hemodialysis has some previous exposure to the concept of fluid exchange. Teaching that begins by comparing the old, known process and the new, unknown one will allow the patient to grasp new information quicker.

Move from simple to complex

The patient will also find learning more rewarding if he has the opportunity to master simple concepts first and then apply these concepts to more complex ones. Remember, however, that what one patient finds simple, another may find complex. A careful assessment will take these differences into account and help you plan the starting point for your teaching.

Accommodate the patient's preferred learning style

Learning styles and rates vary from one person to another. Besides being influenced by a person's intelligence and educational training, they're also influenced by preferences. *Visual* learners learn best by *seeing* or *reading* what you're trying to teach. *Auditory* learners learn best by *listening* to what you're teaching. *Tactile*, or *psychomotor*, learners learn best by *doing*.

You can improve your chances for teaching success if you assess your patient's preferred learning style, then plan teaching activities and use teaching tools appropriate to that style. To assess his learning style, you can observe him or simply ask him how he learns best. You can also experiment with different teaching tools, such as printed material, illustrations, videotapes, and actual equipment, to assess learning style. However, never assume that your patient can read well.

Sort goals by learning domain

You can combine your knowledge of the patient's preferred learning style with your knowledge of learning domains. (See *Understanding Learning Domains*, page 16.) Categorizing what he needs to learn into the proper domains helps identify and evaluate the behaviors you expect him to show.

Learning behaviors fall into three domains: cognitive, psychomotor, and affective. The *cognitive* domain deals with tasks that primarily reflect intellectual abilities. The *psychomotor* domain deals with tasks that are accomplished through physical or motor methods. The *affective* domain covers expression of feelings, attitudes, and values.

Most learning involves all three domains but isn't equally weighted. In teaching a patient about subcutaneous injection sites, recognize that the cognitive domain has the essential task: identifying the sites. The psychomotor and affective domains have less important tasks: finding the best site for

PROMOTING YOUR PATIENT'S INVOLVEMENT IN LEARNING

Your patient will learn best when he's actively participating in the learning process. And he'll be most active when your teaching plan uses materials that simultaneously involve as many of his five senses as possible. You can review the illustration here to identify materials and the senses they involve.

SIGHT	SOUND	SMELL	TOUCH	TASTE
Written material Illustrations Slides	Lectures Audiotapes Records	Treatment solutions Oils Perfumes	Anatomic models Equipment	Food Spices

SIGHT AND SOUND

Role play
Videotapes
Television
Motion pictures

SIGHT, SOUND, AND TOUCH

Working anatomic models

SIGHT, SOUND, TOUCH, AND SOMETIMES TASTE OR SMELL

Demonstration
Return demonstration

ALL SENSES

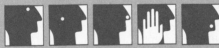

Repeated sensory learning experiences

UNDERSTANDING LEARNING DOMAINS

During the teaching process, you'll be carefully identifying what you want the patient to learn and evaluating if he's actually learned it. Understanding the learning domains can ease both steps.

Every task you want the patient to learn, such as ostomy care (shown in italics in the example here), falls primarily into one of three learning domains—cognitive, psychomotor, or affective. And within each domain, a task can be accomplished or learned on any of several progressively complex levels. Understanding the degree of ability and comprehension each level demands can help you identify the steps you'll have to take in guiding your patient toward his learning goals.

Understanding this, you'll find it easier to clarify learning goals, plan teaching strategies, and focus your evaluation.

COGNITIVE DOMAIN

Knowledge: Recalling information. *(Patient can list equipment needed for pouch change.)*

Comprehension: Understanding. *(Patient can state relation between ostomy care and skin integrity.)*

Application: Applying old information to new situations. *(Patient can recognize skin breakdown by recalling signs of past infection.)*

Analysis: Breaking down whole into parts. *(Patient can pinpoint problem, such as pouch leak.)*

Synthesis: Putting parts together to create a new whole. *(Patient can identify a solution, such as applying more pouch adhesive.)*

Evaluation: Judging the value of material for a given purpose. *(Patient can rate effectiveness of his solution to problem.)*

PSYCHOMOTOR DOMAIN

Perception: Becoming aware of a stimulus through the senses. *(Patient knows what equipment is needed for pouch change.)*

Set: Readiness for a particular physical action. *(Patient can handle equipment and ask questions.)*

Guided response: Performing overt behavior under supervision. *(Patient can follow pouch application instructions.)*

Mechanism: Learning a behavior to the point of habit. *(Patient can apply pouch correctly without instructions.)*

Complex overt response: Performing a complex motor pattern. *(Patient can incorporate local skin care into pouch application.)*

Adaptation: Altering a learned motor response to meet new problems. *(Patient can use same principles to apply different type of pouch.)*

Origination: Creating new motor patterns. *(Patient can cut pouch to fit.)*

AFFECTIVE DOMAIN

Receiving: Attending to and allowing continuation of a stimulus. *(Patient can look at stoma.)*

Responding: Responding voluntarily to a stimulus. *(Patient can ask and answer questions about stoma and pouch application.)*

Valuing: Accepting the value of a behavior to the point of acting it out. *(Patient's willing to perform pouch application.)*

Organization: Organizing behavioral framework based on values. *(Patient's willing to make time for stoma care.)*

Characterization: Expressing feelings that portray view of life. *(Patient shows self-esteem despite altered body image.)*

a particular injection and expressing how the patient feels about this.

Make material meaningful

Another way to facilitate learning is to relate material to the patient's lifestyle—and to recognize incompatibilities. For example, teaching a hypertensive patient how to take his blood pressure may be futile if he perceives this as something his spouse ought to be doing. Similarly, discussing the need for a low-sodium diet with a traveling salesman may also be futile if he eats regularly in restaurants and feels unable to control the ingredients in his diet.

Allow immediate application of knowledge

Giving the patient the opportunity to promptly apply his new knowledge and skills reinforces learning and builds his confidence.

For instance, when you teach a mother how to perform postural drainage for her infant, you'll find that she'll learn better if she can quickly transfer what she's practiced on a doll to her own child (under your supervision, of course). This immediate application lets her translate her learning to the "real world" and provides an opportunity for problem solving, feedback, and emotional support.

Another example: providing sample menus to the diabetic patient helps reinforce his cognitive skills of food selection. This type of rehearsal reinforces his ability to select foods correctly on his own.

Plan for periodic rests

While you may want the patient to push ahead until he's learned everything on your teaching plan, remember that periodic plateaus occur normally in learning. When your instructions are especially complex or lengthy, your patient may feel overloaded and appear unreceptive to your teaching. Be sure to recognize these signs of mental fatigue and let the patient relax. (You,

too, can use these periods—to review your teaching plan and make any necessary adjustments.)

Tell the patient how he's progressing

Learning's made easier when you make the patient aware of his progress. This feedback can often motivate him to greater effort because it makes his goal seem attainable.

Also remember to ask your patient how he feels he's doing. He probably wants to take part in assessing his own progress toward learning goals. And his input can guide your feedback, since his reactions are often based on what "feels right."

Reward desired learning with praise

Praising desired behavior improves the chances of the patient's repeating that behavior. For example, a child with cystic fibrosis may have difficulty learning how to perform breathing exercises. But praising his success associates the desired learning goal with a feeling of growing competence in an appreciative atmosphere. It can reassure him that he's learned the technique, can help him refine it, and can motivate him to practice.

A FINAL WORD

For your teaching to be effective, the learning process must be dynamic, with your patient involved every step of the way. The extent of his involvement will depend greatly on how well you've identified his learning needs. And this, in turn, will depend on how completely and accurately you've assessed his developmental level, his ability to learn, and his receptivity to your teaching.

2 Assessing Learning Needs

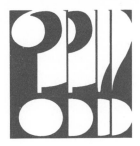

Assessing
Learning Needs

Introduction

Like most nurses who've conscientiously tried to teach patients, you've probably been disappointed with the results at one time or another. Maybe you've felt that your message just wasn't getting through—for example, when a patient didn't follow your explicit instructions for taking his medication. Or perhaps you've felt that your teaching somehow missed its mark—for example, when you tried to teach a patient how to change a dressing but found that he just couldn't do it.

Assess before you teach
Often, you can avoid frustrations like these by carefully assessing your patient before you begin teaching. By assessing first, you can determine what your patient wants and needs to know. And you can determine what he's ready, willing, and able to learn. Knowing this information can make your teaching faster, easier, and more effective.

Careful assessment *saves you valuable teaching time*. It helps you pinpoint a patient's specific learning needs and evaluate his receptivity to learning, so you'll know what—and when—to teach. It also helps you establish your patient's learning priorities, so you'll know where to devote most of your teaching time.

Careful assessment *facilitates your teaching*. It allows you to discover possible barriers—physical, emotional, behavioral, or environmental—that may interfere with your teaching and inhibit learning. With this information, you can decide which teaching methods and tools are best to include in your teaching plan. Then you can modify your teaching techniques to meet your patient's individual needs.

Finally, careful assessment *makes your teaching more effective*. Once you've identified your patient's needs, you can tailor your teaching plan to make learning more meaningful to him. The result? He'll learn faster, retain the information longer, and be more likely to follow directions or change his behavior accordingly.

How to proceed
Your preteaching assessment begins with collecting information about the patient. Then, you'll need to assess the various factors that influence his readiness to learn—for example, his emotional state and personal learning goals. Next, you'll need to assess his willingness to learn and the factors that may affect it—for example, his health and religious beliefs. You'll also need to assess his ability to learn by identifying any factors that may enhance or impede learning—for example, his physical condition, intellectual abilities, and learning style.

THE TECHNIQUES

Collecting Assessment Data

Your preteaching assessment is an ongoing process—it won't be completed in one session. Each time you talk to a patient, check his chart, or attend a meeting with other members of his health care team, you gather information that can help you assess the patient's learning needs and abilities. When collecting assessment data, consider the following sources of information:
• interviews with the patient and his family
• written records, such as the patient's medical chart
• meetings with members of the health care team.

Interviewing the patient
You'll gather most of the information you need to complete a preteaching assessment during formal and informal interviews with the patient. *Formal interviews,* such as the health history you take when the patient's admitted to the hospital, provide a structured format for obtaining data. *Informal interviews* are the conversational exchanges that usually occur while you're providing routine care—for example, when you ask a postoperative patient how he's feeling while you change his dressing. Because they're less structured, informal interviews tend to be less threatening to the patient and often elicit his true thoughts and feelings. During both formal and informal interviews, remember to ask about the patient's past health experiences, current illness, and health expectations.

• *Ask about the patient's past health experiences—both positive and negative.* Is it unusual for the patient to be ill, or is he often bothered by health problems? When he's ill, does he like others to care for him, or does he prefer to care for himself? The patient's answers to these questions may reveal his customary reaction to illness—information that can help you choose the best approach for planning care and teaching. What's more, asking the patient about his past health experiences helps you assess his compliance with past care instructions.
• *Ask about the patient's current illness.* How much does the patient already know about his illness and its symptoms, and what additional information would he like to learn? By knowing the patient's perceived need for further learning, you can decide what to include in the teaching plan.
• *Ask about the patient's health expectations.* Try to find out how the patient thinks his present illness will affect his future health. This information helps you determine how well the patient has adjusted to his diagnosis and prognosis. It may also provide clues about the condition's impact on the patient and his family, and help point out the need for additional teaching and support measures.

Interviewing the patient's family
During your preteaching assessment, be sure to interview the patient's family or any close friends or companions who'll be involved in your teaching plan. The patient's family and close acquaintances not only help you validate and clarify the patient's history but also may point out a need for additional teaching—especially if they'll be involved in caring for the patient after he leaves the hospital.
• *Assess the family's reaction.* Try to determine how well the patient's family is coping with his hospitalization. Their reaction may color his response to learning. For example,

FOUR STEPS TO TAKE BEFORE TEACHING

Before you begin teaching, you'll need to take four important steps. Your first step entails setting standards for what a patient should learn. And your last step entails formulating a statement of the patient's readiness, willingness, and ability to meet those standards—in effect, your teaching diagnosis. Between these steps, you'll collect and evaluate information. You'll probably also discover additional areas for teaching, based on what your patient and his family want to learn about his condition. If so, you'll need to reassess the patient or modify your teaching standard to create the best possible teaching plan.

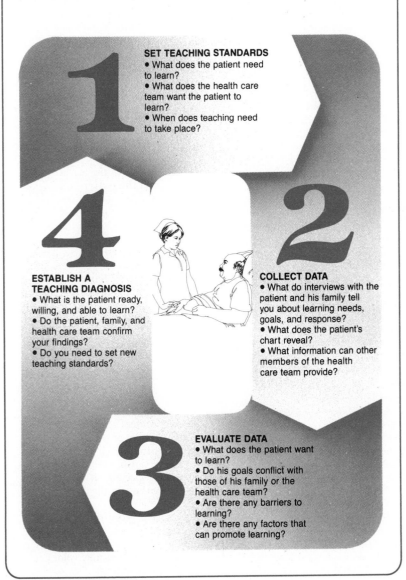

SET TEACHING STANDARDS
- What does the patient need to learn?
- What does the health care team want the patient to learn?
- When does teaching need to take place?

COLLECT DATA
- What do interviews with the patient and his family tell you about learning needs, goals, and response?
- What does the patient's chart reveal?
- What information can other members of the health care team provide?

EVALUATE DATA
- What does the patient want to learn?
- Do his goals conflict with those of his family or the health care team?
- Are there any barriers to learning?
- Are there any factors that can promote learning?

ESTABLISH A TEACHING DIAGNOSIS
- What is the patient ready, willing, and able to learn?
- Do the patient, family, and health care team confirm your findings?
- Do you need to set new teaching standards?

suppose your patient's family is eager for him to "hurry up and get well," so he can return home and resume his customary role and responsibilities. Their eagerness may pressure the patient to tackle learning tasks before his condition permits. This could prolong the teaching process and spell frustration for both the patient and his family.

When the family understands the reason for a patient's treatment, they're more likely to support him as he acquires new information and skills. Generally, a patient's most likely to learn effectively when his family supports his efforts and shares a positive, realistic attitude.

When you interview the family, you'll also need to assess their understanding of the patient's diagnosis and prognosis. Are they well-informed, or do they have misconceptions that could interfere with your teaching? Have they accepted the diagnosis or are they unable to face it? Find out their goals for the patient's recovery and their perception of the patient's ability to learn. Are their expectations geared toward the patient's true capabilities?

Also ask the family about the patient's usual coping mechanisms. Often, they can provide insights into the patient's daily activities and coping mechanisms that the patient himself may overlook. Finally, assess the family's willingness to learn and participate in the patient's care. Do they ask pertinent questions about the patient's illness and need for care, or do they "tune out" during your explanations?

• *Identify emotional needs.* Sometimes you'll need to identify—and try to meet—some specific emotional need before you can effectively teach the patient's family. For example, if a patient's wife seems *hostile* during the interview, you may realize it's because she feels she's in the way—or because members of the health care team have pushed her away. These feelings are especially likely to surface if the patient needed her care at home, before his hospitalization. Once you've identified

the wife's need to play a larger role in her husband's care, you can try to meet it while you teach—for example, by asking her to perform basic care techniques while you're explaining them.

Guilt can also interfere with the family's understanding of the patient's illness—especially if they think something they did or didn't do was responsible for the hospitalization. You can sometimes recognize this emotion by a family member's inattentiveness and questions. For example, suppose you're interviewing a woman whose elderly mother fell and struck her head, causing formation of a cerebrovascular clot, which required surgery. During the interview, you realize that the daughter clearly isn't paying attention. When you ask if there's anything else she'd like to know about her mother's condition, she asks several seemingly unimportant questions and then asks the "big" one: could she have kept the clot from forming if she'd put an ice bag on her mother's head? In cases like this, you'll need to relieve a family member's guilt before she'll be ready to learn what you need to teach her.

Conducting a successful interview

Successful interviewing involves listening, posing questions, and choosing words with care. It also requires you to assess nonverbal cues and to recognize how your attitudes and the environment affect the interviewing process.

• *Be a good listener.* The way you talk and listen to your patient and his family can enhance communication—or hinder it. For example, if you frequently interrupt the patient, you force him to reinitiate the conversation. The result? Not only will the patient feel you aren't listening but the message you receive will be disjointed.

• *Pose questions carefully.* By posing your questions carefully, you can encourage the patient and his family to continue talking, so you can learn as much as possible. You can also direct their responses to provide the type of information you need.

Asking an *open-ended question* generally garners the most information, since this type of question allows many possible answers. It also allows a person to clarify his thoughts and feelings or elaborate on them. For example, suppose a patient tells you that he hasn't felt comfortable since beginning a new treatment schedule. By responding with an open-ended question—such as "What is it about your schedule that makes you uncomfortable?"—you allow the patient to expound on his original statement. His response may also provide clues about his approach to problem solving, since open-ended questions often require a person to form a judgment.

In contrast, by responding with a *closed question*—such as "When did you begin your new treatment?"—you direct the patient toward providing specific information. Unlike an open-ended question, a closed question can usually be answered in just one or two ways. This type of question may require the patient simply to recall information or also to translate, interpret, and rephrase that information. His response may help you determine how well he remembers and understands what he's been taught.

• *Watch your language.* During the interview, keep in mind that your choice of words may keep you from getting the information you need. For example, using unfamiliar medical terms or jargon—such as *enuresis*, *stat*, and *NPO*—when readily understandable lay expressions exist can confuse the patient. Similarly, using familiar terms that have a double meaning, such as *dirty* and *sterile*, can also confuse him. However, if you must use a special term, such as *EKG* or *catheter*, be sure to explain it—or at least ask the person if he knows what it means. Remember, however, some people may be reluctant to admit they don't understand.

Using vague language can also hinder communication, create confu-sion, and sometimes result in an incorrect assessment. For example, suppose you're interviewing a patient who's receiving anticoagulant therapy. If you ask him whether he has experienced any "excessive or prolonged bleeding," he may say "no" simply because he doesn't understand how much bleeding is "excessive" or how long the bleeding must persist to be considered "prolonged."

• *Watch the patient's language, too.* By listening carefully to your patient's choice of words, you can adjust your vocabulary to his level of understanding. For example, if a patient says "pee" and you insist on using the word "urinate" or "void," the patient may not grasp your meaning. Having to constantly explain yourself will make both of you feel foolish. On the other hand, you may be led to believe a patient or family member who uses specialized medical terms is knowledgeable when he really isn't. In both situations, you must determine the person's level of understanding so you can communicate clearly with him.

Sometimes, you may have difficulty understanding what your patient or his family says—especially if they use slang or "street talk." This can keep you from developing a trusting relationship and completing your preteaching assessment. If a patient or a family member uses unfamiliar words, ask him to explain them. Or ask an appropriate colleague to help you communicate with the patient. (Some hospitals provide staff with special vocabulary lists that translate local slang into common language.)

• *Assess nonverbal cues.* Pay attention to the nonverbal cues—such as behavior, facial expressions, and gestures—that a patient sends during an interview. Sometimes, the nonverbal message a patient conveys may conflict with his verbal message. For example, a blank look may mean he hasn't understood what you've told him, even if he says he has.

Similarly, a patient's nonverbal ac-

> ## KNOW YOURSELF:
> ## ASSESSMENT'S FIRST COMMANDMENT
>
> Like most nurses, you probably find that teaching certain patients—or certain topics—makes you feel anxious or uneasy. Why? Possibly because they challenge your self-confidence as a nurse. Or perhaps because they trigger an emotional response based on your values or biases.
>
> Your life experiences help shape your values, opinions, and expectations. But as a nurse, you can't allow them to interfere with the objective preteaching assessment each patient deserves. Do you, for example, disapprove of certain kinds of people, such as alcoholics or drug abusers? If so, you may unconsciously make careful assessment a lower priority for them than you would for other patients. Or you may omit certain assessment information or interpret it to match your preconceptions.
>
> Do you dislike teaching certain procedures, such as stoma care? If so, your negative attitude may surface when you assess a patient who needs this teaching.
>
> Do you find yourself agreeing with sweeping statements about:
> - ethnic background, such as "The Irish are so stubborn; you can't teach them anything."
> - sex, such as "Men don't need to talk about their problems the way women do."
> - aging, such as "Old people can't learn new things or care for themselves."
> - physical appearance, such as "If he weren't so fat, he'd have learned to walk with a cane by now."
> - the effect of an unfavorable prognosis, such as "He has AIDS, so what's the point in teaching him about maintaining good nutrition?"
>
> To keep biases like these from coloring your assessment, think about patients or teaching topics that have been challenging for you. What kind of person do you most dislike finding in your patient assignments? Which procedures are you uncomfortable teaching? Why do you think you feel this way?
>
> Of course, you can't change the way you feel overnight. But you can learn to put your feelings into perspective and try to prevent them from compromising the way you assess—and teach—your patients.

tions can give very different meanings to the same words. For example, a patient who meets your eyes with a steady, determined look and says, "I'm just not getting any better," may be telling you that he's ready to learn about new treatment options. Another patient who says these same words but shrugs his shoulders, looks away, and begins to weep is communicating a very different message. He may be telling you that he thinks his situation is hopeless and that nothing you teach him will make a difference.

A patient's nonverbal cues can also indicate when a particular topic needs to be addressed in more detail—or when it needs to be shelved temporarily. For example, when you raise a sexually related topic, does the patient avoid eye contact or develop nervous mannerisms? If so, he's telling you with his actions that the topic is sensitive. By being aware of both verbal and nonverbal responses, you can determine if you need to probe further, change the subject, or stop asking questions.

• *Be aware of your attitude.* Your own feelings and values may influence not only the information you collect during the interview but also your interpretation of the patient's learning needs. Like everyone else, your feelings and values have been shaped by your past experiences. But as a nurse, you can't allow any biases to interfere with the objective assessment each patient deserves. Being aware of your own biases can help you recognize, anticipate, and avoid problems. During the interview, try to look at how your personal response to the patient is influencing the interviewing process. If it seems to be influencing it negatively, check your assessment findings with other members of the health care team. (See *Know Yourself: Assessment's First Commandment.*)

• *Be aware of the hospital environment.* Keep in mind that the hospital environment can also affect the accuracy of your preteaching assessment. For example, a room that's crowded or noisy is distracting and may prevent you and the patient or his family from concentrating. One that's too cold, too hot, or poorly lit also impedes assessment by causing discomfort. Lack of privacy may make the patient or his family reluctant to reveal personal or intimate details.

You may not always be able to create the ideal setting for an interview—an environment that's quiet, comfortable, and private. But do make an effort, especially to reduce distractions and to provide privacy. For example, if the patient's in a semiprivate room but ambulatory, take him to a quiet area outside the room. If he isn't ambulatory, draw the curtains around the bed and speak in a low tone to convey respect for his privacy. Or conduct the interview when his roommate's gone.

Reviewing written records

The patient's medical chart provides the data base for your preteaching assessment. His health history reveals his general physical and emotional state and educational level—factors that can greatly affect his readiness, willingness, and ability to learn. The patient's chart also outlines basic information about his diet, living situation, support systems, and usual daily activities—details that can affect his health practices after he leaves the hospital. Social service records and consultation sheets may also provide information about any family difficulties, emotional problems, or use of support services that can influence the patient's approach to learning. By regularly checking laboratory and radiology reports, nurses' change-of-shift notes, and progress reports, you can continually update your assessment.

Meeting with the health care team

Formal and informal interviews with the patient's doctor and other health care team members expand and validate your preteaching assessment. Find out what your colleagues have learned from their interviews with the patient and his family. Do their impressions support or contradict your findings? Also find out what other health care team members have told the patient and his family about the patient's diagnosis, prognosis, and treatment plan. By clarifying these facts, you can avoid dispensing conflicting information to the patient and his family.

You can further enhance your preteaching assessment by attending regular multidisciplinary conferences with other members of the patient's health care team—his dietitian, physical therapist, or social worker, for example. If possible, also include the patient and his family in these meetings. Group conferences allow the health care team to share information about the patient and to set goals for his recovery or rehabilitation. They also provide a forum for resolving conflicts about teaching priorities.

THE LEARNER

Assessing Readiness to Learn

Various factors influence a patient's readiness to learn. During your assessment, consider the patient's current *emotional state*, his *stage of adaptation to his illness*, his *emotional maturity*, his *past life experiences*, and the *goals* he and his family want to reach. Assessing a patient's readiness to learn involves answering these questions:

• What information, if any, is the patient emotionally ready to learn at this time?

• How well has the patient adapted to his illness?

• Is the patient emotionally mature enough to take responsibility for learning?

• Have the patient's experiences helped prepare him to learn the concept or skill you're planning to teach?

• Do the patient and his family have realistic learning goals?

Most patients show that they're ready to learn by asking questions or by participating in care. If possible, plan to time your teaching to take advantage of your patient's readiness to learn. Not only will learning be more effective but your teaching task will be easier.

Emotional state

During your assessment, find out if the patient has any pressing emotional needs or any emotional problems that will require you to adapt your teaching techniques. A patient's emotional state affects not only the way he looks at the world but also his readiness to learn. For example, an overwhelming health problem can crush a patient's confidence in his ability to control his life, leaving him *depressed* about his illness and *apathetic* about learning. If he can't do anything about his illness, he feels, why should he bother learning about it? Another patient who feels *happy* about his progress and *hopeful* about his recovery will more likely be ready to learn how to achieve his goals.

A patient typically feels a variety of emotions that can affect his readiness to learn. Often, mild emotional responses speed learning. *Mild anxiety,* for example, occurs normally during learning and can sharpen a patient's attention, increasing his readiness to learn and understand. More intense emotional responses can overwhelm him and make him less receptive to teaching. Here are some common emotions hospitalized patients feel:

• *Anxiety.* A patient who feels threatened by his illness often reacts with anxiety. As his anxiety worsens, his perception of what's going on around him narrows; his goals become oriented toward gaining immediate relief rather than toward learning.

Often, a hospitalized patient's family experiences severe anxiety that can increase the patient's stress and create a barrier to learning. For example, suppose you're assessing the learning needs of a couple whose 5-year-old daughter has been admitted for possible leukemia. Naturally, their anxiety level is high. The father is impatient and abrupt when he speaks; he paces up and down and often becomes hostile during the interview. The mother acts nervous and edgy; she appears to have been crying and is on the verge of tears frequently during the interview. The daughter sits on her mother's lap throughout the interview, stroking her mother's arm and staring at her father. She seems bewildered and frightened. At this time, neither parent is ready to learn about their daughter's suspected illness. What's more, their anxiety heightens their daughter's stress, decreasing her readiness to learn on her own.

Some people try to protect themselves from anxiety through various coping mechanisms, such as denial or regression. You'll need to recognize when your patient's using coping mechanisms—they can make him less receptive to learning. (See *Recognizing Coping Mechanisms.*)

• *Anger.* A patient commonly becomes angry when he has unrealistic expectations of medical care. For example, he may express anger if he believes that he's not receiving sufficient care or not recovering quickly enough.

• *Fear.* A hospitalized patient may be prone to a variety of fears. For example, a patient who's especially dependent on his family or friends may fear *loneliness.* Another patient may fear *financial instability* if his illness forces a realignment of family roles—such as when the homemaker must seek employment to support the family. And a patient who hasn't been fully informed about (or doesn't fully understand) his

RECOGNIZING COPING MECHANISMS

A patient may use coping mechanisms to protect himself from anxiety by changing, concealing, or falsifying the threat he believes a stressful event or condition poses. As you know, coping mechanisms aren't always harmful. But because they can interfere with a patient's learning, you need to recognize and understand them. This chart defines and describes some of the coping mechanisms patients commonly use.

COPING MECHANISM	DEFINITION	BEHAVIOR TRAITS	REASONS FOR USE
Denial	Refusing to recognize some aspect of reality	Denies known facts or reality of illness; refuses responsibility for learning self-care	Protects patient from painful reality
Rationalization	Justifying behavior by using a plausible excuse	Intensely defends own position	Maintains patient's self-respect and wards off guilt feelings
Displacement	Redirecting an emotion or impulse to another person or object	Focuses on teaching inconsistencies of health care team	Allows patient to express repressed feelings
Conversion	Translating psychological problems into physical complaints	Claims physical problems that have no clinical cause; requests self-care information related to physical problems	Helps patient avoid anxiety-producing situation because he's "ill"; gives patient legitimate reason for seeking help and support or removes focus from psychological problems
Regression	Returning to a previous, immature way of behaving	Refuses to participate in learning; performs previously learned tasks at a lower level of ability	Permits patient to avoid anxiety of real situation
Projection	Transferring unwanted thoughts and tendencies to others	Minimizes own guilt by making others feel guilty; blames others for own problems; makes others responsible for learning tasks or for own failure to learn	Provides an outlet for patient's repressed thoughts and tendencies

ASSESSING YOUR PATIENT'S STAGE OF ADAPTATION

When you interview your patient, try to determine how he feels about his illness. Does he deny its existence? Does he blame it on himself or others? Does he seem willing to accept it and modify his life-style?

Your patient may be experiencing any of these feelings about his illness. In fact, he may experience all of them, but at different times. By recognizing his response—or stage of adaptation—to his illness, you can avoid teaching him something he's not ready to learn. For example, if he's still in the initial stage of disbelief, you'll need to postpone teaching until he's ready to face the existence of his illness. This chart will help you recognize the six stages of adaptation patients commonly experience.

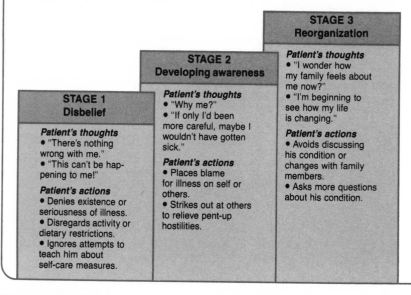

STAGE 3
Reorganization

Patient's thoughts
• "I wonder how my family feels about me now?"
• "I'm beginning to see how my life is changing."

Patient's actions
• Avoids discussing his condition or changes with family members.
• Asks more questions about his condition.

STAGE 2
Developing awareness

Patient's thoughts
• "Why me?"
• "If only I'd been more careful, maybe I wouldn't have gotten sick."

Patient's actions
• Places blame for illness on self or others.
• Strikes out at others to relieve pent-up hostilities.

STAGE 1
Disbelief

Patient's thoughts
• "There's nothing wrong with me."
• "This can't be happening to me!"

Patient's actions
• Denies existence or seriousness of illness.
• Disregards activity or dietary restrictions.
• Ignores attempts to teach him about self-care measures.

illness or treatment regimen may fear *the unknown.*

Sometimes, fear prevents a patient from hearing or understanding what you say. This frequently happens when words such as *cancer* or *heart surgery* frighten the patient so much that he fails to hear your message. When you see that a patient's frightened, don't go any further with your teaching. Wait until he starts asking questions—the signal that he's ready to hear more.

• *Mistrust.* A patient who shows signs of mistrust may be influenced by previous unpleasant experiences with hospitalization. He may also be mistrustful if he doesn't understand the roles of the many professionals involved in his care or if he receives conflicting information from them. For example, suppose you

tell a patient during preoperative teaching that he'll be able to get up and walk the day after surgery, but his doctor tells him that he'll be allowed to get out of bed only to go to the bathroom. This discrepancy can be extremely upsetting for the patient. It can foster feelings of mistrust that may interfere with both your ability to teach and the patient's readiness to learn.

Stage of adaptation

A patient may go through various stages before successfully adapting to his illness, including disbelief, developing awareness, reorganization, resolution, and identity change. (See *Assessing Your Patient's Stage of Adaptation.*) Most patients don't progress in an orderly way from one stage to the next:

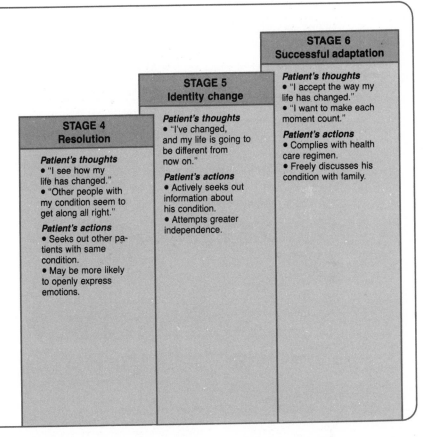

STAGE 6
Successful adaptation

Patient's thoughts
• "I accept the way my life has changed."
• "I want to make each moment count."

Patient's actions
• Complies with health care regimen.
• Freely discusses his condition with family.

STAGE 5
Identity change

Patient's thoughts
• "I've changed, and my life is going to be different from now on."

Patient's actions
• Actively seeks out information about his condition.
• Attempts greater independence.

STAGE 4
Resolution

Patient's thoughts
• "I see how my life has changed."
• "Other people with my condition seem to get along all right."

Patient's actions
• Seeks out other patients with same condition.
• May be more likely to openly express emotions.

a patient may skip one or two stages or regress to an earlier stage during a health crisis. During your assessment, be aware of the patient's stage of adaptation. This will help you understand his coping strategies, so you can avoid teaching him something he's not ready to learn. For example, suppose you're assessing a teen-aged patient whose neck was broken when he was thrown from a horse. The patient tells you what the doctor's said about his condition: he'll probably be permanently paralyzed from the neck down. But when you try to talk with him about rehabilitation, he responds by talking about going back to school and riding his horse again. This patient isn't ready to learn about rehabilitation; he hasn't accepted his condition.

A patient who denies his condition presents a paradoxical problem: you need to discuss the reality of his condition with him, but he isn't ready to acknowledge it. When a patient denies his condition, respect his response as a necessary coping mechanism. Then, gradually begin to talk with him about realistic plans for the future.

Emotional maturity
When you assess a patient's emotional maturity, try to determine his *developmental level* and his *self-esteem*. These factors affect a patient's ability to make decisions, take responsibility for their consequences, and manage his life—hallmarks of emotional maturity.
• *Determine developmental level.* Try to determine whether the patient

RELATING GROWTH AND DEVELOPMENT TO ASSESSMENT CONCERNS

INFANT
Trust vs. mistrust

DEVELOPMENTAL TASKS
• Develops attachment to primary care giver
• Develops awareness of self as separate person
• Begins developing communication skills

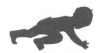

WHAT TO ASK
• Does the infant respond to the physical presence of his parents?
• How does he communicate his needs and feelings?

WHAT TO LOOK FOR
• Shows distress when family leaves
• Uses motor and verbal skills to communicate needs and feelings

TODDLER
Autonomy vs. shame and doubt

DEVELOPMENTAL TASKS
• Develops sense of autonomy
• Further develops sense of self
• Begins developing socialization skills

WHAT TO ASK
• Does the toddler prefer certain foods or activities?
• How does he acknowledge parental distress or approval?
• Does he play with other children or adults?

WHAT TO LOOK FOR
• Willing to follow whims
• Plays alongside others or interacts with them
• Approaches others with show-and-tell items

has mastered the tasks of each developmental stage he's passed through. (See *Relating Growth and Development to Assessment Concerns.*) Whether or not he's mastered these tasks can affect his ability to cope with the stress of illness and hospitalization. To reduce stress, a patient sometimes regresses to less difficult levels he's already passed.

Also recognize developmental tasks that are in a state of transition or stagnation. These tasks can affect a pa-

tient's readiness to learn by influencing his motivation to try out new behaviors. For instance, suppose your patient is a 15-year-old boy with insulin-dependent diabetes. Self-consciousness about his appearance and a desire to be "one of the gang"—typical adolescent concerns—may make it difficult for him to accept the change in body image his diabetes produces. Nevertheless, before your patient leaves the hospital, you'll need to teach him how

PRESCHOOLER
Initiative vs. guilt

DEVELOPMENTAL TASKS
- Develops sense of purpose
- Masters self-care skills
- Develops sense of self, gender, identity, and family relationship

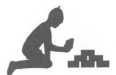

WHAT TO ASK
- Which self-care skills does the child perform at home?
- How does he keep busy at home?
- What's his reaction to schedules and routines?
- What would the child like to be when he grows up?
- What's his favorite activity?
- Can he state his name and identify family members?

WHAT TO LOOK FOR
- Occupies free time independently
- Participates in self-care activities
- Evaluates disapproval of others
- Initiates activities rather than just imitating others' actions

SCHOOL-AGE CHILD
Industry vs. inferiority

DEVELOPMENTAL TASKS
- Further develops sense of self through achievement
- Develops sense of right and wrong
- Shows more interaction with peers

WHAT TO ASK
- What does the child do best?
- What's his favorite subject in school?
- Who's his best friend? What kinds of things do they do together?
- What would he do if he found a lost item in the playground?

WHAT TO LOOK FOR
- Talks about friends, family, and activities
- Interacts with others and initiates conversation
- Participates in self-care activities
- Attempts to improve his skills

(continued)

to give himself insulin injections. But you know he may not be ready to learn the procedure because it sets him apart from his peers—one of the major fears of adolescence. Knowing your patient's developmental level helps you plan teaching strategies that compensate. For example, because adolescents develop their identity in relation to their peers and in opposition to their parents, this patient's readiness to learn self-injection techniques may improve if you conduct your teaching without his parents present.

• **Assess self-esteem.** A patient's self-esteem—his judgment of how he rates as a person—influences how he responds psychologically to illness. If a patient considers himself to be a good person, he can adapt to illness with an intact ego and will more likely be ready to learn. On the other hand, a patient who views himself as bad or worthless may feel overwhelmed by his illness

RELATING GROWTH AND DEVELOPMENT TO ASSESSMENT CONCERNS *(continued)*

ADOLESCENT
Identity vs. role confusion

DEVELOPMENTAL TASKS
• Establishes self-identity
• Prepares for independent role in society
• Continues to develop relationships with peers of both sexes

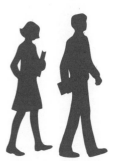

WHAT TO ASK
• Is he in school? Does he want to attend college or learn a trade?
• Who are his friends? Will they be visiting or calling while he's hospitalized?

WHAT TO LOOK FOR
• Expresses individuality through appearance or activities
• Interacts with significant peers and hospital staff
• Willing, if able, to continue school work

YOUNG ADULT
Intimacy vs. isolation

DEVELOPMENTAL TASKS
• Establishes independence from parental figures
• Initiates a permanent life-style
• Adjusts to companionship style
• Integrates values into career and socioeconomic constraints

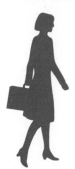

WHAT TO ASK
• Does he live at home with his parents? Or does he have his own family?
• Is he employed or in school?

WHAT TO LOOK FOR
• Forms role-appropriate relationships with staff and others
• Copes with hospital regulations
• Assists and directs care
• Forms intimate relationship with another person

and will less likely be ready to learn.

Past life experiences
As a person matures, he acquires certain skills and experiences that help prepare him for learning new tasks. A patient's experiences—not only with health care procedures but also with hobbies or work-related activities—can increase his readiness to learn by making learning more meaningful and familiar. For example, suppose you

need to teach a patient how to apply adhesive paste around his ileostomy. If he's ever performed a task that required a similar skill—such as caulking a window—he'll be ready to learn this new task sooner than if he weren't familiar with the technique.

Patient and family goals
The goals of the patient and his family determine the patient's priorities for learning. Realistic goals can motivate

MIDDLE-AGED ADULT *Generativity vs. stagnation*	OLDER ADULT *Integrity vs. despair*
DEVELOPMENTAL TASKS • Establishes socioeconomic status • Helps younger and older persons • Finds satisfaction through his work, as a citizen and family member, or as a care provider	**DEVELOPMENTAL TASKS** • Forms mutually supportive relationships with grown children • Adjusts to change in or loss of friends and relatives • Prepares for retirement • Uses leisure time in satisfying way • Adapts to aging
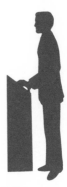	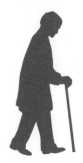
WHAT TO ASK • What's the most satisfying thing in his life? • Who are the important people in his life? • Is he active in community affairs?	**WHAT TO ASK** • Does he have any financial concerns? • What are his retirement plans? • What does he do in his leisure time? • Does he have friends his own age? • How does he feel about getting older?
WHAT TO LOOK FOR • Copes with hospital regulations • Directs and participates in care	**WHAT TO LOOK FOR** • Shows concern for children and grandchildren • Keeps current on world events • Forms adult relationships with hospital staff • Participates in care and decision making

a patient to learn, but "impossible dreams"—expectations beyond the patient's current capabilities—can discourage him in his efforts to learn.

• *Recognize the patient's goals.* The first step in recognizing the patient's learning goals is to discover what, if anything, he wants to know. Until the patient meets his goals, he'll be unable to meet the expectations of his family or the health care team. Similarly, a patient can't concentrate on learning if

other goals are more important to him. Consider this example: a man in his early sixties undergoes a bowel resection for colon cancer, has complications, and faces prolonged hospitalization. His doctor encourages him to increase his activity to prevent further complications. His nurse wants him to take a more active role in learning, so he can become self-sufficient. His wife urges him to cooperate, so he can come home as soon as possible: she's worried about shouldering his responsibilities while he's hospitalized. But the patient's apathetic about learning self-care procedures. Why? There are several possible answers: first of all, he probably feels overwhelmed by the expectations of those involved in his care. Second, he may feel that he hasn't received enough information to make decisions about his future or to take positive action. And finally, he may be using all of his energy to meet his own immediate goal—survival.

When a patient feels overwhelmed by the goals others have set for him, he may react with frustration, anger, or even despair—barriers to effective learning. To help avoid this, you'll need to assess his goals accurately and to share your information with his family and health care team. After you've determined what the patient's ready to learn, work with him, his family, and other members of the health care team to set realistic teaching goals.

• **Recognize the family's goals.** Does the patient's family have confidence in his ability to achieve his learning goals? Or do they believe he'll never be able to learn a particular skill or concept? Families often have expectations of what the hospitalized family member should accomplish. Are their goals realistic? If so, their support can increase the patient's readiness to learn. If not, their unrealistic expectations can make the patient feel uneasy or hesitant about learning.

The family's goals also reveal their willingness to take an active part in the learning process. Find out what they'd like to learn about the patient's illness. If the patient's family will be caring for him after he leaves the hospital, determine their goals for learning about home care procedures.

• **Help the patient and his family set realistic goals.** Many patients and families are unfamiliar or uncomfortable with goal setting. You can ease the process by asking them well-focused questions and by encouraging them to discuss their expectations with you as well as among themselves.

Encourage the patient and his family to develop goals geared toward the patient's true capabilities. For example, suppose your patient's had a cerebrovascular accident (CVA), with resulting right-sided hemiplegia. In this situation, a realistic goal might be to learn to walk with a cane. But, if your patient's had a total T6 spinal transection, such a goal would be impossible. Instead, a realistic long-term goal might be to learn how to function independently while using a wheelchair.

Working with both the patient and his family, write down their goals. Remember, each patient will achieve his goals at his own pace, so avoid setting an inflexible time limit for when he should learn a particular skill or concept. Otherwise, he may feel unnecessarily frustrated or depressed if he fails to meet the schedule. If possible, leave the list of goals with the patient and his family so they can review them, make changes, and set new priorities as the patient's condition changes.

Assessing Willingness to Learn

A patient becomes willing to learn when he recognizes a gap between what he knows and what he wants to know. Conversely, if a patient doesn't want to learn about and comply with a particular health care regimen, he won't—especially if it means giving up long-held habits without any evident reward. For example, an overweight diabetic patient who "feels fine" may be unwilling to learn and follow a modified diet to control his illness.

During your assessment, try to determine the patient's attitude about the subject you're planning to teach. Does he think this information is important for him to learn, or does he consider it a waste of time? Also consider the pa-

HOW HEALTH BELIEFS AFFECT WILLINGNESS TO LEARN

Research shows that a patient learns better when he wants to learn. That's why it's important to assess your patient's health beliefs—they often reveal what he wants, or is willing, to learn. Knowing his health beliefs helps you predict his response to illness or the threat of illness, so you can tailor your teaching plan to meet his needs. In the chart below, an example illness—breast cancer—helps clarify how health beliefs affect a patient's willingness to learn.

PATIENT'S STATEMENT	PATIENT'S HEALTH BELIEF	NURSE'S ASSESSMENT
"I worry a lot about getting breast cancer. It runs in my family."	Believes in greater than average likelihood of getting breast cancer.	Patient's perceived *susceptibility* to breast cancer increases her willingness to learn about it.
"If I had breast cancer, my whole life would change."	Believes that breast cancer would affect all aspects of her life.	Patient's perception of the *seriousness* of breast cancer and its impact on her life increases her willingness to learn preventive measures and early treatments.
"Breast self-examinations can help me find lumps in my breasts."	Believes that breast self-examination is a helpful and important self-care procedure.	Patient's perception of the *benefit* of the procedure increases her willingness to learn and perform it.
"I don't have time to perform a breast self-examination each month."	Believes that performing breast self-examination would create burdensome life-style changes.	Patient's perception that the procedure would interfere with her routine indicates a *barrier* that may decrease her willingness to learn it.

tient's health beliefs, sociocultural background, and religious beliefs—factors that can affect his willingness to learn by influencing his attitude toward health and illness.

Health beliefs

A patient's health beliefs determine his response to illness or the threat of illness. For example, a patient who says, "A yearly checkup is important to me," may believe his actions can help prevent certain health problems. His health beliefs tend to increase his willingness to learn. Another patient who says, "I'm afraid to see my doctor; he might find that something's wrong with me," may believe that his actions can have a negative effect by forcing him to confront a condition that frightens or confuses him.

By assessing your patient's health beliefs, you can determine how he makes health care decisions and predict his compliance with the treatment plan—essential information for planning an effective teaching strategy. (See *How Health Beliefs Affect Willingness to Learn.*) Generally, a patient's willingness to learn increases if he believes he's susceptible to a specific illness or that the illness would have a serious effect on his life-style. In addition, if a patient believes his actions can prevent the illness or that taking action is less dangerous than incurring the illness, he'll be more willing to learn about and comply with the treatment plan.

• *Assess locus of control.* A patient's perception of his ability to bring about change—his *locus of control*—often determines his health beliefs. During your assessment, try to find out how the patient feels about his condition. Generally, a patient who believes he's in control of his illness is more willing to learn than a patient who feels powerless to alter it.

• *Examine health practices.* During your assessment, find out where the patient gets most of his health information and how he puts this information to use. A person's health practices often reflect his health beliefs. For example, a patient may include high-fiber foods in his diet if he believes this can help reduce the risk of colorectal cancer. Another patient may believe he can ward off arthritis by wearing a copper bracelet or drinking an herbal preparation.

Keep in mind that many people follow the advice of nonprofessionals— neighbors, relatives, friends—to treat illness. A patient who distrusts established medicine or uses folk remedies may be unwilling to learn about traditional treatments. To help this patient respond openly to your assessment questions, find out what nontraditional remedies he's been using. When you plan your teaching strategy, try to combine these nontraditional remedies with his prescribed regimen (provided, of course, that they don't interfere with legitimate medical and nursing care). For example, a patient could wear a copper bracelet while also taking prescribed medications.

Sociocultural background

From one generation to the next, families pass on specific values, beliefs, and customs that help determine how their members react to various circumstances. In many cultures, for example, women are more free to express their emotions than men. Ask your patient about his sociocultural background: where were his parents or ancestors born? How long has his family lived in this country? Does he speak a second language at home?

During your assessment, consider how the patient's sociocultural background has shaped his response to illness. For example, suppose your hypertensive patient is a 55-year-old American man whose parents immigrated to the United States from Ireland. In this patient's family, men are expected to present a strong, rugged image—a factor that may influence his willingness to learn the relaxation techniques his doctor prescribes.

When you assess a patient's sociocultural background, try to determine its impact on his current life-style. Does he still hold the values and customs of his ethnic group? If not, what changes has he made? Usually, the impact is less dramatic when several generations separate a patient from his family's country of origin.

• *Avoid stereotyping.* If you're familiar with accepted behavior within your patient's sociocultural group, you can assess his learning needs with greater insight. At the same time, however, you must remember that each patient is an individual, not a stereotype. Contrary to popular belief, for example, not all Italian-Americans are highly emotional, and not all Americans of Anglo-Saxon origin are stoic. Despite cultural influences, each patient is unique—and so is his response to learning.

Religious beliefs

A patient's religion can also affect his willingness to learn by influencing his attitudes toward illness and traditional medicine. For example, a patient who regards his CVA as a test of his faith or a divine punishment for wrongdoing may be unwilling to learn about rehabilitation techniques.

During your assessment, determine the nature and strength of your patient's religious beliefs. Does he have any religious beliefs about treating illness? Many Christian Scientists, for example, shun traditional medical treatment, believing that a person can cure illness by altering his thought processes. What role does religion play in the patient's daily routine? If his religion prohibits certain foods, for example, he may resist learning about dietary changes that conflict with his beliefs. By trying to accommodate the patient's religious beliefs and practices in your teaching plan, you can increase his willingness to learn and comply. (See *Reviewing Religious Beliefs and Practices*, pages 38 and 39.)

Assessing Ability to Learn

A patient's ability to learn depends on his current physical and mental status. Generally, a patient who is physically and mentally able to learn can master the skills and understanding necessary to manage his health problems. On the other hand, a patient who has a physical or mental deficit—such as a disabling illness or severe stress—may be temporarily or permanently unable to do so.

During your assessment, focus on examining the patient's current status. Does he have any problems that could interfere with his ability to learn? Assess his physical condition, intellectual level, and preferred learning style. Also consider his support system and socioeconomic status—factors that could affect his ability to learn by causing or reducing stress.

Physical condition
Examine the patient for any physiologic barriers to learning. For example, a patient's likely to be unresponsive to your teaching if he's in pain. A patient who's fatigued or weak may find it difficult or impossible to respond fully to your teaching. Similarly, fever, nausea, or vomiting can make a patient temporarily unable to learn.

A *sensory-impaired* patient will probably need teaching sessions aimed at his unimpaired senses. During your assessment, explore the extent of his deficit and his method of compensating. If the patient has a hearing loss, for example, find out whether he uses a hearing aid, whether deafness is unilateral or bilateral, whether he can lip-read, and whether he can speak. This information not only allows you to plan an effective teaching strategy but also helps you to complete your assessment.

A *physically handicapped* patient may be unable to learn certain skills. If your patient has rheumatoid arthritis, for example, he may be unable to perform self-care procedures that require precise hand movements. However, he may still overcome his disability if he's strongly motivated.

A patient's reaction to the *stress of hospitalization* can create or heighten barriers to learning. When you assess your patient's physical condition, consider the following barriers:

• **Sensory underload and overload.** Some patients experience an overall lack of stimulation—*sensory underload*—while in the hospital. For example, a patient who's on bed rest won't receive the variety of stimulation available to an ambulatory patient. Other patients experience a heightened state of sensory awareness—a condition called *sensory overload*. This results when a patient perceives sensations more intensely than normal or when he receives sensory input simultaneously from a variety of sources.

Sensory underload and overload produce similar effects—among the most common are anxiety, restlessness, decreased attention span, and somnolence. Both can interfere with the patient's ability to learn by causing confusion and affecting his receptivity to teaching.

• **Disorientation.** Remember to evaluate your patient's orientation to time, person, and place—even if his condition doesn't normally warrant such an assessment. A hospitalized patient of-

REVIEWING RELIGIOUS BELIEFS AND PRACTICES

RELIGION	BIRTH AND DEATH RITUALS	DIETARY RESTRICTIONS	PRACTICES IN HEALTH CRISIS
Adventist (Advent Christian Church, Seventh-Day Adventist, Church of God)	None (baptism of adults only)	Alcohol, coffee, tea, narcotics, and stimulants prohibited; in many groups, meat prohibited also	Communion and baptism performed. Some members believe in divine healing, anointing with oil, and prayer. Some regard Saturday as Sabbath.
Baptist (27 different groups)	At birth, none (baptism of believers only); before death, counseling by clergy and prayer	Alcohol prohibited; in some groups, coffee and tea prohibited also	Some believe in healing by laying on of hands. Resistance to medical therapy occasionally approved.
Church of Christ	None (baptism at age 8 or older)	Alcohol discouraged	Communion, anointing with oil, laying on of hands, and counseling by minister.
Church of Christ, Scientist (Christian Scientist)	At birth, none; before death, counseling by Christian Science practitioner	Alcohol, coffee, and tobacco prohibited	Many members refuse all treatment, including drugs, biopsies, physical examination, and transfusions. Vaccination only when required by law. Alteration of thoughts believed to cure illness. Hypnotism and psychotherapy prohibited. (Christian Science nursing homes honor these beliefs.)
Church of Jesus Christ of Latter-day Saints (Mormon)	At birth, none (baptism at age 8 or older); before death, baptism and gospel preaching	Alcohol, tobacco, tea, and coffee prohibited; meat intake limited	Divine healing through the laying on of hands; communion on Sunday; some members may refuse treatment. Many wear special undergarment.
Eastern Orthodox Churches (Albanian, Bulgarian, Cypriot, Czechoslovakian, Egyptian, Greek, Polish, Romanian, Russian, Syrian, Turkish)	At birth, baptism and confirmation; before death, last rites. For members of the Russian Orthodox Church, arms are crossed after death, fingers set in cross, and unembalmed body clothed in natural fiber.	For members of the Russian Orthodox Church and usually the Greek Orthodox Church, no meat or dairy products on Wednesday, Friday, and during Lent.	Anointing of the sick. For members of the Russian Orthodox Church, cross necklace replaced immediately after surgery and no shaving of male patients except in preparation for surgery. For members of the Greek Orthodox Church, communion and Sacrament of Holy Unction.
Episcopalian	At birth, baptism; before death, occasional last rites	For some members, abstention from meat on Friday, fasting before communion (which may be received daily)	Communion, prayer, and counseling by minister.

Note: Because religious beliefs may vary within particular sects, individual practices may differ from those described here.

RELIGION	BIRTH AND DEATH RITUALS	DIETARY RESTRICTIONS	PRACTICES IN HEALTH CRISIS
Islam (Muslim)	If abortion occurs before 130 days, fetus treated as discarded tissue; after 130 days, as a human being. Before death, confession of sins with family present; after death, only relatives or friends may touch the body.	Pork prohibited; daylight fasting during ninth month of Islamic calendar	Faith healing for the patient's morale only; conservative members reject medical therapy.
Jehovah's Witnesses	None	Abstention from foods to which blood has been added	Generally, no blood transfusion; may require court order for emergency transfusion.
Judaism	Ritual circumcision after birth; burial of dead fetus; ritual washing of dead; burial (including organs and other body tissues) occurs as soon as possible; no autopsy	For Orthodox and Conservative Jews, kosher dietary laws (for example, pork and shellfish prohibited); for Reform Jews, usually no restrictions	Donation or transplantation of organs requires rabbinical consultation. For Orthodox and Conservative Jews, medical procedures may be prohibited on Sabbath—from sundown Friday to sundown Saturday—and on special holidays.
Lutheran	Baptism usually performed 6 to 8 weeks after birth	None	Communion, prayer, and counseling by minister.
Orthodox Presbyterian	Infant baptism; scripture reading and prayer before death	None	Communion, prayer, and counseling by minister.
Pentecostal (Assembly of God, Foursquare Church)	None (baptism only after age of accountability)	Abstention from alcohol, tobacco, meat slaughtered by strangling, any food to which blood has been added, and sometimes pork	Divine healing through prayer, anointing with oil, and laying on of hands.
Roman Catholic	Infant baptism, including baptism of aborted fetus without sign of clinical death (tissue necrosis); before death, anointing of the sick	Fasting or abstention from meat on Ash Wednesday and on Fridays during Lent; this practice usually waived for the hospitalized	Burial of major amputated limb (sometimes) in consecrated ground; donation or transplantation of organs allowed if benefit to recipient is proportional to the donor's potential harm.
United Methodist	None (baptism of children and adults only)	None	Communion before surgery or similar crisis; donation of body parts encouraged.

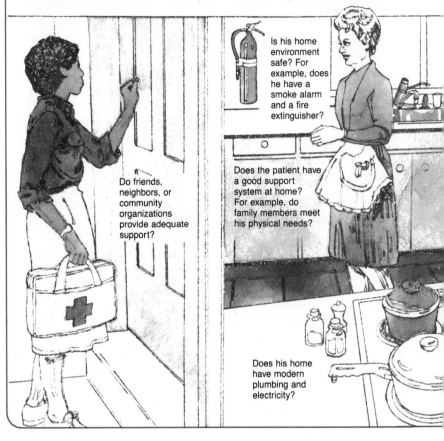

THE HOME ENVIRONMENT: KEY TO COMPLIANCE

One of the biggest frustrations of patient teaching occurs when a patient learns a self-care procedure in the hospital but doesn't comply with it at home. How can you help prevent this? By considering your patient's home environment when you assess his learning needs. This illustration shows some common examples of factors that may influence compliance.

Is his home environment safe? For example, does he have a smoke alarm and a fire extinguisher?

Do friends, neighbors, or community organizations provide adequate support?

Does the patient have a good support system at home? For example, do family members meet his physical needs?

Does his home have modern plumbing and electricity?

ten experiences some disorientation— possibly resulting from the unfamiliar surroundings. This blocks learning because a disoriented patient can't think quickly or coherently. So remain alert for signs of disorientation while you're assessing or teaching the patient. The clue may be a vague expression or a look of fear. In a few patients, signs include anger and refusal to cooperate.

• *Sleep deprivation.* A common effect of hospitalization, sleep deprivation saps a patient's ability to learn. Assess your patient for fatigue, muscle weakness, malaise, or apathy—possible indications of sleep deprivation. A patient who also seems irritable, suspicious, or confused may be deprived of rapid eye movement sleep—the type needed for mental well-being.

• *Pain.* The anxiety of hospitalization often heightens a patient's response to pain, which can hinder his ability to learn by disrupting his concentration and causing fatigue. Be sure to assess your patient for pain before you attempt

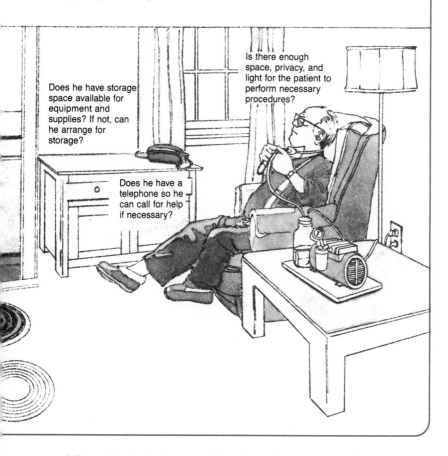

If you can identify barriers to compliance before you teach, you can modify your teaching plan to overcome them. The result? Not only will your patient be more likely to comply but your teaching will be easier.

Does he have storage space available for equipment and supplies? If not, can he arrange for storage?

Is there enough space, privacy, and light for the patient to perform necessary procedures?

Does he have a telephone so he can call for help if necessary?

to teach him. Also check for nonverbal expressions of pain, such as grimacing, unusual posture or body position, or nervousness. Remember that some patients respond to pain with increased activity.

If your patient suffers from chronic pain, assess his ability to cope. Over time, a patient with chronic pain may develop coping mechanisms that permit him to continue functioning but that also interfere with learning. For example, a patient who can't control his pain may compensate by attempting to control his environment and could become manipulative or uncooperative.

Intellectual status

A patient must have adequate intelligence to learn. Of course, your assessment of his intellectual status won't be definitive, but it should determine his basic abilities and identify potential barriers to learning.

• *Estimate intelligence.* You can estimate a patient's intelligence by the vocabulary and language skills he uses, the amount of detail with which he describes his illness, and the extent to which he recalls past events. In addition, you can estimate his intelligence by assessing his understanding and compliance with past medical instructions. Note the extent of his schooling, such as the highest grade completed and courses of study taken. Also note what type of job the patient has.

Conversations with the patient may also reveal his ability to understand abstract or concrete ideas and to solve problems. To determine if the patient understands what you're saying, ask him to repeat—in his own words—what you've said. The patient's re-sponses to questions involving general knowledge may provide additional insight.

Keep in mind that a patient's apparently limited intellectual functioning may be caused by disorientation. Of course, a patient who is critically ill or has a language barrier may also be unable to participate actively in learning.

• *Consider learning barriers.* Check the patient's chart for information about any learning disabilities, such as dyslexia, or language disorders, such as aphasia. If you plan to use written instructions to teach the patient, be sure to assess his literacy. Also check for such conditions as mental retardation or senility, which will directly affect ability to learn. If your patient's mentally retarded, he may be able to learn skills but probably won't be able to understand concepts or become proficient in decision making. A senile patient usually isn't receptive to teaching and learns poorly, if at all. When assessing a patient with either of these barriers, be sure to explore your own feelings; don't let them affect your impression of the patient's learning abilities.

Learning style

A patient's ability to learn increases when teaching incorporates his preferred learning style. During your assessment, try to determine if your patient's primarily a visual learner, a tactile learner, or an auditory learner. (See Chapter 1 for more information on learning styles.)

The support system

A patient can receive emotional support from a variety of sources—including family, friends, the community, and church or religious groups. Together, these sources comprise a patient's *support system*—the group he turns to for comfort, aid, and information to help him cope with life. Having a strong support system reduces stress and may raise a patient's self-confidence and self-esteem, allowing him to concentrate on learning.

IS YOUR PATIENT'S FAMILY INTERFERING?

Your patient's relationship with his family can make learning easier—or more difficult. Properly directed, family members can greatly improve a patient's willingness and ability to learn. But when family members upset your patient, create stress, or undermine your teaching efforts, learning suffers. How can you tell if your patient's family is interfering? These behaviors may be telltale signs.

HOW YOUR PATIENT ACTS

• Refuses to see his family or asks that no one be allowed to visit
• Argues with his family or shows anger toward them
• Experiences signs of stress, such as tachycardia, agitation, perspiration, or flushed skin, when his family visits
• Becomes depressed, uncooperative, or aggressive.

HOW HIS FAMILY ACTS

• Doesn't visit the patient or doesn't interact with him during visits
• Argues with the patient or shows anger toward him
• Avoids physical contact with the patient
• Contradicts your teaching or encourages the patient not to cooperate.

During your assessment, explore the nature and adequacy of the patient's support system. Observe how *family* members talk with the patient and with each other, and note who they turn to, among themselves, for guidance and emotional support. Do they seem to communicate openly and to respect each other's feelings and opinions? Observing the interaction between the patient and his family may give you clues to his role and responsibilities in the family and to the strength and character of his relationships with family members.

Ask the patient about his *friendships,* and note which of his friends visit him during his hospitalization. Does he seem to get along better or talk more freely with his friends than with certain family members?

Also assess the patient's reliance on *community services,* such as independent health care providers, community agencies, and self-help groups. Has the patient rejected any resources that are available to him? If so, why?

Finally, assess the patient's reliance on *church or religious groups.* Such groups may provide the patient with much-needed comfort and support after he leaves the hospital.

Socioeconomic status

During your assessment, be sure to consider your patient's socioeconomic status. After all, research shows that patients with higher incomes suffer less anxiety about hospitalization, and so are better able to learn, than those with lower incomes. A patient who's financially secure tends to view illness more as a minor inconvenience than as a major disruption of his life and livelihood. This patient often has job security, good health insurance coverage, and easy access to appropriate health care. For all of these reasons, he's less threatened by pain and illness than is a patient with a lower income. This increases his sense of control over his condition and, as a result, improves his ability to learn.

CHECKLIST

WHAT TO ASSESS

- [ ] The patient's current emotional state
- [ ] His stage of adaptation to illness
- [ ] His emotional maturity
- [ ] His developmental stage
- [ ] His self-image
- [ ] His past life experiences
- [ ] His learning goals—and his family's
- [ ] The patient's health beliefs
- [ ] His sociocultural background
- [ ] His religious beliefs
- [ ] His physical condition
- [ ] His intellectual status
- [ ] His learning style
- [ ] His socioeconomic status
- [ ] Family support system and availability of support groups

THE OUTCOME

By assessing your patient before you begin teaching, you can identify a wide range of factors that enhance or impede learning. Because assessment is characteristically an ongoing process, you'll be able to recognize how these factors change as your patient's condition changes.

After you've gathered your assessment data, you're then ready to formulate a "teaching diagnosis"—in effect, your evaluation of the patient's readiness, willingness, and ability to learn. Your teaching diagnosis, in turn, serves as the springboard for planning and implementing truly effective patient teaching.

3

Planning and Teaching

Planning and Teaching

Introduction

Having completed your assessment and identified your patient's learning needs, you're probably eager to get on with your teaching. Or perhaps you're a little nervous, wondering where you should begin. Whether you're eager or nervous, taking the time now to develop a well-thought-out teaching plan can facilitate your teaching and improve your skills.

Certainly no one has to convince you of the overwhelming importance of patient teaching. Most likely, you've been doing your share of teaching since your first day on nursing duty and have naturally become better and better at it. You may nevertheless tend to dismiss a teaching plan as an extra for which you have neither the time nor the need. This, however, would be a serious mistake.

Why develop a teaching plan?
As any good teacher will certainly tell you, planning lies at the root of effective teaching. Even though your planning probably won't be evident to your patient, it will make you seem organized, competent, and confident to him. That's important because a patient's impression of you as a teacher can greatly influence his willingness to learn and, thus, your teaching effectiveness.

Your attention to planning now, before you start to teach, may also result in one of those *spontaneous* interchanges between pupil and teacher that rests at the heart of the best teaching. What's more, a teaching plan has other proven advantages for you. For example, a teaching plan will simplify your actual teaching by providing a model you can follow so you don't constantly have to redirect your efforts. It will provide you with an objective basis for evaluating the patient's learning and allow you to get better results. A teaching plan will also save time for you and your colleagues.

When you veer from your teaching plan
Naturally, no matter how painstakingly you put together any teaching plan, you still may have to abbreviate and modify it when other demands impinge on your time. And sometimes, changes in the patient's condition or some other unforeseen circumstances may diminish the importance of following the plan. There will be times, also, when your plan is more honored in the breach.

Don't let the inevitability of veering from your teaching plan dissuade you from preparing one. Always keep in mind that the act of thinking through a formal, *ideal* plan is likely to enhance even the most impromptu bedside teaching session.

LEARNING ABOUT PLANNING

What's in a Teaching Plan?

Simply stated, a *teaching plan* is a carefully organized, written presentation of what the patient must learn and how you'll provide the instruction. It establishes the standards for later evaluating the results of your teaching. Broadly, it should be based on the patient's learning needs, as he's identified them and as you and other members of the health care team have pinpointed them. It should be undertaken in close collaboration with the patient, and it should be realistic enough for you to carry out during a short hospital stay. (Or it must include appropriate provisions for fol-

low-up home teaching.) It should also allow you to be flexible in your teaching and to accommodate the demands of hospital life, such as a patient's sleepless night (which characteristically will make him unreceptive to your teaching the next day) or your limited time for teaching.

Of the many types of teaching plans you'll come across, you'll probably have the most experience with these three: the standard teaching plan, developed by an institution or a commercial company for use with patients having similar learning needs; the individual teaching plan you yourself devise for a patient; and the cardex, which becomes a shorthand version of the plan's intent and content. The ready-made cardex and standard plans can be handy, time-saving resources, but they must always be adapted to your patient's specific needs.

While the scope of these plans differs, each should contain the same elements: a statement of the patient's learning goals, an outline of the content to be taught, a selection of teaching tools

---

POLISHING YOUR TEACHING SKILLS

Your teaching skills, like any other skills you've acquired in nursing, can be refined with practice and direction. And that's especially important today with the growing emphasis on shorter hospital stays and cost containment. After all, effective and timely teaching can improve a patient's understanding of his condition and the prospects for his compliance with treatment. To improve your teaching skills, use these tips:

• Expand your knowledge base by reading professional publications, attending inservice and continuing-education programs, and maintaining a broad range of professional contacts.

• Ask your institution's staff development department to schedule inservice classes that can benefit your entire unit. Then follow up with conferences on your unit for more detailed discussion about what you learned.

• If you're not up to date on a subject you must teach, ask the staff development

department to supply the names of specialists in that subject. Then call one for an appointment.

• Observe more experienced nurses while they're teaching patients. What makes their teaching effective? What kind of rapport do they have with their patients? How do they reach difficult-to-teach patients? Which of their methods could you use effectively?

• If you have a patient who's unusually difficult to teach, ask a colleague or a nursing consultant to do the teaching while you observe.

• Ask a colleague whom you consider an especially good teacher to sit in while you teach. Ask her to review your teaching tools and techniques and offer pointers for your next teaching session. If you're uncomfortable having a third person present while you teach, try role-playing the session beforehand; this can smooth any rough edges in your presentation and help put you at ease for the actual session.

and methods, and some provision for evaluating the results.

Learning goals

When stating the patient's learning goals, make them specific enough so that other members of the health care team will readily understand what is to be taught, why it should be taught, and how it's to be evaluated. (See *Writing Learning Goals Clearly*, page 48.) State these goals in terms of patient behaviors that can be observed and can therefore indicate whether learning has taken place.

Be sure to consider the domains of learning when setting goals. Approached from this viewpoint, learning falls into three domains: the *cognitive,* dealing with tasks that primarily reflect thought processes; the *psychomotor,* dealing with learning in the physical and motor areas; and the *affective,* dealing with attitudes, expressions of feelings, and an individual's value system.

In much of what a patient learns, all three domains can be involved—although not equally. Let's say you're teaching a patient about subcutaneous injection sites. The cognitive task of identifying the site correctly will be primary. Also important will be the patient's use of the needle at the site, which is a psychomotor task. Lastly, his reaction to using the needle, which could be one of anxiety or lack of confidence, falls into the affective domain.

In the course of clarifying the patient's learning goals, take a moment to think about how you'll evaluate whether and what the patient has learned. Deciding at the outset what evaluation techniques, such as question-and-answer or return demonstration, will best reveal the patient's progress can help you find the precise words to phrase his learning goals. This is particularly true when you're establishing learning goals in the affective domain, because attitudes are difficult to measure behaviorally and learning in this domain generally takes place

slowly over time. How, for example, can you be sure your patient has overcome his anxiety about subcutaneous injections? Certainly, you could ask him if he still feels anxious. You could also assess his willingness to perform the procedure. Or you could observe for hesitation or signs of stress as he's doing it. By selecting evaluation techniques like these during your planning, you can formulate precise, measurable learning goals.

• *Involve the patient in setting goals.* Your teaching and the patient's learning are so intricately involved that sharing responsibility with him is essential if your teaching is to be effective. This mutuality begins with step one in your teaching plan—setting learning goals—and comes into play at each succeeding step. It might seem quicker and easier just to set down what you expect or wish your patient to achieve. But when you work closely with the patient to establish learning goals, you give him a chance to add his concerns and expectations to your professional expertise. This will promote cooperation and compliance with treatment.

You may need some practice at first in eliciting the patient's contributions. One technique you might find useful is the reflective method. For example, you might say to your patient with emphysema, "You seem concerned about your activity level and returning to work. How much energy does your job require?" Or, "As I see it, you want to know how to recognize when you're overextending yourself and what to do to recover. What signs have you noticed and what have you tried before?"

Content

The content of your teaching plan represents what you, the doctor, and the other members of the health care team determine the patient *needs* to know, blended with what the patient *wants* to know. Whether you're working with a ready-made or an individualized plan, you'll need to organize its content.

Start by recording your main points

WRITING LEARNING GOALS CLEARLY

To clearly express your patient's learning goals, you'll need to focus on what aspects of his behavior you're aiming to change. His learning behaviors, and your goals for him, fall into the three learning domains: cognitive, psychomotor, and affective.

Your patient may have learning goals in all three domains. For example, understanding his dietary changes would fall into the cognitive domain, while complying with these changes would fall into the affective domain. Taking his blood pressure would fall into the psychomotor domain.

With these domains in mind, you can write clear and concise learning goals for your patient. These goals should clarify what you're going to teach, indicate the behavior you expect to see, and clearly set criteria for later evaluating how successfully the patient has learned.

Review the two sets of sample learning goals below for a patient with chronic renal failure. Notice that the goals in the well-phrased set start with a precise action verb, confine themselves to one task, and describe learning that is measurable and observable. In contrast, the poorly phrased goals may encompass many tasks. They also describe learning that is difficult or even impossible to measure.

WELL-PHRASED LEARNING GOALS	POORLY PHRASED LEARNING GOALS
Cognitive domain	
The patient with chronic renal failure will be able to:	
• state when to administer each drug. • describe symptoms of elevated blood pressure. • list allowed and prohibited foods on his diet.	• know his medication schedule. • know when his blood pressure is elevated. • realize his dietary restrictions.
Psychomotor domain	
The patient with chronic renal failure will be able to:	
• take his blood pressure accurately, using a stethoscope and a sphygmomanometer. • read a thermometer correctly. • collect a urine sample, using sterile technique.	• take his blood pressure. • use a thermometer. • bring in a urine sample for laboratory studies.
Affective domain	
The patient with chronic renal failure will be able to:	
• comply with dietary restrictions to maintain normal electrolyte values. • verbalize adjustments to be made in the home environment. • keep scheduled doctor appointments.	• appreciate the relationship of diet to renal failure. • adjust successfully to limitations imposed by chronic renal failure. • realize the importance of seeing his doctor regularly.

and then supply the detailed, supporting information for each point. Be sure to begin with simple concepts and work toward more complex ones. These cardinal principles of organization will prove especially helpful when you're teaching a patient with little education or one who doesn't learn well through listening.

Teaching methods

Most of your teaching will probably be done on a one-on-one basis, giving you an opportunity to learn about your patient, to build a relationship with him, and to tailor your teaching to his particular needs. But sometimes you'll need to teach a group of patients. First, a word about these situations. Group teaching works well when the patients have experienced, or are about to experience, a common medical situation. They may be facing the prospect of a mastectomy or recovering from a myocardial infarction.

Whatever the group's common experience, it usually results in some valuable pluses. Patients who share a condition tend to support and motivate one another. At times, they learn as much from each other as they do from you. From your point of view, teaching a group of patients obviously saves time for the nurses on your unit.

When you have the responsibility for helping a group develop a sense of identity and cohesiveness, take advantage of certain proven ways to make the group session more successful. (See *Setting the Stage for Successful Group Teaching,* page 50.)

Besides group teaching, other methods and tips for successful, efficient teaching are legion. But you may benefit from reviewing some of the more fundamental methods of teaching.

• *Discussion.* Whether used in individual or group teaching, discussion allows for the open exchange of ideas and information between you and your patient—rather than assuming that you have all the answers. As the discussion moves back and forth between you and the patient, the very act of asking questions or making comments involves the patient more actively in the problem-solving process: he begins, in a small, informal way, to take some responsibility for his own learning.

In addition, discussion can be a valuable follow-up to a lecture, a group-teaching session, or an audiovisual presentation.

• *Demonstration, practice, and return demonstration.* This technique, related to the show-and-tell in a child's classroom, is especially useful after a one-on-one discussion with your patient. There, you've set the stage for demonstrating a treatment or the use of equipment unfamiliar to the patient. Here, you demonstrate step-by-step, so

your patient can imitate what you do. The demonstration can be impromptu, at the patient's bedside, or can be given during a scheduled teaching session. One isn't necessarily superior to the other. Your choice depends on the circumstances.

For instance, an impromptu demonstration is in order if an ostomy patient asks you to show him how to apply his pouch. He wants to know *now*—not later at the formal teaching demonstration you were planning. By taking time now to show him the correct procedure, you're also offering him support in a tense new situation.

A scheduled demonstration usually takes advance planning, since you'll want to be both knowledgeable and confident as you teach the patient. So assemble your materials in advance, and rehearse your presentation until you can convey an air of quiet authority to your patient.

After the demonstration, you'll want to give the patient time to practice, to "do it himself" in private—especially if the need for the procedure results from some major change in body maintenance or image, such as a colostomy.

If it seems advisable, provide the patient with a sheet of written guidelines to the steps he's learning. After allowing time for practice, reinforce your original demonstration with a review that gives the patient ample opportunity for active participation.

Occasionally, you'll encounter a patient who's resistant to, or uncomfortable with, such direct teaching methods. In that case, you'll have to work an abbreviated demonstration into your bedside care. This seemingly casual presentation can be drawn directly from your planned, full-scale demonstration; hence the need for careful planning in your teaching.

• *Role playing.* This teaching technique, which seems simple and spontaneous, becomes a powerful tool for learning. In role playing, your patient acts out an assigned but unrehearsed role in a hypothetical situation. In this

SETTING THE STAGE FOR SUCCESSFUL GROUP TEACHING

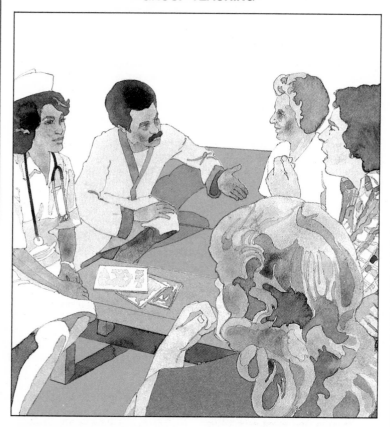

When you're teaching a group, you'll want to enhance the learning process by helping the patients develop a group identity and cohesiveness. Here are some useful techniques:

Shape the environment
• Hold the meeting at a round table, or arrange chairs in a circle. This increases interaction by making participants feel equal to each other and to the teacher.
• Limit the group to 5 to 7 patients to allow for maximum personal exchange and discussion.
• Check the temperature and lighting of the meeting room to be certain that neither is uncomfortable or distracting.
• Serve coffee, tea, or cold drinks to keep the atmosphere informal and relaxed.

Initiate discussion and maintain an overview
• Introduce yourself.
• Ask patients to introduce themselves and to share a bit of personal information.
• Explain the meeting's purpose.
• Invite the group to identify the meeting's goals and ground rules.
• Encourage everyone's participation and be gracious about allowing anyone to leave who isn't comfortable or doesn't wish to participate.
• Use a light rein, yet keep the group close to the agreed-upon areas for discussion.
• Act as a resource, providing information and clarification when necessary.
• Summarize at the end of the discussion, and lead the group to agree on what has been learned.

way, he can prepare himself for a similar but real situation.

Role playing provides a safe environment in which to try out new behaviors or explore alternatives. The patient can take the opportunity to project himself into a situation that's likely to happen—and to plan ahead. If you have an adolescent patient who has just learned he has cancer, role playing can help him "practice" how to tell his friends and teachers about his illness and how to deal with their reactions. Role playing typically works best when a patient really puts himself into the part. He's then better able to transfer what he's learned from the imagined situation to the reality of his everyday life.

A follow-up discussion can enhance the benefits of the role-playing session if you guide the patient to examine his responses with such questions as "What was right about what you did?" "What was wrong?" "How did it feel?" "What would you do differently the next time?"

● *Case study.* A case study is a simulated situation, either written or spoken, very much like one the patient is currently facing. Using this approach, like using role playing, involves the patient in sample problem solving. However, the focus of the problem solving differs. Role playing casts the patient into a situation and emphasizes how he feels and responds in it. In a case study, the patient deals with the sample problem more objectively, as an observer and evaluator of someone else's behavior.

Your responsibility also varies slightly. In role playing, once you've established a situation, the patient more or less takes over, and the outcome is unpredictable. In a case study, you provide direct guidance through your questions and assistance. You might, for example, present your hypertensive patient with the case of a person with the same condition who's experiencing headaches and lack of energy. You'd ask your patient, "What could be causing

his headaches?" "What can he do to alleviate them?" "At what point should he call his doctor?" Then you'd have him come up with possible courses of action for the case patient and weigh the pros and cons of each.

● *Self-monitoring.* In this teaching technique, the patient or his family—rather than you, as his nurse—becomes responsible for collecting the relevant data.

The patient who monitors himself ideally gains a heightened awareness of the aspects of his behavior or environment that call for correction. Let's say you have a patient with vascular headaches who begins to chart their occurrence and characterize the setting and emotional climate in which they occur. The patient might record that a headache began after eating a meal or drinking several glasses of wine, while in a stressful situation at home, or while in a smoke-filled conference room at work. His aim, of course, is to discover the factors that trigger his headaches so he can take corrective action.

The format for self-monitoring should encourage the patient to chart random factors that could prove significant, as well as the more accepted and acknowledged causative factors. Together, you and the patient decide the duration of self-monitoring. Once the patient has collected information for the agreed-upon period, you and he can then sift through what seem to be related or suspicious factors.

● *Lecture.* This traditional form of teaching is usually geared to larger groups of patients. A somewhat formal approach to teaching, a lecture is usually given in a classroom or conference room at a scheduled time. While lecturing seems like a logical means for conveying a large body of information to a group with similar concerns, it has serious drawbacks for patient teaching.

For the patient, the lecture is a passive form of learning. And since it depends almost solely upon language, it can shortchange patients with limited vocabulary or verbal skills or impaired hearing. Lecturing to patients for whom English is a second language is not usually a good teaching bet. And it has yet another drawback. As a one-way process for delivering information, lecturing can lead to misunderstanding and misinterpretation. And you may not discover the problem until it surfaces later in some medical complication.

If you do find yourself lecturing to patients, use some proven ways to counter a lecture's built-in drawbacks and to increase patient participation. First, prepare patients ahead of time for what the lecture will cover. If possible, ask about their specific concerns beforehand. And when you're planning your lecture, spend some time thinking of fresh ways to make it lively and thought-provoking. If appropriate, plan to use audiovisual aids to add interest and try to incorporate some form of audience participation.

During the lecture, change the pace and tone of your talk to maintain audience interest. Invite questions and comments during as well as after the lecture. Repeat each question for those who may not have heard the original question clearly.

Teaching tools

You can use a variety of teaching tools to spur the patient's interest and to reinforce learning. These tools—whether printed pamphlets, special cassettes, or closed-circuit television programs—help familiarize the patient with a topic.

Although some hospitals prefer to develop their own teaching materials, this can be a time-consuming and expensive process. Using already existing materials is certainly more practical. When you're looking for available materials, try the inservice instructors on your unit, the hospital library, or specialists on the staff. (Of course, you can also use the many teaching aids found in this book. Keep in mind that these aids can be reproduced free of charge

for distribution to patients.)

Other good sources for patient-teaching materials include the pharmaceutical and medical supply companies in your community. You can reach the sales representatives of these companies through your hospital's pharmacy department and purchasing agents.

In addition, the large national associations and foundations, such as the American Heart Association, generally have large supplies of patient-education materials written with the lay person in mind. Many of these materials are provided free of charge; some are offered at a nominal cost.

Obviously, these prepackaged references can save you time. But of course, they in no way substitute for your own teaching; they only supplement it. Put your personal imprint on such auxiliary reference materials by marking passages that have significance for your patient and by discussing the information with him.

Some of the tools mentioned here will be available to you; some will not. But you should become familiar with the wide range of tools you can use to enhance your teaching.

• *Printed material.* Books, brochures, and other printed materials are invaluable tools for presenting background information and explaining procedures. Print has the advantage of allowing the patient to read and reread the information at his convenience.

When you recommend printed materials, be sensitive to a patient's ability or inability to read and absorb information. A patient may be too embarrassed to admit he's not a skilled reader and so will pretend he can read and comprehend what you give him. If the material proves too complex or difficult, he may quickly lose the motivation to learn. Actually, the printed word tends to work best not only with the patient who reads competently, but also with the patient who has taken an active interest in his own treatment from the start.

Also determine if the patient can see well enough to read. If he has reading glasses, remind him to use them. If he doesn't have them, suggest using a magnifying glass.

The more pictures the printed materials contain, the better the patient will retain what he's learning. But take a minute to consider the best form. While actual photographs of, say, a step-by-step technique may seem to offer the most accurate illustration, remember that substituting abstract pictures, graphics, or diagrams can sometimes make a concept clearer by eliminating superfluous detail. And of course, if your patient's a child, you'll find that cartoons and pictures that use rock, sports, or movie stars will create interest and help get your message across.

● *Audio cassette tapes.* These tapes can be especially useful for teaching auditory and performance skills. For example, if you're teaching a parent about the care of an asthmatic child, use a tape to record normal breath sounds and wheezing sounds. The parent can then play the tape back and learn to differentiate the sounds. Also, if you're teaching a patient who's uncomfortable with printed materials, you can tape-record the steps of the procedures he's to follow. He can listen to the tape with you; then, once he understands it, he can go over it by himself.

A word of caution if you're planning to use cassette tapes or any other electrical audiovisual equipment: check your equipment beforehand to be sure you can operate it smoothly—without any mechanical hitches. With some equipment, this can take a bit of preparation and practice.

● *Physical models.* Anatomic models and actual equipment convey both visual and tactile information. Besides making your instruction seem more realistic than pictures, they can also reduce the patient's anxiety by familiarizing him with equipment he'll be seeing or using later.

● *Posters and flip charts.* Adaptable enough to be used in teaching a group of patients or a single patient at his bedside, posters and flip charts can be supported by an easel or, when necessary, propped against the back of a chair. If you're planning to use these aids repeatedly, try laminating them. This will make them easy to clean and will prevent them from becoming shabby and discolored with use.

● *Transparencies.* You can augment a lecture or demonstration by using an overhead projector and transparencies to project images onto a screen or wall. Transparencies can be used in a normally lighted room and thus permit you to maintain eye contact with your audience.

● *Slides and filmstrips.* A familiar part of lectures, demonstrations, and even individual teaching sessions, slides are displayed through a carousel projector onto a screen. The most commonly used slides are 35 mm and 2″ square. Slides can be synchronized with an audiotape when a slide-tape projector is used.

Similar to a slide and tape show, filmstrips are merely slide frames that are connected in a continuous strip. They can prove awkward and difficult to change when you want to bring your material up to date or show only a portion of your slides. For this reason, they're being used less and less.

● *Videotapes.* If your hospital has a centralized hookup, a videotape can be shown on the patient's own television screen. He can use earphones so other patients won't be disturbed.

Blank videotapes can also be used to record a patient while he's role-playing or practicing an unfamiliar procedure. Later, he can replay the tape and get an idea of how he's progressing.

● *Closed-circuit television.* Prepared teaching programs can be shown on closed-circuit television by prearrangement if your hospital has the facilities. This can provide important background teaching for a group of patients with a similar problem.

WATCH YOUR LANGUAGE!

Your language can improve or impair your teaching effectiveness. So be sensitive to its effect and adapt it to each patient. Follow these suggestions for making your words help your teaching efforts:

Use language appropriate to your patient's educational level or fluency with English. You're usually on safe ground if you select simple words with few syllables, make your sentences short, and use action verbs.

For clarity, break your information into large, distinct categories. You might say to the patient, "I have three important things to tell you. Number one is ...." This is a good teaching technique whether you're in the patient's room or in a lecture room.

Express complex medical and scientific concepts in layman's terms. Use analogies to make your meaning clear. Whenever possible, avoid complex clinical terms and abbreviations.

Choose specific rather than general words when giving instructions. This applies particularly to directions for the patient's medications and self-care.

Give plenty of examples and hypothetical cases to humanize your teaching.

State your most important points first and last. It's a given in teaching that the first and last points will be remembered best.

Repeat your important points. And don't be afraid to repeat them again if you feel the patient hasn't grasped them.

● *Computer-assisted instruction.* If your hospital has a computerized patient-teaching program like the ones being developed and used in many institutions, you'll have to make arrangements for your patient to have access to the computer. If he needs instruction or orientation, you'll need to provide for that, too.

Empathy: Not to be overlooked

Teaching tools are no substitute for your personal teaching. No matter how colorful, stimulating, and novel your tools may be, your patient still needs further personal orientation and follow-up. Your personal touch will add a meaning and emphasis that no aid can provide—particularly when you supply the empathy he needs.

Empathy isn't listed here as a "tool," but it is indeed a subliminal teaching device that makes your patient comfortable, builds his confidence in you, and generally fosters his readiness to learn. If you don't feel instinctively empathetic toward a patient, you can cultivate this emotion by following this approach. First, show an interest in the patient and a willingness to help him. Make an active effort to see the situation through his eyes and to imagine what he must be feeling. Keep your body relaxed and maintain eye contact. Soon enough, you'll find yourself sharing some of the patient's feelings.

PREPARING A TEACHING PLAN

Now it's time to prepare an actual teaching plan, making use of the tools and methods just explored. (See *Understanding the Components of a Teaching Plan,* pages 56 and 57.)

As you approach this task, don't think of a teaching plan as a lengthy, written document. Whatever format you use—outline, checklist, flowchart—aim to make your plan complete enough to be helpful, yet concise enough to be practical.

Preparing a teaching plan may seem like just one more thing for you to do. But this step in the teaching process can actually save you time and will certainly make your teaching more effective. Even when you can't carry out the plan to the letter—which may be the case more often than not—the organization and thought you put into the plan will pay dividends in the quality and depth of your teaching.

Tailoring the Plan to Fit Your Patient

Let's see how you'd go about preparing a teaching plan for a specific patient. Suppose your patient is Mr. Fleming, a 70-year-old retired salesman with a 9-year history of congestive heart failure. On admission he told the nurse that he "ran out of medicine." This lack of his medicine undoubtedly contributed to the episode that led to his hospitalization.

Since you discover that Mr. Fleming ran out of his medicine because of financial and transportation problems, you won't want to bother teaching him the importance of taking his medication regularly. He was doing this until he developed financial difficulties. This aspect of Mr. Fleming's problem, you realize, could be better managed by a hospital resource outside of nursing—in this case, the social services department. Knowing and using your hospital's resources will save you time and promote your patient's well-being.

Before you design a teaching plan for Mr. Fleming, you'll need to consider the goals the entire health care team has set for him. So, after investigation, you find the goals are to have Mr. Fleming learn to manage his diet, his medications, and his activities at home. Since these goals are more likely to be achieved with Mr. Fleming's cooperation and understanding than without them, you'll want to work with him from the start to make the learning goals mutual. Approach this in a casual, conversational manner, rather than in a formal interview. Determine first whether he understands that he's in the hospital because his heart isn't pumping efficiently. Then you might say, "I'd like to talk with you about taking your medications and following your diet at home. Are there some things you'd like to know more about?

Have you had any problems in the past that I can help you with now?" You may find that Mr. Fleming responds well to your approach: that he's reasonable, cooperative, and willing to learn.

But you can't always count on your patient's responding positively. So for the moment, let's say Mr. Fleming is *not* eager to learn and participate in his own care. What then? There's little point in going ahead with the plan you'd normally use for his situation.

Form a contract

Establishing a contract with a noncompliant and resistant patient doesn't guarantee that effective learning and a change in attitude will take place. However, a contract *does* give the patient control over what is to be learned and allows you to make concessions—without losing sight of your overall teaching objectives.

Whether written or oral, a contract spells out each item of learning that is to be accomplished, describes your obligation as well as that of the patient, and gives a timetable. It also provides for an evaluation afterward of what learning has taken place.

How would a contract work in the case of Mr. Fleming's diet? You know he understands that salt is bad for him; yet he doesn't limit his salt intake. "I can't taste food without it," he says. Giving Mr. Fleming a lesson about the harmful effects of salt in his diet would be a waste of your time and his. You'd be going over information he already knows and chooses to ignore. But contracting with him to try other spices as salt substitutes could be the beginning of the behavioral changes you're trying to bring about.

As background information, you might explain to Mr. Fleming that as he ages, the number of his taste buds decreases; this tends to make tasting more difficult. Some of the spices included in his contract—thyme, basil, paprika, marjoram, and tarragon—are strong enough to give food some taste, thus making salt unnecessary.

UNDERSTANDING THE COMPONENTS OF A TEACHING PLAN

Whether your teaching plan is a comprehensive outline or a concise checklist, it should include a statement of your assessment findings and the patient's learning goals. What's more, it should include the activities, methods, and tools needed to accomplish these goals. Lastly, it should include the methods you'll use to evaluate the outcome of your teaching.

The chart below sets out part of a teaching plan for a diabetic patient.

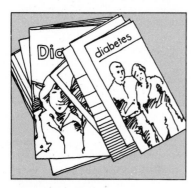

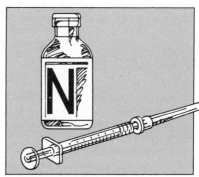

Assessment findings
Mr. Jones needs to understand the timing and action of his insulin.

Learning goals
Mr. Jones will be able to state the action, onset, peak, and duration of effect for NPH insulin.

Activities
• Present written brochures.
• Discuss content.
• Check the patient's understanding.

Teaching methods
• One-on-one discussion

Teaching tools
• Printed materials describing the timing and action of NPH insulin

Evaluation methods
• One-on-one discussion
• Written test

Assessment findings
Mr. Jones needs to learn how to give himself a subcutaneous injection of insulin.

Learning goals
Mr. Jones will correctly demonstrate self-injection of insulin.

Activities
• Show Mr. Jones the videotape on drawing up and injecting insulin.
• Have him study printed materials.
• Demonstrate each step of the procedure. Provide feedback and practice time.
• Have Mr. Jones demonstrate the procedure.

Teaching methods
• Demonstration
• Practice
• One-on-one discussion

Teaching tools
• Videotape
• Printed materials
• Photographs or illustrations of key steps in the procedure
• Physical objects

Evaluation methods
• Return demonstration
• One-on-one discussion

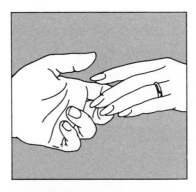

Assessment findings
Mr. Jones reports a loss of interest in sex. He needs to learn how to cope with this and to discuss sexual concerns with his wife.

Learning goals
Mr. Jones will share his concerns about his decreased libido with his wife.

Activities
• Explore with Mr. Jones how diabetes affects his libido. If appropriate, present case studies of how other patients have dealt with the situation.
• Encourage positive responses.
• Verify that Mr. Jones has discussed sexual concerns with his wife.

Teaching methods
• One-on-one discussion
• Group discussion
• Role playing
• Case study
• Self-monitoring

Teaching tools
• Printed materials

Evaluation methods
• One-on-one discussion
• Interview

Determine your teaching priorities

When you're ready to outline the content of your teaching plan, you'll need to decide on your teaching priorities. Your patient may well have complex medical problems that will require considerable teaching time. You'll have to decide at the start what the patient needs to know for his protection, safety, and well-being, and what would be nice for him to know for his comfort and convenience. The reality is that what's necessary may be all you'll have time to accomplish in your teaching plan. By establishing your priorities early, you'll be better able to organize your teaching time.

One aid you can use to determine your teaching priorities is Maslow's classic hierarchy of needs. Maslow theorized that human behavior is dominated by certain basic needs that, though interrelated, are hierarchical. The lower-level needs must be satisfied before other, higher-level needs can be met. According to Maslow, the most basic needs are physiologic. During an illness, these fundamental physiologic needs are usually in jeopardy. (See *Relating Learning Needs to Maslow's Hierarchy*, pages 60 and 61.)

Applying Maslow's hierarchy to Mr. Fleming's learning needs, you'll see that teaching Mr. Fleming the proper positioning for relief of the dyspnea resulting from his congestive heart failure attends to a basic and immediate physiologic need—maintaining his supply of oxygen. Breathing is necessary for his survival and therefore comes first. Teaching Mr. Fleming about salt substitutes doesn't qualify as an immediate survival skill, but rather as a long-term need.

In short, make your teaching priorities reflect the patient's survival priorities. That way, if you don't have time on your shift to teach about salt substitutes, you can be comfortable letting the staff on the next shift handle that part of the plan. If necessary, any lessons addressing Mr. Fleming's long-

FITTING A STANDARD TEACHING PLAN TO YOUR PATIENT'S NEEDS

Your institution may have developed standard teaching plans for some of the most common disorders you teach about. Here's how to adapt such a plan to meet your patient's specific learning needs.

Let's say your patient, Mrs. Porter, is a 47-year-old mother of three teenagers. She works as a housekeeper to augment her husband's salary as a school custodian.

Mrs. Porter has been hospitalized many times with chronic renal failure, caused initially by a streptococcal infection. Her disease is progressing, and the health care team feels that she'll soon require dialysis. Adjustments have been made in her diet and medications, and she needs further instruction in these areas.

In your assessment, you find Mrs. Porter depressed about her advancing disease. She agrees to be taught about diet and medication changes but has no questions. She avoids eye contact and her face seems expressionless. Her comments indicate concern about the impending dialysis.

What are Mrs. Porter's learning needs? What, if anything, will you teach her today? What tools will you use?

With the standard teaching plan as your guide, start by assessing Mrs. Porter's knowledge and skills in the areas listed. This will tell you which points to delete from

STANDARD TEACHING PLAN FOR CHRONIC RENAL FAILURE

CONTENT	TOOLS/ACTIVITIES	EVALUATION METHODS
Kidney function • Anatomy • Fluid balance • Electrolytes	• Discussion • Pamphlet #27 • Model of kidney	• Question/ answer • Discussion
Renal failure • Causes • Stages • Complications • Signs/symptoms of complications	• Discussion with MD/RN • Pamphlet #32 • Videotape #16	• Question/ answer • Discussion
Diagnostic tests • Sodium, potassium, creatinine, BUN • Radiographic studies	• Brochure #17 • Discussion	• Question/ answer
Dialysis options • Peritoneal (intermittent or continuous) dialysis • Hemodialysis	• Discussion of process (peritoneal dialysis or hemodialysis), photos 33 to 37 (peritoneal), 66 to 100 (hemodialysis) • Visit to dialysis unit with equipment preview and demonstration • Discussion of life-style changes • Identification of support services	• Return demonstration
Other treatments • Activity • Diet • Medication	• Discussion of activity • Videotape #5 • Discussion by dietitian • Pamphlet #7 • Discussion of medications by MD/RN • Medication cards for each drug	• Question/ answer • Menu selection • Medication management • Discussion

the teaching plan, which ones to include, and which ones to modify.

For example, Mrs. Porter already seems to understand renal anatomy and function, but you decide to check the extent of her knowledge and refresh her memory when you describe how dialysis works. And when you teach her about diagnostic tests, you'll explain just the ones she hasn't experienced before.

Consequently, you draw up individualized learning goals for Mrs. Porter (see below) and then determine your teaching priorities. You decide that Mrs. Porter's emotional adjustment to the progression of her disease poses a barrier to her learning at this time, but you decide to address her concerns about dialysis. Because Mrs. Porter won't be especially receptive to your teaching, you may only be able to familiarize her with the process and perhaps dispel any misconceptions. But doing this today may make future teaching sessions more productive. You decide to describe the process, using photos and diagrams, and leave some pamphlets for her to read. You also decide to discuss the life-style changes that dialysis requires and Mrs. Porter's concerns about those changes. After today's session, you'll reevaluate to see what else you may want to use from the standard teaching plan.

Mrs. Porter's learning goals: Chronic renal failure

Mrs. Porter and her family will be able to:

1. describe basic kidney functions.

2. relate personal symptoms to the process of chronic renal failure.

3. list symptoms of impending pulmonary edema and pericarditis.

4. state the reason for the necessary diagnostic tests (serum studies, urinalysis, CT scans, IVP, arteriograms, and biopsy).

5. select a form of dialysis that's compatible with her desired lifestyle.

6. state dietary and fluid restrictions as they relate to Mrs. Porter's particular stage of failure.

7. state correct administration method of medications.

8. state side effects of medications that should be reported to the doctor.

term needs can even be taught when he gets home.

Most likely, Mr. Fleming isn't the only patient whose learning needs you must address. When you're spreading your teaching time among a number of patients, you'll find that ranking learning needs first by the individual patient and then across all of your patients will help you make the most effective use of your limited teaching time.

Accommodate the patient's learning strengths

Before selecting the teaching methods and tools for your plan, try the direct approach: ask the patient how he learns best. If he tells you he learns by watching and imitating, or perhaps by reading and figuring out the instructions for himself, you'll have gained a useful insight for your teaching plan. When you're ready to put this information to work, your plan stands a chance of saving time and energy for you, the patient, and other members of his health care team.

Knowing your patient's preferred learning style, you can then select complementary methods and materials. If, for example, Mr. Fleming sees himself as a visual learner, you would ideally make generous use of films, photographs, and even cartoons to illustrate the concepts you're teaching him. If he learns best by reading and figuring out the instructions and procedures for himself, you'd supply him with suitable printed materials to supplement your initial explanation. Remember to take a few minutes to come back to him afterward and ask if he had any problems with or questions about the material.

But don't ever feel that your patient's learning preference eliminates other tools and methods that seem suitable or valuable to you. You'll want to achieve as varied a teaching "menu" as possible to stimulate the patient's curiosity and to enable him to view a problem from more than one perspective.

RELATING LEARNING NEEDS TO MASLOW'S HIERARCHY

If your patient has complex medical problems that require extensive teaching, you may find it difficult to put his learning needs into proper order. Maslow's hierarchy of physiologic and psychological needs can help you establish the sequence and priority of your teaching.

The diagram here shows how, in Maslow's terms, you might rank learning needs for a patient with chronic obstructive pulmonary disease. At the foundation lie the patient's basic physiologic needs, which take precedence over his need for safety and, in turn, his needs for psychological well-being and self-actualization. Your teaching should follow a similar pattern, beginning with the topics that relate to physiologic needs and progressing to teaching for higher levels of need.

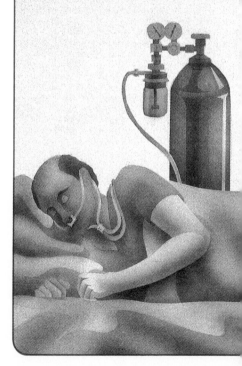

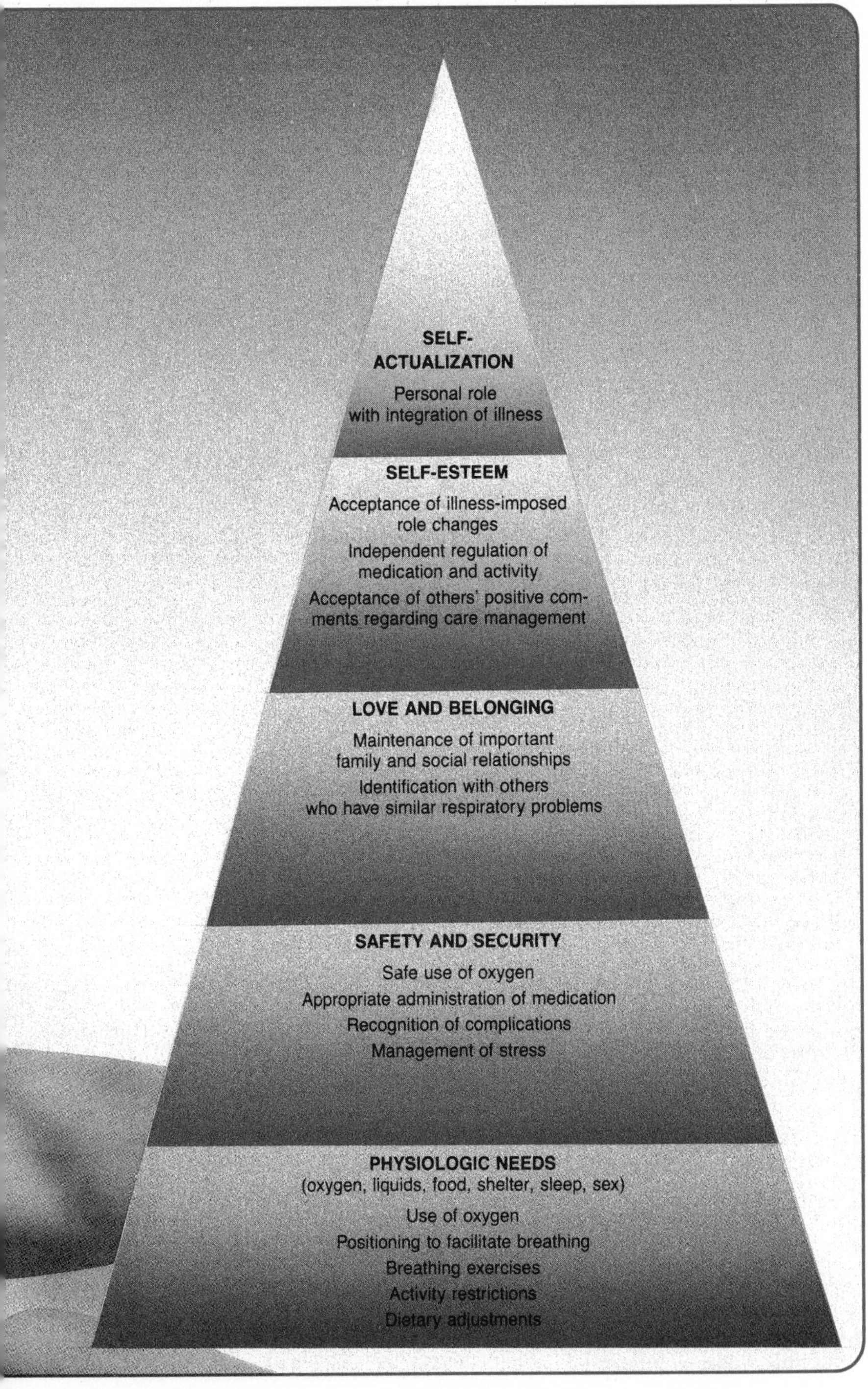

**SELF-
ACTUALIZATION**

Personal role
with integration of illness

SELF-ESTEEM

Acceptance of illness-imposed
role changes

Independent regulation of
medication and activity

Acceptance of others' positive comments regarding care management

LOVE AND BELONGING

Maintenance of important
family and social relationships

Identification with others
who have similar respiratory problems

SAFETY AND SECURITY

Safe use of oxygen

Appropriate administration of medication

Recognition of complications

Management of stress

PHYSIOLOGIC NEEDS
(oxygen, liquids, food, shelter, sleep, sex)

Use of oxygen

Positioning to facilitate breathing

Breathing exercises

Activity restrictions

Dietary adjustments

TEACHING

Implementing Your Plan

The true challenge comes when you're ready to put your plan to work. In planning stages, all things seem possible. But when the time comes to implement your plan, you may have to take off the rose-colored glasses and become as creative as you can with the materials—and the time—you have.

Sidestepping obstacles
In short, if the wide variety of resources we've described aren't available when lesson time arrives, you'll have to get down to teaching without them. You still have the most important tool at hand: an active interchange between you and your "student."

Another major obstacle to the best-laid teaching plans is time. A staff shortage can easily sabotage your planned time for teaching. At other times, you'll have time for teaching, but your patient will be out of his room for tests. Or he'll be in too much discomfort to be receptive to your teaching. Or he'll have visitors. And so on.

As a nurse, you've learned to expect the unexpected. So circumvent the unexpected that steals your teaching time: use any moment you're with the patient to do some teaching. Don't think your planning is wasted. Your most spontaneous teaching will be better for the work that went into your plan.

Incorporating teaching into your patient care can be done in a number of ways. You can talk the patient through a new procedure, such as learning to take his own blood pressure, as you're performing that part of his care.

If the material to be taught is complicated, such as medication schedules, or comes in several parts, such as dressing changes or tracheostomy care, save time by explaining one part at a time. Do this especially when you detect a low point in the patient's attention span.

Explain what you're doing as you do it. If you're teaching Mr. Fleming how to position himself for breathing ease and comfort, encourage him to ask questions and to repeat what you've just told him. Review the procedure with him the next time you're in his room; in subsequent visits, allow him to do more and more of the task by himself. This technique, called *chaining*, allows for learning and practicing in a series of sessions.

You can also give your patient written instructions that he can refer to between teaching sessions and after his discharge. When he's on his own, these instructions can help to diminish his anxiety and to remind him of the things you stressed in your teaching. They can also serve as a hedge against backsliding that requires repeat teaching. Keep the written instructions brief and close to the information and advice you gave him in person. Refer to things you talked about—or even laughed about—in teaching sessions; this will help to refresh his memory and make the material more personal. Group the information under topical headings, which you can emphasize with large, bold letters. Add magazine pictures or your own illustrations to make the material memorable. Check your instructions carefully for accuracy, then go over them with the patient to ensure that he can read and understand what you've written. Encourage him to refer to the instructions until he's sure of the contents.

Gear your teaching to the patient's social, emotional, and cognitive needs to gain maximum benefit from his developmental capabilities (see *Relating Developmental Stages to Teaching Approaches,* pages 64 and 65).

If you identify a patient who seems unmotivated to learn and you're convinced he's resistant to your teaching, document this on his chart, explaining objectively the basis for your conclusion. Inform the doctor of the problem, and then spend your time elsewhere. Although he may be the very patient who needs your teaching and guidance the most, he's also the one who will benefit the least from your efforts. Come back to this patient later to try again—perhaps with a fresh approach. His situation and attitude can change, making him a more willing learner. However, if he remains unwilling to listen and learn, you're responsible for noting this on the chart and arranging for the required teaching to be done at discharge.

Promoting compliance

Your best teaching will prove meaningless if your patient doesn't apply what you've taught him. If you've been working closely with him from the start, chances are greater for approaching the ideal two-way teaching-learning dynamic that promotes compliance. But now, when you're implementing your plan, you're especially anxious to have an "A" student.

Working toward compliance begins early with soliciting the patient's reaction to the teaching plan as you're formulating it. Keep his concerns in mind, and be willing to consider his criticisms of the plan or his suggestions for improvement. All of this will contribute to agreement not only on the plan, but also on what the patient's rightful participation should be.

You'd be wise to limit the number of tasks you expect of a patient at a given time. If too much is expected of him, he's in danger of doing nothing. Also, when you're attempting to reach a behavioral goal with your patient, try approaching the problem by *adding* new behaviors rather than by *phasing out* established ones.

To make the teaching process work, keep the patient as active a participant as possible. Also stress the importance of his practicing what he's learned.

Giving the right feedback

The feedback you give your patient has the potential for helping or hurting him. In giving him the information he needs to correct, improve, or continue what he's doing, you're providing concrete help. On the other hand, feedback that describes the patient himself—whether praising him as smart and cooperative or criticizing him as slow and unmotivated—isn't typically helpful and could even be harmful.

Reinforcing the gains

Success, we know, breeds success. The patient who is learning successfully is the patient likely to continue learning. The opposite is also true: lack of success can lead to discouragement and can quickly end a patient's efforts to learn.

Patient teaching, though, isn't necessarily a foregone success or failure. After all, you can influence its outcome by using reinforcement and reward. As adjuncts to your teaching, reinforcement and reward will increase the probability of your patient's learning and following his prescribed therapy.

Reinforcers vary from person to person and from situation to situation. They can be verbal or nonverbal, material or intangible. They can range from a book or a piece of candy to a smile or a hug; from extra privileges to an expression of appreciation.

Some reinforcers are external, coming to the patient from you and others; some are internal, coming to the patient from within himself. The latter would include a sense of accomplishment, improved sleeping patterns, greater self-esteem, and improved body image. Sometimes, external reinforcers are added to internal ones; this happens when the patient gets comments and compliments on, for example, improving interpersonal relationships, achieving desired weight loss, or increasing his mobility.

RELATING DEVELOPMENTAL STAGES TO TEACHING APPROACHES

STAGE OF DEVELOPMENT	TYPICAL BEHAVIOR DURING HOSPITALIZATION	TEACHING APPROACHES
Infant	*Under 7 months:* • Responds well to nurse • Allows parents to leave *Over 7 months:* • Anxious and unhappy • Clings to parents and cries when they leave	• Teach the parents to participate in their infant's care. • Handle the infant gently and speak in a soft, friendly tone of voice. • Use a security toy or pacifier to reduce the infant's anxiety and elicit cooperation.
Toddler	• Commonly experiences separation anxiety • May show anger by crying, shaking crib • Rejects nurse's attention • May become apathetic, crying intermittently or continuously • May reject parents and respond to nurse	• Teach the parents to participate in their child's care. • Give the child simple, direct, and honest explanations just before treatment or surgery. • Use puppets or coloring books to explain procedures. • Let the child play with equipment to reduce anxiety. • Let the child make appropriate choices, such as choosing the side of the body for an injection.
Preschooler 	• Experiences separation anxiety; may panic or throw tantrums, especially when parents leave • Often regresses (enuresis) • Commonly shows eating and sleeping disturbances	• Teach the parents to participate in their child's care. • Use simple, neutral words to describe procedures and surgery to the child. • Encourage the child to fantasize to help plan her responses to possible situations. • Use body outlines or dolls to show anatomic sites and procedures. • Let the child handle equipment before a procedure. • Use play therapy as an emotional outlet and a way to test the child's sense of reality.
School-age child 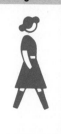	• May have insomnia, nightmares, enuresis due to anxiety about the unknown • Alternately conforms to adult standards and rebels against them	• Use body outlines and models to explain body mechanisms and procedures. • Explain logically why a procedure is necessary. • Describe the sensations to anticipate during a procedure. • Encourage the child's active participation in learning. • Praise the child for cooperating with a procedure.

STAGE OF DEVELOPMENT	TYPICAL BEHAVIOR DURING HOSPITALIZATION	TEACHING APPROACHES
Adolescent 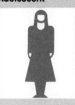	• Fluctuates in willingness to participate in care because of need for both independence and approval • Shows concern about how procedure or surgery may affect appearance	• Ask the patient if she wants her parents present during teaching sessions and procedures. • Give scientific explanations, using body diagrams, models, or videotapes. • Encourage the patient to verbalize her feelings or express them through artwork or writing. • Offer praise appropriately.
Adult 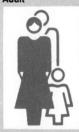	• Directs and participates in her own care • Complies with hospital regulations • Freely asks questions when she has concerns or uncertainties • Demonstrates continued interest in personal roles • Shows concern for family and economic results of hospitalization	• Negotiate learning goals with the patient. • Include family members in teaching. • Use problem-centered teaching. • Provide for immediate application of learning. • Let the patient test her own ideas, take risks, and be creative. Allow her to evaluate her actions and change her behavior. • Use the patient's past experiences as a learning resource.
Older adult 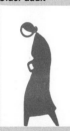	• Demonstrates anxiety over new procedures or a change in routine • Often forgets new material or ideas or takes a long time to make decisions • Maintains interest in personal matters • Asks for instructions to be repeated • Participates in care and decision making • Requires frequent rest periods	• Negotiate learning goals with the patient. • Include family members in teaching. • Schedule frequent, short teaching sessions (15 minutes maximum) at times of peak energy. Avoid holding sessions after the patient has bathed, ambulated, or taken medications that affect learning ability. • Check for memory deficit by asking for verbal feedback. • Present one idea at a time. • Use simple sentences, concrete examples, and reminders, such as calendars or pillboxes. • Speak slowly and distinctly in a conversational tone. • Use large-print materials and equipment with oversized numbers. Avoid using teaching materials printed on glossy paper.

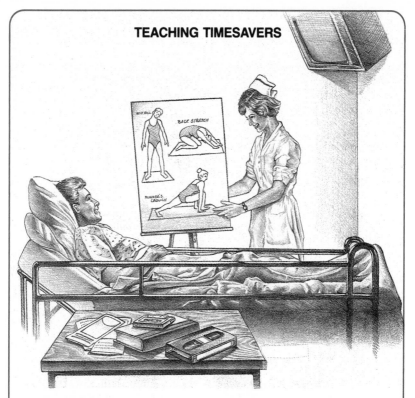

TEACHING TIMESAVERS

Saving your time

Consider these ways to save time in your patient teaching:
• Before you begin teaching, have the patient review written materials, audio cassettes, or videotapes to gain a basic understanding of his disorder.
• Use diagrams, charts, and other visual aids in your teaching sessions to speed comprehension.
• Rely on support staff to augment your teaching. For example, have the dietitian discuss meal plans with your patient, the respiratory technician explain spirometry, and the physical therapist teach crutch walking.
• If the patient's family will be participating in his care at home, schedule your teaching sessions during their visits.
• Teach the patient while you're providing routine nursing care. Let his questions guide your teaching.
• If you're teaching a short-stay patient and a home health nurse has been selected for him, you may want to emphasize the major points in your teaching and leave the minor points for the home health nurse.

• Document your teaching to avoid duplication of instruction.
• Document a patient's repeated resistance to teaching, and move on to teach another patient.
• Give the patient preprinted information and instructions to take home, rather than write new ones yourself.
• Once you've developed a teaching plan for a specific disorder, keep it filed for reuse or adaptation.
• Constantly evaluate your teaching to find the methods that work best for you. Then use those methods.

Saving staff time

To save time for your colleagues, suggest implementing timesaving programs that have worked in other institutions:
• Use group-teaching sessions for patients with similar teaching needs, such as diabetes, hypertension, cardiac rehabilitation, and postnatal care.
• For same-day surgery patients, add a nurse to the preadmission testing staff and make preoperative and postoperative teaching that nurse's responsibility.

The value of a reinforcer varies from patient to patient. For a patient who has been on an inflexible diet, a less restrictive one can become a powerful reinforcer. However, what seems like a liberalized diet to this patient could feel like a punitive one to another patient who hasn't been subject to any restrictions.

If a patient's basic physiologic needs have been met, reinforcers that help meet his needs for love, belonging, and esteem are likely to be effective.

• *Reward the positive.* Because reinforcement can dramatically influence a patient's behavior, you'll want to use it selectively and cautiously. Try a guideline that applies to many teaching situations: recognize what's desirable and ignore what's undesirable—unless the undesirable behavior is dangerous, disruptive, or illegal. So, if you have a demanding patient who seems to use the call bell more often than all the other patients on the floor combined, refrain from remarking about his annoying habit as much as you can. But do give him ample attention when he's not ringing the bell. He should get the idea eventually that his desirable behavior brings more rewards and attention than his undesirable behavior.

It's axiomatic that when the attention paid to undesirable behavior exceeds the attention paid to desirable behavior, the undesirable behavior is reinforced. Complaining or demanding patient behavior, noncompliance with prescribed regimens, and other negative responses can and should be overlooked. The emphasis and attention should be focused on positive responses and behaviors.

In your use of reward and reinforcement, you can't always afford to wait until a task is learned or accomplished. The patient can become discouraged along the way and stop trying. "What's the use?" he tells himself. "I'll never make it." When the goal seems particularly difficult or far away, encouragement and recognition of intermediate progress are crucial. A patient who's learning to walk with crutches or use a prosthesis needs this ongoing encouragement and reinforcement.

• *Be specific, appropriate, and prompt.* If you nod and say "great" or "good" to a patient, he may sense approval on your part; but you haven't succeeded in reinforcing any *specific* behavior. Make your comments specific, and indicate whether you're approving (and reinforcing) progress toward an agreed-upon teaching goal, a change in attitude, or his first attempt at a difficult task.

Use reinforcement or reward only when it's justified. Contrived enthusiasm and unfounded praise have no place in the process of reinforcement. Only genuine acknowledgment of a desired behavior will work.

Try to vary the words and change your approach from time to time. A single phrase or response repeated with unwavering regularity has virtually no power as a reinforcer. Let's say you have a patient who should be walking more. In addition to the usual encouragement, why not try a little humor or have a coffee break with him?

Give the patient his rewards and reinforcement promptly. Even a short delay can make a reward ineffective, especially if you're dealing with a young patient or a patient whose memory or time sense is impaired. The delayed reward may still be pleasing, but it won't have the same strength to influence the patient's behavior.

A FINAL WORD

While you're teaching, don't overlook the importance of the feedback you get from the patient, his family, and your colleagues. You'll find it an important stimulus to adapting, modifying, and improving your teaching.

4

Evaluating Your Teaching

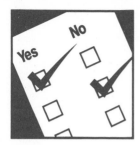

Evaluating Your Teaching

Introduction

Can the patient tolerate sitting still in a chair for 5 more minutes? Is the wound healing? Is the product doing its job?

More often than not, you ask yourself questions like these every day you're on duty. And as you answer them, you're making judgments. You're evaluating.

However, if you're like many nurses, you may not always remember to evaluate your patient teaching. Nonetheless, legislators and consumers today demand greater accountability from the health care system than ever before, and this accountability extends to patient teaching. You must demonstrate results in your teaching as surely as you do in your other responsibilities.

Evaluation is the tool you'll use to show those results. It helps you individualize your teaching and improve your skills. (See *How Evaluation Improves Your Teaching,* pages 70 and 71.) What's more, thorough evaluation helps you promote patient compliance and competent self-care at home.

What is evaluation?

Evaluation refers to the continuous and systematic appraisal of the patient's learning progress during and after your teaching. By comparing the results of your evaluation with the learning goals that you and the patient have agreed upon, you'll be able to judge the effec-

tiveness of your patient teaching. Obviously, the more clearly defined and objective the learning goals, the more accurate and useful your evaluation will be.

Let's look at an example of a well-defined learning goal, one that lets you measure the patient's progress precisely: "The patient will list the five common symptoms of excessive cardiac work load." This goal gives you a clear-cut standard for evaluating the patient's success; his answer will tell you whether he knows the five symptoms or not. Accurate evaluation requires learning goals as precise as this one.

Compare this with an example of a poorly defined learning goal, which makes evaluation difficult if not impossible: "The patient will recognize unusual chest pain." This vague goal doesn't explain how the patient can recognize this pain or how different "unusual" is from "usual." How could you possibly evaluate this goal when you and the patient wouldn't be sure what it means?

As you can see, you need to clearly define your patient's goals, so that you can collect the information you need to evaluate your teaching—whether it's cognitive information, motor skills, or attitudes. With precise data and standards, you'll know how well the patient

HOW EVALUATION IMPROVES YOUR TEACHING

Evaluation of your effectiveness as a teacher can—and should—draw on many sources. Use feedback from the patient and his family to judge how well you've carried out the process of teaching and achieved the product, the patient's learning. Of course, you'll also want to evaluate your own performance.

This dynamic system of feedback and evaluation will help you identify the changes needed to improve your teaching effectiveness.

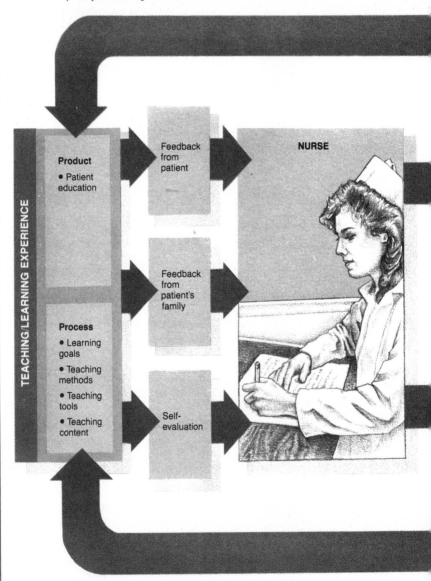

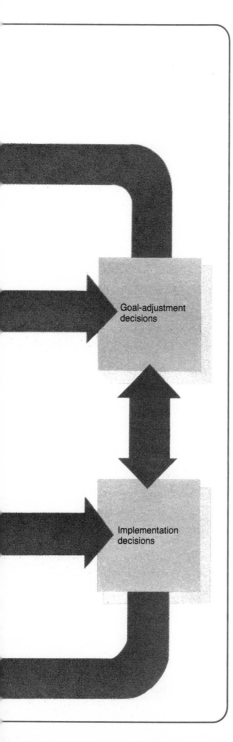

Goal-adjustment
decisions

Implementation
decisions

has learned, which is a good indicator of how well you've taught.

Not an exact science

Of course, evaluation isn't an exact science. Your good judgment is another important ingredient. For example, if you're evaluating a patient's skill at giving himself a subcutaneous insulin injection, you know that there isn't just one "right" way to do it. Your knowledge and experience provide the criteria for you to judge whether the patient's injection technique is safe and effective.

Perspectives on evaluation

You can evaluate your teaching from several perspectives. As a nurse, you'll of course be evaluating the learning of your individual patient. And you'll be evaluating your own skill and technique as a teacher. But you may also be asked for feedback that others can use to evaluate the overall worth of your institution's patient-education program. In some cases, you yourself may be the person who'll be evaluating that program.

Why evaluate patient teaching?

In the teaching/learning process, your ongoing evaluation constantly redirects your planning and teaching. What are some of the main advantages of this ongoing evaluation?

• *Reinforcing desirable behavior.* Continuous evaluation provides the basis for feedback to the patient, so you can reinforce desirable behavior.

• *Redirecting undesirable behavior.* Ongoing evaluation can also help you correct flaws early. For example, if your patient is contaminating his sterile eye dressing, you'll probably discover this early enough to help him learn the correct technique and speed his recovery.

• *Measuring the patient's progress in meeting learning goals.* Can the patient do a full dressing change or just part of it? Can he select his menu for a whole day or for just one meal? Knowing the answers to questions like these lets you determine how much progress the patient's making and how much he has yet to learn. And it addresses your foremost concern: can the patient survive on his own? Has he learned the skills and coping mechanisms he'll need to manage his condition at home?

• *Avoiding pitfalls.* Ongoing evaluation helps you avoid common pitfalls. For example, if a patient has trouble with tracheal suctioning in the hospital, he may not even try the procedure when he gets home. Your prompt evaluation will alert you in time to reteach him or to include additional home instruction in his discharge plan.

• *Justifying costs.* In a time of cost containment, evaluation can justify the time, materials, and staff used in teaching. For example, your evaluation may show that many patients benefit from physical therapy. You can use this information in a new patient's hospitalization to schedule timely, efficient use of staff.

• *Providing necessary documentation.* Even if you clearly and completely document your patient's learning goals and your teaching sessions, you still need to document the results. This documentation, required by the Joint Commission for the Accreditation of Hospitals, serves as a legal safeguard: it provides a permanent record of the extent and success of teaching. And it could serve as your defense against charges of insufficient patient care even years later.

Clear documentation also has other advantages. For instance, it helps other members of the health care team gauge the overall worth of a patient's education program. This keeps all caregivers on the same wavelength, ensuring continuity of care and further saving time and money. Documentation can also give you "ammunition" to back up any of your requests for improving patient care or to demonstrate cost effectiveness.

• *Identifying effective teaching strategies.* You may not know what

you're doing right unless you check up on yourself. When you know which teaching techniques work well, you can develop a blueprint for productive teaching.

Where does evaluation begin?

Evaluation represents a kind of ongoing follow-up assessment. You should start by planning how you're going to evaluate as you plan what you're going to teach. For instance, if you plan to teach the steps of tracheostomy care, plan for each step's evaluation as you go along. Decide what data you'll need to determine if the patient's learned the step and what method you'll use to get that data.

Don't save your entire evaluation for the end of your teaching. Plan for brief, periodic evaluations throughout the teaching process. This serves a double purpose: it lets the patient immediately try out what he's learned, and it gives you immediate feedback for deciding the next step in your teaching—either reteaching the last step or moving ahead. For example, if you've just explained the types of high-cholesterol foods and their risks to a patient, let him try selecting low-cholesterol foods from a menu. This gives him a chance to try his new knowledge. And it gives you a chance to evaluate his learning, to reinforce his correct responses, and to redirect any incorrect ones. If you postpone evaluation at this point, you may later find yourself reteaching information you mistakenly assumed he'd already learned.

Immediate evaluation has another advantage. It lets you see if you're the one who needs redirection, especially if the patient doesn't seem to be making any headway. In that case, you may need to try a different tack. For example, if your patient can't correctly care for his colostomy, you may discover he felt awkward and embarrassed during your teaching session and only half-heard what you were saying. Perhaps you should try using an audiovisual teaching aid that lets the patient become familiar with the procedure in private before you rehearse it with him.

Although evaluation lets you discover which teaching strategies work best in specific situations, bear in mind that no one strategy works best for all patients in all situations.

Let your patient participate in his evaluation, just as you include him in other phases of teaching. And don't forget to give yourself time for evaluation. After all, evaluation isn't something you can sandwich between your other duties. It requires its own allotted time in your teaching schedule.

THE PROCESS

What to Evaluate

Effective evaluation assesses the learner, the teacher, and the teaching strategies and media.

Evaluating the learner
You'll be evaluating your patient against the yardstick of his learning goals: the more goals he's achieved, the better he's learned. Still, although the patient may have helped set these goals and have agreed to them, he may not be as goal-oriented as you. You must provide the motivation and direction. (See *Giving Feedback,* page 74.)

Start by letting the patient know how and when you'll evaluate his learning. Tell him the sort of questions you'll be asking and explain that you'll be asking them throughout the teaching sessions.

Structure your evaluation around the patient's successes, not around his failures. Ask him to tell you what topics *he* feels he's mastered. This lets him begin the process of self-evaluation and helps him take responsibility for his

learning. For example, to evaluate the patient's grasp of your instructions about menu planning, you might say, "Let's talk about choosing foods for your diet. Why don't you tell me what you'd select for breakfast—or, for that matter, for any other meal?" Or, to determine another patient's grasp of a new procedure, you might say, "Before we look at this procedure as a whole, show me the parts of it you feel most comfortable about."

Such a learner-centered approach to evaluation lets you quickly know what the patient has learned. It also lets him start off successfully, which can go far in cushioning any future setbacks.

When your patient meets with a failure, as he undoubtedly will, discuss with him what *the two of you as a team* are going to do about it. Promoting teamwork and feedback at this early stage helps you set the stage for handling future problems and decisions. For example, suppose your patient can't apply his ostomy bag with a good seal. Without your guidance and encouragement, he might become frustrated and discouraged. With it, he might opt to use a different method of application or a different type of pouch. This way, you'll have handled a failure positively and turned it into a success.

Evaluating the teacher
While you're evaluating the patient's progress, don't forget to evaluate your own teaching skills. You can use several methods to evaluate them, but you'll probably find that getting feedback from as many sources as possible provides better data than does a solitary approach. Here are some teacher-evaluation methods that work well:
• *Patient-family satisfaction reports.* These short, simple questionnaires can be completed by the patient and his family at the end of a teaching session or, if necessary, at home after discharge. However, reports that go home may not be returned. (Bear in mind that patients may give only the answers they believe you want to hear

GIVING FEEDBACK

Evaluation of patient teaching rests on a foundation of helpful feedback. The patient tells or shows you what he's learned, and you point out his successes as well as any areas needing improvement. Obviously, this exchange of information should help build the patient's confidence and improve his competence. To achieve this, though, and to avoid confronting and frustrating the patient, you'll need to adopt a positive, constructive attitude in these ways:

BE HELPFUL

Make your comments helpful, not hurtful. Share information and present alternatives, rather than dictate rules. And avoid using absolute words, such as "always" and "never."

Be sure to focus on the patient's behavior, not on his progress or personality. And discuss his *current* behavior, not his past. For instance, don't say, "That's the third time you've made this incorrect diet selection. Try it again." Instead, say some-

thing like, "Remember, carrots are high in carbohydrates. If you eat them at noon you'll have to leave them out of your evening meal, to maintain your carbohydrate restrictions."

Give the patient positive feedback first to reinforce desired behavior. Then discuss the points that he still needs to master. Otherwise, the negative comments are probably all he'll hear and remember.

BE PROMPT

Give feedback as soon as possible after you observe the patient's behavior. The longer the patient continues with an undesirable behavior, thought, or attitude,

the more comfortable he'll become with it and the greater difficulty he'll have changing it.

BE SPECIFIC

Offer specific suggestions for improvement along with the rationale. If the patient understands why something needs to be done, he'll more easily remember to do it— and do it correctly. For example, you might say, "The angle at which you're holding the needle makes it go too deep. Hold the needle at a 45-degree angle instead of perpendicular to your skin."

And make sure the patient understands

the feedback you've given him. If he's perfecting a technique, have him repeat it immediately, so you can check his corrections. If he's attempting something less tangible, such as changing an attitude, you might ask him to rephrase your feedback, to see if he's really listening. Also, observe other clues in his facial expressions and his offhand remarks.

BE PRACTICAL

Comment on situations that the patient can change, not ones beyond his control. For instance, if your colostomy patient has

limited financial resources, don't emphasize the advantages of using more expensive disposable equipment.

BE FLEXIBLE

Move at the patient's pace, not yours. Keep in mind his needs and abilities and the amount of information he can handle. For example, instead of discussing the patient's entire drug regimen all at once, you might

say, "Your medication schedule is complex. Let's talk today about just the one thing that's giving you the most trouble. We can cover the rest at our next session."

when they give face-to-face feedback.)

In these reports, phrase your questions clearly and directly. Avoid negative or ambiguous questions, since they produce negative or ambiguous answers. Here are some useful questions:

☐ Was the material well organized?

☐ Was the presentation clear?

☐ Did you find the session interesting?

☐ Was the teacher's approach satisfactory?

☐ Did she use a pleasant tone of voice?

☐ Was the presentation paced properly or was it too fast or slow?

☐ Was humor used effectively?

☐ What, if anything, would improve the presentation?

Don't expect unanimous opinions and do expect some unfavorable ones. However, use the majority opinion to guide you in improving your presentation.

• *Self-evaluation.* As a teacher, you can teach yourself. Write down what you think are the strengths and weaknesses of your instruction. If possible, use a tape recorder to capture your teaching session. Or videotape the session, if possible, to give you an audiovisual record for later evaluation. Let your recording or written review sit for a few days; then go over it again. You'll have a fresher, more objective approach when you return to it.

Start your self-critique by asking yourself questions similar to those you asked your patient:

☐ Were you comfortable with all aspects of your presentation?

☐ What kind of questions did the patient and his family ask?

☐ Do they point to the need for more information or a clearer presentation?

☐ How well did the patient achieve his learning goals?

Accentuate the positive as you did in evaluating the patient's learning. The negative aspects can point toward improvements; don't be discouraged by them.

• *Peer evaluation.* Your colleagues can be some of your best teachers. Ask a nurse whose opinion you respect, or ask several nurses, to observe your teaching. If possible, show her your teaching goals and content outline. Then ask her to comment on your teaching approach and to suggest improvements.

Evaluating your teaching strategies and media

Are your teaching strategies the most effective and efficient means of instruction you can provide, given the resources available to you? To find out, you must examine how your strategies work on individual patients:

☐ Are my strategies well implemented, considering the constraints of time and space?

☐ Is the patient enthusiastic?

☐ Am I individualizing my teaching?

If you answer "no" to most of these questions, you need to revise your teaching strategy.

To help you evaluate the media used in teaching, ask yourself these questions:

☐ Can I use media well and easily in the space I have?

☐ Does the patient have time to view the filmstrip or the videotape?

☐ Can I easily integrate media into my teaching plan?

If you answer "no" to most of these questions, the media probably aren't worthwhile and should be discarded.

Preparing for Evaluation

Once you've committed yourself to evaluation, begin by focusing clearly on what you want to evaluate. Narrow your goals and set priorities for the outcomes to be measured. Otherwise, you'll waste time collecting more data than you can possibly evaluate.

Then consider what types of questions and instruments are most apt to provide you with answers. Throughout your own education, tests were probably used as the main measure of your learning. Naturally, you may want to rely on them to evaluate your patient's learning. Resist the urge. Although tests are useful in some situations, they evaluate knowledge, not behavior. To evaluate behavior, you must observe it. Watching the patient change a dressing is better than giving him a test on the steps involved.

Think about where and when to best evaluate specific types of learning. For example, you can evaluate a patient's abstinence from smoking in the hospital, but a truer evaluation may come after the patient's discharged. Similarly, some outcomes may be evaluated effectively in a single test, while others—such as techniques to lower blood pressure or cholesterol levels—will require repeated evaluation over time. Remember, too, that factors interfering with the learning process can also interfere with evaluation of learning. If you evaluate the patient when he's tired, upset, or in pain, the results may not be accurate.

THE METHODS

Gathering Data

In carrying out your evaluation, you have a mix of data-gathering techniques at your disposal—and you should use a mix to provide the broadest possible view. Let's look closely at the most useful techniques.

Direct observation
In this method, often called *return demonstration*, you watch the patient demonstrate a skill or act out a simulated situation. This method works well in evaluating motor skills, such as giving an injection, changing a dressing, or bathing a newborn. It doesn't work as well in evaluating attitudinal changes since these are more difficult to observe. You might, however, become adept at reading the subtle body-language cues that signal a patient's changing attitude about doing his own ostomy irrigation or changing an amputation dressing.

You can save time with this type of evaluation by incorporating it into the patient's routine care. For instance, you can have him change his dressing while you observe for correct equipment collection, establishment of a sterile field, gloving, and handling of dressing materials using sterile techniques. You may also observe the patient's nonverbal reactions as clues to his feelings about this aspect of his care.

Besides actively involving the learner and providing for immediate feedback, observation also helps you make the patient aware of inappropriate behavior that occurs outside your teaching sessions. For example, suppose your postsurgical patient can accurately describe how to use correct body mechanics when picking up his slippers. Only by direct observation will you find out if he's applying what he has learned.

Written tests
You can use written tests before, during, and after teaching. Use them before teaching to measure what the patient already knows and what he needs to learn. Use them during teaching to measure his progress and after teaching to measure what he's learned.

Although they're useful, written tests have several disadvantages. Obviously, they work only with literate patients. They're also difficult to construct, and that's a job best left to the patient-education specialist. In addition, written tests may intimidate some patients—especially if you're using an untried test that still has flaws. Perhaps the biggest drawback is that written tests are indirect indicators of learning. As you've

CREATING TOP-NOTCH TESTS

Written and oral tests are among your most valuable evaluation tools, but they're most effective when they least seem like tests. In effect, tests that seem too "testlike" may intimidate the patient and impair his performance. Here are some guidelines for making tests informative for you but less threatening for your patient.

GETTING THE INFORMATION YOU NEED

- Make tests comprehensive enough to cover all aspects of what you taught. Do not, however, focus on insignificant details.
- Emphasize understanding, interpretation, and application of the material taught— the how, why, and what questions.
- Choose questions that range from easy to hard. Test items at all levels of difficulty.
- Use questions whose answers are plausible but not obvious. Eliminate questions whose answers are suggested by other questions.
- Avoid questions with answers that follow set patterns.

REDUCING YOUR PATIENT'S ANXIETY

- Word questions as simply as possible, using language that's familiar to the patient.
- State questions clearly, so only one correct answer is possible.
- Group related questions together.
- Number the questions consecutively from beginning to end.
- Use different types of questions—multiple choice, true or false, and fill in the blanks—and give clear directions for answering each type.
- Don't ask "catch questions," which only confuse the patient.
- Give the patient plenty of time to finish the test.
- Explain how the test will be scored.
- If patient after patient seems confused by certain questions, revise these questions before you use the test again.

seen, a patient may say as you say, but not do as you say.

The redeeming aspect of written tests is that they save time. They can also measure each level of the patient's learning, from recall to synthesis.

Oral tests

Questioning the patient can evaluate his learning better than either direct observation or written tests. It lets you individualize evaluation for specific patients and situations. Like direct observation, this technique offers the advantage of allowing you to give instant feedback. Its main drawback is that it takes considerable time.

Oral tests, like written tests, demand careful preparation. (See *Creating Top-*

Notch Tests.) You have to do a lot more than just ask a few pertinent questions. Here are good tips to follow for oral tests:

☐ Make your questions specific to the patient's particular life situation.

☐ Pose your questions tactfully so the patient won't feel he's being grilled.

☐ Phrase your questions objectively to avoid giving away particular answers. (See *How to Ask Open-Ended Questions,* page 78.)

☐ Try to ask hypothetical questions about how the patient will respond to situations after he's out from under your wing. For instance, you might ask, "Mr. Allen, many people who've had a heart attack feel depressed after they go home. How do you think you might

HOW TO ASK OPEN-ENDED QUESTIONS

Phrasing questions to get the answer you expect is natural. However, you need to resist this natural inclination in order to get accurate data for evaluation.

Review the following examples of leading and open-ended questions. Leading questions suggest a "yes" or "no" response and can limit the scope and accuracy of your evaluation. In contrast, open-ended questions encourage an accurate, complete response. You'll want to use them for collecting information for your evaluation.

LEADING QUESTIONS	OPEN-ENDED QUESTIONS
Are you physically active during the day?	What sort of activities do you perform during a typical day?
Do you have episodes of pain during the day?	What type of activity makes the pain start?
Do you eat a lot of foods that are high in cholesterol?	Tell me about your eating patterns. When do you usually eat and what sorts of foods do you usually have?
Do you shovel snow?	How often do you shovel snow in winter?
Have you quit smoking?	How much are you smoking now? When do you usually smoke?
Do you know how you got this disease?	What do you know about your disease?
Do you know how to give yourself an insulin injection?	Could you show me how you give yourself an insulin injection?

handle this feeling?" Or, "Mr. Allen, if you were watching TV at home and had an uncomfortable feeling in your chest, what would you do?"

Interviews
Like oral tests, interviews are most effective when you ask sharply focused questions. Use a written outline to make your questions relate to each other, and use follow-up questions to elicit more information.

Interviews require creative listening—as important a technique as proper focusing of your questions. Try to restate each of your patient's answers. This pays dividends by assuring him that you understand his answers. It also gives him the chance to change his answers if he feels they need clarification after he hears you restate them.

Checklists
The most commonly used evaluation tool, the checklist enumerates specific characteristics or activities the patient should have mastered from the teaching session. With it, you can check off those the patient has mastered as you observe or interview him. (See *Devising Useful Checklists*, pages 80 and 81.)

Rating scales
Rating scales are practical devices for gathering evaluation data—if they're thoughtfully conceived and constructed. They have two strong points: they save time and they don't require writing. You simply check the appropriate response.

Rating scales also have weaknesses. For example, you may tend to choose the middle-scale values because you don't like to use the extremes. Or you may find yourself rating patients higher or lower than is appropriate because of your feelings toward them. Be forewarned. When you use a rating scale, try not to be swayed by your biases.

Good rating scales include definitions that explain the value or weight of each of the multiple choices. They

may be "anchored" by numbers (the higher the number, the higher the value) or by adjectives or adverbs (bipolar terms anchor each end of a continuum and you rate the patient's performance somewhere between the two). Commonly used bipolar terms include accurate/inaccurate, complete/incomplete, and always/never.

A rating scale may also be anchored by descriptions of patient behavior. For example, you may rate the patient who performs cardiac rehabilitation exercises by using the following descriptions for points on a continuum: needs prompting to correctly perform exercises; performs some exercises accurately with assistance or occasionally loses count and performs more or fewer exercises than recommended; consistently performs exercises independently and accurately.

Anecdotal notes
When behaviors can't be rated easily by scales or checklists, you can describe them as objectively as possible in anecdotal notes. You can later review these notes to evaluate behavior change or lack of it.

Physiologic measurements
In many cases you can evaluate teaching by the patient's physiologic status, using such measures as blood pressure level, serum cholesterol level, and activity tolerance. Obviously, changes in these measures aren't commonly seen during a brief hospitalization. Rather, they're usually the long-term results of patient education and compliance, characteristically seen on return visits or in the home. Nevertheless, researchers have demonstrated the usefulness of physiologic measures in the hospital. One study showed that short, intensive hospital teaching sessions can dramatically reduce errors in patients' self-monitoring of blood glucose levels.

Simulation
In a simulation session, you present a typical problem for the patient to solve.

DEVISING USEFUL CHECKLISTS

Checklists provide a simple, quick way of obtaining information for your evaluation. You can use them to gauge your patient's progress at various stages during your teaching.

Using checklists will give you and the patient clear evidence of what learning goals he's achieved and what goals need further work. To devise a useful checklist, follow these tips:

• Make the list concise, but wide-ranging enough to cover all aspects of the skill or activity being evaluated.

• Limit the items on the checklist to a group of related activities, such as the steps in tracheostomy care or the segments of a cardiac rehabilitation plan. Arrange the items in a logical order—sequentially, chronologically, or in order of importance.

• Identify the *essential* steps of the activities or behavior you're evaluating.

• Make the checklist items relate to the patient's learning goals and to your teaching methods.

• Use only one idea or concept in each item.

• Phrase each item succinctly and accurately.

• Test your checklist on at least two patients before adopting it permanently.

• Use the checklist along with other evaluation tools to avoid giving it undue importance.

The illustration on the right shows a sample checklist for evaluating how well a patient has learned to draw up insulin.

For example, you might say to a diabetic patient, "Before taking a 2-week vacation to Hawaii, what plans would you make to manage your condition?"

Simulation has the advantage of actively involving the patient in applying knowledge and skills to realistic situations. It's also nonthreatening. Unfortunately, simulation requires considerable time for planning and execution.

AN ONGOING ACTIVITY

Evaluation may seem like the final phase of your patient teaching, but it's not. It's something you'll be doing con-

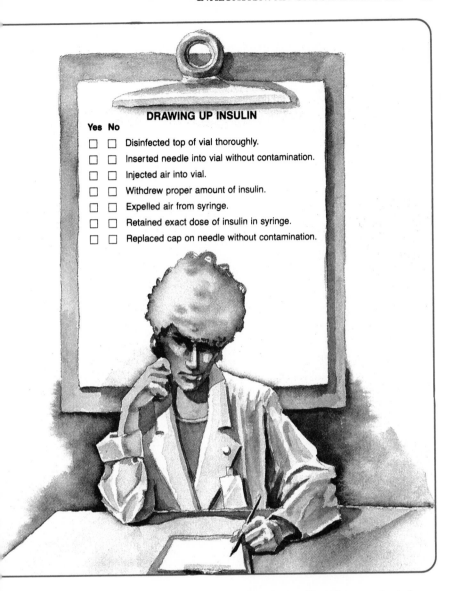

DRAWING UP INSULIN

Yes No

- ☐ ☐ Disinfected top of vial thoroughly.
- ☐ ☐ Inserted needle into vial without contamination.
- ☐ ☐ Injected air into vial.
- ☐ ☐ Withdrew proper amount of insulin.
- ☐ ☐ Expelled air from syringe.
- ☐ ☐ Retained exact dose of insulin in syringe.
- ☐ ☐ Replaced cap on needle without contamination.

stantly from the moment you begin to teach.

Evaluation will help you set better learning goals for your patient at the start, determine his progress in meeting these goals, and redirect your planning and teaching as needed to achieve these goals. Evaluation will also help you recognize the skills you have that make you a good teacher and identify the ones you'll need to acquire to be an even better one.

If you strive to make evaluation a part of your patient teaching, you won't be disappointed. In fact, you'll achieve three valued goals: teaching the patient to manage his own condition, bolstering his confidence by showing him evidence of his success, and improving your teaching skills.

5 Core Teaching Topics

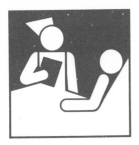

Core Teaching Topics

Introduction

All patients have questions about their disorders, about the diagnostic tests they'll undergo, and about the treatments their doctors have ordered. As a nurse, you're in the unique position to answer these questions from admission through discharge. And, in some instances, you're in a position to answer them in the patient's home. You're an invaluable provider of patient education, responsible for seeing that the patient's learning needs are met.

This chapter will provide general information that will help you teach your patient what he needs to know about his condition and the care he'll be receiving. Such knowledge will help diminish his anxiety and improve his ability to cope with hospitalization.

TEACHING UPON ADMISSION

The learning process for the patient and his family begins during the patient's admission to the hospital. Admission procedures can affect the patient positively or negatively and can set the tone for the rest of his stay.

During the admission procedure, you should introduce yourself to the patient and his family. Also introduce other members of the health care team whom they'll be seeing. Try to establish an early rapport and trust. This is essential to the therapeutic relationship and the learning process. If you appear concerned, caring, and efficient, the patient will feel less initial anxiety about being in a hospital.

Your initial teaching responsibilities include orienting the patient to his new environment, explaining safety measures, and reviewing everyday hospital routines. (See *Hospital Safety Measures*, page 84, and *Hospital Routines*, page 85.) Because a hospital can seem foreign to a newly admitted patient, think of the practical things he needs to know—the location of the bathroom, where to store his belongings, how to operate the bed and the call bell, and when he's allowed to have visitors. If the patient is admitted to a double room, be sure to introduce him to his roommate.

During these early encounters with the patient, take advantage of the opportunity to do a quick, focused, pre-teaching assessment. How much does the patient seem to understand about his condition? Does he seem anxious? What's your impression of his general intelligence? His ability to speak and understand English?

TEACHING ABOUT THE DISORDER

Typically, a patient wants to know what's wrong with him and what he has to do to feel better. Before he can gain this understanding, he's going to have some questions.

"What's my condition?"
Although the doctor will usually tell the patient his diagnosis and prognosis, the

responsibility for actually *explaining* what it all means most often falls to the nurse. A good place to begin is with a clear, concise definition of the patient's condition. Without overwhelming him with clinical details, try to give him some understanding of basic anatomy and physiology as they relate to his condition. Using diagrams or anatomic illustrations may be helpful. Just remember to keep these teaching tools simple and to label them with terms the patient will understand.

"What causes it?"
When discussing the cause of your patient's disorder, try to relate it to your previous explanation of anatomy and physiology. Again, keep your explanation simple.

"What can be done about it?"
Inform the patient of the expected benefits of treatment. Explain how treatment will most likely affect his symptoms. Remember, the patient has the right to determine the type and amount of treatment. You can help him decide by discussing alternative treatments.

When discussing treatment, explain how it relates to anatomy and physiology. For example, when discussing coughing and deep breathing after surgery, explain why expelling mucus from the lungs is so important.

"What can I do?"
One of your most important responsibilities is teaching the patient *his* responsibilities for managing his condition. Make sure he knows what signs and symptoms to look for to detect a relapse. If he has a chronic disorder, teach him what to expect during an exacerbation. Show him how to record the duration, location, and severity of his signs and symptoms. And tell him to call his doctor whenever they occur.

"What about home remedies?"
Well-meaning friends, family members, or acquaintances often pass on to

---

CHECKLIST

HOSPITAL SAFETY MEASURES

Use this checklist to review hospital safety measures with the patient. To prevent injuries from falls, tell him to:

☐ wear slippers with low heels and non-slip soles.

☐ avoid walking on freshly washed or waxed floors.

☐ keep the bed in a low position so he can get into it and out of it easily and safely. Mention that the side rails will be kept up at night.

☐ keep the telephone, call bell, and personal belongings, such as eyeglasses, within reach.

☐ use the call bell to summon help if he can't walk to the bathroom.

☐ use the handrails in the bathroom.

To prevent electrical or fire hazards, tell the patient to:

☐ plug personal appliances (such as electric shavers or hairdryers) into approved outlets only.

☐ restrict smoking to designated areas. Always use an ashtray. Observe *No Smoking* signs.

☐ stay in his room during fire alarms and drills until instructed otherwise by hospital staff.

a patient certain myths or misconceptions concerning the cause or treatment of his condition. For example, a patient may have heard that arthritis can be cured by wearing a copper bracelet over the inflamed joint. By explaining the pathophysiology of arthritis and the way in which treatments work, you should be able to dispel this myth.

"Can any groups help me?"
Give the patient a list of organizations that he can contact for financial or psychological support. If he needs further assistance, put him in touch with your social service worker. If appropriate, arrange to have a member of a support group visit him in the hospital.

TEACHING ABOUT TESTS

CHECKLIST

HOSPITAL ROUTINES

Use this checklist when discussing hospital routines with the patient. Tell him:

☐ the time at which meals will be delivered to the unit.

☐ hospital visiting hours (including who may visit, how many visitors he may have in his room at one time, any age restrictions on visitors).

☐ special precautions (such as isolation procedures), if appropriate.

☐ scheduled times for taking vital signs and giving medications.

☐ information about newspapers, TV rental, telephone procedures, smoking regulations, and use of the hospital safe for storing money or valuables.

☐ information about his rights. Provide him with your hospital's own patient's bill of rights or the American Hospital Association's Patient's Bill of Rights.

When explaining a diagnostic test to the patient, tell him exactly what will happen before, during, and after the procedure. This will promote his cooperation during the test and help ensure accurate results.

Just make sure that you understand the test yourself before you attempt to teach the patient. You'll need to have the answers to the following questions clear in your own mind first.

"What is the test?"
Refer to the test by its full name, not an abbreviation, and give a clear definition for the patient, using layman's terms. For example, don't say "lumbar puncture"; say "spinal tap." Avoid acronyms that only you and other health care professionals would understand. If a test is so well-known by an acronym, however, that using its full name would be awkward—for example, "CAT" for "computed tomography"—then explain the acronym fully the first time you use it.

"What is the test's purpose?"
Explain the general purpose of the test in words the patient can understand. For example: "A complete blood count—you might hear us refer to it as a 'CBC'—shows the number and type of blood cells circulating in your bloodstream. We only have to take a small amount of blood to do this test, and it can tell us a lot of important things about your condition..."

A clear and complete explanation of the test's purpose can relieve patient anxiety, confusion, and embarrassment. If appropriate, give the patient any available literature that will amplify what you have told him. Don't rely on pamphlets alone, however, to do your job for you.

"Does anything have to be done before the test?"
Explaining pretest responsibilities—both yours and the patient's—will help ensure the patient's cooperation and the

validity of the test results. For example, you would explain to a patient scheduled for a bronchoscopy that he shouldn't eat or drink after midnight before the test. (If the patient asks, explain the rationale for this: food or fluid in the stomach increases his risk of aspirating gastric contents should he vomit while under anesthesia.) Also let him know that you'll be emptying his water pitcher and calling the dietary department to have his breakfast canceled because of this restriction.

"Who'll perform the test—and where?"

Before the test, tell the patient who will be performing the test. Identify this person by name and position or title, if known. Also tell him where the test will be done. Describe the room and the equipment that will be used. This will relieve his apprehension about being taken to a part of the hospital where he's never been before.

"What will happen during the test?"

Naturally, you'll need to explain exactly how the test is conducted. First, tell the patient about how long it will take. To help explain positioning during the test, you can use sketches or have the patient practice the actual positions.

If the patient has to take a drug before the test, tell him its purpose, route of administration, and possible adverse reactions. Also explain any necessary nursing measures, such as putting up the side rails. At this time you can describe in more detail any special equipment that will be used during the test.

Think in terms of the patient's five senses when you're trying to explain the test to him. The closer you can come to giving him a clear picture of what he'll see, hear, feel, smell, and possibly even taste during the test, the less anxiety he'll experience. For example, describe what a CT scanner looks like, the clacking sound made by an X-ray machine, or the pinprick of EEG electrodes as they're attached.

Outline the patient's responsibilities during the test. If appropriate, have him practice things he'll be asked to do during the test—lying perfectly still for a CT scan, for example, or holding his breath and then exhaling fully for pulmonary function studies.

Finally, advise the patient of any adverse reactions he might experience during or after the test.

"When will results be available?"

Remember that the patient has the legal right to be informed of the test results within a reasonable amount of time. Letting him know beforehand when test results should be available can minimize his anxiety.

TEACHING ABOUT TREATMENTS

Drug Therapy

Your responsibilities in teaching the patient about drug therapy will vary, depending on the setting in which you're practicing. In most cases, however, the nurse is the health care professional who sees the patient most often. So you'll probably be in the best position to teach him what he needs to know about drug therapy.

Begin by assessing the patient's understanding of his condition, his general knowledge of drug therapy, and his ability and desire to comply with the prescribed therapy.

When teaching the patient about drug therapy, be sure to cover each drug's names, purpose, appearance, dosage, and form. Also cover any special precautions or directions, adverse effects, and storage instructions. (See *Taking Medications Correctly*, pages 88 and 89.)

The drug's names

Tell the patient both the generic and brand names of each drug he'll be taking. Brand names, which tend to be shorter and catchier than generic names, are often easier for the patient to remember. Use the name that you think the patient is more likely to recognize and remember, whether it's "penicillin" (generic) or "Lasix" (brand). If the patient is being discharged with a prescription, tell him that he may be able to buy the drug at a cheaper price if he asks for it by its generic name. Knowing this, the patient may be more likely to comply with his regimen. Tell him he'll need to talk to his doctor about generic substitutions.

The drug's purpose

The patient should know why the drug was prescribed and its desired effect. Once again, use simple language. For example, if furosemide (Lasix) is prescribed because the patient has swollen ankles, explain that the desired effect of this diuretic, or "water pill," is to help him eliminate excess fluid through urination.

The drug's appearance

Teach the patient to recognize the distinctive characteristics of his medication, such as color, size, shape, and identification code (in the case of pills). If the patient knows exactly what his medication should look like, he's less likely to get confused when taking several different drugs during the day. Once he's home by himself, his ability to recognize the right drug to take may be the final safeguard against a serious drug error.

If a generic drug is prescribed on discharge, the patient should ask the pharmacist to inform him of any difference in appearance between the new drug and a previous brand name he may be used to. When generic drugs are prescribed in the hospital, you should provide the patient with this information.

Dosage and form

Because many drugs are manufactured in various strengths, the patient must understand the dosage he's taking. This is especially important if the doctor adjusts the dosage after the patient goes home. A patient taking warfarin, for example, may be given a prescription for 5-mg tablets at discharge. Based on the results of a prothrombin time test performed a week later, he may be instructed to reduce the dose to 2.5 mg, half of a tablet.

Tell the patient how often he should take the prescribed drug. Be sure to explain whether the doses should be spaced at equal intervals over a 24-hour period or whether he can take all the doses during waking hours. Try to work out times when the patient can take his medications without changing his everyday routine. For example, taking medications just before or after meals—provided that food won't interfere with the absorption of the drug—will help the patient remember his schedule. Since patients often misinterpret prescription labels, be sure to explain what they mean in layman's language.

The patient's strict compliance with drug therapy is always desired, of course. But if a patient misses one or more doses—and patients *will* miss doses from time to time—discuss the best way to get his drug therapy back on track. If the patient misses one or more doses and is uncertain what he should do, instruct him to call his doctor or pharmacist immediately for instructions.

Tell the patient how long he can expect his drug therapy to last. This will encourage him to comply with short-term therapy for its full duration or will prepare him to accept long-term treatment. If appropriate, discuss the danger of abruptly stopping some drugs, such as cortisone or antibiotics.

Also advise the patient to inform his pharmacist, doctor, or nurse if he has any problems swallowing certain forms of a drug. Let him know that many

TAKING MEDICATIONS CORRECTLY

Dear Patient:

Your doctor has prescribed medication for you to help treat your condition. In order for your medication to be beneficial, however, you must take it *as prescribed.*

Safety tips

• Keep your medication in its original container or in a properly labeled prescription bottle. If you're taking more than one medication, do *not* mix them together in a pillbox.

• Store your medication in a cool, dry place or as directed by your pharmacist. *Don't* keep it in the bathroom medicine cabinet, where heat and humidity may cause it to lose its effectiveness. All containers should have childproof caps and should be kept out of the reach of children. (The top shelf of a closet is a good storage place.)

• Always take your medication in a well-lit room. Read the label to make sure you're taking the right medication. If you don't understand the directions, ask your pharmacist or doctor for clarification.

• Don't take medication whose expiration date has passed. Not only will it be ineffective, but it may be harmful. Discard the medication by flushing it down the toilet.

• If you miss a dose or several doses, ask your doctor or pharmacist for further directions (unless you were given specific instructions beforehand.)

• Refill all prescriptions promptly so you don't run out of medication when the pharmacy is closed.

• Have all prescriptions filled at the same store so that the pharmacist can keep a complete record of your medications. Inform him of any medication allergies and any nonprescription drugs you're taking.

• Don't start taking any nonprescription drugs without first checking with your pharmacist about potential interactions with other drugs you're taking. (Remember, nonprescription drugs can be harmful, too, if not taken correctly.) If you're taking a nonprescription drug, call your doctor if your condition doesn't improve after a few days.

• If you're pregnant or breast-feeding, speak to your doctor before taking any medication or home remedy. Some drugs may be harmful to the fetus.

• Your medication has been prescribed specifically for you. Do *not* share it with other members of your family or with friends; they could have a serious allergic reaction.

Administration tips

• Make a medication calendar. To do this, use a calendar with enough space to write in the names of the drugs and the times you should take them each day. Then put a check mark next to the drug when you take it.

• Set your alarm clock to go off when it's time to take your medication. Or ask a friend or relative to remind you.

• Write down the following information about each of your medications on index cards or on a chart: its name, its purpose, its appearance, directions for taking it, special cautions or side effects, and when to take it.

• Don't forget that most drugs cause side effects. Make sure you know the potential side effects that your medication can cause, especially those that must be reported to your doctor or pharmacist. If you have any questions about symptoms you're experiencing while taking your medication, call your doctor immediately.

Additional information for your prescribed medication

_____

_____

_____

_____

_____

_____

_____

_____

_____

_____

_____

_____

drugs are available or can be prepared as liquids rather than as tablets or capsules.

Special precautions and instructions

Inform the patient of any special precautions he must observe—for example, not driving or using power tools when taking a drug that causes dizziness or drowsiness until he's familiar with the drug's effects. Typically, the patient will be able to drive or use power tools once he becomes accustomed to the drug.

You may have to give the patient special instructions before he starts taking his prescribed drug. For example, some drugs—such as ophthalmic, otic, and nasal preparations; sublingual and buccal tablets; respiratory inhalants; and vaginal tablets or creams—have to be administered or applied a certain way to be effective. Use diagrams, demonstrations, or practice sessions with the patient (and his family) to reinforce these special instructions.

If the patient must avoid alcohol or certain foods or drugs during therapy because of the risk of toxicity or inactivation of the therapeutic drug, explain the reasons and the possible reactions. Discuss any special procedures he must perform before he takes his prescribed drug. For example, he may need to test his urine or blood glucose level before taking insulin or to take his pulse rate before taking digoxin.

If a patient is seeing more than one doctor for various medical problems, instruct him to tell each doctor the names of all the drugs he's taking. This precaution may prevent potentially harmful interactions between prescription drugs. Also inform him that most pharmacies have patient-profile systems that keep track of a patient's prescriptions as another precaution against hazardous interactions. For this reason, advise the patient to have all his prescriptions filled at the same pharmacy.

Adverse reactions

The patient has a right to know the adverse reactions his prescribed drug might cause before he begins drug therapy. So give him a list of signs and symptoms to look for; underline the ones that he should report to his doctor immediately. Also, tell him what he can do to relieve or prevent certain adverse reactions, such as sucking on a piece of hard candy to relieve a dry mouth. As a precaution, advise the patient to always call his doctor if he's not sure about the seriousness of a sign or symptom that has developed during drug therapy.

Storage instructions

Tell the patient to store his medication in its original container, with the label clearly visible. He should keep it in a cool, dry place, out of the sun. If the medication must be refrigerated, the label will say so. Some drugs require special storage instructions—nitroglycerin, for example. If the patient is taking such a drug, tell him to ask his pharmacist about storing it. Make sure the patient knows the expiration date of his medication. Remind him that a drug whose expiration date has passed will no longer be effective and may even be unsafe. Such a drug should be discarded.

Diet Therapy

Patients on a prescribed diet need to have the rationale for their diet fully explained. They may also need your help in planning acceptable meals. The dietitian will usually talk to the patient first about a new diet, but you'll probably have to clarify some points for the patient and his family.

In planning this aspect of your patient teaching, first assess the patient's current diet, eating habits, likes and dislikes, and any cultural or socioeconomic factors that have influenced his diet. Knowing what the patient usually eats and helping him see how his new diet can accommodate these preferences will promote compliance.

Most diet therapy revolves around the four basic food groups. In your teaching, you should impress on the patient the importance of following a diet that is well balanced among these food groups. Explain such dietary terms as "calories," "carbohydrates," "grains," and "protein" in relation to the foods in the patient's new diet.

Dietary instructions
Your instructions to the patient and his family should include the following information:
- *Name of the diet.* Refer to the patient's new diet by its proper name. If necessary, clarify the name in layman's language.
- *Rationale and duration.* Explain the rationale behind the patient's diet as it relates to his condition. Tell the patient how long he should stay on the diet. Generally, patients will comply most readily with short-term diets. Patients who must stay on their diets for longer periods will need more encouragement and counseling.
- *Allowed and prohibited foods.* Tell the patient which foods he'll be allowed to eat, keeping his preferences in mind. Of course, food restrictions must also be pointed out. Again, relate the pathophysiology of the patient's disorder to his dietary regimen. Writing out a list of allowed and prohibited foods is a good idea.
- *Sample meal plans.* A sample meal plan should also be put into writing and given to the patient and his family. Describe how meals should be prepared and specify the size of each portion, using common household measuring units. Define different methods of cooking, such as boiling, broiling, and frying.
- *Important phone numbers.* Give the patient the phone number of a dietitian or organization to call if he has any questions.

Surgery

Physically and psychologically, surgery must rank as one of the most stressful experiences a person can undergo. The stress results from what the person sees as a threat to his body, perhaps even to his life, and from the instinctive fear of pain. In preparing a patient, your goal should be to help him cope with this stress through preoperative teaching addressed to both him and his family. Studies show that patients who've been prepared through careful teaching feel less anxious about their operations, experience less pain and fewer complications postoperatively, and spend less time in the hospital than those who haven't been prepared.

You can be sure that your surgical patients will have many questions on their minds. Before surgery, patients usually want to know how long they'll have to wait before they can return to normal activities. They may even appear eager to participate in their preoperative and postoperative care. Some, however, may suddenly become anxious when you start to explain the surgery itself. If a patient seems uncomfortable talking about his operation and changes the subject, stop and think about how much he really needs to know. He may want to know only so much about his surgery—and no more.

With shorter hospital stays and same-day surgeries on the rise, preadmission and preoperative teaching has become more important than ever. But it must be structured to accommodate a short time period. Patterning your teaching along the following lines will help you do it better and faster.

Providing an overview
Your preoperative teaching should provide an overview of what needs to be done before, during, and after surgery to make it successful and free of complications. Your teaching should be

PREOPERATIVE TEACHING FOR CHILDREN

Structured preoperative teaching is as essential for children as for adults. It can reduce a child's anxiety and help him cope with the stress of an operation. Here are some tips and methods you can use during your preoperative teaching for children:
• Convey concrete information using simple language. Supplement this with pictures, books, and films.
• Arrange for group tours of the surgical suite and a discussion of the surgery.

• Show pictures of doctors and nurses in surgical dress.
• Use puppets to play the parts of doctor, nurse, and patient in the operating room.
• Promote hands-on play with equipment, including stethoscopes, I.V. tubing and bottles, dressings, oxygen masks, and surgical gowns, caps, and masks. Or use life-size dolls that have incisions, dressings, I.V. lines, or casts.

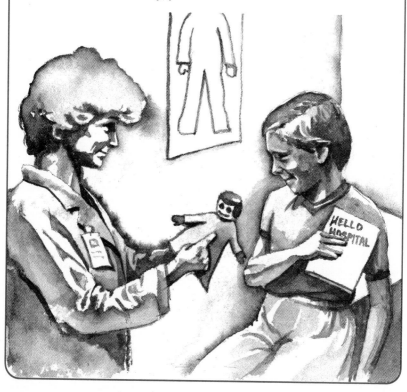

carried out the day before surgery—even earlier, if possible—to give the patient time to practice techniques. On admission, he should be assessed to determine how much he knows about surgery in general and the operation he'll undergo in particular. As part of this assessment, you'll need to gather information about:
• past operations (type and purpose)
• the patient's understanding of the scheduled surgery
• his knowledge of preoperative routines, such as diagnostic tests and physical preparation for surgery
• his knowledge of immediate postoperative care, such as recovery room procedures and I.V. therapy
• his knowledge of postoperative exercises, such as deep breathing, coughing, and leg exercises
• his psychological readiness for sur-

gery, fears about the proposed operation, coping mechanisms, and support systems.

Explaining preoperative tests to the patient and his family is your first teaching priority. Review the rationale for chest X-rays, a CBC, urine studies, an EKG, and other diagnostic tests. Tell the patient when and where the tests will be done. Describe any sensations he'll experience, and assure him that the test results will help determine his readiness for surgery. If the patient smokes, advise him to stop for at least 12 hours before surgery. Explain that this will decrease the risk of postoperative respiratory or circulatory complications.

Discussing preoperative routines that apply to your patient will allay some of his anxiety. For example, you may need to cover anesthesia, dietary and bowel preparation, and medication.

• *Anesthesia.* No matter what kind of surgery your patient is scheduled for, he'll need an anesthetic. Tell him the name of his anesthesiologist. Explain that the anesthesiologist is responsible for his care until he leaves the recovery room.

Tell the patient that his anesthesiologist will visit him before surgery and answer all of his questions. Encourage the patient to jot down any questions he has beforehand, so he doesn't forget them. If he prefers one type of anesthetic over another, advise him to discuss this with his anesthesiologist, too.

Keep in mind that your patient may have special concerns that he's reluctant to mention. For example, if he's supposed to receive a general anesthetic, he may worry that he'll suddenly awaken in the middle of the operation. Or he may be concerned about possibly never awakening at all. Try to anticipate these concerns. Assure your patient that the anesthesiologist will monitor his condition carefully throughout surgery. He'll get just the right amount of anesthetic.

• *Diet.* Explain the importance of a nutritious diet up to 8 hours before surgery. At that time food and fluids will be withheld. Make sure the patient understands that he can't eat or drink anything after this time. Remind the family, too.

• *Bowel preparation.* This procedure is usually done only if the patient is having lower abdominal surgery. Explain the procedure and rationale.

• *Medication.* Tell the patient what medication he'll be given before surgery and why he'll need it. Let him know the approximate time the medication will be given and describe any sensations he may feel. Explain that the side rails must be kept up and that he must stay in bed. The preoperative medication will help him relax but he won't fall asleep. Explain that the medication will make his mouth feel dry.

• *Voiding.* Instruct the patient to void immediately before preoperative medications are given. For some surgical procedures, the patient will need to be catheterized before the operation. Explain the procedure to the patient.

• *Skin preparation.* Preoperative skin preparation and hair removal may have a negative effect on the patient's body image. Carefully explain the rationale—to prevent surgical wound infection by cleansing the skin of microorganisms, some of which are found in body hair.

• *I.V. therapy.* Discuss I.V. therapy in terms of the site and technique to be used. Tell the patient if an I.V. will be started before he goes to surgery or after he gets to the operating room. Explain that fluids and nutrients, given during surgery, help prevent postoperative complications.

• *Clothing.* Instruct your patient to remove jewelry, eyeglasses or contact lenses, prostheses (including dentures), wigs, makeup, and nail polish. Explain that you can tape a plain wedding band to his finger. Give the patient a gown and surgical cap to put on. Assure him that his privacy will be respected with proper draping.

• *Family waiting area.* Show the patient's family where they can wait dur-

HOW TO REDUCE INCISIONAL PAIN

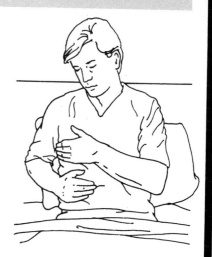

Dear Patient:

To help reduce pain when you move, cough, or breathe deeply, you'll need to observe precautions and, perhaps, learn how to splint your incision.

Observing precautions
• Use the bed's side rails for support when you move and turn.
• Move slowly and steadily. Don't move quickly or jerkily.
• Whenever possible, wait to move until *after* your pain medication has taken effect.
• Frequently move those parts of your body that weren't affected by surgery to prevent them from becoming stiff and sore.
• If you have difficulty moving by yourself, ask the nurse or a family member to help.

Splinting your incision
If you've had chest or abdominal surgery, splinting the incision may help reduce pain when you cough or move.

You can do this by placing one hand above and the other hand below your incision, then pressing gently and breathing normally when you move. (The patient shown in the illustration at the top of the next column has a chest wall incision.)

Or you can place a small pillow over the incision. Hold it in place with your hands and arms, as shown below. Press gently, breathe normally, and move to a sitting or standing position.

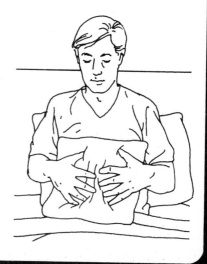

ing the operation. If they want to visit the patient preoperatively, tell them to arrive 2 hours before the surgery.

• *Operating room.* Transfer time, procedures, and techniques also need to be explained to the patient. Once again, describe sensations the patient will experience. Warn him that he may have to wait a short time in the holding area before he's taken into the operating room. Explain that the doctors and nurses will be in surgical dress and that even though they'll be observing him closely, they probably won't talk to him. Tell him that this will allow the medication to take effect.

Advise the patient that he'll be taken to the operating room on a stretcher and transferred from the stretcher to the operating room table. For his own safety, he'll be strapped securely to the table. The operating room nurses will check his vital signs frequently.

Warn the patient that the operating room may feel cool. Electrodes may be put on his chest to monitor his heart rate during surgery. Describe the drowsy, floating sensation he'll feel as the anesthetic is administered. Tell him it's important that he relax at this time.

• *Recovery room.* To allay the patient's anxiety, briefly describe the sensations he'll experience after the anesthetic wears off. Let him know how long he'll be in the recovery room. Tell him that the recovery room nurse will call his name, then ask him to answer questions and follow simple commands, such as wiggling his toes. He may feel pain at the surgical site, but the nurses will try to minimize it.

Describe the oxygen delivery device, such as a nasal cannula, that he'll need after surgery. Once he's recovered from the anesthesia, he'll be taken back to his room. Tell him that he'll be able to see his family, but that he'll probably feel drowsy and may want to nap for the rest of the day. Make sure he knows that you'll be taking his blood pressure and pulse frequently as a routine precaution. That way he won't become alarmed and think something's wrong.

Controlling pain
A surgical patient is usually anxious about how much pain he'll feel after his operation. You can help reduce his anxiety by advising him of pain-control measures that you'll be using. You can also teach him when to ask for pain medication and how to use certain pain-control measures on his own.

Briefly, point out to him that pain usually occurs after surgery because of stimulation of nerve endings in the skin, as well as from tissue swelling and organ manipulation. Postoperative pain typically lasts 24 to 48 hours but may last longer with extensive surgery.

Now discuss specific measures that can be used to prevent or relieve incisional pain. (See *How to Reduce Incisional Pain.*)

Explain that the doctor will order pain medication to be given every 3 to 4 hours, if needed. Instruct the patient to describe his pain in terms of its quality, severity, and location. Encourage him to let you know as soon as he feels any pain instead of waiting until it becomes intense. Pain can be controlled better if it's managed early. Discuss how the medication will be administered—whether by injection or orally (once the patient resumes eating, usually 48 hours postoperatively). Identify the type of medication to be given (for example, a narcotic or an analgesic), and explain how it works to control pain.

Tell the patient which nursing measures you'll use to relieve pain and promote comfort, such as positioning, diversional activities, and splinting.

Preventing complications
The best way to prevent postoperative complications is by teaching the patient *preoperatively* the techniques of early mobility and ambulation, coughing and deep breathing, use of an incentive spirometer, and leg exercises.

Tell the patient that early mobility and ambulation increase the rate and depth of breathing, preventing atelectasis and hypostatic pneumonia. With

96

HOW TO COUGH AND DEEP-BREATHE

Dear Patient:

Coughing and deep-breathing exercises will speed your recovery and reduce the risk of respiratory complications.

How to cough

Practice coughing exercises before surgery. After it, you'll need to do them at least every 2 hours to help keep your lungs free of secretions.

1

If your condition permits, sit on the edge of your bed. Ask for a stool if your feet don't touch the floor. Lean slightly forward.

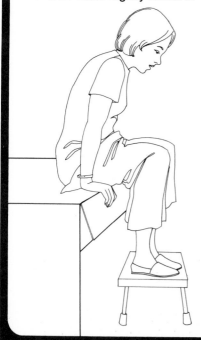

(After surgery, you can perform this exercise while lying in a comfortable position instead of sitting on the edge of the bed.) Bend your legs to support your abdominal muscles.

If you're scheduled for chest or abdominal surgery, splint your "incision" before you cough.

2

To help stimulate your cough reflex, take a slow, deep breath. Breathe in through your nose and concentrate on fully expanding your chest. Breathe out through your mouth, and concentrate on feeling your chest sink downward and inward. Then take a second breath in the same manner.

3

Now take a third deep breath, but this time hold your breath. Then cough two or three times in a row (once is not enough). This will clear your breathing passages. As you cough, concentrate on feeling your diaphragm force out all the air in your chest. Then take three to five normal breaths, exhale slowly, and relax.

Repeat this exercise at least once. Don't worry about your stitches splitting. They're very strong.

How to deep-breathe

Performing deep-breathing exercises several times an hour helps keep your lungs fully expanded.

To deep-breathe correctly, you must use your diaphragm and abdominal muscles—not just your chest muscles. This exercise teaches you how. Practice it two or three times a day before surgery, as follows:

1

Lie on your back in a comfortable position. Place one hand on your chest and the other over your upper abdomen, as shown in the illustration below. Bend your legs slightly and relax.

Exhale normally. Then close your mouth and inhale deeply through your nose. Concentrate on feeling your abdomen rise. Don't expand your chest. If the hand on your abdomen rises as you inhale, you're breathing correctly.

Hold your breath and slowly count to five.

2

Purse your lips as though about to whistle, then exhale completely through your mouth. Don't let your cheeks puff out. Using your abdominal muscles, squeeze all the air out. Your ribs should sink downward and inward. Try not to take intermittent shallow breaths during this full exhalation.

3

Rest several seconds, then repeat the exercise until you've done it 5 to 10 times.

Note: You can also do this exercise while lying on your side, sitting, or standing, or as you're turning in bed.

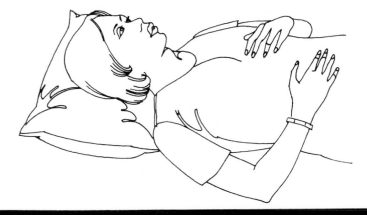

LEARNING ABOUT SPIROMETERS

Preoperatively, your patient may understand why deep-breathing exercises are important. But after surgery, when he's weak, sedated, or in pain, he may need some encouragement to do them regularly. Incentive spirometry, which provides instant feedback, may give him the encouragement he needs.

Before you teach your patient how to use incentive spirometers, compare and review the two different types. Even though all spirometers are designed to encourage slow, sustained maximal inspiration, they can be divided into *flow incentive* and *volume incentive* types. A flow incentive spirometer measures the patient's inspiratory effort (flow rate) in cubic centimeters per second (cc/second). A volume incentive spirometer goes one step further. From the patient's flow rate, it calculates the *volume* of air the patient inhales. Because of this extra step, many volume incentive spirometers are larger, more complicated, and more expensive than flow incentive spirometers.

If the patient is to use a volume incentive spirometer, the doctor or respiratory therapist will order a *goal volume* (in cubic centimeters) for the patient to reach. This will be the amount of air the patient should inspire when he takes a deep breath.

With one type of volume incentive spirometer, the goal volume will be displayed on the machine. As the patient inhales, the volume of air he's taking into his lungs will also be shown, climbing a scale until he reaches or surpasses the goal volume. This will not only help him fully expand his lungs, but will also provide immediate feedback as to how well he's doing.

The patient will usually do this exercise five times each day. Between exercises he should rest. Each morning he should reset the goal-volume-achieved display so he can try to do even better.

With another type of volume incentive spirometer, smaller and easier to use, the patient inhales slowly and deeply as a piston inside a cylinder rises to meet the preset volume. The number of exercises the patient should do each day remains the same.

Flow incentive spirometers have no preset volume. These spirometers usually have three cylinders, each containing a colored ball. As the patient inhales, the balls rise, one at a time. The patient's flow rate is measured in cc/second. For example, when the first ball rises, the flow rate may be 600 cc/second; the second ball, 900 cc/second; and the third ball, 1,200 cc/second. The number of exercises the patient should do each day is the same as with volume incentive spirometers.

Which type of spirometer is better for your patient?

That depends. For low-risk patients, a flow incentive spirometer would probably be better. Lightweight and durable, it can be left at the bedside for the patient to use even when you're not there to supervise.

But if your patient is at high risk for developing atelectasis, a volume incentive spirometer may be preferred. Because it measures lung inflation more precisely, this type of spirometer helps you determine whether your patient is inhaling adequately.

FLOW INCENTIVE SPIROMETER　　　　**VOLUME INCENTIVE SPIROMETER**

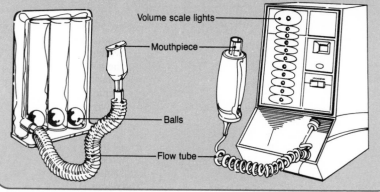

Volume scale lights

Mouthpiece

Balls

Flow tube

increased cerebral oxygenation, he'll feel more alert and more optimistic about his recovery. Circulation will improve as a result of early mobility, promoting renal perfusion and urine production. Thrombophlebitis from venous stasis may also be prevented.

Early ambulation quickens peristalsis, which usually slows to a halt during surgery from the effects of the anesthetic. Postoperative constipation and abdominal distention can thus be diminished. Finally, early ambulation increases metabolism and prevents loss of muscle tone.

Coughing and deep breathing prevent atelectasis after surgery. Explain to the patient that to deep-breathe correctly, he must use his diaphragm and abdominal muscles and not just his chest muscles. Tell him to practice two or three times a day before surgery, if possible. Maneuvers should be done 30 minutes after pain medication is administered and should be repeated every 1 to 2 hours. (See *How to Cough and Deep-Breathe*, pages 96 and 97.)

Incentive spirometers encourage the patient to deep-breathe and provide feedback on how well he's doing. (See *Learning about Spirometers*.)

Simple leg exercises—such as alternately contracting and relaxing the calf and thigh muscles—will prevent venous pooling.

DISCHARGE TEACHING

Effective discharge teaching begins immediately after admission and takes into account the initial assessment of the patient's understanding of his condition, surgery or other treatment, and postoperative care. Your discharge teaching must include the patient's family or other caregivers to ensure that the patient receives proper home care.

Home Care Requirements

Begin determining the patient's home care requirements by finding out how much walking he'll have to do at home. What's the floor plan of his house or apartment, for example? Will he need to climb stairs? Let the patient know how soon he should be able to drive a car or return to work.

If the patient has had surgery, inform him or a family member to observe the incision daily for warmth, redness, and swelling. Unless he's been given other instructions, explain that he should use clean water to wash the incision. Tell him to keep the incision clean and dry and to discard dressings in a plastic trash bag. Teach proper hand-washing technique. Discuss when the patient can take a shower or bath, and make a point of specifying whether he should shower or bathe.

Discuss the doctor's recommendations concerning activity and exercise level, relating them to the patient's everyday routine. After surgery, patients are often advised not to lift a heavy weight, such as a basket of laundry. Make sure the patient and his family understand such restrictions.

Review dietary restrictions and meal plans. Recommend a good diet book, and refer the patient to a dietitian for further information.

If the patient needs to rent or purchase special equipment, such as a hospital bed or walker, give him a list of suppliers in the area.

Finally, teach the patient and his family about emergency care procedures. Provide written instructions on reportable signs and symptoms, such as bleeding or discharge from an incision or acute incisional pain. Advise the patient to keep his follow-up medical appointments and to call the doctor with any questions.

6

Cardiovascular System

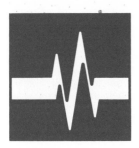

Cardiovascular System

Introduction

Cardiovascular disorders rank as the leading cause of illness and death in the United States—ahead of both cancer and accidents. Obviously, you'll encounter patients with such disorders day in and day out. As a result, you're in a key position to teach them not only about their condition and treatment but also about recognizing and modifying possible risk factors.

Risk factors

One of your chief teaching goals is to explain risk factors that can precipitate or exacerbate cardiovascular disorders. Typically, these risk factors include stress, obesity, a sedentary lifestyle, smoking, high blood pressure, and a diet high in sodium, cholesterol, and saturated fats. By helping the patient identify and modify his risk factors, your teaching can significantly reduce his chance of cardiovascular complications—namely, myocardial infarction. What's more, it may even help reverse the course of his cardiovascular disorder. For example, research suggests that modifying risk factors may promote regression of the atherosclerotic buildup in coronary artery disease.

Preparation for diagnostic tests

Besides teaching about risk factors, you'll bear much of the responsibility for preparing the patient for various diagnostic tests. Because many patients associate the heart with life itself, your teaching must always address their often intense psychological needs. Diagnostic tests for cardiovascular disorders range from routine analysis of serum cardiac enzymes to complex studies, such as cardiac blood pool imaging and cardiac catheterization. The latter require complicated, often intimidating equipment that could frighten the uninformed patient.

Preparation for treatments and home care

Cardiovascular treatments are equally diverse. For example, you may need to teach the patient how to change his leg ulcer dressings or how to safely resume activity after open-heart surgery.

Frequently, you'll teach the patient how to perform treatments at home. Occasionally, he'll need to learn special skills, such as measuring his blood pressure or taking his pulse rate. Or he may need directions for taking certain drugs, such as nitroglycerin or anticoagulants. Sometimes, your teaching aims to help the patient manage specialized equipment, such as a pacemaker, at home. Clearly, achieving the patient's long-term compliance with home care ranks among your chief teaching goals.

DISORDERS

Chronic Arterial Occlusive Disease

Most commonly affecting the elderly, chronic arterial occlusive disease often goes undetected until symptoms of arterial insufficiency—typically, painful intermittent claudication from leg artery occlusion or transient ischemic attack from carotid artery occlusion—force the patient to seek treatment. Unfortunately, by the time symptoms

appear, arterial damage is often extensive, limiting the effectiveness of treatment. Nevertheless, your teaching can help the patient cope with the demands of his chronic disorder. For example, you'll need to teach him about relieving symptoms through proper exercise, nutrition, and positioning. If necessary, you'll also need to teach him about arterial bypass grafting or other surgical procedures. To reduce the risk of long-term complications, you'll need to emphasize scrupulous skin care, correct use of anticoagulant drugs, and appropriate life-style changes.

Describe the disorder

Explain the vascular changes—primarily arteriosclerotic and atherosclerotic—that produce chronic arterial occlusive disease. Tell the patient that one or both of these vascular changes may cause his condition. In arteriosclerosis, calcification and occlusion of the arteries stem from a progressive loss of vessel elasticity due to such factors as aging, hypertension, and diabetes. Atherosclerosis, the gradual buildup of fatty, fibrous plaques on the inner arterial walls, results from lipoprotein abnormalities, arterial wall injury, and platelet dysfunction. Both disorders produce varying degrees of arterial occlusion.

Next, explain how intermittent claudication results from these arterial changes. Insufficient blood flow through occluded arteries leads to oxygen deficiency in the leg muscles—usually in the calves, the most distal leg muscles—causing a painful cramp. The patient usually feels no symptoms while resting; pain and weakness develop in the calf muscle after he walks a certain distance without resting. When he does rest, his symptoms disappear as the supply of blood to the calf muscle is restored.

Point out possible complications

Stress the importance of strict compliance with treatment in helping prevent

---

CHECKLIST

TEACHING TOPICS IN ARTERIAL OCCLUSIVE DISEASE

- ☐ Major causes of reduced arterial blood flow—atherosclerosis and arteriosclerosis
- ☐ How intermittent claudication and arterial ulcers develop
- ☐ Preparation for arteriography, Doppler ultrasonography, blood clotting studies, and possibly serum lipid and lipoprotein measurements
- ☐ Relief of intermittent claudication with rest or by placing leg in a dependent position
- ☐ Regular exercise to prevent further occlusion and to develop collateral circulation
- ☐ Anticoagulant drugs—proper use and precautions
- ☐ Preventing infection and ulcers
- ☐ Caring for ulcers, including dressing changes
- ☐ Preparation for possible surgery: sympathectomy, endarterectomy, arterial bypass grafting, revascularization

complications of arterial occlusive disease, such as painful and slow-healing arterial ulcers. (However, because vascular changes from underlying arteriosclerosis and atherosclerosis are irreversible, the patient is still susceptible to complications even with compliance and successful surgery.) Arterial ulcers can form wherever a blocked or constricted artery produces ischemia in distal tissues. As ischemia worsens, capillary perfusion drops, metabolic exchange decreases, and the skin becomes increasingly fragile and susceptible to disruption and eventual infection from direct injury, pressure, and irritation.

Extremely dangerous, though rare, complications of arterial occlusive disease include embolism and aneurysm.

Teach about tests

Explain to the patient all diagnostic tests, such as arteriography and Doppler ultrasonography to determine the extent of arterial occlusion and collateral circulation. (See *Teaching Patients about Cardiovascular Tests*, pages 143 to 147, for more information on these tests.)

Prepare the patient for blood coagulation studies, such as partial thromboplastin time and prothrombin time, to investigate possible clotting abnormalities or to evaluate the effectiveness of anticoagulant therapy. Tell him who will collect the blood samples and when. Also, if ordered, prepare the patient for serum cholesterol, triglyceride, and lipoprotein studies to assess for atherosclerosis. Instruct him to abstain from alcohol for 24 hours and from exercise for 12 hours before the tests. If ordered, tell the patient to discontinue all thyroid, antilipemic, and oral contraceptive drugs.

Teach about treatments

• *Activity.* Tell the patient that regular exercise is essential to prevent further arterial occlusion and to promote development of collateral circulation, which helps reduce intermittent claudication and formation of arterial ulcers. Depending on the patient's age and capabilities, encourage him to walk, swim, or bicycle daily. Instruct him to exercise until claudication forces him to stop; then to rest; and then to resume exercising when the pain subsides. Daily, progressive exercise of this type may gradually reduce the severity of claudication and increase the distance the patient can walk without pain.

Unless contraindicated, teach the postoperative patient's family passive range-of-motion exercises: alternately flexing and extending the patient's legs, wiggling his toes, and rotating and flexing his feet. Then, as the patient's condition allows, have him begin active exercises.

If the patient's ambulatory, instruct him to walk for about 10 minutes each hour and to rest the remainder of the time. Reinforce the need to balance exercise and rest. Explain that overly vigorous exercise generates excessive heat in the leg muscles and places inordinate demands on already compromised leg circulation, increasing the risk of infection and exacerbating leg pain. For the same reasons, instruct him to avoid crossing his legs and elevating or applying heat to the affected leg.

Teach the patient to relieve persistent leg pain by periodically placing his legs in a dependent position, such as dangling them over the side of the bed. This position improves blood flow to the legs and relieves symptoms. Advise him to report any excessive leg or ankle swelling resulting from this practice.

• *Diet.* Depending on the underlying cause of arterial occlusive disease, you may need to review previously specified dietary restrictions on cholesterol, saturated fats, and sodium. (See "Coronary Artery Disease," pages 112 to 119, for information on necessary dietary changes in atherosclerosis.)

To help maintain skin integrity and reduce the chance of infection and ulceration, stress the importance of adequate intake of protein, vitamin B_{12}, and vitamin C. Be sure to point out good sources of these nutrients. For example, nutritional yeast is high in vitamin B_{12} and protein; it comes in a powder form that can easily be added to various foods. Sources of vitamin C include citrus fruits, strawberries, cantaloupe, tomatoes, bean sprouts, broccoli, cabbage, peppers, and brussels sprouts. Because traditional protein sources—meats, dairy products, and eggs—also contain high levels of cholesterol and/or saturated fats, teach the patient good alternative sources of protein: legumes, nuts, seeds, and grains.

• **Medication.** Explain to the patient the purpose of prescribed anticoagulant therapy. Tell him that an anticoagulant reduces his blood's ability to clot. Emphasize the need for precautions while taking anticoagulants. Give the patient a copy of the home care aid *Do's and Don'ts of Anticoagulant Therapy,* page 122, and discuss the guidelines with him. Tell him what pain medications will be available to him. (See *Teaching Patients about Cardiovascular Drugs,* pages 150 to 163, for more information.)

As appropriate, teach the patient how to apply topical antibiotics to areas of skin breakdown and ulceration.

• **Procedures.** Stress the importance of meticulous skin care to prevent infection. Advise the patient to avoid any activity that could cause injury or irritation to the skin or that could apply pressure or heat to it.

Daily foot and leg care is also essential to prevent infection and ulceration. Provide the patient with a copy of the home care aid *Taking Care of Your Feet* in Chapter 13, and go over it with him until you're sure he understands all the instructions.

Also essential is proper care of any arterial ulcers that develop. Explain to the patient that wet-to-dry dressings will mechanically debride the ulcer and help it heal. Instruct him to take his prescribed pain medication about ½ hour before changing dressings. Give

him a copy of the home care aid *How to Change Leg Dressings.* Remember to tell him what supplies he'll need to care for his ulcers at home and where he can get them.

As ordered, prepare the patient for percutaneous transluminal angioplasty to reopen a stenosed artery. (Refer to "Coronary Artery Disease," pages 112 to 119, for more information on this procedure.)

• **Surgery.** Point out to the patient that surgery is usually performed for chronic arterial occlusive disease when claudication interferes with ambulation, when carotid artery occlusion produces neurologic deficits, or when the procedure will improve blood supply to an ulcerated area. Surgical procedures include sympathectomy, endarterectomy, and bypass grafting for revascularization. Patient teaching varies slightly, depending on the procedure. (See "Surgery," pages 148 and 149, for general teaching points applicable to all patients undergoing cardiovascular surgery.)

Explain some additional considerations for these vascular surgeries. For example, if the patient's scheduled for an aortofemoral bypass, explain that he may have two or three incisions: one midline abdominal and one groin site for each femoral graft done. Tell him he'll receive a general anesthetic and that the graft will be sutured to the aorta and then to the femoral artery or arteries to create a bypass around a femoral artery occlusion.

If the patient's scheduled for an axillofemoral bypass, he may also have up to three incisions: one axillary and one or two groin sites. Explain that he'll receive a general anesthetic and that the graft will be sutured to his axillary artery and then threaded down along his side, in a tunnel created just under his skin, to the femoral artery or arteries. Postoperatively, tell the patient not to lie on the side of the graft; this could result in graft occlusion. Also advise him to avoid heavy lifting, carrying, any sudden or forceful use of the

HOW TO CHANGE LEG DRESSINGS

Dear Patient:

To treat your leg ulcers, you'll apply wet-to-dry or dry-to-dry dressings. Wet-to-dry dressings remove dead tissue and allow new tissue to grow. Dry-to-dry dressings keep the ulcer clean and dry.

1
Gather equipment: one pair of sterile gloves, one pair of unsterile gloves, plastic bag with twist-tie closure, fine-mesh sterile 4″ x 4″ gauze pads, wetting solution for wet-to-dry dressings or cleansing solution for dry-to-dry dressings, sterile absorbent pad, elastic bandage, mirror, and clean towel. Place equipment on the towel.

2
Wash your hands with soap and water. Now, open the packages of sterile gauze and the absorbent pad *without touching* the gauze or absorbent pad. If you're applying a wet-to-dry dressing, dampen the gauze with wetting solution.

3
To remove the old dressing, unwrap the elastic bandage or carefully cut it off. Then, put on unsterile gloves and remove

the dressing's top layer. Next, gently remove the contact layer. Check the ulcer for changed appearance, odor, and drainage. Place old dressing and gloves in plastic bag.

4
Put on sterile gloves. If you're applying a wet-to-dry dressing, lift the wet gauze from its package and wring out excess moisture over the plastic bag. Before applying a dry-to-dry dressing, saturate a piece of gauze with cleansing solution, and gently clean the ulcer.

5
Gently apply the new dressing, keeping the layers even. Remove and discard sterile gloves. Then secure the new dressing with an elastic bandage. Afterward, wash your hands.

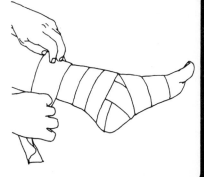

arm on the affected side, and reaching high overhead—these maneuvers could dislodge the graft from the donor site. Help the patient gradually regain use of the affected arm by teaching a member of his family how to perform passive range-of-motion exercises. Instruct the patient not to wear any tight or restrictive garments (belts, girdles, or suspenders) over the graft. Demonstrate how to check the graft pulse, placing the patient's index and middle fingers on the graft where it passes over the rib cage into the femoral area. Instruct the patient to notify the doctor promptly if he can't detect a graft pulse or if he experiences intermittent claudication.

If the patient's scheduled for sympathectomy, explain that he'll receive a general anesthetic and that selected sympathetic nerve fibers will be surgically excised. If successful, this surgery will allow arterial dilation and increased blood flow to the limbs. Tell him that sympathectomy may be done in conjunction with other revascularization procedures.

If the patient's scheduled for an endarterectomy (to relieve cerebral ischemia due to carotid artery occlusion), tell him that this surgery will improve cerebral circulation by removing the atherosclerotic plaque that has built up in the artery and occluded blood flow. Explain that he'll remain in the critical care unit for at least 24 hours and that he'll have a bulky dressing and, possibly, a drain on his neck for the next 24 to 48 hours. Tell him that frequent neurologic checks will be done to assess nerve function near the surgical site. Before he's discharged from the hospital, instruct the patient to call the doctor immediately if he experiences any changes in speech or level of consciousness, difficulty swallowing, hoarseness, paralysis or weakness in the extremities, or facial drooping— these could be early signs of developing neurologic damage.

Tell the patient undergoing revascularization of the femoral-popliteal-tibial area that he'll have an indwelling catheter, but probably not a nasogastric tube. Explain that this procedure can be done under general or spinal anesthesia. Tell him he'll have a few small incisions from ankle to groin, depending on the specific surgical procedure.

Postoperatively, teach the patient proper incision care and advise him to promptly report any early signs of infection, such as fever and pain, redness, swelling, warmth, or drainage at the incision site. Explain that he'll probably be up and walking within 1 to 5 days after surgery, depending on the extent of the procedure. Ambulation will begin gradually, and he may need to use a cane or walker at first. He'll also need to avoid sitting or standing for prolonged periods to prevent graft occlusion.

Stress that, although surgery may relieve symptoms, it won't cure chronic arterial occlusive disease. The patient will still need to follow prescribed treatment measures to prevent further progression.

● *Other care measures.* Counsel the patient about long-term management of arterial occlusive disease. If his job involves standing for prolonged periods or being outdoors in cold weather, he may want to consider changing to an indoor, sedentary type of job or, if possible, retiring early. If the patient agrees, refer him to available social service agencies for counseling.

Also advise the patient of other steps he can take to reduce risk factors for this and other cardiovascular diseases: controlling his weight, minimizing his dietary intake of salt and cholesterol, quitting smoking, learning to reduce stress, and, if applicable, receiving proper treatment for hypertension and diabetes.

Finally, teach him to recognize and report early warning signs of embolism and aneurysm: sudden onset of excruciating pain, mottling or pallor, loss of pulse, and paralysis in the affected extremity.

Congestive Heart Failure

Like the prognosis in so many cardiovascular disorders, the prognosis in congestive heart failure (CHF) depends not only on the disorder's severity and underlying cause but also on the patient's compliance with prescribed treatment. Although you can't guarantee compliance, you can improve its likelihood by teaching the patient about the pathophysiology of CHF, the reasons for prescribed treatments, and the importance of strict adherence to the treatment plan. Your teaching will need to cover sodium and fluid restrictions, a suggested activity plan, use of diuretics to reduce fluid retention, and other measures to relieve symptoms and prevent complications. And, to be truly effective, your teaching must emphasize the relationship between CHF and other cardiovascular disorders and provide the patient with the information he needs to help minimize common risk factors and improve his cardiovascular fitness.

When teaching about CHF, you'll encounter two groups of patients: those with acute CHF, commonly triggered by myocardial infarction, and those with chronic CHF, associated with renal retention of sodium and fluids. Of course, you'll have to tailor your teaching plan to each patient's needs and condition.

Describe the disorder

Tell the patient that CHF is characterized by myocardial dysfunction that leads to impaired pump performance or to frank heart failure and abnormal circulatory congestion. Explain the cyclical nature of CHF—how impaired pump performance sets into motion compensatory mechanisms that attempt to maintain blood flow to body tissues and how, if these mechanisms

fail, they can actually end up contributing to the problem—a phenomenon known as decompensation. (See *What Happens in Congestive Heart Failure,* pages 108 and 109, for a review of compensation and decompensation.)

Explain the type of heart failure the patient has. Although heart failure usually originates in the left ventricle (left heart failure), it sometimes originates in the right ventricle (right heart failure). In left heart failure, a large volume of blood remains in the dilated left ventricle, thereby reducing its ability to accept blood from the left atrium. This, in turn, causes atrial dilation and, eventually, pulmonary congestion, which may precipitate life-threatening pulmonary edema. In right heart failure, which often follows left heart failure, fluid backs up in the systemic circulation, eventually producing such effects as peripheral edema, distended neck veins, hepatomegaly, and weight gain. Sometimes, left and right heart failures develop simultaneously.

WHAT HAPPENS IN CONGESTIVE HEART FAILURE

Congestive heart failure (CHF) begins when the heart fails to pump sufficient blood to meet the body's needs. This lowers cardiac output, elevates venous pressure, and reduces arterial pressure, triggering a series of *compensatory* mechanisms (shown graphically here) to ensure perfusion of vital organs. However, these mecha-

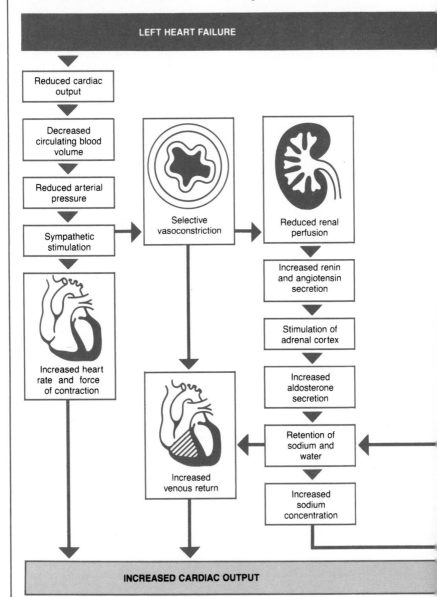

LEFT HEART FAILURE

Reduced cardiac output

Decreased circulating blood volume

Reduced arterial pressure

Sympathetic stimulation

Selective vasoconstriction

Reduced renal perfusion

Increased renin and angiotensin secretion

Stimulation of adrenal cortex

Increased aldosterone secretion

Increased heart rate and force of contraction

Retention of sodium and water

Increased venous return

Increased sodium concentration

INCREASED CARDIAC OUTPUT

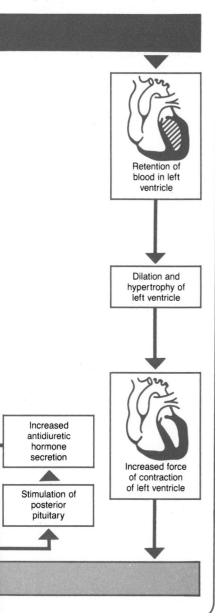

nisms can't sustain themselves indefinitely. When they begin to fail (a phenomenon known as *decompensation*), CHF progresses.

Retention of blood in left ventricle

Dilation and hypertrophy of left ventricle

Increased antidiuretic hormone secretion

Stimulation of posterior pituitary

Increased force of contraction of left ventricle

Point out possible complications

Emphasize the need for strict adherence to the prescribed treatment plan. Explain that noncompliance can cause serious cardiovascular and respiratory complications—including pulmonary edema, susceptibility to pneumonia and other respiratory infections, thromboembolism, and exacerbation of CHF. It can also result in damage to other organs, notably the liver, kidneys, and brain.

Teach about tests

Prepare the patient for expected diagnostic tests, such as a chest X-ray to detect fluid in the lungs or cardiac enlargement, electrocardiography to reveal conduction abnormalities, echocardiography or cardiac blood pool imaging to evaluate valvular and ventricular function, and cardiac catheterization to assess coronary artery blood flow and valvular and ventricular function. (See *Teaching Patients about Cardiovascular Tests*, pages 143 to 147, for more information on these tests.)

Arterial blood gas analysis may be ordered to evaluate oxygenation; if so, tell the patient who will perform the arterial puncture and when. Also tell him which site—radial, femoral, or brachial artery—will be punctured. Instruct the patient to breathe normally during the test, and warn him that he may experience brief cramping or a throbbing pain at the puncture site.

Teach about treatments

• *Activity.* Explain to the patient that excessive physical activity can further weaken his already weakened heart, possibly exacerbating CHF. For this reason, he must avoid overexertion.

To help the patient function as normally as possible and maintain independence, teach him to gradually increase his activity level and to pace himself. To help the patient avoid excessive fatigue, instruct him to conserve energy by alternating light and heavy tasks and by resting frequently.

If the patient's on bed rest, instruct him to alternately flex and extend his toes several times an hour or to perform range-of-motion leg exercises as scheduled. These exercises can help prevent deep vein thrombosis due to vascular congestion.

● **Diet.** Tell the patient he'll need to restrict sodium intake to prevent excessive fluid retention. Instruct him to avoid high-sodium foods, such as many processed foods, canned soups and vegetables, snack foods, and condiments. Advise him to check the sodium content on package labels, and suggest he use alternatives to table salt, such as herbs, spices, and commercially prepared salt substitutes.

If the doctor orders fluid restrictions, discuss them with the patient and arrange a mutually acceptable schedule for allowable fluids. Tell him he can relieve mouth dryness with rinses, hard candy, or gum; adding humidity to room air can also help.

● **Medication.** If appropriate, teach the patient about drugs used to reduce cardiac workload during the acute stage of CHF. These drugs typically include a rapid-acting I.V. diuretic, such as furosemide, to reduce salt and water retention, and I.V. morphine to reduce anxiety and induce vasodilation. After the acute stage passes, teach him about drugs prescribed to increase cardiac output, relieve symptoms, and prevent complications. These may include various combinations of oral diuretics, digoxin, antiarrhythmics, angiotensin-converting enzyme inhibitors (such as captopril), and anticoagulants (see *Teaching Patients about Cardiovascular Drugs*, pages 150 to 163). If the doctor has instructed the patient to check his pulse to monitor the effects of these drugs, teach him the proper technique. Give him a copy of the home care aid *How to Take Your Pulse*, page 130, and review it with him.

● **Procedures.** Explain the need for supplemental oxygen, if ordered. Endotracheal intubation and mechanical ventilation may be required for the patient with severe pulmonary involvement; if so, reassure him that this is only temporary and won't be needed once his respiratory status stabilizes. Provide him with pencil and paper to help him communicate while intubated; explain that he'll be able to speak once the tube is removed.

If pulmonary artery (PA) catheterization is ordered to measure hemodynamic pressures and cardiac output, explain that the procedure will help evaluate his heart function and will allow the doctor to tailor treatment accordingly. (See "Coronary Artery Disease," pages 112 to 119, for further teaching considerations in PA catheterization.)

If rotating tourniquets are necessary, explain to the patient that these reduce venous return and relieve pulmonary congestion, which will help him breathe more easily. Warn him that the skin on his extremities may become slightly discolored during this procedure.

Because unexplained weight gain may be an important early sign of recurrent CHF, teach the patient how to take accurate daily weights. Instruct him to weigh himself at the same time each day, on the same scale, and while wearing the same amount of clothing. Tell him to keep an accurate record of daily weights and to notify the doctor if he notices a gain.

● **Surgery.** Although surgery isn't generally indicated for CHF, the patient may need open-heart surgery for associated coronary artery disease or structural abnormalities. (See "Surgery," pages 148 and 149, for specific teaching points.)

● **Other care measures.** Teach the patient other measures to help relieve symptoms. Explain that he can help ease severe dyspnea by sitting up, leaning forward, and dangling his legs. Advise him to place extra pillows under his head to prevent orthopnea and paroxysmal nocturnal dyspnea.

Tell the patient he can minimize leg

LIVING WITH CONGESTIVE HEART FAILURE

Dear Patient:

Congestive heart failure impairs your heart's ability to pump blood. Follow these guidelines to help minimize your symptoms.

Take prescribed drugs
The doctor will order digitalis to strengthen your heart and improve its pumping ability. Do not substitute one brand of digitalis for another without first consulting him. Notify him promptly if you develop any loss of appetite, nausea and vomiting, diarrhea, fatigue, visual disturbances, headache, or muscle weakness.

Take prescribed diuretics to reduce your body's total volume of water and salt. If you're taking a potassium-wasting diuretic, eat plenty of high-potassium foods—such as citrus fruits, tomatoes, and bananas. Call your doctor if you develop dizziness, bloating, weakness, fatigue, leg cramps, confusion, or a persistent headache.

Restrict sodium intake
Limiting your sodium intake helps decrease water retention and ease your heart's work load. Don't add salt to your food. Avoid salted snack foods, canned soups and vegetables (unless labeled "low sodium"), prepared foods (such as frozen dinners), luncheon meats, cheeses, and pickles or other foods preserved in brine. Check food package labels for sodium content before buying.

Balance rest and exercise
Get adequate rest. If possible, shorten your workday and set aside a daily rest period. Prop your feet up with pillows for 20 minutes each evening to ease swelling. Also, try to avoid emotional stress.

Gradually increase walking and other physical activities. Stop if you feel short of breath, palpitations, or unusually tired. Also, notify your doctor if these symptoms get worse; he may need to adjust your medication.

Avoid temperature extremes
When possible, stay in a comfortable environment. In hot weather, perform your activities in the cooler part of the day. In cold weather, dress warmly but avoid restrictive clothing, which interferes with circulation. Wrap a scarf over your nose and mouth to warm incoming air and ease breathing.

and ankle edema by elevating his legs. Also, advise him to change positions slowly to prevent dizziness. Because extreme heat can make breathing difficult, tell him to stay in a cool environment whenever possible. And because extreme cold interferes with circulation, instruct him to dress warmly in cold weather.

Teach the patient measures to prevent complications—for example, relaxation techniques to help reduce anxiety, which can increase arterial pressure and heart rate and possibly reduce urine output. Instruct him to watch for and report early signs of pulmonary edema: cough, difficulty breathing, fatigue, restlessness, anxiety, and increased pulse rate. Also tell him to report signs of recurrent CHF, such as weight gain, anorexia, dyspnea on exertion, nocturia, or leg and ankle edema. And since CHF makes the patient more susceptible to pneumonia and other respiratory infections, warn him to limit his exposure to crowds and to people with infections. Suggest that he ask his doctor about the advisability of pneumonia and influenza vaccinations.

Before discharge, give the patient a copy of the home care aid *Living with Congestive Heart Failure*, page 111, which explains the essentials of home care. Refer him to a local chapter of the American Heart Association for more information and support.

Coronary Artery Disease

Year after year, coronary artery disease (CAD) claims more lives in the United States than any other disorder. However, research has shown that modifying significant risk factors can limit or even reverse the course of CAD. These risk factors include obesity, smoking, a high-cholesterol diet, a sedentary life-style, stress, and hypertension. Because many of these factors are within the patient's control, your teaching must focus on helping him identify them and develop a strategy for remedying them. It must also cover other treatment measures to relieve angina or, if necessary, to reopen or bypass occluded coronary arteries.

Angina, in fact, often prompts patients to seek medical help. After all, many patients confuse this classic symptom of CAD with the chest pain of myocardial infarction (MI). And they'll often turn to you for advice on its significance and on preventing or relieving it. How can your teaching help them? By pointing out angina-provoking activities and by teaching them how to take prescribed nitroglycerin.

Describe the disorder

Tell the patient that CAD is characterized by narrowing or blockage of one or both of the coronary arteries, resulting in diminished blood flow to the heart. This deprives the heart of vital oxygen and nutrients, causing tissue damage. Point out that the heart doesn't get oxygen from the blood it pumps through its chambers—it needs its own blood supply, which is provided by the coronary arteries. Use an illustration of the heart, if available, to clarify your teaching.

Explain that CAD usually results from atherosclerosis—the buildup of fatty, fibrous plaques on inner arterial walls. These plaques narrow the vessels and reduce the volume of blood that can be pumped through them. Discuss the risk factors linked to atherosclerosis. Have the patient complete the *CAD Risk Factor Survey*, pages 114 and 115, and discuss the results with him. This survey shows where you'll need to focus your teaching and allows you to develop an individualized plan for each CAD patient.

Next, discuss how lack of oxygen triggers the classic symptom of angina by stimulating the pain fibers surrounding the heart. Angina is typically described as a burning, squeezing, or crushing sensation in the chest. This pain may also radiate to the arm, shoulder blades, neck, or jaw. Inform the patient that angina doesn't always herald an MI, although it's a significant warning symptom. Tell him that certain activities tend to precipitate angina: physical exertion, exposure to extreme heat or cold, emotional stress, and even eating a large, heavy meal. (Keep in mind, though, that one type of angina occurs during rest and isn't related to stress. This variant, known as Prinzmetal's angina or the nocturnal variant, is associated with coronary artery spasm rather than atherosclerosis.)

Point out possible complications

Emphasize that strict adherence to the treatment plan can reduce the patient's risk of serious complications, including MI, dysrhythmias, and congestive heart failure.

Teach about tests

Prepare the patient for diagnostic tests to evaluate his heart and coronary arteries, including EKG, exercise EKG, thallium scan, coronary angiography, and, possibly, cardiac catheterization. (See *Teaching Patients about Cardiovascular Tests*, pages 143 to 147, for more information.)

Also prepare the patient for blood tests to detect and classify hyperlipemia, including serum triglycerides, total cholesterol, lipoprotein phenotyping, and lipoprotein-cholesterol fractionation. Instruct him not to eat for 12 to 14 hours and not to drink alcohol for 24 hours before the tests. Also instruct the patient to refrain from exercising for 12 hours before the tests and to discontinue thyroid, antilipemic, and oral contraceptive medications, as ordered by the doctor. Explain that these blood tests will be done regularly to help evaluate the effectiveness of dietary therapy aimed at reducing serum lipid levels.

CHECKLIST

TEACHING TOPICS IN C.A.D.

☐ An explanation of disease mechanisms: atherosclerosis and coronary artery spasm

☐ Risk factor analysis

☐ How angina develops and how to treat and prevent it

☐ Importance of treating CAD to prevent complications, such as myocardial infarction, dysrhythmias, and congestive heart failure

☐ Preparation for diagnostic tests, such as electrocardiography, angiography, and serum lipid studies

☐ Recommended exercise program

☐ Dietary restrictions to lower serum low-density lipoprotein levels and control hypertension

☐ Use of prescribed drugs

☐ Preparation for percutaneous transluminal coronary angioplasty or coronary artery bypass grafting, if ordered

☐ Other measures to reduce risk factors: reducing stress, controlling weight, quitting smoking

---

Teach about treatments

● *Activity.* Explain how a sedentary life-style contributes to CAD. Tell the patient that it encourages overeating, leads to obesity and hypertension, and unfavorably alters the ratio of high-density lipoprotein (HDL) to low-density lipoprotein (LDL).

Next, discuss the benefits of regular exercise. Tell him that it increases serum HDL levels, enhances weight loss, lowers blood pressure, and tones the entire cardiovascular system. Encourage aerobic exercises, such as jogging, bicycling, or swimming. Advise against isometric exercises, such as weight lifting, which elevate blood pressure and tax the heart and coronary arteries. Warn that occasional strenuous exercise may be more dangerous than no exercise at all.

C.A.D. RISK FACTOR SURVEY

Researchers recognize certain factors that can increase the risk of developing CAD and its complications. To assess your patient's risk, help him complete this survey. In each category, circle the number that applies to him; then add the circled numbers to get his score. Compare his score to the ranges at right to get an idea of his overall risk. Explain that some factors can be controlled if he's willing to make changes in his life-style.

Score	1	2
Age	10 to 20	21 to 30

Score	1	2
Heredity Include parents, grandparents, and siblings	No known history of cardiovascular disease	One relative with cardiovascular disease after age 60

Score	0	1
Weight	More than 5 lb below standard weight	−5 to +5 lb of standard weight

Score	0	1
Smoking Add 1 point if you inhale deeply and smoke cigarettes to the end. (*Don't* subtract any points if you do not inhale or if you smoke only part of a cigarette.) Subtract 1 point if you smoke but exercise regularly.	Nonsmoker	Smoke cigar and/or pipe

Score	1	2
Exercise	Intensive occupational and recreational exertion	Moderate occupational and recreational exertion

Score	1	2
Serum cholesterol level and percentage of fat in diet Use your cholesterol level if you know it. Otherwise, estimate your intake of dietary fats—primarily animal fats. The U.S. average, 40%, is too high for good health.	Cholesterol level of 180 mg or less. Diet contains no animal or solid fats.	Cholesterol level of 181 to 205 mg. Diet contains 10% animal or solid fats.

Score	1	2
Blood pressure	Systolic pressure of 100 mm Hg or less	Systolic, 101 to 120 mm Hg

Score	1	2
Sex/physique	Female under age 40	Female aged 40 to 50

SCORE	RISK	SCORE	RISK
6-11	Well below average	**25-31**	Above average
12-17	Below average	**32-40**	Well above average
18-24	Average	**41-62**	Exceptionally high—see your doctor now

3	4	6	8
31 to 40	41 to 50	51 to 60	61 and over

3	4	6	7
Two relatives with cardiovascular disease after age 60	One relative with cardiovascular disease before age 60	Two relatives with cardiovascular disease before age 60	Three relatives with cardiovascular disease before age 60

2	3	5	7
6 to 20 lb overweight	21 to 35 lb overweight	36 to 50 lb overweight	More than 50 lb overweight

2	4	6	10
Smoke 10 cigarettes or less a day	Smoke 20 cigarettes a day	Smoke 30 cigarettes a day	Smoke 40 or more cigarettes a day

3	5	6	8
Sedentary work and intense recreational exertion	Sedentary work and moderate recreational exertion	Sedentary work and light recreational exertion	Complete lack of exercise

3	4	5	7
Cholesterol level of 206 to 230 mg. Diet contains 20% animal or solid fats.	Cholesterol level of 231 to 255 mg. Diet contains 30% animal or solid fats.	Cholesterol level of 256 to 280 mg. Diet contains 40% animal or solid fats.	Cholesterol level of 281 mg or higher. Diet contains 50% or more animal or solid fats.

3	4	6	8
Systolic, 121 to 140 mm Hg	Systolic, 141 to 160 mm Hg	Systolic, 161 to 180 mm Hg	Systolic pressure over 180 mm Hg

3	5	6	7
Female over age 50	Male	Stocky male	Bald, stocky male

INQUIRY

QUESTIONS PATIENTS ASK ABOUT C.A.D.

Why is coronary artery bypass surgery done on some patients but not on others?

Candidates for coronary artery bypass usually fall into one of three groups: patients with severe angina that doesn't respond to medication or other treatments; patients who've developed complications of CAD, such as myocardial infarction; and patients who are scheduled for artificial heart valve replacement. However, bypass surgery isn't always appropriate for everyone in these groups. In some patients, the number and degree of arterial blockages precludes bypass surgery; in others, the risk of the surgery outweighs its possible benefits. The doctor will consider all available information on your condition before deciding on bypass surgery; he may try a relatively new procedure known as percutaneous transluminal coronary angioplasty (PTCA) as an alternative to surgery.

Will bypass surgery cure me?

No, surgery can't cure CAD. The vein grafts can develop atherosclerosis just like your arteries did. You should feel relief from angina, though, and have more energy. But you'll need to carefully follow postoperative and long-term care instructions to reduce the risk of developing new blockages.

What happens to fatty arterial deposits after a PTCA?

Although we don't know for sure, we do know that they don't float "downstream" to lodge somewhere else. Inflation of the balloon inside the artery breaks up the hard protective coating of the fatty plaque deposits and flattens the deposits against the arterial wall. Then, over the course of several months, "scavenger" cells in the bloodstream presumably remove most of the debris.

Teach the patient to take his prescribed medication before engaging in any activity that normally provokes angina, including exercise and sex. If angina occurs, he should stop the activity immediately, sit or lie down with his head elevated, breathe deeply and slowly to relax, and take his prescribed medication. Tell him to notify the doctor if angina persists for more than 10 minutes after he takes three spaced doses of his medication.

• *Diet.* Tell the patient that diet may affect one important risk factor of CAD—hyperlipemia, or high serum levels of cholesterol, triglycerides, and saturated fatty acids. Encourage the patient to modify his intake of fat. For example, tell him to use margarine instead of butter. Advise him to limit his intake of red meats, organ meats, luncheon meats, whole-milk dairy products, and egg yolks. Encourage him to eat fruits and vegetables, poultry, seafood, and high-fiber foods. Recommend use of polyunsaturated fats, such as vegetable oils, for cooking.

Explain the difference between desirable HDL and undesirable LDL, and point out that an unfavorable HDL:LDL ratio is a recognized risk factor for CAD. Make sure the patient knows his levels of these cholesterol fractions. Mention that recent research has linked intake of omega-3 fats, found mostly in cold-water fish such as salmon and mackerel, to reduced LDL levels and elevated HDL levels. If the patient drinks alcohol, advise him that up to two drinks a day can also raise HDL levels but that more than this amount can adversely affect the heart.

Because hypertension is a major risk factor for CAD, instruct the patient to control his blood pressure by limiting his salt and caffeine intake. Encourage him to lose weight, if necessary, by following a balanced diet and a regular exercise program. Advise against fad diets or pills. Refer him to a weight control group for additional information and support.

• *Medication.* Explain all prescribed

medications, including nitrates, calcium channel blockers, beta-adrenergic blockers, antilipemics, and certain anticoagulants. (See *Teaching Patients about Cardiovascular Drugs*, pages 150 to 163, for more information.) Also teach him how to use nitroglycerin to prevent or treat angina (see *How to Use Nitroglycerin*, pages 118 and 119).

To help manage hypertension, tell the patient to check labels on food and over-the-counter drug packages for sodium and caffeine content.

● *Procedures.* If drug therapy fails to relieve angina, the doctor may order percutaneous transluminal coronary angioplasty (PTCA) to dilate an obstructed coronary artery. If he does, explain that the doctor will numb an area on the patient's groin with a local anesthetic, then insert a thin, balloon-tipped catheter into a peripheral artery. Guided by fluoroscopy, he'll thread the catheter into the narrowed coronary artery to the site of obstruction. After verifying the catheter's placement by instilling contrast dye, the doctor will inflate the balloon tip. This compresses the obstruction against the arterial walls, expanding the vessel to increase blood flow. Tell the patient that the doctor will then deflate the balloon but may leave the catheter in place temporarily to repeat the procedure, if necessary, or to administer drugs.

Inform the patient that he'll be given a sedative before the procedure to help him relax and that he'll be asked to cough several times during the procedure to help clear contrast dye from his heart. Warn him that he may feel flushed and experience angina when the contrast dye's instilled; reassure him that these effects are transient. Explain post-PTCA procedures: the patient will be on bed rest for 1 or 2 days and will require periodic blood tests to evaluate blood coagulation, cardiac enzymes, and electrolytes. He'll receive I.V. nitroglycerin (to prevent coronary artery spasm) and/or anticoagulants (to prevent clot formation). Tell the patient that some short tubes or sheaths

may be left in his groin until the next day. Instruct him to keep the affected leg straight to prevent tube kinking. Reassure him that he'll be able to bend his leg and then stand a few hours after the tubes are removed.

Make sure the patient understands that PTCA doesn't cure CAD. The expanded artery can eventually reocclude if he fails to modify his risk factors.

● *Surgery.* If the doctor schedules coronary artery bypass grafting to relieve angina and, possibly, to prevent MI, explain the surgery to the patient, and teach him about pertinent preoperative and postoperative care measures. Provide encouragement by mentioning that surgery may improve the patient's life expectancy. (See "Surgery," pages 148 and 149, for more information.)

● *Other care measures.* Tell the patient that smoking and stress are also CAD risk factors. Explain that smoking reduces serum HDL levels, constricts his arteries (thereby elevating blood pressure), and reduces the blood's oxygen-carrying capacity. Encourage him to quit by noting that most of these effects will cease shortly after he quits. Refer him to a support group, such as a local chapter of the American Lung Association or the American Cancer Society, if necessary.

Also discuss how stress aggravates hypertension and overstimulates the heart. Help the patient identify stressors in his life and develop strategies to cope with them. No one can eliminate stress altogether, but the patient can learn to reduce it by avoiding noise and crowds; by modifying aggressive, hard-driving ("type A") behavior; by changing a stressful job; by learning to relax through such measures as yoga, walking, or deep-breathing exercises; by getting adequate exercise and rest; and by taking up an enjoyable hobby. If appropriate, consider referring the patient to an assertiveness training workshop to help him reduce aggression and frustration. Also refer the patient to a local chapter of the American Heart Association.

HOW TO USE NITROGLYCERIN

Dear Patient:

Your doctor has prescribed nitroglycerin to control angina. By temporarily widening your veins and arteries, nitroglycerin brings more blood and oxygen to your heart when it needs it most. This drug is available in ointment, disk, tablet, and spray forms. To ensure its effectiveness, follow these directions for the form of medication you're taking.

Ointment

1

Measure the prescribed amount of nitroglycerin ointment onto the special paper.

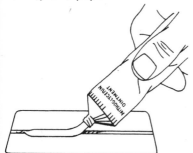

Spread it lightly over the area specified by the doctor—usually the upper arm or chest. Don't rub it into your skin. For best results, spread the ointment to cover an area about the size of the application paper (roughly 3½" by 2¼").

2

Cover the ointment with paper and tape it in place. If you experience persistent headache or dizziness while using the ointment, notify your doctor.

Disk

1

Apply the disk to any convenient skin area—preferably on the upper arm or chest, but never below the elbow or knee—touching only the back of the disk. If necessary, shave the site first.

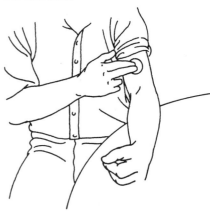

Avoid applying the disk to skin folds, scars, calluses, and any damaged or irritated skin. Use a different site every day.

2

After application, wash your hands. Avoid wetting the disk. If the disk should leak or fall off, throw it away and apply a new disk at a different site.

To ensure 24-hour coverage, set a routine for applying a new disk each day. Also, apply the new disk 30 minutes before removing the old one. If you experience persistent headache or dizziness while using the disk, tell your doctor.

Sublingual tablets

1

Place one tablet under your tongue and let it dissolve. Avoid swallowing while the tablet's dissolving.

2

If angina lasts for more than 5 minutes after taking the first tablet, take another one. Then take a third one after 5 more minutes, if necessary.

3

If three tablets don't provide relief, call your doctor and have someone take you to the nearest hospital. *Never* take more than three tablets. Get new tablets after 3 months, even if you have some left.

Spray

1

Hold the spray canister upright as close as possible to your open mouth.

2

Press the button on the canister's top to release the spray onto or under your tongue.

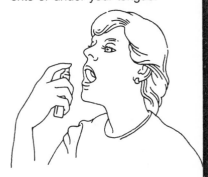

Release the button and close your mouth. Avoid swallowing immediately after spraying.

3

If angina lasts for more than 5 minutes, spray again. Then spray a third time after 5 more minutes, if necessary. Do not take more than three sprays within any 15-minute period. If angina persists, call your doctor and have someone take you to the nearest hospital.

Deep Vein Thrombosis

Sudden, often excruciating, deep muscle pain will initially motivate the patient with deep vein thrombosis (DVT) to respond to your teaching. You'll need to prepare him for immediate anticoagulant drug therapy and, perhaps, surgery to relieve pain and avoid potentially life-threatening pulmonary embolism. As the patient recovers from DVT, your teaching must then focus on preventing or managing long-term complications of chronic venous insufficiency—edema, varicose veins, and skin infection and ulceration. It's here that your major work lies. For example, you'll need to teach the patient how to apply antiembolism stockings and encourage him to wear them, as directed. You'll also need to teach him to periodically elevate his legs to improve venous return. To prevent skin infection, you'll need to teach him meticulous skin care and the importance of good nutrition. If the patient already has skin ulcers, he'll need your instruction to care for them at home.

Describe the disorder
Explain that DVT occurs when a blood clot, or thrombus, occludes a vein, blocking blood flow. More than half of all thrombi develop in the deep veins of the leg; other sites include the veins of the pelvis, kidneys, liver, right heart, and arm. Thrombi may form as a result of venous stasis, hypercoagulability of the blood, and/or injury to the vascular wall. Recurrent venous inflammation, as in thrombophlebitis, may also play a role in their formation.

Point out possible complications
Describe the complications that may develop if the patient doesn't adhere to the treatment plan. The thrombus may break loose into the systemic circulation and eventually lodge in the lungs, causing pulmonary embolism—a potentially life-threatening occlusion of the pulmonary arterial bed. Or the thrombus may remain immobile and eventually destroy venous valves, causing chronic venous insufficiency. Straying from the treatment plan then increases the patient's risk of developing local skin infections, dermatitis, and venous stasis ulcers.

Teach about tests
Prepare the patient for expected diagnostic tests, such as Doppler ultrasonography and impedance plethysmography to assess venous blood flow, and venography to determine the affected vessel. (See *Teaching Patients about Cardiovascular Tests*, pages 143 to 147, for more information.)

Also prepare him for blood clotting studies, such as prothrombin time or partial thromboplastin time, to screen for a coagulation disorder as the cause of DVT or to monitor the effectiveness of anticoagulant drug therapy.

Teach about treatments
• *Activity.* Explain to the patient how bed rest reduces the oxygen and nutrient demands of the affected leg. Instruct him to keep the leg elevated to reduce swelling and pain, and to alternately flex, extend, and rotate each foot several times an hour to enhance venous return.

Later, once the acute stage subsides, tell the patient to resume his daily activities, according to his doctor's instructions. Point out that regular exercise helps develop collateral circulation and improves venous return. However, caution him not to overdo it. Also caution him to periodically rest the affected leg.

• *Diet.* Your dietary teaching has two basic goals: to minimize complications—particularly skin ulcers—and to improve overall cardiovascular health. To achieve the first goal, instruct the patient to include adequate amounts of protein and vitamins B_{12} and C in his diet. These nutrients help maintain skin integrity.

To achieve the second goal, you'll need to investigate the patient's eating habits. Then, review the basics of good nutrition with him, stressing general restrictions that promote cardiovascular health. For example, tell him to limit his intake of salt and saturated fats. If appropriate, also encourage the patient to lose weight.

• **Medication.** Stress the importance of taking anticoagulant drugs exactly as prescribed to help prevent expansion of an existing thrombus or formation of any new ones. In acute DVT, the patient may receive parenteral anticoagulants; once his condition stabilizes, he'll be given an oral form of the drug.

Before discharge, teach about precautions the patient should take while on anticoagulants (see *Do's and Don'ts of Anticoagulant Therapy*, page 122).

• **Procedures.** Teach the patient how to prevent skin breakdown and ulceration on his legs and feet. Give him a copy of the home care aid *Taking Care of Your Feet* in Chapter 13, which discusses specific guidelines for skin care that he should follow.

To minimize venous stasis, instruct the patient to wear antiembolism stockings whenever he's up and about. Show him how to apply these stockings (see *Applying Antiembolism Stockings*, page 123); then have him give a return demonstration. Inform the patient what size stockings to buy and tell him where he can get them.

Promote meticulous care of existing ulcers to prevent infection and aid healing. Teach the patient how to change his leg dressings (see *How to Change Leg Dressings*, page 105).

• **Surgery.** If ordered, prepare the patient for thrombectomy, or excision of the thrombus. Usually, this surgery is reserved for an acute thrombus in a large vein.

If anticoagulant therapy fails or is contraindicated in the patient, the doctor may surgically place a tiny filter or

---

CHECKLIST

TEACHING TOPICS IN D.V.T.

☐ An explanation of how a thrombus occludes blood flow through a vein

☐ The importance of prompt treatment to prevent potentially fatal pulmonary embolism or debilitating chronic venous insufficiency

☐ Preparation for diagnostic tests, such as Doppler ultrasonography, impedance plethysmography, venography, and blood clotting studies

☐ The need for rest and limb elevation during the acute stage of DVT, and for regular exercise after the acute stage has passed

☐ Increased intake of protein and vitamins B_{12} and C to maintain skin integrity; other dietary modifications to improve overall cardiovascular health

☐ Anticoagulant drug use and precautions

☐ Application of antiembolism stockings to prevent venous stasis and embolism

☐ Skin care to prevent venous ulcers

☐ Care of existing ulcers

☐ Preparation for thrombectomy, if ordered

☐ Warning signs of pulmonary embolism and chronic venous insufficiency

---

"umbrella" in the inferior vena cava to intercept migrating thrombi and prevent pulmonary embolism. Explain this surgery to the patient, including where he should expect the incision (usually under the right clavicle) and how to care for it postoperatively.

• **Other care measures.** Because life-threatening pulmonary embolism can develop suddenly, teach the patient to watch for and immediately report warning signs: acute shortness of breath or severe chest pain, and cough with blood-tinged sputum. Also teach him to report early signs of chronic venous insufficiency, including leg pain, edema, skin changes (scaling, brown pigmentation), and dilated superficial veins.

DO'S AND DON'TS OF ANTICOAGULANT THERAPY

Dear Patient:

To hinder your blood's ability to clot, your doctor has prescribed an anticoagulant drug. Follow this list of do's and don'ts when taking this drug.

Do:
• Carry Medic Alert identification stating you're taking an anticoagulant.
• Use an electric razor to shave or a depilatory to remove unwanted hair.
• Place a rubber mat and safety rails in your bathtub to prevent falls.
• Wear gloves while gardening.
• Use a soft-bristled toothbrush.
• Ensure adequate intake of foods high in vitamin K: green leafy vegetables, tomatoes, bananas, fish.
• Avoid sharp objects, rough sports, and blunt trauma. Report abdominal or joint pain or swelling to your doctor.
• Draw a line around the margins of new bruises. If the bruise extends outside of the line, notify your doctor.
• Maintain pressure on all cuts for 10 minutes. If you cut your arm or leg, also elevate it above heart level. If the bleeding doesn't stop, call for help immediately.
• Check your urine and stool for any signs of blood.

• Notify your doctor of bleeding gums, nosebleed, bleeding hemorrhoids, reddish or purplish skin spots, or excessive menstrual flow. Also report vomiting, diarrhea, or fever that lasts longer than 24 hours.
• Keep all appointments for blood tests.
• Refill your prescription at least 1 week before your supply runs out.
• Take your medication at the same time each day, as prescribed. Change your dosage only as directed by the doctor.
• Store your medication away from extreme heat or cold.

Don't:
• Take aspirin, drugs containing aspirin, or any other drug (including over-the-counter cough and cold remedies and vitamins) without checking with your doctor or pharmacist.
• Take an extra dose of your anticoagulant. If you forget to take a dose, just take your next dose at the scheduled time. If you miss two doses, call your doctor.
• Put toothpicks or sharp objects into your mouth.
• Walk barefoot.
• Trim calluses and corns. Consult a podiatrist.
• Use power tools.
• Drink alcohol heavily.

APPLYING ANTIEMBOLISM STOCKINGS

Dear Patient:

To improve circulation in your lower legs, the doctor wants you to apply antiembolism stockings in the morning before getting out of bed and to remove them at night once you're in bed. Follow these steps to apply the stockings.

1

Lightly dust your ankle with powder to ease stocking application.

2

Insert your hand into the stocking from the top, and grab the heel pocket from the inside. Turn the stocking inside out so your foot's inside the stocking leg.

3

Hook the index and middle fingers of both your hands into the foot section. Ease the stocking over your toes, stretch-ing it sideways as you move it up your foot. Point your toes to help ease the stocking on.

4

Center your heel in the heel pocket. Then, gather the loose material at your ankle, and slide the rest of the stocking up over your heel with short pulls, alternating front and back.

5

Insert your index and middle fingers into the gathered stocking at your ankle, and ease the stocking up your leg to the knee.

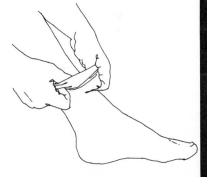

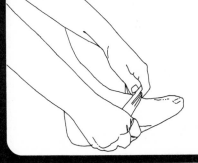

Stretch the stocking toward the knee, front and back, to distribute the material evenly. Make sure the stocking fits snugly, with no wrinkles.

Dysrhythmias

Affecting a broad section of the population, dysrhythmias vary from mild, asymptomatic disturbances like sinus arrhythmia to life-threatening irregularities like ventricular fibrillation, which requires immediate intervention. This greatly complicates your teaching responsibilities. Not only are you teaching about diverse degrees of illness, but you're also teaching patients of diverse learning needs, ages, and health histories. However, no matter what your patient's status may be, your main teaching goal remains the same: to teach the patient about his specific dysrhythmia and its treatment. For some patients, treatment may mean implantation of a temporary or a permanent pacemaker—or both. This adds greatly to your teaching responsibilities, not only for preimplantation preparation and postimplantation care, but also for long-term pacemaker use and maintenance.

Describe the disorder

Tell the patient that a dysrhythmia is an abnormal change in his heart rate and/or rhythm. Explain that normal conduction of the heart's electrical impulses can become disrupted for various reasons (both congenital and acquired). Briefly explain the normal conduction pathway: impulses usually originate in the sinoatrial node, then travel across the right atrium through the atrioventricular node to the bundle of His, and then disperse throughout the ventricles. Tell the patient that any disruption of this pathway can produce dysrhythmias.

As appropriate, discuss the characteristics and significance of the patient's dysrhythmia. (See *Reviewing Common Dysrhythmias*, pages 126 and 127.)

Point out possible complications

Reinforce the need to follow prescribed treatment by pointing out the possible consequences of untreated or improperly treated dysrhythmias. Without causing the patient undue alarm, explain that dysrhythmias alter cardiac output, which can lead to a wide range of complications—from palpitations and dizziness to life-threatening thromboembolism or cardiac arrest.

Teach about tests

Prepare the patient for an EKG to identify and monitor his specific dysrhythmia. Later, prepare him for other possible diagnostic tests, such as exercise EKG, ambulatory EKG, electrophysiologic studies, and cardiac

---

CHECKLIST

TEACHING TOPICS IN DYSRHYTHMIAS

- [ ] An explanation of normal cardiac conduction
- [ ] An explanation of the patient's specific dysrhythmia
- [ ] Preparation for diagnostic tests, such as EKG, serum electrolyte studies, and electrophysiologic studies
- [ ] Activity instructions: regular exercise, appropriate warnings
- [ ] General dietary restrictions: moderate use of alcohol, caffeine, and tobacco; increased or decreased potassium intake, as ordered
- [ ] Antiarrhythmic drug use
- [ ] Applicable treatment methods: carotid sinus massage, Valsalva's maneuver, temporary pacemaker implantation, electrocardioversion
- [ ] Preparation for permanent pacemaker implantation, if necessary
- [ ] Guidelines for pacemaker use and maintenance, if necessary
- [ ] How to take pulse rate
- [ ] Sources of additional information and support

catheterization. (See *Teaching Patients about Cardiovascular Tests*, pages 143 to 147, for information on these tests.)

The doctor may also order blood tests to measure levels of serum electrolytes, such as potassium, or certain drugs, such as quinidine and propranolol. He may even order tests for illicit drugs, such as heroin, amphetamines, and cocaine, if he suspects them as the underlying cause of dysrhythmia. If so, prepare the patient for venipuncture.

Teach about treatments

● *Activity.* Tell the patient that most dysrhythmias, if managed properly, shouldn't interfere with normal activities. Encourage him to establish a regular exercise routine, under his doctor's supervision, to improve his overall cardiovascular fitness. Remind him to avoid overexertion, and warn him to stop exercising immediately if he experiences dizziness, light-headedness, dyspnea, or chest pain. Also warn against driving or operating heavy machinery if his dysrhythmia causes periodic dizziness or syncope.

● *Diet.* Although dietary restrictions aren't usually required in many dysrhythmias, you can give your patient general guidelines to help prevent aggravating his condition. For example, caution him against overeating or over-consumption of alcohol, and advise him to limit intake of caffeine and use of tobacco. Explain the dangers of "holiday heart syndrome": the combination of increased food and alcohol consumption, smoking, and emotional excitement associated with holiday get-togethers can trigger or worsen his dysrhythmia. Because both elevated and depressed serum potassium levels can sometimes contribute to dysrhythmias, teach the patient to increase or decrease his intake of potassium-rich foods, as necessary. Such foods include bananas, citrus fruits, figs, leafy green vegetables, meats, and seafood.

● *Medication.* Stress the importance of strict compliance with the prescribed drug regimen. Such a regimen usually consists of an antiarrhythmic, such as digitalis, verapamil, propranolol, quinidine, or procainamide, possibly given in combination with other drugs to treat an underlying cardiovascular disorder. Point out that medications can only control, not cure, his dysrhythmia. Tell him he must continue taking antiarrhythmics and other prescribed drugs on schedule, even if he's experiencing no symptoms. (See *Teaching Patients about Cardiovascular Drugs*, pages 150 to 163, for additional teaching points.)

● *Procedures.* Depending on the patient's dysrhythmia, teach about various procedures that may be used to manage it. For example, you may need to teach the patient with paroxysmal atrial tachycardia how to quickly restore his heart's regular rhythm by performing carotid sinus massage or Valsalva's maneuver. For carotid massage, show him how to locate the carotid sinus on both the right and left sides of his neck. Next, demonstrate how to *gently* massage the right sinus for no more than 5 seconds. Then, depending on the doctor's orders, show him how to do the same for the left sinus. *Caution the patient never to massage both sinuses at once.* Have him perform the procedure in front of you to ensure that he's doing it correctly. Improper technique, such as use of excessive pressure or overly long massage, can block blood flow to the brain, possibly causing cerebrovascular accident. Or it can trigger new, more dangerous dysrhythmias.

To teach the patient Valsalva's maneuver, simply tell him to inhale deeply, hold his breath, and strain hard for at least 10 seconds before exhaling. Explain that the resulting increase in intrathoracic pressure converts the dysrhythmia to a normal rhythm.

If the patient is scheduled for temporary pacemaker implantation (usually done for patients with sick sinus syndrome or certain conduction blocks), prepare him for the procedure. Tell him that the doctor will in-

REVIEWING COMMON DYSRHYTHMIAS

DYSRHYTHMIA	DESCRIPTION

Atrial fibrillation

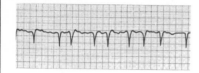

- Impulse forms in atrial ectopic areas.
- Atrial rate exceeds 400 beats/minute.
- Ventricular rate varies, and ventricular rhythm is grossly irregular.

First-degree AV block

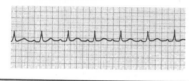

- Slowed AV node conduction with normal rate and rhythm.
- Usually no treatment needed.

Second-degree AV block, Mobitz Type I (Wenckebach)

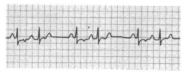

- Every second, third, or fourth impulse from the atria is fully blocked, creating a discrepancy between atrial and ventricular rates.
- Ventricular rhythm is irregular; atrial rhythm, regular.
- Second-degree heart block may progress to third-degree heart block.

Second-degree AV block, Mobitz Type II

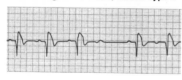

- Every second, third, or fourth impulse from the atria is fully blocked, creating a discrepancy between atrial and ventricular rates.
- Ventricular rhythm may be irregular with varying degrees of block.
- Second-degree heart block may progress to third-degree heart block.

Third-degree AV block (complete heart block)

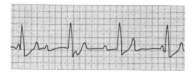

- Atrial impulses are blocked at AV node; atrial and ventricular impulses dissociated.
- Atrial rhythm is regular; ventricular rhythm, slow and regular.
- Onset may initiate pause before ventricular pacemaker activates. During this pause, cardiac output decreases, causing syncope or ventricular standstill (asystole) characterized by convulsions (Stokes-Adams syndrome). Sudden death will result if an artificial pacemaker isn't used.

DYSRHYTHMIA	DESCRIPTION

Paroxysmal atrial tachycardia (PAT)

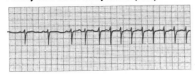

- Heart rate exceeds 140 beats/minute; rarely exceeds 250 beats/minute.
- Onset and termination of dysrhythmia occur suddenly but may be prevented by tachycardia. Such tachycardia often begins during sleep and awakens the patient.
- PATs may cause palpitations, light-headedness, and exhaustion.
- When atrial rate is exactly twice the ventricular rate, patient is said to have PAT with 2:1 block (common in digitalis toxicity).

Premature ventricular contraction (PVC)
Interpolated PVCs

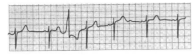

- Most common dysrhythmia.
- PVC may be interpolated—falling exactly between two normal beats.
- Focus can be unifocal (same appearance in every lead) or multifocal (in serious organic heart disease).

Multifocal PVCs

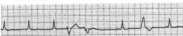

- PVCs are most ominous when clustered and multifocal, with R wave on T pattern (may precipitate ventricular tachycardia or fibrillation).

R-on-T phenomenon

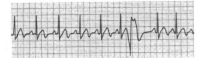

- Beat occurs prematurely, usually followed by a complete compensatory pause after PVC; irregular pulse.
- Dysrhythmias can occur singly, in pairs, or in threes, and can alternate with normal beats, as in ventricular bigeminy (one normal beat followed by PVC) or trigeminy (two normal beats followed by PVC).
- Coupling interval—time between normal beat and PVC—is usually fixed but may vary, especially if ectopic focus is parasystolic.

Sick sinus syndrome

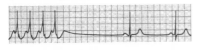

- Tachycardia and bradycardia may alternate and be interrupted by long sinus pauses, resulting in Stokes-Adams syndrome.

Ventricular tachycardia

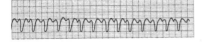

- Ventricular rate ranges from 140 to 220 beats/minute; rhythm may be regular.
- Because of dangerously low cardiac output, ventricular tachycardia can produce chest pain, anxiety, palpitations, dyspnea, shock, coma, and death. It can lead to ventricular fibrillation.

sert a long, thin electrode lead wire into a peripheral vein and, guided by fluoroscopy, will advance it through the vena cava into the right atrium and perhaps into the right ventricle. Explain that once the electrode lead is in place, the doctor will attach its other end to a battery-powered pacemaker pulse generator that will control his heart rate. Tell the patient that he may feel transient pain at the catheter insertion site and possibly palpitations as the pacemaker is activated or adjusted, but reassure him that otherwise he'll feel no discomfort. Explain that the pacemaker will remain in place for up to several days until his dysrhythmia is controlled or until other measures, such as permanent pacemaker insertion or cardiac surgery, are taken. Tell him that he'll wear the temporary pacemaker on his chest, waist, or upper arm and that he'll be able to move around fairly normally.

Electrocardioversion may be ordered for the patient with atrial fibrillation or certain other unstable dysrhythmias; if so, explain the procedure to the patient. Tell him that cardioversion uses an electric current to restore normal heart rate and relieve symptoms. Instruct him to abstain from food and fluids for at least 8 hours before the procedure. If applicable, tell him that a blood sample will be taken to check serum potassium level. Explain that he'll be given an I.V. sedative to induce sleep and that while he's asleep, electric current will be delivered to his heart through paddles placed on his chest. Reassure him that he'll feel no pain or discomfort from the procedure and that he'll be able to eat and move about once the sedative wears off.

● *Surgery.* If the patient's dysrhythmia can't be controlled by medications or other conservative measures, the doctor may order surgery. Depending on the specific dysrhythmia and possible underlying cardiovascular problems, surgical procedures can range from complex open-heart surgery to correct structural defects (see "Surgery," pages 148 and 149) to relatively uncomplicated permanent pacemaker implantation. Prepare the patient scheduled for pacemaker surgery by explaining the implantation procedure and by making sure he understands all preoperative and postoperative instructions. (See *Living with Your Pacemaker* for detailed postoperative instructions.) Tell him that he'll receive a sedative and local anesthetic before the procedure. Explain how the pacemaker pulse generator will be implanted under his skin in an unobtrusive area and how electrodes will be threaded through a vein into his heart's right chamber. Mention that cardiac monitoring will evaluate pacemaker function before his discharge. Tell the patient that once the pacemaker's in place, he'll be able to resume most normal activities without fear of damaging it. Instruct him to avoid manipulating the pacemaker through his skin (a behavior known as "twiddler's syndrome")—he may dislodge an electrode. If the patient had a temporary pacemaker implanted before permanent implantation, explain that it will be left in place for up to 24 hours after permanent implantation to serve as a backup. And, if thoracotomy was done during implantation to attach electrodes directly to the epicardium, teach him proper postthoracotomy care. (See "Surgery" in Chapter 7.)

● *Other care measures.* Teach the patient—especially one with a pacemaker—how to take his pulse. (See *How to Take Your Pulse*, page 130.) Remind him to accurately record all daily pulse readings and to notify the doctor of any significant abnormalities—a rate 5 or more beats lower than his pacemaker's preset rate, a rate exceeding 100 beats/minute, or any unusually irregular rhythm. If ordered by the doctor, teach the patient with atrial fibrillation how to take his carotid pulse rather than his radial pulse.

Teach the patient measures to reduce long-term complications of his dysrhythmia. Suggest that at least one fam-

LIVING WITH YOUR PACEMAKER

Dear Patient:

Your doctor has inserted a pacemaker in your chest to produce the electrical impulses needed to keep your heart working correctly. Follow these guidelines to ensure that your new pacemaker functions effectively.

Check your pacemaker daily

To do so, count your pulse for 1 minute after you've been at rest for at least 15 minutes—a good time to count it is the first thing in the morning. Call the doctor if you detect an *unusually fast or slow* rate or if you experience chest pain, dizziness, shortness of breath, prolonged hiccups, muscle twitching, nausea, vomiting, or diarrhea.

Check the implantation site each day. Normally, the implantation bulges slightly. If it reddens, swells, drains, or becomes warm or painful, call the doctor. Remember to wear loose clothing to avoid putting pressure on the site.

Follow doctor's orders

Take your heart medication as prescribed to ensure a regular heart rate. Also follow the doctor's orders concerning diet and physical activity. You should exercise every day, but *don't overdo it.* Be especially careful not to stress the muscles near the pacemaker. Also, avoid contact sports.

Keep all scheduled doctor's appointments. Usually, periodic hospitalization is necessary for battery changes or pacemaker replacement.

Take precautions

Don't get too close to gasoline engines, electric motors, or poorly shielded microwave ovens; these may interfere with your pacemaker. Also stay away from high-voltage fields created by overhead electric lines.

Avoid driving until 1 month after implantation, and avoid long trips for at least 3 months. If you're traveling by plane, you must pass through an airport metal detector. Before doing so, let the authorities know you have a pacemaker.

If you need dental work or surgery, tell the care provider that you have a pacemaker. You may need an antibiotic to prevent infection.

Always carry your pacemaker emergency card. The card lists your doctor, hospital, type of pacemaker, and date of implantation.

HOW TO TAKE YOUR PULSE

Dear Patient:

The doctor wants you to take your pulse—the number of times your heart beats per minute. Take your pulse at rest and during exercise. By comparing these two pulse rates, the doctor can evaluate how well your heart is pumping.

Taking your pulse at rest

Don't check your resting pulse right after exercising, eating a big meal, or taking your prescribed antiarrhythmic drugs. When you're ready to take your *resting* pulse rate, be sure you have a watch or a clock with a second hand. Sit quietly and relax for 2 minutes. Then place your index and middle fingers on your wrist just above the thumb, as shown here.

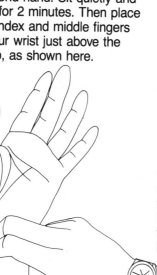

Count the pulse beats for 30 seconds and multiply by 2. (Or count for 60 seconds, but do not multiply, if your doctor has so instructed because of your irregular heart rhythm.) Record this number and the date.

Taking your pulse during exercise

By taking your pulse during exercise, you can help ensure the most benefit from your exercise program. As soon as you stop exercising, find your pulse as instructed above. Count the beats for 6 seconds; then add a zero to that figure. This gives you a reliable estimate of your *working* heart rate for 1 minute. (Don't count your pulse for a whole minute. Because your heart rate slows quickly when you rest, that figure won't be accurate.) Record this number and the date.

If your working heart rate is 10 or more beats above the target rate specified by your doctor, don't exercise so hard the next time. But if your working heart rate is lower than your target rate, exercise a little harder next time.

ily member learn cardiopulmonary resuscitation; this training could make the difference between life and death in a patient who develops sudden cardiac arrest or myocardial infarction.

Also make the patient aware of other cardiovascular disorders that can either contribute to or result from uncontrolled dysrhythmias. Discuss general risk factors for these disorders—stress, obesity, smoking, and sedentary life-style, among others. Refer the patient to a local chapter of the American Heart Association for more information.

Hypertension

Affecting as many as one in every five adults, hypertension often goes undetected until revealed by a routine checkup. Because the patient is typically asymptomatic, your first teaching session may involve convincing him that hypertension is a serious disorder and, most important, that he must take steps to control it. You'll need to define blood pressure simply, then review how hypertension taxes the heart and its vessels.

However, achieving long-term patient compliance will be the major goal of your teaching. You'll need to stress the importance of adhering to the prescribed medication regimen, dietary restrictions, and exercise program. For many patients, these measures demand difficult life-style changes. For instance, restrictions on sodium and caffeine may force the patient to give up his favorite junk foods and his morning cup of coffee. His exercise program may compel him to change his leisure-time schedule.

Because stress has been linked to hypertension, you'll need to teach the patient relaxation techniques and how to modify his response to daily stressors. You may also need to teach him how to take his blood pressure, thereby

---

CHECKLIST

TEACHING TOPICS IN HYPERTENSION

- [ ] An explanation of the patient's type of hypertension: primary or secondary
- [ ] An explanation of how high blood pressure develops, including significant risk factors
- [ ] Normal blood pressure readings
- [ ] The importance of adhering to treatment measures to prevent potentially fatal complications, such as myocardial infarction
- [ ] Exercise program and precautions
- [ ] Dietary restrictions
- [ ] Use of antihypertensives, diuretics, and other prescribed medications
- [ ] Home blood pressure monitoring, including an explanation of systolic and diastolic pressures
- [ ] Other measures to reduce long-term complications, such as controlling weight, quitting smoking, and reducing stress
- [ ] Sources of information and support, such as the American Heart Association

---

helping to ensure his active role in self-care.

Describe the disorder
Tell the patient that hypertension is another name for high blood pressure. Then explain that blood pressure is the force blood exerts against the arterial walls as it's pumped through the body by the heart. High blood pressure simply means that this force is greater than it should be. Explain the two numbers that comprise a blood pressure reading: the systolic figure indicates arterial pressure during the heart's contractions, or beats; the diastolic figure, arterial pressure when the heart momentarily relaxes between beats. Normal systolic pressure ranges from 100 to 135 mm Hg; normal diastolic pressure, from 60 to 80 mm Hg. Tell the patient that blood pressure normally

VASCULAR DAMAGE IN HYPERTENSION

Sustained hypertension can cause pathologic changes in the entire vascular system.
Vascular damage begins with alternating
areas of dilation and constriction in the
arterioles. Here, increased intraarterial
pressure damages the epithelium. Independently, angiotensin induces contraction of
endothelial walls, allowing plasma to
leak through interendothelial spaces. Eventually, deposition of plasma constituents
in the vessel walls causes medial necrosis.
Such damage may eventually produce
occlusion, aneurysm, or rupture of the vessels.

NORMAL VASCULAR STRUCTURE

Normal arteriole

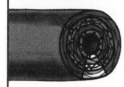

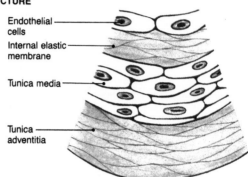

Endothelial cells

Internal elastic membrane

Tunica media

Tunica adventitia

VASCULAR DAMAGE

Increased blood pressure damages endothelial cells

Deposition of plasma constituents

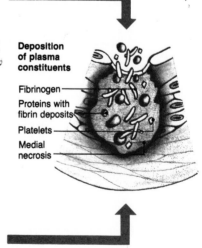

Fibrinogen

Proteins with fibrin deposits

Platelets

Medial necrosis

Angiotensin migrates to site of endothelial damage

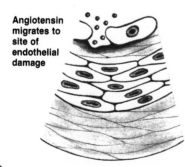

fluctuates with age, activity, and emotional stress. For example, blood pressure rises during exercise and returns to normal with rest. In hypertension, though, blood pressure remains elevated all the time.

Explain the type of hypertension the patient has. More than 90% of cases have no known cause, although certain factors (notably diet, stress, and heredity) contribute to its development. This type—known as primary (or idiopathic or essential) hypertension—is incurable but can be controlled with proper treatment. Less often, hypertension results from an identifiable—and often curable—cause. Causes of secondary hypertension include renal arterial or parenchymal disease, various endocrine disorders, coarctation of the aorta, and pheochromocytoma.

Point out possible complications
Help the patient understand the importance of strict compliance with treatment by explaining the dangers of untreated or improperly treated hypertension. Sustained hypertension eventually causes pathologic changes in the blood vessels, reducing the amount of blood they can deliver to tissues (see *Vascular Damage in Hypertension*). This can lead to widespread organ damage, especially to the heart, brain, kidneys, and eyes. Cardiovascular damage increases the risk of potentially fatal congestive heart failure, myocardial infarction, or cerebrovascular accident.

In hypertensive crisis, a rare but life-threatening complication, blood pressure rises sharply to more than 200/120 mm Hg. Untreated hypertensive crisis can lead to brain damage and death.

Teach about tests
Although hypertension is confirmed by consistently elevated blood pressure readings, the doctor may order various blood studies to rule out secondary causes, including plasma renin activity and serum aldosterone, plasma corti-

sol, serum calcium, and serum parathyroid hormone levels. Tell the patient who will draw the blood sample and when. Also tell him that his urine may be tested for vanillylmandelic acid (VMA), aldosterone, catecholamines, and 17-hydroxycorticosteroids. If ordered, teach him how to collect a 24-hour urine specimen to measure VMA levels. Instruct him to restrict foods and beverages containing phenolic acid, such as coffee, tea, bananas, citrus fruits, chocolate, and vanilla, for 3 days before urine collection, and to avoid physical and emotional stress during the collection period.

Prepare the patient for other tests to confirm secondary causes or detect complications of hypertension. For example, angiography can reveal renal artery stenosis or coarctation of the aorta; electrocardiography, echocardiography, and cardiac catheterization can detect cardiac complications, such as ventricular hypertrophy. (See *Teaching Patients about Cardiovascular Tests*, pages 143 to 147.)

Teach about treatments
● *Activity.* Encourage the patient to engage in regular exercise to help lower his blood pressure. Tell him that the doctor will prescribe an exercise program based on his medical history, age, and medication regimen. The program will emphasize aerobic exercise, such as walking, jogging, or swimming, which helps tone the cardiovascular system and lowers blood pressure. However, it won't include isometric exercise, such as weight lifting, which raises blood pressure by elevating serum catecholamine levels. Explain that exercise should be frequent (at least three times a week), vigorous (sufficient to raise heart rate to 70% to 80% of maximum capacity), and sustained (gradually building up to 20 to 30 minutes per session) for best results.
● *Diet.* Because excessive sodium intake contributes to hypertension, instruct the patient to avoid or limit foods high in sodium, such as most processed

foods, luncheon meats, canned soups and vegetables, and many snack foods and condiments. Tell him to examine package labels for sodium content. Sug-

INQUIRY

QUESTIONS PATIENTS ASK ABOUT HYPERTENSION

How does salt raise my blood pressure?

Most experts agree that large amounts of salt absorbed into your blood from your diet "trick" your kidneys into thinking that you're dehydrated. So your kidneys retain water, increasing the force blood exerts against the arterial walls—your blood pressure. They also respond to antidiuretic hormone, a chemical secreted by the pituitary that makes you retain more salt and water.

Now that my blood pressure is normal, why can't I stop taking my medication?

Even though your blood pressure falls within acceptable limits, it's not really normal—it's just controlled. If you discontinue your medication, it will surely rise again. You'll probably always need to take some medication. Of course, other measures may also help keep your blood pressure in check—for example, regular exercise, stress reduction, and a low-salt diet.

Can my blood pressure get too low?

Yes, but this is very unlikely, especially if you have your pressure checked regularly. You'll be able to tell that it's too low if you feel dizzy when you sit up in bed from lying flat or when you first stand up. You're more likely to develop low blood pressure if you've been vomiting or had diarrhea, or if you've been drinking less fluid than usual. Be sure to notify your doctor if you suspect your blood pressure is too low.

gest that he use alternatives to table salt, such as herbs, spices, or sodium-free salt substitutes.

Also instruct the patient to limit his caffeine and alcohol intake. (He may need to avoid alcohol entirely, depending on his prescribed medications.)

When teaching about diet, make sure you include the patient's family, especially if the patient doesn't usually do the grocery shopping and cooking for his household.

• *Medication.* If dietary restrictions and exercise fail to lower blood pressure sufficiently, drug therapy may be necessary. Initial therapy usually consists of a diuretic, a beta blocker, or an angiotensin-converting enzyme inhibitor. Later, a combination of these drugs may be prescribed if blood pressure still isn't under control. (See *Teaching Patients about Cardiovascular Drugs*, pages 150 to 163, for more information on these drugs.)

Stress the importance of strict compliance with the prescribed drug regimen to treat primary hypertension. Make sure the patient understands that these drugs can only control, not cure, his hypertension and that he'll probably have to take some antihypertensive drug for the rest of his life. Remind him that reducing or discontinuing his prescribed drugs without his doctor's guidance can lead to severe rebound high blood pressure, possibly precipitating hypertensive crisis.

Also remind him to check the labels on all over-the-counter drugs for sodium content—particularly antacids, laxatives, diet pills, and cold and allergy medications.

• *Procedures.* If appropriate, teach the patient and his family how to monitor blood pressure at home. Give the patient a copy of the home care aid *How to Take Your Blood Pressure,* page 135, or give a family member a copy of *How to Take Another Person's Blood Pressure,* page 136. Remind the patient to keep a written record of all blood pressure readings.

• *Surgery.* If the patient has secondary

HOW TO TAKE YOUR BLOOD PRESSURE

Dear Patient:

To take your own blood pressure, you can use a digital blood pressure monitor. (You can also use a standard blood pressure cuff and stethoscope. Typically, though, you need help from a family member or another caregiver to do so.)

Before you begin, review the instruction booklet that comes with the blood pressure monitor. Operating steps vary with different monitors, so be sure to follow the directions carefully. Keep these guidelines in mind.

1

Sit in a comfortable position and relax for about 2 minutes. Rest your arm on a table so it's level with your heart. (Use the same arm in the same position each time you take your blood pressure.)

2

Wrap the cuff securely around your upper arm just above the elbow. Make sure that you can slide only two fingers between the cuff and your arm. Next, turn on the monitor.

3

Inflate the cuff, as the instruction booklet directs. When the digital scale reads 160, stop inflating. The numbers on the scale will start changing rapidly. When they stop changing, your blood pressure reading will appear on the scale.

4

Record this blood pressure reading, with the date and time. Then deflate and remove the cuff, and turn off the machine.

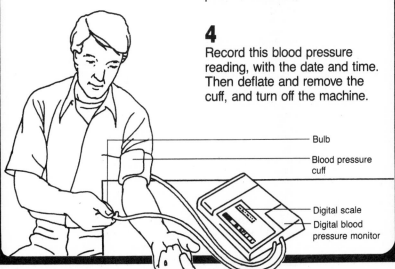

Bulb

Blood pressure cuff

Digital scale

Digital blood pressure monitor

HOW TO TAKE ANOTHER PERSON'S BLOOD PRESSURE

Dear Caregiver:

To take the blood pressure of the person in your care, you can use a standard blood pressure cuff and stethoscope.

1

Ask the person to sit comfortably and relax for about 2 minutes. Tell him to rest his arm on a table so it's level with his heart. (Use the same arm in the same position each time you take his blood pressure.)

2

Push up his sleeve and wrap the cuff around his upper arm so you can slide only two fingers between cuff and arm.

3

Place the stethoscope around your neck. Then, using your middle and index fingers, feel for a pulse in his wrist. When you've found his pulse, turn the bulb's screw counterclockwise to close it; then squeeze the bulb rapidly to inflate the cuff. Note the reading on the gauge when you can no longer feel his pulse. Deflate the cuff.

4

Place the stethoscope's earpieces in your ears. Then place the stethoscope's diaphragm over the brachial pulse, in the crook of the person's arm.

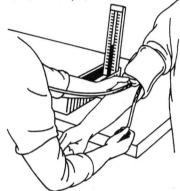

5

Inflate the cuff 30 points higher than the reading you obtained in step 3. Then loosen the bulb's screw to allow air to escape from the cuff. Listen for the first beating sound. When you hear it, note and record the number on the gauge: this is the *systolic* pressure (the top number of a blood pressure reading).

Continue to slowly deflate the cuff. When the beating stops, note and record the number on the gauge: this is the *diastolic* pressure (the bottom number of a blood pressure reading). Now, deflate and remove the cuff. Record the blood pressure reading, date, and time.

hypertension, you may need to prepare him for thyroidectomy, excision of a pheochromocytoma, or renal artery repair.

● *Other care measures.* Because stress has been directly linked to hypertension, teach the patient stress-reducing techniques, such as deep relaxation and biofeedback.

If your patient's overweight, explain how excess weight exacerbates high blood pressure by taxing the cardiovascular system. Encourage him to begin a weight-loss program under his doctor's supervision that emphasizes a balanced diet, regular exercise, and gradual weight reduction. Advise against fad diets and pills. If your patient smokes, encourage him to quit by explaining how nicotine constricts arterioles, further increasing blood pressure. As appropriate, refer him to community programs or agencies that can help him lose weight or stop smoking. Also direct him to the local chapter of the American Heart Association for more information about hypertension.

Myocardial Infarction

Few disorders provoke as much anxiety in a patient as does myocardial infarction (MI). Typically, the MI patient worries not only about his immediate survival but also about the quality of his life after recovery. When severe, his anxiety can interfere with his ability to learn and cooperate. What's worse, it can increase his risk of complications. Obviously, then, helping ease the patient's anxiety ranks among your first nursing priorities. To achieve this and improve the patient's receptivity to your teaching, you'll need to recognize anxiety even when it's masked by coping mechanisms—most commonly, denial.

Shortly after the patient's hospitalized with an MI, you'll need to interpret for him the intensive care environment, with its bewildering array of equipment. What's more, you'll need to teach him about immediate treatment measures to help ensure his compliance. For example, the doctor may schedule intracoronary or intravenous thrombolytic therapy or percutaneous transluminal coronary angioplasty (PTCA) to restore cardiac blood flow. Or the doctor may elect immediate open-heart surgery. Your teaching must be carefully timed and sensitive to see the patient through this acute period.

To promote a successful recovery, you'll need to emphasize the importance of resuming activity gradually to give the heart time to heal. Besides reviewing the prescribed exercise program, you'll need to discuss daily activities with the patient. For example, he may be afraid to resume sex after his MI. Your teaching can help him understand that having an MI doesn't mean he should stop living; he must simply be careful not to overexert himself.

Because MI usually occurs as a complication of coronary artery disease, you'll need to discuss the risk factors common to both conditions—hypertension, obesity, a diet high in saturated fats, stress, a sedentary life-style, and smoking. One of your chief teaching goals will be helping the patient modify these factors to reduce his risk of another MI.

Describe the disorder
Tell the patient that an MI results from blocked coronary arterial flow, which reduces the supply of oxygen to the affected area of the heart. This results in chest pain—ranging from mild discomfort to burning or crushing pain—that may radiate to the arm, jaw, neck, or shoulder blades. If blood flow isn't restored, the affected area of the heart becomes necrotic. Later, scar tissue forms but isn't able to contract. This reduces the heart's ability to pump blood, placing the patient at risk for another MI.

CHECKLIST

TEACHING TOPICS IN M.I.

- [ ] An explanation of how atherosclerosis, thromboembolism, or coronary artery spasm occludes cardiac blood flow
- [ ] The area of infarction
- [ ] The importance of following the prescribed treatment plan to aid recovery and forestall complications
- [ ] Preparation for serial EKGs, blood enzyme studies, and other scheduled tests
- [ ] Importance of bed rest
- [ ] Exercise program and precautions
- [ ] Dietary restrictions
- [ ] Drugs and their administration
- [ ] Preparation for percutaneous transluminal coronary angioplasty, pulmonary artery catheterization, or other necessary procedures
- [ ] Preparation for open-heart surgery, if scheduled
- [ ] Other measures to reduce long-term complications, such as controlling weight, quitting smoking, and reducing stress
- [ ] Availability of support groups, such as the American Heart Association

Discuss the causes of MI with the patient. By far the most common cause is atherosclerosis in one or more coronary arteries. This disorder is characterized by the buildup of fatty, fibrous plaques that narrow or occlude the arterial lumen. Thrombosis, or clot formation, often occurs in atherosclerotic arteries and is a contributing factor in many MIs.

Not all MIs result from atherosclerosis or thrombosis. Tell the patient that a sudden smooth-muscle contraction or spasm in a coronary artery can block blood flow to part of the heart as well. Coronary artery spasm can occur in both normal and atherosclerotic arteries, although its causes aren't well understood.

Point out possible complications

Stress to the patient that his compliance with prescribed treatment can significantly reduce the risk of another MI. *Important:* Use your nursing judgment when pointing out this complication. Above all, you don't want to exacerbate the patient's anxiety.

Teach about tests

Prepare the patient for tests during the first few days of hospitalization, including serial EKGs to detect conduction abnormalities and serial blood tests (once or twice daily) for isoenzymes of creatine phosphokinase and lactic dehydrogenase to help reveal the extent of heart muscle damage. Other early tests may include a technetium scan to identify the location and extent of infarction and echocardiography to assess the structure and function of cardiac walls and valves.

If the doctor orders cardiac catheterization to evaluate heart function, prepare the patient for this procedure as well. Tell him that when his condition stabilizes, he may also undergo such tests as exercise EKG, ambulatory EKG, and electrophysiologic studies. (See *Teaching Patients about Cardiovascular Tests,* pages 143 to 147, for more information on these tests.)

Teach about treatments

• *Activity.* Explain to the patient that bed rest for the first 24 to 48 hours after an MI greatly reduces the demands on his heart and improves his chances for recovery. While he's in bed, encourage him to regularly wiggle his toes to reduce the risk of thromboembolism. However, caution against pressing his feet against the footboard, raising his legs off the bed, and any other activity that strains his heart.

Teach the patient about his prescribed activity program. Emphasize the need to resume activities gradually. For example, he'll progress from sponge baths in bed to unsupervised showers. Help the patient plan his daily activities so that he alternates light and heavy tasks and rests between tasks. Encourage him to share tasks with a family member, when necessary, to avoid overdoing it.

Before discharge, give the patient a copy of the home care aid *Walking the Road to Recovery,* pages 140 and 141, and explain it to him and his family. Warn the patient not to exercise in extreme heat or cold. (Walking in an enclosed shopping mall is a good alternative to outdoor exercise in inclement weather.) He should stop exercise immediately if he feels dizzy, faint, or short of breath or if he develops chest pain. Note that exercise may bring on angina, which he may mistake for the chest pain of MI. Teach him how to treat angina (see *How to Use Nitroglycerin,* pages 118 and 119).

• *Diet.* Usually, the MI patient receives clear fluids only during the first days of hospitalization; explain that this is because digesting solid foods places a greater strain on his heart. Tell the patient to avoid caffeine, which also stimulates his heart. (See "Coronary Artery Disease," pages 112 to 119, for more information on dietary teaching for patients with atherosclerosis.)

• *Medication.* Tell the patient about prescribed parenteral medications as you administer them. For example, explain that I.V. nitroglycerin and morphine will help relieve chest pain by increasing the oxygen supply to his heart; nitroprusside will lower his blood pressure, reducing the demand on his heart; lidocaine will control dysrhythmias; and dopamine or dobutamine will strengthen cardiac contractions.

Also teach him about other drugs that he may receive during hospitalization or be instructed to take after discharge. Common ones include a stool softener to prevent straining during defecation, sedatives to decrease anxiety, and hypnotics to promote rest. Later, such drugs as calcium channel blockers, beta-adrenergic blockers, digoxin, antiarrhythmics, diuretics, antilipemics,

_____ INQUIRY

QUESTIONS PATIENTS ASK ABOUT POST-M.I. ACTIVITY

When can I safely resume sex?

Usually, the doctor will give his okay for you to resume sex several weeks after your heart attack. Sex uses up about as much energy as climbing two flights of stairs or completing a session in week 3 or 4 of your walking program. To avoid placing too much strain on your heart during sex, you should follow certain precautions. For example, don't have sex right after a big meal—wait a few hours. Also avoid sex when you're tired or upset. Choose a quiet, familiar setting for sex, and avoid positions that require you to use your arms to support yourself or your partner.

Remember, it's normal for your pulse and breathing rates to rise during sex. But they should return to normal within 15 minutes. If angina occurs during sex, rest a few minutes and take your prescribed nitroglycerin; then resume sex.

When can I start driving again?

Wait 3 to 4 weeks before driving, and then start out with short trips. Driving increases stress and makes you tense your arm muscles—neither of which is good for your healing heart.

How will I know if I'm overdoing my exercise program?

You're overdoing it if you feel chest pain, dizziness, or extreme shortness of breath during exercise, or if you're tired for more than 45 minutes after exercise. To monitor your heart during exercise, take your pulse. If your pulse exceeds 110 beats/minute or if you notice a new irregularity, you're probably overdoing it. (If you're taking a beta blocker, though, your pulse rate may not rise this high during exercise.) If your pulse rate changes or you develop the symptoms above, just go back to a more comfortable exercise level.

140

WALKING THE ROAD TO RECOVERY

Dear Patient:

To help strengthen your heart and speed your recovery, follow this simple daily walking program. Be sure to allow the full times for warm up and cool down.

To limber up your muscles, do stretching exercises, such as calf and shoulder stretches. For the calf stretch (shown below), place both hands on a wall, about shoulder height. Step with one foot toward the wall and lean against it, keeping your palms flat on the wall and your feet flat on the floor. Push against the wall until you feel a pull. For the shoulder stretch, clasp your hands over your head and pull your shoulders backward.

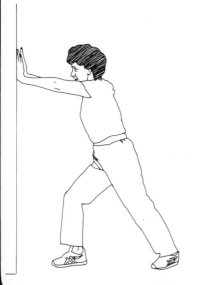

WEEK	WARM UP
1	Stretch 2 min. Walk slowly 3 min.
2	Stretch 2 min. Walk slowly 3 min.
3	Stretch 2 min. Walk slowly 3 min.
4	Stretch 2 min. Walk slowly 3 min.
5	Stretch 2 min. Walk slowly 3 min.
6	Stretch 2 min. Walk slowly 3 min.
7	Stretch 2 min. Walk slowly 3 min.
8	Stretch 2 min. Walk slowly 5 min.
9	Stretch 2 min. Walk slowly 5 min.
10	Stretch 2 min. Walk slowly 5 min.
11	Stretch 2 min. Walk slowly 5 min.
12	Stretch 2 min. Walk slowly 5 min.
13 and after	Continue like week 12.

EXERCISE	COOL DOWN	TOTAL TIME
Walk briskly 5 min.	Walk slowly 3 min. Stretch 2 min.	15 min
Walk briskly 7 min.	Walk slowly 3 min. Stretch 2 min.	17 min
Walk briskly 9 min.	Walk slowly 3 min. Stretch 2 min.	19 min
Walk briskly 11 min.	Walk slowly 3 min. Stretch 2 min.	21 min
Walk briskly 13 min.	Walk slowly 3 min. Stretch 2 min.	23 min
Walk briskly 15 min.	Walk slowly 3 min. Stretch 2 min.	25 min
Walk briskly 18 min.	Walk slowly 3 min. Stretch 2 min.	28 min
Walk briskly 20 min.	Walk slowly 5 min. Stretch 2 min.	34 min
Walk briskly 23 min.	Walk slowly 5 min. Stretch 2 min.	37 min
Walk briskly 26 min.	Walk slowly 5 min. Stretch 2 min.	40 min
Walk briskly 28 min.	Walk slowly 5 min. Stretch 2 min.	42 min
Walk briskly 30 min.	Walk slowly 5 min. Stretch 2 min.	44 min

antihypertensives, and even aspirin may be prescribed to help regulate the patient's cardiovascular function and prevent complications. (See *Teaching Patients about Cardiovascular Drugs,* pages 150 to 163, for more information.)

• **Procedures.** Tell the patient that he'll receive supplemental oxygen through a nasal cannula for the first 24 to 48 hours and as needed after that to keep his heart and other tissues well-oxygenated.

Also prepare him for procedures to help restore blood flow in an obstructed coronary artery, as ordered. For example, the patient may be scheduled for intracoronary thrombolytic therapy—usually in the first few hours following an MI, before much permanent heart damage has occurred. Explain that a catheter will be threaded through his aorta into the obstructed coronary artery. Then, the drug streptokinase or urokinase will be infused through the catheter to dissolve the obstruction, or clot, and reopen the artery. Instruct him to keep the catheterized limb straight and still, and tell him that frequent blood tests will be done to monitor blood levels of the infused drug. (Alternatively, streptokinase or urokinase may be infused intravenously. While less complicated than direct intracoronary infusion, this method is also usually less effective—a finding confirmed by cardiac catheterization to assess the artery's patency. Although still experimental, I.V. infusion of tissue plasminogen activator shows great promise in dissolving coronary artery thromboses.)

As an alternative or adjunct to open-heart surgery, the patient may be scheduled for PTCA. If so, explain that this procedure involves threading a thin, balloon-tipped catheter into the narrowed coronary artery. By injecting contrast dye through the catheter, the doctor can pinpoint the site of arterial narrowing under a fluoroscope. He then inflates the balloon catheter to expand and reopen the artery. Tell the

patient that he'll receive a local anesthetic to numb the catheterization site, a sedative to promote relaxation, an anticoagulant to prevent embolism, and nitroglycerin to prevent coronary artery spasm. Warn the patient that he may feel flushed and experience brief chest pain as the contrast dye is infused. (For more information on PTCA, see "Coronary Artery Disease," pages 112 to 119.)

If the patient develops congestive heart failure, hypotension or hypertension, or oliguria, the doctor may order pulmonary artery catheterization to assess cardiac function. This procedure may also be done to monitor the effects of drug therapy. Explain to the patient that a sheath will be inserted into the subclavian, jugular, or femoral vein under local anesthesia, then sutured in place. Next, a thin, balloon-tipped catheter will be introduced through the sheath. This balloon-tipped catheter will be carried by the circulation through the right atrium and right ventricle into the pulmonary artery. There, certain pressures will be measured until the patient's condition stabilizes.

• **Surgery.** If appropriate, prepare the patient for surgery. The doctor may perform coronary artery bypass grafting to treat acute MI or complications associated with cardiac catheterization or PTCA. He may also repair abnormalities, such as papillary muscle rupture or ventricular aneurysm, during open-heart surgery. (See "Surgery," pages 148 and 149, for more information.)

• **Other care measures.** Educate the patient about the importance of correcting certain risk factors for MI, such as obesity, excessive stress, and smoking. (These major risk factors are also closely associated with coronary artery disease; see "Coronary Artery Disease," pages 112 to 119, for specific teaching points.) In addition, refer the patient to support and information groups, such as the American Heart Association.

TEACHING PATIENTS ABOUT CARDIOVASCULAR TESTS

TEST AND PURPOSE	TEACHING POINTS
Abdominal ultrasonography • To detect an abdominal aortic aneurysm	• Explain that this test evaluates the major blood vessel in the abdomen for aneurysm formation. Mention who will perform the test and where, and that it takes about 30 minutes. • Explain what happens during the test: the patient will lie on his back on the examining table. A transducer covered with conductive jelly will be placed directly on his skin and will be moved slowly around his abdomen. The patient will feel only mild pressure. He may be asked to breathe deeply or hold his breath briefly to obtain a clear image.
Ambulatory electrocardiography (Holter monitoring, ambulatory monitoring) • To detect cardiac dysrhythmias • To evaluate chest pain • To evaluate the effectiveness of antiarrhythmic therapy	• Explain that this test records the heart's electrical activity while the patient goes about his normal activities. Tell him that the test takes 24 hours and causes no discomfort. • Describe the physical preparation for the test: the technician will cleanse, dry, and possibly shave different sites on the patient's body, such as his chest and arms, and will apply a conductive jelly over them. Then the technician will attach electrodes at these sites. • If the patient will be taking the test at home, tell him he'll wear a small 2-lb (0.9-kg) tape recorder with a belt or shoulder strap. Instruct him to continue his routine activities during the test period and to log all activities and emotions in a diary: walking, stair climbing, urinating, sleeping, sexual activity, emotional upsets, physical symptoms (such as dizziness, palpitations, fatigue, chest pain, and syncope), and ingestion of medications. Show the patient a sample diary. If applicable to the monitor, teach the patient how to mark the tape at the onset of symptoms. (With a patient-activated monitor, he'll need to know to press the event button to activate the monitor if he experiences any unusual sensations.) Instruct him not to tamper with the monitor or disconnect lead wires or electrodes. Tell him to avoid magnets, metal detectors, high-voltage areas, and electric blankets, to prevent spurious findings. However, you'll need to demonstrate how to check the recorder for proper function. Light flashes, for example, may indicate a loose electrode; the patient should test each one by depressing its center and should call the doctor if one comes off.
Angiography • To examine arteries or veins for suspected abnormalities, such as aneurysms, thrombi, atherosclerotic obstructions, and arteriovenous malformations • To detect vessel compression from an extravascular tumor • To evaluate patency of arterial grafting and reconstruction	• Explain to the patient that this test evaluates arteries and veins for abnormalities. Tell him who will perform the test and where, and that it may take 30 minutes to 4 hours, depending on the blood vessels examined. • Describe the physical preparation for the test: an area on the patient's groin or armpit or on another location will be shaved and cleansed. After a local anesthetic is injected, a catheter will be inserted into a vessel and advanced as necessary. • Explain what happens during the test: a contrast dye will be injected into the blood vessels; then several X-rays will be taken to follow the dye's passage. The patient may feel flushed or nauseated or may have an unusual taste, but these feelings will pass quickly. He may be asked to turn on

(continued)

TEACHING PATIENTS ABOUT
CARDIOVASCULAR TESTS *(continued)*

TEST AND PURPOSE	TEACHING POINTS
Angiography *(continued)*	one side or to elevate an arm or leg for the X-rays. Tell him to remain perfectly still when asked, to avoid distorting the X-ray image. • Describe what happens after the test: when the catheter is removed, pressure is applied over the insertion site for 15 to 30 minutes; then a bulky dressing is applied and a sandbag is rested against it. The patient must keep his arm or leg extended and immobile for 4 to 24 hours after the test. The pulse and circulation in this limb will be checked often.
Cardiac blood pool imaging • To assess left ventricular function • To detect motion and structural abnormalities of the ventricular wall	• Explain to the patient that this test evaluates how well the main chamber of his heart pumps. Tell him who will perform the test and where, and that it takes 30 to 45 minutes. • Mention that a technician will attach electrodes to various sites on the patient's body before the test begins. • Explain what happens during the test: the patient will be placed in a supine position, and a mildly radioactive contrast dye will be injected into a vein. The scintillation camera will record the dye's passage through the heart and then will be synchronized with the EKG to correlate subsequent images with EKG waveforms. The patient must remain still during scanning.
Cardiac catheterization • To assess valve and cardiac wall function • To diagnose various abnormalities, such as valvular insufficiency or stenosis, septal defects, and congenital anomalies • To evaluate coronary artery and bypass graft patency • To detect pulmonary artery hypertension • To evaluate the effectiveness of drug therapy	• Explain to the patient that this test evaluates the function of his heart and its vessels. Tell him who will perform the test and where, and that it takes 2 to 3 hours. • Instruct the patient not to eat or drink anything for 6 hours before the test. • Describe the physical preparation for the test: the patient will be placed on a padded table, and his groin area will be shaved and cleansed. The technician will start a peripheral I.V. line and attach electrodes to various sites. The patient will receive a mild I.V. sedative to help him relax. • Explain what happens during the test: after a local anesthetic is injected into the patient's groin, a catheter is inserted and threaded up through an artery to the left side of his heart or through a vein to the right side of his heart and to his lungs. Next, the doctor will inject a contrast dye through the catheter. When he does so, the patient may feel flushed or nauseated or may experience chest pain; reassure him that these sensations should pass quickly. Instruct him to follow directions to cough or breathe deeply. Tell him that he may receive nitroglycerin during the test to dilate coronary vessels and aid visualization. • Describe what happens after the test: when the catheter is removed, pressure and a bulky dressing are applied to the site to control bleeding. The nurse will check the site frequently for swelling. The patient must keep his leg straight for several hours. Once he's allowed to resume his diet, he should drink plenty of fluids. To monitor the patient's response to therapy, the doctor may leave the pulmonary catheter in place for a few days.

TEACHING PATIENTS ABOUT
CARDIOVASCULAR TESTS *(continued)*

TEST AND PURPOSE	TEACHING POINTS
Doppler ultrasonography • To aid diagnosis of chronic venous insufficiency, superficial and deep vein thromboses, peripheral artery disease, and arterial occlusion • To detect abnormalities of carotid artery blood flow associated with such conditions as aortic stenosis • To monitor patency of arterial grafting and reconstruction	• Explain to the patient that this painless test evaluates circulation in his blood vessels. Tell him who will perform the test and where, and that it takes 10 to 20 minutes. • Describe the physical preparation for the test: the patient will be asked to uncover his leg, arm, or neck and to loosen any restrictive clothing. • Explain what happens during the test: a transducer coated with conductive jelly will be placed on the patient's skin and moved along the vessel to be examined.
Echocardiography • To diagnose and evaluate valvular abnormalities • To aid diagnosis of cardiomyopathy • To detect atrial tumors • To evaluate cardiac function after myocardial infarction • To detect pericardial effusion	• Explain to the patient that this test evaluates the size, shape, and motion of various cardiac structures. Tell him who will perform the test and where, that the test takes 15 to 30 minutes, and that it's safe and painless. Mention that other tests, such as an EKG and phonocardiography, may be performed simultaneously. • Describe the physical preparation for the test: conductive jelly will be applied to the patient's chest. • Explain what happens during the test: a transducer will be angled over the patient's chest to observe different parts of the heart, and the patient may be repositioned on his left side. He may be asked to breathe in and out slowly, to hold his breath, or to inhale a gas with a slightly sweet odor (amyl nitrite) while changes in heart function are recorded. Amyl nitrite may cause dizziness, flushing, and tachycardia, but these effects quickly subside. Tell the patient to remain still during the test, since movement may distort results.
Electrocardiography (EKG) • To help identify primary conduction abnormalities, dysrhythmias, cardiac hypertrophy, pericarditis, electrolyte imbalance, myocardial ischemia, and the site and extent of myocardial infarction • To evaluate the effectiveness of cardiac drugs • To monitor pacemaker performance	• Explain to the patient that an EKG evaluates the heart's function by recording its electrical activity. Tell him who will perform the test and where. Also tell him the test takes about 15 minutes and usually causes no discomfort. • Describe the physical preparation for the test: the technician will cleanse, dry, and possibly shave different sites on the patient's body, such as his chest and arms, and will apply a conductive jelly over them. Then the technician will attach electrodes at these sites. • Describe what happens during the test: the patient will be asked to lie still, to relax and breathe normally, and to remain quiet. Explain that talk or limb movement will distort the EKG recordings and require additional testing time.

(continued)

TEACHING PATIENTS ABOUT
CARDIOVASCULAR TESTS *(continued)*

TEST AND PURPOSE	TEACHING POINTS
Electrophysiologic studies • To diagnose dysrhythmias • To evaluate the effects of antiarrhythmic drugs	• Explain to the patient that these tests evaluate electrical activity in his heart and the effect of medication he takes for an irregular heart rhythm. Tell him who will perform the tests and where, and that they take 2 to 5 hours. • Instruct him to avoid food, fluids, and nonprescription drugs for 6 hours before the test. Explain that a catheter insertion site on his groin will be shaved and cleansed. • Explain that after injection of a local anesthetic, a catheter will be inserted into the femoral vein and advanced into the right side of the heart. The patient will receive an I.V. sedative to help him relax. Tell him he may feel mild pressure at the groin site but that he should report any other discomfort. Explain that the doctor may try to induce extra heartbeats with the catheter. • Explain that after the catheter is removed, pressure and then a heavy dressing are applied to the site to control bleeding. The nurse will check the site frequently for swelling. The patient may need to lie with his leg straight for a few hours after the test.
Exercise electrocardiography (stress test) • To help diagnose the cause of chest pain or other possible cardiac pain • To identify dysrhythmias that develop during physical exercise • To evaluate the effectiveness of antiarrhythmic or antianginal therapy	• Explain that the stress test records the heart's electrical activity while the patient walks a treadmill or pedals a bicycle. Tell him who will perform the test and where, that it takes about 30 minutes, and that a doctor will be present in the testing area at all times. Inform him that he mustn't eat, smoke, or drink alcohol for 3 hours before the test. However, he should continue any drug regimen, as ordered. • Tell the patient to wear comfortable shoes and loose, light-weight shorts or slacks; men usually don't wear a shirt during the test, and women usually wear a bra and a lightweight short-sleeved blouse or a patient gown with front closure. Also tell the patient that a technician will cleanse, shave (if necessary), and abrade sites on the chest and, possibly, back. Then he'll attach electrodes at these sites. • If the patient's scheduled for a multistage treadmill test, tell him that the treadmill speed and incline increase at predetermined intervals and that he'll be told of each adjustment. If he's scheduled for a bicycle ergometer test, tell him that resistance to pedaling gradually increases as he tries to maintain a specific speed. Inform the patient that he may receive an injection of thallium during the test. After this injection, the doctor will evaluate coronary blood flow on a scanner. Reassure him that the injection involves negligible radiation exposure. Be sure to tell the patient that he can stop the test if he experiences severe fatigue or chest pain. Typically, he'll feel tired, out of breath, and sweaty. However, he should report any feelings during the test. He'll have his blood pressure and heart rate checked periodically during the test. • Describe what happens after the test: the patient's blood pressure and EKG will be monitored for 10 to 15 minutes. Explain that he should wait at least 1 hour after the test before showering, and then he should use warm water.

TEACHING PATIENTS ABOUT
CARDIOVASCULAR TESTS *(continued)*

TEST AND PURPOSE	TEACHING POINTS
Impedance plethysmography • To detect deep vein thrombosis in the legs	• Explain to the patient that this test helps detect blood clots in his leg veins. Tell him that the test takes 30 to 45 minutes to examine both legs. Assure him that it's painless and safe. • Tell the patient that he'll put on a hospital gown and lie on his back on an examining table or bed. The technician will cleanse, dry, and possibly shave sites on his lower legs and then attach electrodes with conductive jelly. • Explain that during the test a pressure cuff will be wrapped around the patient's thigh and inflated for 1 or 2 minutes. Then the cuff will be quickly released. Usually, the test is repeated to confirm initial tracings.
Technetium scan • To confirm the presence, size, and location of an acute myocardial infarction	• Explain to the patient that this test detects any damaged areas of his heart muscle. Tell him who will perform the test and where, and that it takes 45 minutes. • Tell the patient that the doctor will inject technetium pyrophosphate into an arm vein about 3 hours before the test. Reassure him that the injection causes only transient discomfort and that it involves negligible radiation exposure. • Explain what happens during the test: the patient will be placed in a supine position. A series of scans will be taken at different angles. Instruct the patient to remain still.
Thallium scan • To assess myocardial perfusion • To locate and estimate the size of an acute or old myocardial infarction • To diagnose coronary artery disease • To evaluate the patency of coronary artery bypass graft • To evaluate the effectiveness of percutaneous transluminal coronary angioplasty	• Explain to the patient that this test assesses his heart's blood supply. Tell him who will perform the test and where, and that it takes 45 to 90 minutes. Reassure him that a doctor will be present during the test. Tell him to avoid alcohol, tobacco, and nonprescription drugs for 24 hours, and food and fluids for 4 hours before the test. • Advise the patient to wear comfortable shoes and loose, lightweight shorts or slacks; men usually don't wear a shirt during the test, and women usually wear a bra and a lightweight short-sleeved blouse or patient gown with front closure. Tell the patient that a technician will cleanse, shave (if necessary), and abrade several sites on the patient's chest and, possibly, back, then attach electrodes at those sites. • If the patient's scheduled for a multistage treadmill test, tell him that the treadmill speed and incline increase at periodic intervals and that he'll be told of each adjustment. If he's scheduled for a bicycle ergometer test, explain that resistance to pedaling gradually increases as he tries to maintain a specific speed. His heart rate and blood pressure will be monitored during the test. At peak stress, contrast dye will be injected into his arm and he'll be asked to lie on his back under the scintillation camera. Additional scans may be taken after he has rested for 3 to 6 hours. Be sure to tell the patient that he can stop the test if he experiences severe fatigue or chest pain. Typically, he'll feel tired, out of breath, and sweaty. • Describe what happens after the test: the patient's blood pressure and EKG will be monitored for 10 to 15 minutes. Explain that he should wait at least 1 hour after the test before showering, and then he should use warm water.

SURGERY

Open-heart surgery includes various procedures that involve opening the chest cavity and incising the heart muscle or its vasculature. These procedures include valve replacement, septal repair, and aneurysm or thrombus excision. However, open-heart surgery most commonly refers to coronary artery bypass grafting (CABG). This section will focus on CABG, but you can easily adapt the information here to teach patients about other open-heart procedures as well.

Who's a candidate for CABG?

About 50,000 patients undergo CABG each year. Prime candidates for this procedure include patients with severe angina from atherosclerosis in one or more coronary arteries and those with coronary artery disease at high risk for myocardial infarction. By circumventing blocked coronary arteries and restoring myocardial blood flow, CABG eliminates anginal pain, improves heart function, and may increase life expectancy.

The patient scheduled for CABG will undoubtedly have many questions and concerns. You'll need to carefully explain the procedure itself as well as outline preoperative and postoperative care measures to help speed his recovery and prevent complications.

Explain the procedure

Tell the patient that CABG will restore normal blood flow to his heart. As necessary, clarify and reinforce what the doctor has told him. Explain that the doctor will excise a portion of a healthy vessel from another part of the body (usually a portion of a saphenous vein or a mammary artery), then graft it above and below the blocked coronary artery. Tell him that his circulation will then be diverted through the graft. Reassure him that circulation won't be disrupted in the area from which the graft was excised.

Next, tell the patient where he'll be taken to recover after the procedure. If possible, arrange a tour for the patient and his family before surgery. Explain the complex, and often frightening, equipment that will support the patient's vital functions after surgery. For example, prepare the patient for intubation and mechanical ventilation. Mention that he won't be able to speak while intubated but will be able to communicate by gesturing or writing.

Explain to the patient that an intraaortic balloon pump may be inserted to provide circulatory support for several hours postoperatively. He'll also have a nasogastric tube, a mediastinal chest tube, and an indwelling catheter in place for the first day or two. What's more, he'll be connected to a cardiac monitor.

Describe preoperative care

The afternoon before surgery, teach the patient about preoperative care measures. Explain that he'll be asked to shower with a special antiseptic soap and may be shaved from his neck to his toes. Tell him that he won't be allowed to eat or drink anything after midnight, although he can request a sleeping pill. Inform him that he may receive a sedative the morning of surgery to help him relax.

If indicated, prepare the patient for preoperative pulmonary artery catheterization. Explain that the catheter will remain in place after surgery, but reassure him that the catheter, arterial lines, and epicardial pacing wires will cause minimal or no discomfort.

Teach about postoperative care

After surgery, teach the patient about short- and long-term postoperative care measures and his role in them. Start with the expected course of his hospital stay—how many days he'll spend in the critical care area, step-down unit, and regular room before discharge.

Emphasize that his first priority is to relax and rest; stress and anxiety will only hinder his recovery. Encourage him to request pain medication to promote relaxation. When the endotracheal, nasogastric, and chest tubes are removed, he'll be able to sit up and swallow liquids. Tell him that, after that, solid foods will be reintroduced gradually.

To help prevent pulmonary complications, encourage the patient to perform coughing and deep-breathing exercises. Teach him how to splint his incision to minimize pain and how to use an incentive spirometer. Reassure him that coughing won't loosen or damage the graft or reopen his chest incision.

Next, discuss other self-care measures. About 6 days after surgery, the patient will probably be allowed to shower. Instruct him to use warm, not hot, water and to wash all incision sites gently. Explain that complete healing takes time and that he'll always have a scar (although it will fade). Suggest that he wear soft, loose clothing, such as cotton T-shirts, at first for maximum comfort.

To enhance circulation and reduce swelling in a leg from which a saphenous vein graft was taken, he may also need to wear support stockings, elevate the leg frequently, and avoid crossing his legs. Tell him to watch for and report any new tenderness, redness, swelling, or drainage from his chest and leg incisions.

As the patient gains strength, begin teaching him about long-term care measures. Review his prescribed exercise program. Emphasize the need to increase his activity gradually, and encourage him to set realistic goals. Teach him to alternate light and heavy tasks and to rest between tasks. Reinforce the doctor's restrictions on such activities as lifting, working, and driving, as appropriate.

Address the patient's concerns about sex after surgery. Reassure him that once the doctor has given his okay, sex is no more dangerous to his heart than other forms of moderate exercise, such as walking up a couple flights of stairs. Point out that a satisfying sex life can help speed his recovery. Advise him to reduce strain on his heart by avoiding sex right after eating a big meal or drinking alcohol, when he's fatigued or emotionally upset, or when he's in an unfamiliar and stressful situation— in a strange environment or with a new partner, for example. Tell him to choose a position that doesn't restrict his breathing; he should also avoid any position in which he has to support himself or his partner with his arms. Explain that impotence occurs fairly commonly but that it's almost always temporary and is no cause for concern.

Because medications form an important part of postoperative care, make sure the patient understands their administration schedules and possible adverse effects.

Discuss long-term dietary restrictions with the patient. Tell him he can reduce the chance of reocclusion in his arteries by sticking to a diet that's low in cholesterol and saturated fats. With his doctor's permission, the patient can have up to two alcoholic drinks per day beginning 2 or 3 weeks after surgery. (Refer to "Coronary Artery Disease," pages 112 to 119, for more information on dietary and other measures.)

Before discharge, teach the patient to watch for and report warning signs of reocclusion or other serious complications: angina, persistent fever, swelling or drainage at the incision site, dizziness, shortness of breath at rest, rapid or irregular pulse, or prolonged recovery time from exercise or sex. Also prepare him for postoperative depression, which may not set in until he's home. Reassure him that depression is usually temporary.

Finally, refer the patient to local chapters of the Mended Hearts Club and the American Heart Association for more information and support.

TEACHING PATIENTS ABOUT CARDIOVASCULAR DRUGS

DRUG	ADVERSE REACTIONS	INTERACTIONS*
Antiarrhythmics		
amiodarone (Cordarone)	*Reportable:* diaphoresis, dyspnea, lethargy, tingling in the extremities, weight loss or gain *Other:* corneal microdeposits, photosensitivity, and bluish pigmentation	• Tell the patient that foods, beverages, and over-the-counter drugs don't influence the safety or effectiveness of amiodarone.
disopyramide (Norpace)	*Reportable:* ankle edema, dizziness, drowsiness, excessive hunger, hypotension, impotence, irregular heart rate, rapid weight gain, shortness of breath, urinary retention, weakness *Other:* anorexia; constipation; mouth, nose, and eye dryness	• Tell the patient that over-the-counter drugs don't influence the safety or effectiveness of disopyramide. • Advise him to avoid alcohol, which can further reduce blood pressure. • Instruct him to take the drug on an empty stomach—1 hour before or 3 hours after a meal.
flecainide (Tambocor)	*Reportable:* ankle edema, chest pain, dizziness, irregular heart rate, shortness of breath, visual disturbances, weight gain *Other:* fatigue, headache, nausea, palpitations	• Tell the patient that foods, beverages, and over-the-counter drugs don't influence the safety or effectiveness of flecainide.
procainamide (Procan SR, Pronestyl)	*Reportable:* hypotension, SLE-like syndrome (chills and fever, joint pain, malaise, skin rash) *Other:* anorexia, bitter taste, diarrhea, dizziness, gastric upset	• Instruct the patient to take procainamide on an empty stomach, if possible. • Warn him to avoid antihistamines, which can exacerbate side effects.

*Includes food, beverages, and over-the-counter drugs.

TEACHING POINTS

• Explain to the patient that this drug should control his irregular heart rhythm.
• Tell him that if he misses a dose, he should take that dose as soon as possible, unless the next scheduled dose is less than 4 hours away. He must never double-dose.
• Demonstrate proper instillation of methylcellulose ophthalmic solution, if prescribed, which may reduce corneal microdeposits. Because corneal microdeposits usually don't interfere with vision, advise the patient that an eye examination is necessary only if vision changes occur.
• Tell him that limiting sun exposure is the best way to prevent sunburn and that clothing provides more protection than sunscreens. Also tell him to wear sunglasses if he experiences photosensitivity.

• Explain to the patient that this drug should control his irregular heart rhythm.
• Tell him to take a missed dose as soon as possible, but warn him not to double-dose.
• Because disopyramide may cause hypoglycemia, teach the patient these telltale symptoms: excessive hunger, weakness, drowsiness, and shakiness. If symptoms develop, he should eat sweets, such as candy, or drink a sugar-containing beverage, such as orange juice. Then he should call his doctor immediately.
• Instruct him to rise slowly from a sitting or lying position to prevent dizziness or fainting from hypotension.
• Tell him to avoid operating machinery until he has taken disopyramide for a while without experiencing adverse effects.
• Suggest that he chew gum or ice chips to relieve mouth dryness and use artificial tears or saline eyewash for eye dryness.
• Advise him to increase his dietary fiber and water intake and to use bulk laxatives if he experiences constipation.

• Explain to the patient that this drug should control his irregular heart rhythm.
• Tell him to take a missed dose as soon as possible, but warn him not to double-dose.
• If palpitations accompany the patient's dysrhythmia, teach him how to take his pulse. Advise him to report an unusually low or high rate or a new irregularity.
• Warn against driving or operating machinery if dizziness develops.
• Instruct the patient to weigh himself at least every other day and to report any sudden weight gain.
• If the patient has a permanent pacemaker, explain that its function will be evaluated and possibly modified after flecainide begins to take effect.

• Explain to the patient that this drug should control his irregular heart rhythm.
• Advise him to reduce bothersome GI symptoms by taking procainamide with food. Caution him never to chew, break, or crush an extended-release tablet before swallowing it; this destroys the tablet's coating and releases the full drug dose all at once.
• Tell him to take a missed dose as soon as possible, but warn him not to double-dose.

(continued)

**TEACHING PATIENTS ABOUT
CARDIOVASCULAR DRUGS** (continued)

DRUG	ADVERSE REACTIONS	INTERACTIONS*
Antiarrhythmics (continued)		
quinidine (Cardioquin, Cin-Quin, Duraquin, many other forms and brands)	*Reportable:* blurred vision, severe or prolonged diarrhea, hypotension, irregular heart rate, shortness of breath, syncope, tinnitus *Other:* anorexia, diarrhea, nausea, vomiting	• Tell the patient that foods and beverages don't influence the safety or effectiveness of quinidine. • Warn him to limit his use of antacids, which can raise blood levels of quinidine and exacerbate side effects.
tocainide (Tonocard)	*Reportable:* chest pain, chills, confusion, cough, dyspnea, easy bruising and bleeding, fever, hypotension, irregular heart rate, rash, sore throat, unsteadiness, sudden weight gain, wheezing *Other:* dizziness, fatigue, headache, nausea, numbness, sweating, tremors	• Tell the patient that foods, beverages, and over-the-counter drugs don't influence the safety or effectiveness of tocainide.
Anticoagulants		
warfarin (Coumadin, Panwarfin)	*Reportable:* bleeding nose or gums, chills, dark blue toes, discolored urine, excessive menstrual flow, fatigue, fever, prolonged bleeding from cuts or bruises, prolonged diarrhea, red or black stool, sore throat, vomiting (sometimes bloody) *Other:* bruising, diarrhea, nausea, slight hair loss	• Instruct the patient to avoid over-the-counter drugs containing aspirin or acetaminophen and high doses of vitamins A and E; he may take an occasional dose of ibuprofen with his doctor's permission. • Tell him to limit alcohol consumption to one or two drinks per day. • Because vitamin K counteracts warfarin, stress the need to maintain a consistent intake of vitamin K and of fats, which enhance vitamin K absorption. Explain that this is necessary to adjust his warfarin dosage precisely.

*Includes food, beverages, and over-the-counter drugs.

TEACHING POINTS

• Explain to the patient that this drug should control his irregular heart rhythm.
• Advise him to take the drug with food to reduce gastric upset.

• Tell him to take a missed dose as soon as possible, but warn him not to double-dose.

• Explain to the patient that this drug should control his irregular heart rhythm.
• Tell him to take a missed dose as soon as possible, but warn him not to double-dose.
• Explain that he can reduce nausea by taking the drug with food.

• Tell the patient to weigh himself at least every other day and to report any sudden weight gain.

• Explain to the patient that this drug should prevent blood clots in his legs, lungs, and heart.
• Tell him to take a missed dose within 8 hours, but warn him not to double-dose.
• Tell the patient that he'll need frequent blood tests to monitor the drug's effects.
• Help him obtain a Medic Alert tag or card, identifying him as a warfarin user.
• Teach measures to reduce the risk of

bleeding, such as always wearing shoes, placing a nonslip mat in the bathtub, shaving with an electric razor, using a soft toothbrush, and wearing gloves for yard work.
• If the patient's a female of childbearing age, emphasize the need for practicing birth control. That's because warfarin can adversely affect fetal development and cause placental bleeding.

(continued)

**TEACHING PATIENTS ABOUT
CARDIOVASCULAR DRUGS** *(continued)*

DRUG	ADVERSE REACTIONS	INTERACTIONS*
Antihypertensives		
captopril (Capoten) **enalapril** (Vasotec)	*Reportable:* chest pain, diaphoresis, severe diarrhea, dyspnea, fever, mouth sores, rapid heart rate, skin rash, sore throat, severe vomiting *Other:* altered taste, dizziness, fatigue, headache, palpitations	• Instruct the patient to avoid foods with extremely high potassium levels (low-salt milk and salt substitutes) and to limit his intake of high-potassium foods, such as bananas and citrus fruits. • Tell the patient that alcohol and over-the-counter drugs don't influence the safety or effectiveness of captopril and enalapril.
clonidine (Catapres)	*Reportable:* ankle edema, skin pallor, vivid dreams or nightmares *Other:* constipation, drowsiness, insomnia, mouth dryness, slow heart rate	• Tell the patient that foods and nonalcoholic beverages don't influence the safety or effectiveness of clonidine. • Instruct him to limit his alcohol intake and to avoid over-the-counter sympathomimetics, such as ephedrine-containing nasal sprays.
hydralazine (Apresoline)	*Reportable:* chest pain, numbness, palpitations, rapid heart rate, SLE-like syndrome (fever, joint pain, malaise, skin rash), tingling *Other:* anorexia, diarrhea, headache, nasal congestion, nausea	• Instruct the patient to take the drug on an empty stomach—1 hour before or 3 hours after a meal. • Advise him to avoid over-the-counter sympathomimetics, such as ephedrine-containing nasal sprays.
methyldopa (Aldomet)	*Reportable:* chest pain, depression, edema, fever, impotence, syncope, very slow heart rate, weakness, weight gain *Other:* decreased libido, diarrhea, dizziness, drowsiness, dry mouth, nausea, slightly slow heart rate, stuffy nose, vomiting	• Tell the patient that foods don't influence the safety or effectiveness of methyldopa. • Advise him to limit his alcohol intake and to avoid over-the-counter sympathomimetics, such as ephedrine-containing nasal sprays, and central nervous system stimulants, such as phenylpropanolamine.

*Includes food, beverages, and over-the-counter drugs.

TEACHING POINTS

- Explain to the patient that the prescribed drug should lower his blood pressure and relieve symptoms of heart failure.
- Instruct him to take a missed dose as soon as possible, but warn him not to double-dose.
- Teach him to minimize postural hypotension by rising slowly from a sitting or lying position.
- Tell him to drink 2 to 3 quarts of fluid a day, unless otherwise ordered. This will help prevent hypotension.

- Explain to the patient that this drug should control his hypertension.
- Tell him to take a missed dose within 6 hours, but warn him not to double-dose.
- Suggest that he take one of his scheduled daily doses just before bedtime to take advantage of the drug's tendency to cause drowsiness.
- If the patient experiences constipation, instruct him to increase dietary fluids and fiber and to use bulk laxatives, as needed.
- Tell him to chew gum, suck hard candy, or use mouth rinses to relieve mouth dryness.

- Explain to the patient that this drug should control his hypertension.
- If a four-dose-per-day schedule is prescribed, tell the patient to take a missed dose only up to 2 hours before his next scheduled dose; warn against double-dosing. Help him work out a regular medication schedule.

- Explain to the patient that this drug should control his hypertension.
- Tell him to take a missed dose as soon as possible, but warn him not to double-dose.
- Instruct him to take one of his scheduled daily doses at bedtime to take advantage of the drug's tendency to cause drowsiness.
- Reassure the patient that drowsiness is usually transient. Tell him to notify his doctor if it persists.
- Tell him to rise slowly from a sitting or lying position to minimize postural hypotension.
- Advise him to use chewing gum, hard candy, or mouth rinses to relieve mouth dryness.

(continued)

TEACHING PATIENTS ABOUT CARDIOVASCULAR DRUGS *(continued)*

DRUG	ADVERSE REACTIONS	INTERACTIONS*
Antihypertensives *(continued)*		
minoxidil (Loniten)	*Reportable:* distended neck veins, dyspnea, edema, rapid heart rate, weight gain *Other:* lengthening and darkening of fine body hair	• Tell the patient that foods and beverages don't influence the safety or effectiveness of minoxidil. • Advise the patient to avoid over-the-counter sympathomimetics, such as ephedrine-containing nasal sprays.
prazosin (Minipress)	*Reportable:* chest pain, dyspnea, edema, rapid heart rate, syncope *Other:* drowsiness, gastric upset, headache, slight dizziness	• Tell the patient that foods and nonalcoholic beverages don't influence the safety or effectiveness of prazosin. • Tell him to limit his alcohol intake to prevent dizziness. • Advise him to avoid over-the-counter sympathomimetics, such as ephedrine-containing nasal sprays.
Antilipemics		
cholestyramine (Questran)	*Reportable:* severe constipation, rash, black or tarry stools, severe stomach pain, unusual weight loss *Other:* bloating, diarrhea, flatulence, mild constipation, nausea, vomiting	• Tell the patient that over-the-counter drugs don't influence the safety or effectiveness of cholestyramine. • Instruct him to take the drug 1 hour before or 3 hours after a meal. • If the patient's taking fat-soluble vitamins (A, D, or E), instruct him to stagger administration times, since cholestyramine interferes with vitamin absorption.

*Includes food, beverages, and over-the-counter drugs.

TEACHING POINTS

• Explain to the patient that this drug should control his hypertension.
• Tell him to take a missed daily dose within 8 hours of the scheduled time, but no later. Warn him not to double-dose.
• Tell the patient to remove unwanted hair by shaving or using a depilatory.
• If beta blockers are prescribed to control reflex tachycardia, explain to the patient that he must take both drugs on schedule to ensure their safety and effectiveness. Similarly, if diuretics are prescribed to control sodium and water retention, tell him he must also take them on schedule.
• Instruct him to weigh himself at least every other day and to report any sudden weight gain.

• Explain to the patient that this drug should control his hypertension.
• Tell him to take a missed dose as soon as possible, but warn him not to double-dose.
• Advise him to take the initial dose at bedtime. Dizziness is most pronounced after this dose.
• To reduce dizziness during therapy, instruct him to take this drug with food.
• Caution him not to operate heavy machinery or drive a motor vehicle during the first week of therapy, in case syncope occurs.

• Explain to the patient that this drug should reduce the levels of certain protein and fat combinations in his blood.
• Tell the patient to take a missed dose as soon as possible, but warn him not to double-dose.
• Teach him to mix the powder with liquids, applesauce, or crushed pineapple to prevent gastrointestinal erosion. Also encourage him to increase dietary fluids and fiber and to use a bulk laxative, as needed.
• Point out that he must continue to limit his intake of cholesterol and saturated fats even though he's taking an antilipemic.

(continued)

TEACHING PATIENTS ABOUT
CARDIOVASCULAR DRUGS *(continued)*

DRUG	ADVERSE REACTIONS	INTERACTIONS*
Antilipemics *(continued)*		
clofibrate (Atromid-S)	*Reportable:* bloody or painful urination, chest pain, chills, dyspnea, fever, irregular heart rate, leg and ankle edema, sore throat *Other:* abdominal fullness, decreased libido, diarrhea, flatulence, flulike aches and pains, nausea, weight gain	• Tell the patient that foods, beverages, and over-the-counter drugs don't influence the safety or effectiveness of clofibrate.
Antithrombotics		
aspirin (multiple forms and brands)	*Reportable:* bleeding gums, dyspnea, easy bruising, hearing loss, tarry stools, tinnitus, vomiting blood *Other:* gastric upset, heartburn	• Tell the patient that foods don't influence the safety or effectiveness of aspirin. • Advise him to avoid antacids, which can reduce aspirin's effectiveness. • Warn him not to take aspirin with alcohol to avoid GI bleeding.
dipyridamole (Persantine)	*Reportable:* chest pain or tightness, vomiting, weakness *Other:* dizziness, flushing, gastric upset, headache	• Tell the patient that over-the-counter drugs don't influence the safety or effectiveness of dipyridamole. • Advise against combining dipyridamole and alcohol to avoid dizziness. • Instruct him to take the drug 1 hour before or 3 hours after a meal.
Beta-adrenergic blockers		
acebutolol (Sectral) **atenolol** (Tenormin) **labetalol** (Trandate) **metoprolol** (Lopressor) **nadolol** (Corgard) **pindolol** (Visken) **propranolol** (Inderal) **timolol** (Blocadren)	*Reportable:* depression, dizziness, dyspnea, skin rash, very slow heart rate, wheezing *Other:* decreased libido, diarrhea, fatigue, headache, insomnia, nasal stuffiness, nausea, vivid dreams and nightmares, vomiting	• Tell the patient that over-the-counter drugs don't influence the safety or effectiveness of beta-adrenergic blockers. • Instruct him to take labetalol, metoprolol, and propranolol with foods to increase drug absorption.

*Includes food, beverages, and over-the-counter drugs.

TEACHING POINTS

• Explain to the patient that this drug should reduce the levels of cholesterol and certain protein and fat combinations in his blood.
• Tell him to take a missed dose as soon as possible, but warn him not to double-dose.

• Reassure him that any GI distress is transient.
• Point out that he must continue to limit his intake of cholesterol and saturated fats even though he's taking an antilipemic.

• Explain to the patient that this drug hinders the clotting of his blood.
• To relieve mild GI distress, advise him to take aspirin with food or milk or to use a buffered or enteric-coated form of the drug.

• Tell him to take a missed dose within 12 hours, but warn him not to double-dose.
• Teach him that acetaminophen doesn't have the same antithrombotic effect as aspirin and cannot be substituted.

• Explain to the patient that this drug hinders the clotting of his blood and dilates his coronary arteries.
• Tell him to take a missed dose as soon as possible, but warn him not to double-dose.

• To minimize dizziness, tell the patient to rise slowly from a sitting or lying position.
• Advise him to take dipyridamole with a light snack or a glass of milk to reduce GI distress.

• Explain to the patient why this drug has been prescribed. For example, it can lower his blood pressure, reduce the frequency of angina attacks, control rapid heart rate, and minimize the risk of complications after myocardial infarction by easing cardiac work load.
• If the patient takes one dose daily, instruct him to take a missed dose within 8 hours. If he takes two or more doses each day, instruct him to take a missed dose as soon as possible. However, he must never double-dose.

• Warn him against suddenly discontinuing the drug. He must taper the dosage, as directed, to avoid serious complications.
• Teach him to take his pulse before taking the drug and to notify his doctor if his pulse rate falls below 60 beats/minute.
• If the patient complains of insomnia, suggest that he take the drug no later than 2 hours before bedtime.

(continued)

TEACHING PATIENTS ABOUT CARDIOVASCULAR DRUGS (continued)

DRUG	ADVERSE REACTIONS	INTERACTIONS*
Calcium channel blockers		
diltiazem (Cardizem) **nifedipine** (Procardia) **verapamil** (Calan, Isoptin)	*Reportable:* ankle edema, chest pain, dyspnea, fainting, very slow or fast heart rate *Other:* constipation, dizziness, flushing, headache, nausea	• Tell the patient that foods, nonalcoholic beverages, and over-the-counter drugs don't influence the safety or effectiveness of calcium channel blockers. • Advise him to limit alcohol intake. Alcohol can exacerbate dizziness.
Cardiac glycosides		
digoxin (Lanoxicaps, Lanoxin)	*Reportable:* abdominal pain, anorexia, blurred vision, color vision changes, diplopia, dizziness, drowsiness, fatigue, headache, irregular heart rate, malaise, nausea *Other:* breast enlargement	• Tell the patient to avoid antacids, kaolin and pectin mixtures, antidiarrheals, and laxatives, which decrease digoxin absorption. • Also instruct him to limit his fiber intake, as dietary fiber can decrease digoxin absorption.
Loop diuretics		
bumetanide (Bumex) **ethacrynic acid** (Edecrin) **furosemide** (Lasix)	*Reportable:* fever, hearing loss, increased thirst, jaundice, muscle cramps, nausea, tinnitus, unusual fatigue or weakness, urgent or burning urination, vomiting *Other:* anorexia, blurred vision, diarrhea, dizziness, muscle aches and cramps, weight loss	• Tell the patient that foods and over-the-counter drugs don't influence the safety or effectiveness of loop diuretics. • Advise him to limit his alcohol intake to prevent dizziness.

*Includes food, beverages, and over-the-counter drugs.

TEACHING POINTS

• Explain to the patient that this drug should reduce the frequency and severity of his chest pain and lower his blood pressure.
• Tell him to take a missed dose within 4 hours, but warn him not to double-dose.
• To minimize dizziness, tell the patient to rise slowly from a sitting or lying position.
• Explain that the drug won't relieve acute chest pain. He must continue to use sublingual nitroglycerin, if prescribed.

• Reassure him that he can continue to eat and drink calcium-containing foods in reasonable amounts.
• Teach him to prevent constipation by increasing his fluid and fiber intake and by using a bulk laxative, as necessary.

• Explain to the patient that this drug should strengthen his heart contractions and regulate his heart rate.
• Tell him to establish a regular routine for taking digoxin each day.
• Instruct him to take a missed dose within 12 hours, but warn him not to double-dose.

• Teach him to take his pulse before taking digoxin and to report an unusually low, high, or irregular pulse rate to his doctor.
• Warn him not to take another person's tablets; different generic digoxin tablets are absorbed at different rates.

• Explain to the patient that this drug should help his kidneys filter out excess body fluid, thereby lowering his blood pressure and clearing fluid from his lungs.
• Instruct him to take a missed dose as soon as possible. Warn him against double-dosing.
• If the patient takes the drug twice daily, tell him to take the second dose in late afternoon rather than at night to prevent sleep interruption from nocturia.
• Advise him to take the drug with meals to prevent GI distress.
• Encourage intake of high-potassium foods

(citrus fruits, tomatoes, bananas, dates, and apricots). Also remind him to take potassium supplements, if ordered.
• Instruct the patient to record his weight daily to monitor fluid loss.
• To minimize postural hypotension, tell him to rise slowly from a lying or sitting position.
• Remind the female patient to wipe from front to back after urinating to prevent urinary tract infection (UTI). Teach all patients to report symptoms of possible UTI: burning, fever, or urgency followed by voiding a small amount.

(continued)

TEACHING PATIENTS ABOUT
CARDIOVASCULAR DRUGS *(continued)*

DRUG	ADVERSE REACTIONS	INTERACTIONS*
Nitrates		
erythrityl tetranitrate (Cardilate) **isosorbide dinitrate** (multiple forms and brands) **nitroglycerin** (multiple forms and brands) **pentaerythritol tetranitrate** (Duotrate, Peritrate)	*Reportable:* blurred vision, extreme dizziness, mouth dryness, rapid heart rate, skin irritation or rash *Other:* headache, flushing, mild dizziness, nausea, vomiting	• Tell the patient that foods, beverages, and over-the-counter drugs don't influence the safety or effectiveness of nitrates.
Potassium-sparing diuretics		
amiloride (Midamor) **spironolactone** (Aldactone) **triamterene** (Dyrenium)	*Reportable:* confusion, irregular heart rate, muscle flaccidity, numbness, tingling in hands and feet, weight changes *Other:* decreased libido, diarrhea, headache, nausea, stomach cramps, vomiting, weakness	• Instruct the patient to limit his dietary potassium intake and to avoid foods with extremely high potassium levels, such as salt substitutes and low-salt milk.
Thiazide and thiazide-like diuretics		
chlorothiazide (Diuril) **chlorthalidone** (Hygroton, Thalitone) **hydrochlorothiazide** (multiple brands) **metolazone** (Diulo, Zaroxolyn)	*Reportable:* excessive thirst, fever, irregular heart rate, lethargy, mouth dryness, muscle cramps, skin rash, urgent or burning urination, weakness, weak pulse *Other:* anorexia, diarrhea, dizziness, GI distress, restlessness	• Instruct the patient to avoid large doses of calcium supplements. • Advise him to avoid over-the-counter sympathomimetics, such as ephedrine-containing nasal sprays. • Teach him to increase his intake of foods high in potassium, such as bananas and citrus fruits.

*Includes food, beverages, and over-the-counter drugs.

TEACHING POINTS

• Explain to the patient that this drug should prevent or relieve his chest pain.
• Tell him to take a missed dose as soon as possible, but warn him not to double-dose.
• If nitroglycerin tablets are prescribed for relief of acute angina, instruct the patient to take one tablet every 5 minutes up to a maximum of three tablets. Tell him to hold each tablet under his tongue until it dissolves. Meanwhile, he should sit down and try to relax. If the tablets bring no relief, tell him to call his doctor immediately or have someone take him to an emergency department at once.
• Because nitroglycerin tablets must be fresh to be effective, tell the patient to cap the bottle quickly and tightly after each use and to replace an opened bottle after 3 months, even if several tablets remain.
• Instruct him to shield tablets from light and to avoid handling them except for administration.
• If the patient uses nitrates to prevent angina, teach him to maintain a regular self-administration schedule. He should also take the drug before any activity likely to induce angina, such as exposure to cold, exertion, and sexual activity.
• Advise him to avoid overly hot showers. Why? Vasodilation might make him dizzy and faint.
• To prevent dizziness, tell him to rise slowly from a sitting or lying position.
• Reassure him that headaches should diminish with continued use of nitrates. If they don't, tell him to notify his doctor.
• Provide the patient with a copy of the home care aid *How to Use Nitroglycerin,* pages 118 and 119.

• Explain to the patient that this drug should lower his blood pressure and relieve ankle edema and lung congestion. Unlike other diuretics, this drug avoids potassium loss.
• Tell him to take a missed daily dose within 8 hours. Otherwise, he should skip the missed dose. Warn him against double-dosing.
• Advise him to take the drug with food to relieve GI distress.
• Instruct him to weigh himself at least every other day and to report any unusual weight changes.

• Explain to the patient that this drug should relieve lung congestion and edema, and lower his blood pressure.
• Tell him to take a missed daily dose within 8 hours. Otherwise, he should skip the missed dose. Warn against double-dosing.
• Instruct him not to take an evening dose just before bedtime to prevent sleep interruption from nocturia.
• Caution the diabetic patient that this drug may elevate blood glucose levels.
• Remind the female patient to wipe from front to back after urinating to prevent UTI. Teach all patients to report signs of possible UTI: burning, fever, or urgency followed by voiding a small amount.
• Instruct the patient to record his weight daily to monitor fluid loss.

7

Respiratory System

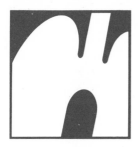

Respiratory System

Introduction

According to the American Lung Association, chronic respiratory disorders account for more lost time from work—exceeding 30 million days per year—than any other illness. What's more, they rank as a major cause of short-term hospitalization. As a result, you'll be expected to teach about them *routinely*. And when you do, you'll find that one key symptom will motivate the patient to respond to your teaching: dyspnea. This frightening symptom occurs in all chronic respiratory disorders whether they limit airflow (obstructive disorders) or lung expansion (restrictive disorders) or interfere with gas exchange across the alveolocapillary membrane (vascular disorders). By forcing the patient to limit his activity, dyspnea can also cause frustration and depression—emotions you'll need to recognize and deal with to teach effectively.

Achieving teaching goals

Your major goals are to help the patient cope with dyspnea and avoid complications that require hospitalization. To achieve these goals, you'll often need to help the patient master special skills. For example, you'll need to teach him how to perform abdominal and pursed-lip breathing exercises and how to control his cough.

Achieving your goals may require more than one-on-one teaching sessions with the patient. For example, if the doctor prescribes chest physiotherapy at home, the patient's family will require equal instruction. You'll need to teach them how to help position the patient for postural drainage and how to perform percussion correctly. Occasionally, you'll also need to coordinate your teaching efforts with other health professionals. For example, to ensure safe and effective use of oxygen at home, you'll need to work with the medical equipment supplier and a visiting nurse.

In all chronic respiratory disorders, you'll need to teach the patient how to recognize and, if possible, prevent complications, such as life-threatening respiratory infection. In some disorders, though, you'll be able to point toward more positive benefits of following your instructions. For example, by encouraging compliance in chronic bronchitis, your teaching may help the patient restore some pulmonary function. For the patient with asthma, your teaching can spell the difference between a normal, active life and one marred by frequent asthma attacks. By helping this patient identify and avoid causative triggers—such as pollen, animal dander, and certain foods—your teaching can prevent or minimize such attacks.

DISORDERS

Asthma

In this chronic disorder, your teaching will focus on helping the patient learn to prevent and control asthma attacks. A host of factors can trigger an attack—from eggs to aspirin to cigarette smoke. Helping the patient identify and then avoid his triggers marks the first step toward preventing attacks. You'll also need to stress the importance of daily compliance with drug therapy. Because the patient usually remains asymptomatic between attacks, he may easily forget to take prescribed medications—or may mistakenly believe he no longer needs them.

CHECKLIST

☑ TEACHING TOPICS IN ASTHMA

☐ An explanation of how asthma triggers elicit bronchospasm, airway edema, and mucous production

☐ Complications such as status asthmaticus

☐ Identification of asthma triggers

☐ Preparation for arterial blood gas (ABG) analysis, pulmonary function tests, and other diagnostic studies

☐ Importance of diet and adequate hydration

☐ Drugs and their administration

☐ How to use an oral inhaler

☐ How to control an asthma attack

☐ Warning signs and prevention of respiratory infection

☐ Availability of support groups, such as the American Lung Association

To help the patient control an asthma attack, you'll need to teach him how to perform pursed-lip breathing and how to use an oral inhaler to take prescribed medications. By helping him master these techniques, your teaching can relieve much of the anxiety associated with asthma attacks. More important, though, it can ensure that the patient's asthma doesn't prevent him from leading a normal, active life.

Describe the disorder

Tell the patient that this chronic, episodic disorder is characterized by acute attacks of dyspnea, wheezing, and productive cough. During an attack, his airways contract (bronchospasm), swell, and clog with mucus. An attack may last from minutes to hours and subside spontaneously or in response to drug therapy. Explain how certain triggers can precipitate an attack (see *Recognizing Common Asthma Triggers*).

Point out possible complications

Warn the patient about possible complications that may occur if he doesn't strictly adhere to the treatment plan. A potentially fatal complication of asthma is status asthmaticus—a prolonged, severe attack that fails to respond to drug therapy. In status asthmaticus, mucous plugs may constrict or block the airways, leading to respiratory arrest.

Teach about tests

Prepare the patient for tests to confirm the diagnosis of asthma and to monitor its treatment. Explain that no one laboratory test can conclusively diagnose asthma. Instead, he'll usually undergo a battery of tests. Typically, the doctor will order sputum and blood samples to check for eosinophils.

If the doctor also orders arterial blood gas (ABG) analysis to detect hypoxemia, explain to the patient that this test evaluates how well his lungs deliver oxygen to blood and eliminate carbon dioxide. Tell him who will perform the

RECOGNIZING COMMON ASTHMA TRIGGERS

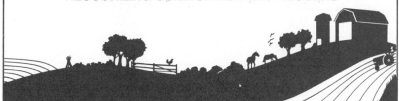

AT HOME

• Foods such as nuts, chocolate, eggs, shellfish, and peanut butter
• Beverages such as orange juice, wine, beer, and milk
• Pollens from flowers, trees, grasses, hay, and ragweed; mold spores
• Animals such as rabbits, cats, dogs, hamsters, gerbils, and chickens
• Feather pillows, down comforters, and wool clothing
• Insect parts such as those from dead cockroaches
• Medicines such as aspirin
• Vapors from cleaning solvents, paint, paint thinners, and liquid chlorine bleach
• Sprays from furniture polish, starch, cleaners, and room deodorizers
• Spray deodorants, perfumes, hair sprays, talcum powder, and scented cosmetics
• Cloth-upholstered furniture, carpets, and draperies that gather dust
• Brooms and dusters that raise dust
• Dirty filters on hot air furnaces and air conditioners that put dust into the air

IN THE WORKPLACE

• Dusts, vapors, or fumes from wood products (western red cedar, some pine and birch woods, mahogany); flour, cereals, grains, coffee, tea, or papain; metals (platinum, chromium, nickel sulfate, soldering fumes); and cotton, flax, and hemp
• Mold from decaying hay

OUTDOORS

• Cold or hot air
• Excessive humidity or dryness
• Changes in seasons
• Smog
• Automobile exhaust

ANYPLACE

• Overexertion, which may cause wheezing
• Lying down, which allows mucus to collect in the airways
• Common cold, flu, and other viruses
• Fear, anger, frustration, laughing too hard, crying
• Smoke from cigarettes, cigars, pipes—either yours or someone else's

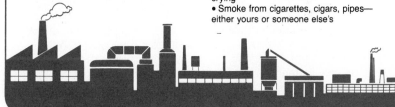

arterial puncture, and when and where it will be done. Inform him about which site has been selected (radial, brachial, or femoral artery) and, if appropriate, whether he should continue his oxygen therapy during the test. Instruct the patient to breathe normally during the test. Warn him that he may experience a brief cramping or throbbing pain at the puncture site.

Inform the patient that he may re-quire a daily venipuncture to monitor theophylline drug therapy; when blood levels reach the desired therapeutic range (10 mcg/ml to 20 mcg/ml), he won't need this test anymore. Tell him who will perform each venipuncture and when.

Prepare the patient for other studies to diagnose asthma or monitor its treatment, such as chest X-rays and pulmonary function tests. (See *Teaching*

HOW TO CONTROL AN ASTHMA ATTACK

Dear Patient:

Usually, an asthma attack is preceded by warning signs that give you time to take action. Be alert for:

- chest tightness
- coughing
- awareness of your breathing
- wheezing.

Once you've had a few asthma attacks, you'll have no trouble recognizing these early warning signs. Above all, *do not ignore them*. Instead, follow these steps:

1

Take your prescribed medicine with an oral inhaler to prevent the attack from getting worse.

2

As this medicine goes to work, try to relax. Although you may be understandably anxious or fearful, remember that these feelings only increase your shortness of breath. To help relax, sit upright in a chair, close your eyes, and breathe slowly and evenly. Then, begin consciously tightening and relaxing the muscles in your body. First, tighten the muscles in your face and count to yourself: one-1,000; two-1,000. Be sure not to hold your breath. Then, relax these muscles and repeat with the muscles in your arms and hands, legs and feet. Finally, let your body go limp.

3

Regain control of your breathing by doing the pursed-lip breathing exercises you've been taught. *Don't gasp for air*. Continue pursed-lip breathing until you no longer feel breathless.

4

If the attack triggers a coughing spell, you'll need to control your cough so that it effectively brings up mucus and helps clear your airways. To do so, lean forward slightly, keeping your feet on the floor. Next, breathe in deeply and hold that breath for a second or two. Cough twice, first to loosen mucus, then to bring it up. Be sure to cough into a tissue.

5

If, even after you've followed these steps, the attack gets worse, call your doctor.

Patients about Respiratory Tests, pages 188 to 194.)

Teach about treatments

• *Activity.* Explain to the patient that exercise promotes a normal, healthy life. However, emphasize that he may need to avoid or curtail certain forms of exercise, especially if they trigger an attack. Encourage him to use trial and error to find the exercise that's right for him. For example, if the patient starts wheezing when he jogs, suggest that he slow his pace or try a different exercise, such as bike riding. Advise him to consult his doctor about taking his prescribed medication before exercise to prevent an attack.

• *Diet.* Stress the importance of a nutritious, well-balanced diet to help prevent infection and fatigue. Tell the patient to drink plenty of fluids daily to keep his mucus thin, which helps reduce bronchospasm. Encourage him to try to associate what he eats with his asthma attacks. Recommend that he compile a list of attack-triggering foods—such as egg yolks, chocolate, and shellfish—and give it to his doctor. Make sure he avoids foods that are known asthma triggers for him.

• *Medication.* The methylxanthines and sympathomimetics are the pharmacologic mainstays of asthma therapy. However, since these drugs cause similar adverse reactions, instruct the patient to keep a written record of when reactions occurred in relation to taking each drug.

Emphasize that the patient mustn't substitute over-the-counter antiallergy preparations for his prescribed drugs. If the methylxanthines and sympathomimetics fail to relieve the patient's symptoms, the doctor may prescribe cromolyn sodium or corticosteroids (see *Teaching Patients about Respiratory Drugs*, pages 196 to 203, for more information).

If appropriate, teach the patient how to use an oral inhaler (see *Using an Oral Inhaler*, page 170) to take nebulized drugs. Warn him not to abuse nebulized drugs, especially those containing concentrated solutions of nonselective beta-adrenergic stimulants—for example, isoproterenol or epinephrine. Explain that such abuse can lead to drug tolerance and potentially serious cardiac side effects, such as dysrhythmias.

Emphasize that the patient must take his prescribed medications even when he feels well. Stopping a medication or changing the dose can make him susceptible to an asthma attack. What's more, if he does so, he may require hospitalization to restore therapeutic levels of the drug. Because the patient's response to medication can change over time, instruct him to notify his doctor if the prescribed medications become less effective.

• *Other care measures.* To help the patient lead a full and active life, teach him to eliminate or reduce his exposure to known asthma triggers, whenever possible. For example, if he's sensitive to aspirin, suggest that he substitute sodium salicylate or acetaminophen.

Because emotions can trigger or worsen an asthma attack, tell the patient to consult his doctor about taking additional medication when he's upset for a prolonged period or ill. Advise him to practice pursed-lip breathing when he becomes fearful, angry, sad, or excited to help prevent an asthma attack (see *Breathing Exercises to Relieve Dyspnea*, page 178).

Teach the patient how to prevent respiratory infection—another common asthma trigger (see *How to Detect—and Prevent—Respiratory Infection*, page 184). However, if the patient does develop a respiratory infection, he and a family member should perform chest physiotherapy at least twice daily to clear mucus from the lungs (see *How to Perform Chest Physiotherapy*, pages 176 and 177).

If appropriate, discuss the link between cigarette smoking and asthma attacks. Also, explain the harmful effects of smoking and refer the patient to a local stop-smoking program.

USING AN ORAL INHALER

Dear Patient:

To use your oral inhaler, just follow these steps:

1

Remove the mouthpiece and cap from the inhaler. Then remove the cap from the mouthpiece. Next, turn the mouthpiece sideways. On one side of the flattened tip you'll see a small hole. Fit the metal

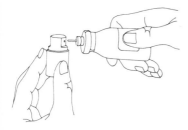

stem on the inhaler into the hole. After it's assembled, shake the inhaler five times.

2

Exhale fully through pursed lips. Hold the inhaler upside down and close your lips and teeth around the mouthpiece.

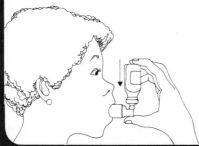

3

Tilt your head back slightly. Take a slow, deep breath. As you do, firmly press the inhaler against the mouthpiece—one time only—to release one dose of medication. Continue inhaling until your lungs feel full.

4

Take the mouthpiece away from your mouth, and hold your breath for three to five counts of one-1,000; two-1,000; three-1,000. Exhale slowly through pursed lips.

5

If your doctor wants you to take more than one dose, wait a couple of minutes before repeating steps 2 through 4.

6

Rinse your mouth, gargle, and drink a few sips of fluid.

Remember to clean the inhaler once a day: take it apart and rinse the mouthpiece and cap under warm running water for 1 minute. Shake off the excess water, allow the parts to dry, and then reassemble them.

When the patient can't possibly avoid known triggers (or allergens), the doctor may attempt hyposensitization, or desensitization. Explain that this involves subcutaneous injection of graded doses of the allergen at regular intervals. Although typically more effective for hay fever, hyposensitization may dramatically improve symptoms for some asthma patients.

Encourage the patient to contact the local chapter of the American Lung Association for more information on asthma and support groups.

Chronic Bronchitis and Emphysema

Whether a patient has chronic bronchitis or emphysema, he'll be highly motivated to respond to your teaching for one reason: to relieve his dyspnea. Typically, dyspnea occurs on exertion in chronic bronchitis but is constant in emphysema. This symptom can dramatically limit the patient's activity, making him feel frustrated and anxious. To help him, your teaching must cover a wide range of topics, especially the use of pursed-lip and abdominal breathing exercises to relieve dyspnea. By mastering these exercises, the patient will have an aid to use whenever—and wherever—he experiences dyspnea. You'll also need to teach him how to use various types of equipment at home, ranging from a simple oral inhaler for prescribed drugs to a more complicated setup for oxygen therapy.

Besides dyspnea, the patient with chronic bronchitis must learn to deal with copious secretions. So, you'll need to stress the importance of adequate hydration to keep secretions thin. Most important, though, you'll need to involve the family in his care by teaching them how to perform chest physiotherapy at home. Because this procedure is especially trying for the

---

CHECKLIST

TEACHING TOPICS IN CHRONIC BRONCHITIS AND EMPHYSEMA

- [ ] An explanation of the disease process: chronic bronchitis and/or emphysema
- [ ] Preparation for pulmonary function tests, chest X-rays, and other diagnostic studies
- [ ] Exercise program
- [ ] Importance of diet and adequate hydration
- [ ] Drugs and their administration
- [ ] How to use an oral inhaler
- [ ] Chest physiotherapy at home
- [ ] Oxygen therapy at home
- [ ] Pursed-lip breathing exercises
- [ ] Importance of avoiding bronchial irritants, such as cigarette smoke
- [ ] How to modify activities of daily living
- [ ] Sexual counseling
- [ ] Warning signs and prevention of respiratory infection
- [ ] Availability of support groups, such as the American Lung Association

---

dyspneic patient, he'll need strong encouragement from both you and his family to ensure compliance.

Both chronic bronchitis and emphysema increase the patient's susceptibility to respiratory infection. As a result, you'll need to teach early signs of infection and key preventive measures. For example, by stressing the importance of good nutrition and adequate exercise, you can help the patient reduce his risk of infection.

Although emphysema is irreversible, chronic bronchitis may partially or completely resolve if the patient eliminates his exposure to the causative irritant. So your teaching must go beyond helping him cope with symptoms and avoid complications. You'll need to urge him to avoid the irritant—usually cigarette smoke—before he develops irreparable lung damage.

WHAT HAPPENS IN CHRONIC BRONCHITIS AND EMPHYSEMA

In chronic bronchitis, repeated exposure to inhaled irritants produces widespread inflammation and increased mucous production, narrowing or blocking the airways. This, in turn, increases airway resistance, causing severe ventilation-perfusion mismatch marked by cyanosis. Because a patient with chronic bronchitis also typically has edema from right ventricular failure, he's often called a "blue bloater."

In emphysema, recurrent inflammation damages and eventually destroys the alveolar walls, thereby creating large air spaces. Alveolar destruction also leads to loss of elastic recoil, causing bronchiolar collapse on expiration and the trapping of air within the lungs. However, associated pulmonary capillary destruction usually allows a patient with severe emphysema to match ventilation to perfusion and thus avoid cyanosis. Because such a patient has a pink color but a dramatically increased expiratory effort, he's sometimes called a "pink puffer."

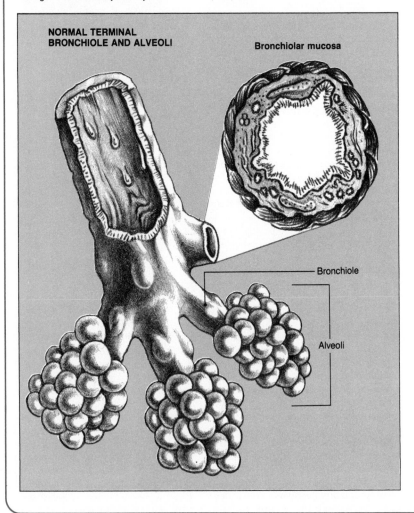

NORMAL TERMINAL BRONCHIOLE AND ALVEOLI

Bronchiolar mucosa

Bronchiole

Alveoli

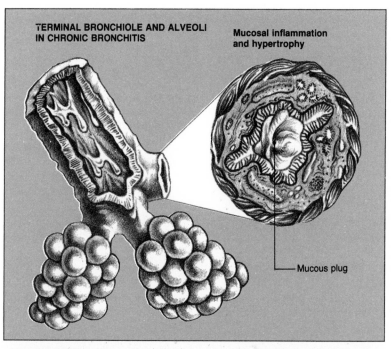

TERMINAL BRONCHIOLE AND ALVEOLI IN CHRONIC BRONCHITIS

Mucosal inflammation and hypertrophy

Mucous plug

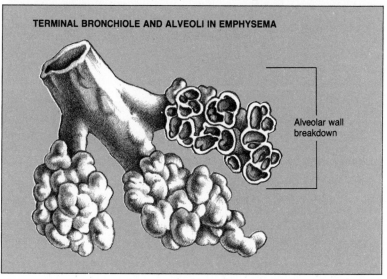

TERMINAL BRONCHIOLE AND ALVEOLI IN EMPHYSEMA

Alveolar wall breakdown

Describe the disorder

Explain to the patient that chronic bronchitis and emphysema are two forms of chronic obstructive pulmonary disease (COPD), one of the most common causes of disability in the United States. Tell him that these disorders may occur separately or together. Chronic bronchitis results from repeated exposure to irritants that inflame the airways, causing them to swell and clog with mucus. In emphysema, such inflammation eventually destroys the alveoli and bronchioles, creating air spaces known as blebs or bullae (see *What Happens in Chronic Bronchitis and Emphysema*, pages 172 and 173). Emphasize that avoiding or removing the causative irritant in chronic bronchitis may improve lung function and ease symptoms of cough, dyspnea, and copious mucous production.

Point out possible complications

Warn the patient with chronic bronchitis that he'll probably develop emphysema if he doesn't adhere to the treatment plan. Whether the patient has chronic bronchitis or emphysema, his limited pulmonary reserve makes him susceptible to respiratory infection. Point out that he can avoid this complication by following preventive measures. Also, make sure he understands the importance of promptly treating infection. Note that untreated respiratory infection can lead to life-threatening acute respiratory failure.

Teach about tests

Prepare the patient for diagnostic tests to assess his degree of impaired respiratory function or to detect possible complications. Typically, the doctor relies on pulmonary function tests and chest X-rays, although he may also order thoracic computed tomography or magnetic resonance imaging. If appropriate, explain how an exercise EKG can help the doctor tailor an exercise program to match the patient's toler-

ance. (See *Teaching Patients about Respiratory Tests*, pages 188 to 194.)

If the doctor orders sputum analysis to screen for infection or malignancy or to detect allergy, teach the patient the proper technique for sputum collection. If he orders ABG analysis, explain to the patient that this test evaluates how well his lungs are delivering oxygen to the blood and eliminating carbon dioxide. Tell him who will perform the arterial puncture, and when and where it will be done. Also tell him which site has been selected (radial, brachial, or femoral artery) and, if appropriate, whether he should continue his oxygen therapy during the test. Instruct the patient to breathe normally during the test, and warn him that he may experience a brief cramping or throbbing pain at the puncture site. If the doctor orders a complete blood count to detect polycythemia, tell the patient who will perform the venipuncture and when.

Teach about treatments

• *Activity.* After evaluating the patient's exercise EKG, the doctor may prescribe an exercise program. Emphasize that this program aims to increase the patient's endurance and strength without causing him severe dyspnea. Also, explain how exercise can improve his sense of well-being. Teach the patient warm-up and cooldown exercises (slow walking, bending, stretching) to perform for several minutes before and after his prescribed program. If the patient needs low-flow oxygen during exercise, teach him and a family member how to use oxygen at home (see *Using Oxygen Safely and Effectively*, pages 186 and 187). Also, show them how to take an accurate radial pulse to monitor the effects of exercise. Warn the patient to stop exercising immediately and notify the doctor if he experiences increased dyspnea, extreme fatigue, nausea, dizziness, or muscle cramps, or develops pale, mottled, or clammy skin. Tell the patient that the doctor will periodically reevaluate his exercise tolerance and modify his program, as necessary.

• *Diet.* Explain to the patient the importance of a well-balanced, nutritious diet to compensate for the extra calories he expends just to breathe. Because dyspnea and increased sputum production can discourage eating and lead to weight loss, teach the patient how to maintain his caloric intake. First, encourage frequent oral hygiene to stimulate his appetite and enjoyment of food. If the patient has severe dyspnea, advise him to eat small, frequent meals to reduce fatigue and air swallowing during eating. Also encourage him to chew his food slowly. Tell him to avoid coffee, tea, alcohol, cola, and spicy foods. If he experiences a bloated feeling at mealtime, advise him to limit intake of gas-producing foods, such as cabbage, brussels sprouts, beans, broccoli, asparagus, cauliflower, apples, watermelon, cantaloupe, onions, and radishes. Recommend nutritious snacks (including fluids like fruit juices) or a liquid enteral supplement for added calories between meals.

Unless contraindicated, encourage the patient to drink plenty of water—at least six glasses daily—to thin his mucous secretions. Adequate fluid intake will also help prevent constipation and avoid breathlessness associated with straining during defecation. Tell the patient to include fresh fruit, vegetables, and bran in his diet to help prevent constipation.

Address any factor that may interfere with the patient's ability to maintain a proper diet. For example, you may need to start by teaching him the basics of good nutrition. Or, if he lacks transportation to the grocery store or has limited financial resources, refer him to the appropriate social service agency. Also, inform him about community programs, such as Meals On Wheels.

If the patient is obese, explain how obesity interferes with diaphragmatic movement and increases cardiac work load. This, in turn, can increase the work of breathing. Provide the obese patient with a weight-reduction diet.

• *Medication.* To treat chronic bronchitis, the doctor will usually prescribe bronchodilators, such as an oral methylxanthine, an inhaled sympathomimetic, and an inhaled anticholinergic (see *Teaching Patients about Respiratory Drugs*, pages 196 to 203). Make sure the patient knows how to use an oral inhaler (see *Using an Oral Inhaler*, page 170). Instruct him to take the sympathomimetic before chest physiotherapy.

• *Procedures.* Explain to the patient that chest physiotherapy helps mobilize and remove mucus from his lungs. Teach him and a family member how to perform this procedure (see *How to Perform Chest Physiotherapy*, pages 176 and 177). Have the family member demonstrate percussion to assure proper technique. If the family member has limited arm strength, show him how to use a mechanical percussor.

If appropriate, also teach the patient and a family member how to use oxygen at home (see *Using Oxygen Safely and Effectively*, pages 186 and 187). When he's planning a trip, instruct the patient to obtain advance information about oxygen regulations on the plane, train, or bus. For example, tell him to call the airline to ensure that enough oxygen will be aboard to make the trip and to circle in a holding pattern. Before takeoff, he should double-check the availability of sufficient oxygen. Make sure he understands that he'll experience the effects of high altitude even in the pressurized cabin of a commercial airliner. Advise him to use his breathing exercises to relieve troublesome dyspnea. Instruct him to get the name of a medical equipment supplier at his travel destination so that any necessary equipment will be ready upon his arrival.

• *Other care measures.* Explain to the patient how inhaled pollutants can aggravate his symptoms—as well as his disorder. Tell him to avoid heavy traffic and smog, whenever possible. Also, advise against using aerosol sprays, such

HOW TO PERFORM CHEST PHYSIOTHERAPY

Dear Patient:

The doctor wants you to perform chest physiotherapy to help make your breathing easier. Chest physiotherapy has three parts: postural drainage, percussion, and coughing. Postural drainage lets the force of gravity drain mucus from the bottom of your lungs. Then percussion helps move thick, sticky mucus from the smaller airways of your lungs into the larger airways. Coughing—the last and most important step—clears mucus from your lungs.

You'll be able to perform postural drainage and coughing yourself, but you'll need a family member's or friend's help to percuss your back. Follow these instructions for each step.

Postural drainage

1

Place a box of tissues within easy reach. Also stack pillows on the floor next to your bed.

2

Next, lie over the side of your bed. Support your head, chest, and arms with the pillows you've placed on the floor. Stay in this position for 10 to 20 minutes, as tolerated.

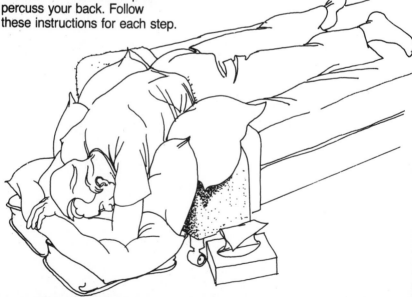

Percussion

1

Remain in the postural drainage position. Have a family member or friend position his hands in a cupped shape, with his fingers flexed and thumbs pressed tightly against his index fingers.

2

Next have him rhythmically pat your back for 3 to 5 minutes, alternating his cupped hands.

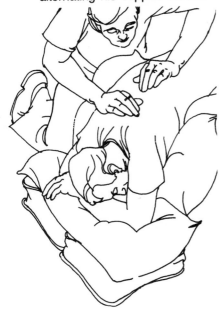

You should hear a hollow sound like a horse galloping.

Coughing

1

While remaining in the postural drainage position, take a slow, deep breath through your nose. Hold the breath as you count to yourself: one-1,000; two-1,000; three-1,000.

2

Briefly cough three times through a slightly open mouth as you breathe out. An effective cough sounds deep, low, and hollow; an ineffective one, high-pitched.

3

Next, take a slow, deep breath through your nose and breathe normally for several minutes. Repeat this coughing procedure, as tolerated.

When to perform chest physiotherapy

Unless the doctor directs otherwise, you should perform chest physiotherapy when you get up in the morning and again in the evening before you have dinner or go to bed. When you have more mucus than usual (for example, during a respiratory infection), try to increase the number of daily treatments.

BREATHING EXERCISES TO RELIEVE DYSPNEA

Dear Patient:

When you experience dyspnea, you can rely on these exercises to help you breathe easier. Practice them each day during your routine activities so they'll become second nature.

Abdominal breathing

1

Lie comfortably on your back and place a pillow beneath your head. Bend your knees to relax your abdomen.

2

Press one hand lightly on your abdomen about 5″ below your sternum, and rest the other hand on your chest.

3

Now breathe slowly through your nose, using your abdominal muscles. The hand on your

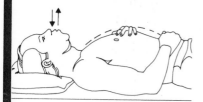

abdomen should rise during inspiration and fall during expiration. But the hand on your chest should remain almost still.

Pursed-lip breathing

1

Breathe in slowly through your nose to avoid gulping air. Hold your breath as you count to yourself: one-1,000; two-1,000; three-1,000.

2

Purse your lips as if you were going to whistle.

3

Then, breathe out slowly through pursed lips as you count to yourself: one-1,000;

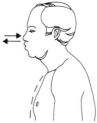

two-1,000; three-1,000; four-1,000; five-1,000; six-1,000. You should make a soft, whistling sound while you breathe out. Exhaling through pursed lips slows down your breathing and helps get rid of the stale air trapped in your lungs.

as paints and cleaners. Encourage him to carefully assess his home and workplace and to make changes to minimize his exposure to toxic inhalants.

Teach the patient about the harmful effects of smoking on respiratory function. In chronic bronchitis, respiratory function may gradually improve if the patient quits smoking. Unfortunately, the same rarely holds true in emphysema. Provide information on stopsmoking programs and refer the patient to the American Cancer Society or the American Lung Association for assistance.

Warn the patient that exposure to blasts of cold or dry air can precipitate airway spasm. Dry air can also cause his mucus to thicken. Suggest that he avoid cold wind or cover his mouth with a scarf or mask when he has to go out in the cold. Also have him maintain environmental humidity between 40% and 50%, whenever possible. A small portable humidifier works well in an enclosed area.

Teach the patient how to plan his daily activities to conserve energy and best cope with dyspnea. Advise him to alternate light and heavy tasks and to rest frequently between tasks. Remind him to use pursed-lip breathing during his activities (see *Breathing Exercises to Relieve Dyspnea*). Also instruct him to minimize body movements. For example, he should pull instead of lift, and sit instead of stand when talking, dressing, or performing other tasks. Tell him to use a cart or wagon to carry groceries and other heavy items.

Since dyspnea may interfere with sexual intercourse, discuss ways to overcome this problem with the patient and his spouse. Advise the patient to use pursed-lip breathing during intercourse to help control dyspnea. Encourage him to assume a comfortable position, such as lying on his side, that doesn't restrict his breathing. Allowing his spouse to take the more active role may also help. Suggest that the patient keep oxygen nearby in case he experiences increasing dyspnea during in-

tercourse. Have him select a time for intercourse that allows him to rest before and afterward. Above all, encourage the patient and his spouse to communicate with each other and to experiment with alternative ways to express affection.

Because the patient is susceptible to respiratory infection, teach him early symptoms of infection and key preventive measures (see *How to Detect—and Prevent—Respiratory Infection*, page 184). Also teach him symptoms of peptic ulcer disease, a complication that strikes about 20% to 25% of patients with COPD. Heartburn and indigestion are the two characteristic presenting symptoms. Instruct him to check his stool every day for occult blood. Tell him to notify the doctor if he has persistent nausea, vomiting, abdominal pain, constipation, diarrhea, or blood in his stool.

If the patient has emphysema, teach him the symptoms of spontaneous pneumothorax, an acute complication that may follow rupture of a bleb or bulla. Tell him to report sudden, sharp pleuritic pain that's exacerbated by chest movement, breathing, or coughing. Also, have the patient watch for signs of cor pulmonale, a complication of chronic bronchitis and emphysema. For example, tell him to observe for and to report increasing dyspnea, dependent edema, and bluish or mottled skin.

Explore with the patient and his family the impact of the illness on their lives. Help them identify coping mechanisms to deal with chronic anxiety and depression. Encourage them to join a support group and to contact the local chapter of the American Lung Association for more information.

Pulmonary Embolism

More than any other pulmonary disorder, pulmonary embolism is likely to complicate the recovery of hospitalized

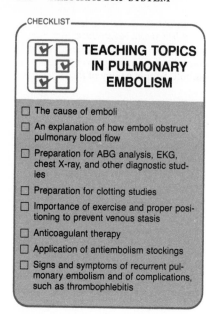

CHECKLIST

TEACHING TOPICS IN PULMONARY EMBOLISM

- ☐ The cause of emboli
- ☐ An explanation of how emboli obstruct pulmonary blood flow
- ☐ Preparation for ABG analysis, EKG, chest X-ray, and other diagnostic studies
- ☐ Preparation for clotting studies
- ☐ Importance of exercise and proper positioning to prevent venous stasis
- ☐ Anticoagulant therapy
- ☐ Application of antiembolism stockings
- ☐ Signs and symptoms of recurrent pulmonary embolism and of complications, such as thrombophlebitis

patients. As a result, you'll often encounter patients who'll need to learn about risk factors and warning symptoms of pulmonary embolism. You'll also encounter patients admitted for an acute pulmonary embolism, who require additional teaching. Because acute pulmonary embolism typically causes dyspnea, you'll be teaching a patient who's understandably anxious about his condition, but willing to comply with therapy. However, once the embolus resolves and the patient becomes asymptomatic, he may become less willing to comply with prolonged anticoagulant therapy to prevent recurrent emboli. Of course, you'll emphasize the need for such therapy. But you'll also have to emphasize the need for periodic blood studies to monitor his anticoagulant drug level, especially during the first weeks of therapy, and close observation for adverse drug effects. Similarly, you'll need to teach about symptoms of drug toxicity and safety measures to follow when taking the drug.

Describe the disorder
Explain that pulmonary embolism is a blood clot lodged in an artery of the lung. Tell the patient that the clot obstructs blood flow to a portion of the lung. As a result, this portion of the lung is ventilated, but not perfused. To compensate for this ventilation-perfusion mismatch, the patient must breathe faster and with more effort to avoid hypoxemia. He may also wheeze in response to distal airway constriction—the body's attempt to shunt ventilation from nonperfused to perfused areas of the lung.

Briefly discuss with the patient the probable cause of the pulmonary embolism: dislodged thrombi, usually originating in the deep leg veins, that form as the result of vascular wall damage, venous stasis, or hypercoagulability of the blood. The thrombi may have embolized spontaneously during clot dissolution or may have become dislodged during trauma, sudden muscular action, or a change in peripheral blood flow.

Point out possible complications
Emphasize that the patient can avoid or minimize atelectasis by strictly adhering to the treatment plan. Explain how atelectasis contributes to hypoxemia and may aggravate tachypnea and dyspnea. Note that the patient's at risk for atelectasis until the embolus resolves.

Teach about tests
Prepare the patient for tests to detect pulmonary embolism and to evaluate his response to anticoagulant therapy. To rule out other disorders, the doctor may order a chest X-ray, white blood cell count, erythrocyte sedimentation rate, fibrin split products, and serum LDH, SGOT, and serum bilirubin levels. To help confirm a pulmonary embolism, he may order a lung perfusion scan, ventilation scan, pulmonary angiography (see *Teaching Patients about Respiratory Tests*, pages 188 to 194), and an EKG. To detect peripheral venous thrombosis, he may order venography and the less specific, though noninvasive, Doppler ultrasonography

or impedance plethysmography (see *Teaching Patients about Cardiovascular Tests* in Chapter 6).

In acute pulmonary embolism, the doctor will monitor clotting time, thrombin time, or activated partial thromboplastin time to evaluate heparin therapy. Once the patient begins oral anticoagulants, the doctor will monitor prothrombin time (PT) until the desired anticoagulant level is achieved. When the patient's discharged on anticoagulant therapy, inform him that he'll need to return for periodic venipunctures to monitor PT. Usually, venipuncture will be performed once a week until PT stabilizes, then every 2 weeks and, eventually, once a month.

If necessary, prepare the patient for ABG analysis. Tell him who will perform the arterial puncture, and when and where it will be done. Also tell him which site will be used—radial, brachial, or femoral artery. Instruct the patient to breathe normally during the test, and warn him that he may experience a brief cramping or throbbing pain at the puncture site.

Teach about treatments

● *Activity.* Explain how prolonged standing, sitting, or inactivity can cause venous stasis, which sets the stage for peripheral venous thrombosis in the legs. Encourage the patient to exercise his legs as frequently as possible to promote blood flow. Show him exercises that he can easily do, such as rocking on his heels or toes. If the patient's disabled or on bed rest, teach his family how to do passive leg exercises by flexing and extending the patient's feet at the ankles.

Instruct the patient to elevate his legs 30 degrees or more whenever possible; for example, while he's watching television or working at a desk. Instruct him not to bend his knees when he elevates his legs.

Also, advise the patient to stop frequently for short walks on long car rides and to periodically stroll up and down the aisles on airplane trips.

● *Medication.* Make sure the patient understands that the prescribed anticoagulants aim to prevent recurrent emboli. Supply a copy of the home care aid *Do's and Don'ts of Anticoagulant Therapy* in Chapter 6. Teach the patient how to detect signs of drug toxicity, such as bleeding gums, epistaxis, bleeding hemorrhoids, reddish or purple skin spots, or excessive menstrual flow. (For more information on anticoagulant therapy, see *Teaching Patients about Respiratory Drugs*, pages 196 to 203.)

If the patient can't tolerate anticoagulants, the doctor may order aspirin and/or dipyridamole instead.

• *Other care measures.* Stress the importance of coughing and deep-breathing exercises to prevent atelectasis. Then, teach the patient how to apply antiembolism stockings or elastic bandage wraps to improve circulation in his legs (see *How to Apply Antiembolism Stockings* in Chapter 6). Emphasize that the stockings must fit properly and be applied smoothly. Tell him to apply them before he gets out of bed in the morning to prevent venous pooling in his feet. Also tell him to remove the stockings before retiring at night.

Advise the patient to remove throw rugs and small objects from floors to help prevent falls. If he does fall, tell him to notify his doctor. The doctor may want to examine him to rule out internal bleeding, especially in the joints.

Instruct the patient to report calf pain and swelling (signs of thrombophlebitis) or lower leg and ankle swelling, hyperpigmentation, and ulceration (signs of postphlebitis syndrome). Show him how to measure his calves to detect nontender swelling (phlebothrombosis). Caution him to report symptoms of recurrent pulmonary embolism, including dyspnea, tachypnea, chest pain, and hemoptysis. Because pulmonary embolism increases pulmonary vascular resistance and taxes cardiac function, tell the patient with underlying cardiopulmonary disease to report signs of ventricular failure: fatigue, dependent edema, unexplained steady weight gain, and chest tightness. And because pulmonary embolism can also precipitate dysrhythmias, such as atrial fibrillation or atrial flutter, tell the patient to report palpitations to his doctor.

Pulmonary Fibrosis

Other than trials of corticosteroids and cytotoxic drugs, no effective treatment exists for pulmonary fibrosis. As a result, your teaching will focus on helping the patient cope with the disorder's characteristic dyspnea and avoid potentially life-threatening respiratory infection.

To achieve the first goal, you'll need to teach the patient abdominal breathing exercises and, if appropriate, how to use oxygen at home. Because dyspnea can interfere with daily activities, you'll also need to help the patient modify his life-style. For example, by teaching him how to pace himself, you can help him to lead a fuller, more active life. To achieve the second goal, you'll need to teach the patient early signs of respiratory infection as well as preventive measures.

Living with a chronic disorder like pulmonary fibrosis will undoubtedly tax your patient's emotional resources. To improve his sense of well-being, encourage him to follow the prescribed exercise program and to eat a nutritious, well-balanced diet to maintain a healthy weight.

Describe the disorder

Explain to the patient that pulmonary fibrosis results from widespread injury to the interstitial spaces of the lung. Although the specific cause of this injury may be unknown, it's usually linked to myriad insults to the lung. To heal the lung injury, the body produces fibrous connective scar tissue. This permanent scarring, or fibrosis, prevents the lung from expanding fully, causing dyspnea, tachypnea, fatigue, and weakness. The patient may also have a dry, nonproductive cough, especially on exertion.

Point out possible complications
Tell the patient that his limited pulmonary reserve makes him susceptible to respiratory infection. By adhering to the treatment plan, though, he can reduce the risk of this complication. Note that untreated respiratory infection can lead to life-threatening acute respiratory failure.

Teach about tests
Prepare the patient for tests to confirm diagnosis of pulmonary fibrosis or to monitor its progression. Explain that the doctor will order ABG analysis to evaluate hypoxemia. Tell the patient who will perform the arterial puncture, and when and where it will be done. Also tell him which site has been selected—radial, brachial, or femoral artery. Remind the patient to breathe normally during the test, and warn him that he may experience a brief cramping or throbbing pain at the puncture site.

Also prepare the patient scheduled for pulmonary function tests or for mediastinoscopy or lung biopsy to diagnose pulmonary fibrosis. Explain that chest X-rays can help detect complications of the disorder. (See *Teaching Patients about Respiratory Tests*, pages 188 to 194, and "Surgery," page 195, for more information about these tests.) Also explain that an exercise EKG may be ordered to help determine the patient's exercise tolerance.

Teach about treatments
• *Activity.* After evaluating the patient's exercise EKG, the doctor may prescribe an individual exercise program. Emphasize that this program aims to increase the patient's endurance and strength without causing him severe dyspnea. Also explain how ex-

---

CHECKLIST

TEACHING TOPICS IN PULMONARY FIBROSIS

☐ An explanation of how diffuse interstitial lung injury results in permanent scarring, or fibrosis

☐ Warning signs of respiratory infection and preventive measures

☐ Preparation for diagnostic mediastinoscopy or lung biopsy, ABG analysis, and pulmonary function tests to monitor the disorder

☐ Exercise program

☐ Importance of well-balanced diet and increased caloric intake, if appropriate

☐ How to use oxygen at home

☐ Life-style changes to cope with dyspnea

☐ Abdominal breathing exercises

☐ Availability of support groups, such as the American Lung Association

---

ercise can improve his sense of well-being. Teach the patient and a family member how to take an accurate radial pulse to monitor the effects of his exercise program (see *How to Take Your Pulse* in Chapter 6).

• *Diet.* Explain to the patient the importance of a well-balanced, nutritious diet to compensate for the extra calories he expends just to breathe. Because dyspnea can discourage eating and lead to weight loss, teach the patient how to maintain his caloric intake. First, encourage frequent oral hygiene to stimulate his appetite and enjoyment of food. If the patient has severe dyspnea, advise him to eat small, frequent meals to reduce fatigue and air swallowing during eating. Also encourage him to chew his food slowly. Finally, recommend that he eat nutritious snacks (including fluids like fruit juices) or drink a liquid enteral supplement for additional calories between meals.

Unless contraindicated, encourage the patient to drink plenty of water—at least six glasses daily—to thin his

184

HOW TO DETECT—AND PREVENT— RESPIRATORY INFECTION

Dear Patient:

Your condition makes you an easy target for respiratory infection. That's why the doctor wants you to be alert for warning signs of infection and to take steps to prevent infection.

Warning signs

Respiratory infection can worsen quickly. Call your doctor immediately if you develop any of these signs:
- fever
- worsening cough or wheezing
- increasing difficulty breathing
- changes in your mucus: thicker, increased or decreased in amount, foul-smelling, or appearing green, yellow, brown, pink, or red
- unusual fatigue or weakness
- swollen ankles
- gain or loss of more than 5 lb in a week
- confusion, decreased alertness, or memory loss.

Preventive steps

To help prevent respiratory infection, follow these steps:
- Eat a well-balanced, nutritious diet.
- Drink at least six glasses of water a day, unless the doctor directs otherwise.
- Get at least 7 to 8 hours of sleep at night, and take frequent, short rest breaks during the day.

- Perform chest physiotherapy and use supplemental oxygen, as directed.
- Take your drugs exactly as prescribed.
- Rinse your oral inhaler after each use.

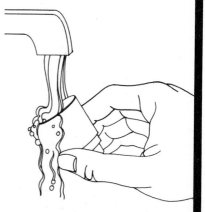

- Avoid people who have a cold or the flu. If you can't avoid them, wear a disposable surgical mask when around them.
- Check with your doctor about flu vaccines.
- Avoid exposure to inhaled pollutants, such as cigarette smoke, noxious industrial fumes, and car exhaust.
- Carefully wash your hands before taking your prescribed drugs or setting up oxygen equipment. Also wash them after handling tissues soiled with mucus, and before and after using the bathroom.

mucus. Adequate fluid intake will also help prevent constipation and avoid breathlessness associated with straining during defecation. Tell the patient to include fresh fruits, vegetables, and bran in his diet to help prevent constipation. If the patient is obese, explain how obesity interferes with diaphragmatic movement and increases cardiac work load. This, in turn, can make breathing even more difficult. Suggest a weight-reduction program, if appropriate.

• *Medication.* Most patients with pulmonary fibrosis do not respond adequately to drug therapy. However, the doctor may attempt a trial of corticosteroids or cytotoxic drugs. Explain that such drugs will be discontinued if the patient's ABG values or pulmonary function tests show no improvement after drug therapy.

• *Procedures.* If appropriate, teach the patient and a family member how to use portable oxygen (see *Using Oxygen Safely and Effectively*, pages 186 and 187). When he's planning a trip, instruct the patient to obtain advance information about oxygen regulations on the plane, train, or bus. For example, tell him to call the airline to ensure that enough oxygen will be aboard to make the trip and to circle in a holding pattern. Before takeoff, he should double-check the availability of sufficient oxygen. Make sure he understands that he'll experience the effects of high altitude even in the pressurized cabin of a commercial airliner. Instruct him to use his breathing exercises to help minimize his dyspnea. Also, advise him to contact a medical equipment supplier at his travel destination so that the necessary equipment will be ready upon his arrival.

• *Other care measures.* Advise the patient to avoid inhaled pollutants—such as cigarette smoke, aerosol sprays, and industrial fumes—which may aggravate his dyspnea. Then teach the patient to organize his daily activities to conserve energy. Suggest that he alternate light and heavy tasks and rest frequently between tasks. Teach him to use abdominal breathing exercises when he performs heavy tasks (see *Breathing Exercises to Relieve Dyspnea*, page 178).

Tell the patient to minimize body movements, whenever possible. For example, he should pull instead of lift and sit instead of stand when talking, dressing, or performing other routine tasks. Instruct him to use a cart or wagon to carry groceries, laundry, and other heavy objects.

Because dyspnea may interfere with sexual intercourse, discuss ways to overcome this problem with the patient and his spouse. Advise the patient to assume a comfortable position, such as lying on his side, that doesn't restrict his breathing. Allowing his spouse to take the more active role may also help. Above all, encourage the patient and his spouse to communicate with each other and to try alternate ways of showing affection.

Warn the patient that untreated respiratory infection can lead to life-threatening respiratory failure. Instruct him to report early signs of infection (see *How to Detect—and Prevent—Respiratory Infection*, page 184). Also instruct him to report symptoms of spontaneous pneumothorax: a sudden, sharp, pleuritic pain that's exacerbated by movement, breathing, or coughing; and shortness of breath. Lastly, instruct the patient to report warning symptoms of cor pulmonale, a chronic complication of pulmonary fibrosis that's marked by progressively worsening dyspnea, leg edema, fatigue, and weakness.

Be sure to explore with the patient and his family the impact of pulmonary fibrosis on their lives. Help them identify coping mechanisms to deal with chronic anxiety and depression. Encourage them to contact the local chapter of the American Lung Association for more information. In addition, you can recommend that the patient join a support group, such as the Better Breathing Club.

USING OXYGEN SAFELY AND EFFECTIVELY

Dear Patient:

To help you breathe easier at home, your doctor wants you to receive extra oxygen. You'll be using an oxygen concentrator, a liquid oxygen unit, or an oxygen tank. Your prescribed oxygen flow rate is _____ liters per minute for _____ hours each day.

When you obtain your home oxygen system from your medical equipment supplier, he'll teach you how to set it up, check for problems, and clean it properly. Your oxygen system will include a humidifier to warm and add moisture to the prescribed oxygen, and a nasal cannula or a face mask to breathe the oxygen. Make sure you keep the supplier's phone number handy in case the system doesn't work. Also arrange to get a backup system—a small portable oxygen tank is usually best. In an emergency (for example, a power failure), this will protect you from being without needed oxygen.

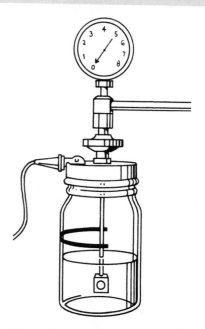

General guidelines
When using an oxygen tank, an oxygen concentrator, or liquid oxygen, be sure to follow these important guidelines:
● Check the water level in the humidifier bottle often. If it's near or below the refill line,

pour out any water remaining in the bottle and refill it with sterile or distilled water.
● If your nostrils become dry or cracked, apply a water-soluble lubricant, such as K-Y brand jelly. Avoid using a petroleum-based lubricant, such as Vaseline.
● Always reorder a new supply of oxygen 2 or 3 days in advance or when the register reads ¼ full so that you don't run out.
● Maintain your oxygen flow at the prescribed rate. If you're not sure whether oxygen is flowing through the system, first check the tubing for kinks or other obstruction. Then, double-

check that the system's turned on. If you're still unsure, try this test: invert the nasal can-

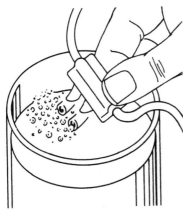

nula in a glass of water. If bubbles appear, oxygen is flowing through the system. Be sure to shake off excess water before you reinsert the cannula.

Safety tips

• Remember that oxygen is highly combustible. Alert your local fire department that oxygen is in the house, and keep an all-purpose fire extinguisher on hand.

• If a fire does occur, turn off the oxygen immediately and leave the house.

• Don't smoke—or allow others to smoke—near your oxygen system. Keep the system away from open flames and heat. If you have a gas stove, stay out of the kitchen when it's on. Don't run oxygen tubing under clothing, bedcovers, furniture, or carpets.

• Keep the oxygen system upright. Make sure the system's turned off when it's not in use.

When to call your doctor

To use oxygen effectively, you need to know when you're not getting enough oxygen—and when you're getting too much.

You may not be getting enough oxygen if you notice these signs:

• difficult, irregular breathing
• restlessness
• anxiety
• tiredness or drowsiness
• blue fingernail beds or lips
• confusion or inability to concentrate.

You may be getting too much oxygen if you notice these signs:

• headaches
• slurred speech
• sleepiness or difficulty waking up
• shallow, slow breathing.

If any of these signs develop, call your doctor immediately. Above all, *never change the oxygen flow rate* without checking with him first.

TEACHING PATIENTS ABOUT RESPIRATORY TESTS

TEST AND PURPOSE	TEACHING POINTS
Bronchography • To help diagnose bronchiectasis, bronchial obstruction, bronchial tumors, and bronchial tears • To help rule out bronchial causes of hemoptysis • To provide guidance while performing a bronchoscopy	• Explain to the patient that this radiologic test helps evaluate abnormalities of the bronchial structures. Tell him who will perform the test, and where and when it will be done. • Describe the pre-test restrictions: the patient mustn't eat or drink for 12 hours before the test. However, he should continue any prescribed drugs unless the doctor orders otherwise. • Explain what will happen before the test: the patient's bronchial hygiene program—including postural drainage and use of expectorants—may be intensified for 24 hours before the test to clear his airways of mucus. Tell him to perform good oral hygiene the night before and the morning of the test. Just before the test, instruct him to remove his dentures, if appropriate, and to void. • Explain what will happen during the test: if the test is being performed under a local anesthetic, tell the patient he'll receive a sedative to help him relax. Prepare him for the unpleasant taste and coldness of the anesthetic spray used to suppress the gag reflex. Assure him that he'll receive enough oxygen during the test, although he may experience increased dyspnea. Emphasize that the catheter or bronchoscope will pass more easily if he's relaxed. Explain that an anesthetic and a radiopaque dye will be instilled after the bronchoscope or catheter is passed into the trachea. Tell him to immediately report hoarseness, dyspnea, wheezing, itching, palpitations, irritability, excitation, or euphoria. These signs may herald an allergic reaction to the dye or anesthetic. As X-rays are taken, the patient will be asked to assume various positions to move the dye into different airways. After the X-rays are taken, the dye will be removed through bronchial hygiene maneuvers. • Describe what will happen after the test: the patient's blood pressure, heart rate, and respirations will be monitored for 10 to 15 minutes. He should lie on his side or sit with his head elevated at least 30 degrees until his gag reflex returns. Explain that food, fluid, and oral drugs will be withheld for about 2 hours after the test or until the gag reflex returns. Reassure him that a sore throat is temporary, and that he can have throat lozenges or a liquid gargle when his gag reflex returns.
Bronchoscopy • To visually examine a possible tumor, secretions, or other obstruction, as demonstrated on an X-ray • To help diagnose the cause of dyspnea and other respiratory symptoms • To help diagnose bron-	• Explain to the patient that this test allows direct examination of his airways. Tell him who will perform the test, where and when it will be done, and that it takes 45 to 60 minutes. • Describe the pre-test restrictions: the patient mustn't eat or drink for 6 hours before the test. However, he should continue taking any prescribed drugs unless the doctor orders otherwise. • Explain what will happen during the test: if the test is being done under a local anesthetic, tell the patient that he may receive a sedative to help him relax. Prepare him for the unpleasant taste and coldness of the anesthetic spray used to

TEACHING PATIENTS ABOUT
RESPIRATORY TESTS *(continued)*

TEST AND PURPOSE	TEACHING POINTS
Bronchoscopy *(continued)* chogenic carcinoma, tuberculosis, interstitial pulmonary disease, or fungal or parasitic pulmonary infection by obtaining a tissue or mucous specimen for examination • To locate a bleeding site in the tracheobronchial tree • To remove foreign bodies, mucous plugs, or excessive secretions from the airways	suppress the gag reflex. • Explain that he'll probably be positioned supinely on a table or bed, although he may be asked to sit upright in a chair. Tell him to remain relaxed, with his arms at his sides, and to breathe through his nose during the test. Mention that the doctor will introduce the bronchoscope tube through the patient's nose or mouth into the airway. Then he'll flush small amounts of anesthetic through the tube to suppress coughing and wheezing. Reassure the patient that although he may experience dyspnea during the test, he won't suffocate and that oxygen will be administered through the bronchoscope. • Describe what will happen after the test: the patient's blood pressure, heart rate, and respirations will be monitored for about 15 minutes. He should lie on his side or sit with his head elevated at least 30 degrees until his gag reflex returns. Food, fluid, and oral drugs will be withheld for about 2 hours or until his gag reflex returns. Reassure him that hoarseness or a sore throat is temporary. He can have throat lozenges or liquid gargle when his gag reflex returns. • Tell the patient to report bloody mucus, dyspnea, wheezing, or chest pain to the nurse immediately. Tell him that a chest X-ray will be taken after the test and that he may receive an aerosolized bronchodilator treatment.
Chest radiography (chest X-ray, chest roentgenography) • To detect pulmonary disorders, such as pneumonia, atelectasis, pneumothorax, pulmonary bullae, and tumors • To detect mediastinal abnormalities, such as tumors, and cardiac disease • To evaluate the effectiveness of therapy	• Explain to the patient that this test detects or monitors the progress of respiratory disorders. Tell him who will perform the test, where and when it will be done, and that it takes only minutes. However, the technician or doctor will need additional time to check the quality of the films. • Describe what will happen before the test: the patient must don a gown without snaps but may keep his pants, socks, and shoes on. Instruct him to remove all jewelry from his neck and chest. • Explain what will happen during the test: if the test is performed in the radiology department, the patient will stand or sit in front of a machine. If it's performed at bedside, someone will help him to a sitting position and place a cold, hard film plate behind his back. He'll be asked to take a deep breath and to hold it for a few seconds while the X-ray is taken. He should remain still for those few seconds. Reassure him that the amount of radiation exposure is minimal. Hospital personnel will leave the area when the technician takes the X-ray because they're potentially exposed to radiation many times a day.
Closed lung biopsy • To confirm diagnosis of diffuse parenchymal disease, such as pulmonary fibrosis, and of pulmonary lesions, such as cancer or abscess	• Explain that this test confirms the cause of his respiratory disorder. Tell him who will perform the test, where and when it will be done, and that it takes 30 to 60 minutes. • Outline the pretest restrictions and describe what will happen before the test. *(For transbronchial biopsy, refer to the information under Bronchoscopy; for needle biopsy, refer to Thoracentesis.)*

(continued)

**TEACHING PATIENTS ABOUT
RESPIRATORY TESTS** *(continued)*

TEST AND PURPOSE	TEACHING POINTS
Closed lung biopsy *(continued)*	• Explain what will happen during the test. (Supplement your teaching from Bronchoscopy or Thoracentesis, as appropriate.) For transbronchial biopsy, the doctor will pass biopsy forceps through the bronchoscope to obtain a tissue specimen. For needle biopsy, he'll make a small incision, then insert the biopsy needle through the incision to obtain a tissue specimen. • Describe what will happen after the test: the patient's blood pressure, heart rate, and respiratory rate will be monitored frequently for the first few hours. Explain that a chest X-ray will be taken after the test to detect complications and that the patient's chest will be assessed frequently. Warn him that he may expectorate pink or blood-tinged mucus for several hours after the test. However, he should notify the nurse or doctor of frank bleeding or large blood clots. (See Bronchoscopy or Thoracentesis.)
Computed tomography scan (CT scan, thoracic computed tomography) • To locate or monitor lesions in the lungs, mediastinum, thoracic lymph nodes, blood vessels, or other tissues	• Explain to the patient that this test uses state-of-the-art computer technology to help diagnose or evaluate respiratory disorders. Tell him who will perform the test, and where and when it will be done. Note whether a radioactive dye will be used to enhance the cross-sectional images of his chest. • Describe the pre-test preparations: if a contrast dye will be used, instruct the patient to fast for 4 hours before the test. Just before the test, have him remove all jewelry. • Explain what will happen during the test: the patient will lie supine on a cold, hard X-ray table that moves into the center of a large, noisy, tunnel-shaped machine. When the dye is injected into his arm vein, he may experience transient nausea, flushing, warmth, and a salty taste. Tell him not to move during the test, but to relax and breathe normally. Movement may invalidate the results and require repeat testing. Reassure him that radiation exposure during the test is minimal.
Exercise electrocardiography (exercise EKG, stress test) • To help diagnose the cause of dyspnea • To help evaluate the effectiveness of bronchodilator therapy • To assess the degree of pulmonary dysfunction • To help plan or evaluate an exercise program	• Explain that this test evaluates cardiopulmonary function while the patient walks a treadmill or pedals a bicycle. Tell him who will perform the test, where and when it will be done, and that it may take several hours. • Describe the pretest restrictions: the patient shouldn't eat, drink alcohol, or smoke for 3 hours before the test. However, he should continue any drug therapy unless the doctor directs otherwise. • Describe the physical preparation for the test: the patient should rest before the test. Advise him to wear comfortable socks and shoes and loose, lightweight shorts or slacks; men usually don't wear a shirt during the test, and women usually wear a bra and a lightweight short-sleeved blouse or a patient gown with front closure. Also tell the patient that a technician will cleanse, shave (if necessary), and abrade several sites on the patient's chest and, possibly, back. Then the technician will attach electrodes at these sites. He will also apply a blood pressure cuff and attach an oximeter ear clip to the patient.

TEACHING PATIENTS ABOUT
RESPIRATORY TESTS *(continued)*

TEST AND PURPOSE	TEACHING POINTS
Exercise electrocardiography *(continued)*	• Explain what will happen during the test: if the patient's scheduled for a multistage treadmill test, tell him that the treadmill speed and incline increase at predetermined intervals and that he'll be told of each adjustment. If he's scheduled for a bicycle ergometer test, tell him that resistance to pedaling gradually increases as he tries to maintain a specific speed. He'll be asked to breathe in and out of a mouthpiece during the test, and may need to wear a noseclip. Be sure to tell the patient that he can stop the test if he experiences severe fatigue or dyspnea. Typically, he'll feel tired, out of breath, and sweaty. However, he should report any feelings during the test. Reassure him that his heart and lung function will be closely monitored. Tell him that he may receive low-flow nasal oxygen during the test to see whether this therapy improves his cardiopulmonary function. • Note that the patient's blood pressure and EKG will be monitored for 10 to 15 minutes after the test.
Lung scan (lung perfusion scan, lung scintigraphy) • To detect and assess pulmonary vascular obstruction, such as pulmonary emboli	• Explain to the patient that this test evaluates blood flow in the lungs. Tell him who will perform the test, where and when it will be done, and that it takes about 30 minutes. • Explain what will happen during the test: the patient will lie supine on a table as a radioactive protein substance is injected into an arm vein. A large camera will take pictures while the patient's supine, then lying on his side, prone, and sitting. More dye will be injected when the patient's on his stomach. Reassure him that the amount of radioactivity in the dye is minimal. However, he may experience some discomfort from the venipuncture and from lying on a cold, hard table.
Magnetic resonance imaging (MRI) (nuclear magnetic resonance [NMR] scan) • To help diagnose respiratory disorders by providing high-resolution, cross-sectional images of lung structures and by tracing blood flow	• Explain to the patient that this painless, noninvasive test relies on a powerful magnet, radio waves, and a computer to produce clear cross-sectional images of the chest. Tell him who will perform the test and when. Mention that it will be done in a special building that shields the MRI scanner's powerful magnetic field. • Describe the preparation for the test: the patient must remove all jewelry and take everything out of his pockets. Emphasize that there must be *no* metal in the test room. The powerful magnet may strip the magnetic stripe off a credit card or stop a watch from ticking. Make sure the patient has notified his doctor if he has any metal inside his body, such as a pacemaker or orthopedic pins or disks. • Explain what will happen during the test: the patient will lie on a table that slides into an 8'-long tunnel inside the magnet. Tell him that he should breathe normally but not talk or move during the test to avoid distorting the results. Warn the patient that the machinery will be noisy, with sounds ranging from an incessant ping to a loud bang. He may feel claustrophobic or bored. Encourage him to relax and try to concentrate on a favorite subject or image, or on his breathing.

(continued)

**TEACHING PATIENTS ABOUT
RESPIRATORY TESTS** (continued)

TEST AND PURPOSE	TEACHING POINTS
Mediastinoscopy • To detect bronchogenic carcinoma, lymphoma, and sarcoidosis • To determine staging of lung cancer	• Explain to the patient that this test allows the doctor to visualize and biopsy the mediastinal area and thereby confirm his diagnosis. Tell him who will perform this surgical procedure, and when and where it will be done. • Describe the preparation for the test: the patient mustn't eat or drink for 8 hours before the test. He'll receive an I.V. sedative before the test and then a general anesthetic. • Explain what will happen during the test: after inserting an endotracheal tube, the surgeon will make a small transverse suprasternal incision. He'll insert a mediastinoscope through this incision to obtain tissue specimens for analysis. • Describe what happens after the test: the patient may remain intubated for several hours or overnight. Tell him where he will go after the test (recovery room, medical/surgical unit, intensive care) and that his vital signs and dressing will be checked frequently for the first 4 hours. Warn the patient that he may have pain or tenderness at the incision site, a sore throat, and hoarseness. He may also experience nausea, vomiting, and a sense of unreality from the anesthetic. Reassure him that the side effects are temporary and that he may request analgesics for pain.
Paranasal sinus radiography • To detect sinus abnormalities, such as cysts or tumors, infection, and fractures	• Explain to the patient that this test helps evaluate sinus abnormalities. Tell him who will perform the test, and where and when it will be done. Mention the need to remove dentures, jewelry, and any hairpins or barrettes before the test. • Explain what will happen during the test: the patient will sit upright between the X-ray tube and a cold, hard film cassette. During the test, the X-ray tube will be positioned at various angles and his head will be placed in several different positions. Emphasize that he must remain still while the X-rays are being taken, to prevent blurring of the image. His head may be immobilized in a foam vise to help him maintain the correct position, but this won't be painful.
Pulmonary angiography (pulmonary arteriography) • To confirm diagnosis of pulmonary emboli	• Explain to the patient that this test allows confirmation of pulmonary emboli. Tell him who will perform the test, where and when it will be done, and that it takes about 1 hour. • Describe the pretest restrictions: the patient must fast for 6 hours before the test, or as ordered. He may continue his prescribed drugs unless the doctor orders otherwise. • Describe the preparation for the test: the patient should remove his clothing, except for socks, and don a gown that fastens in the front. Instruct him to void just before the test. • Explain what will happen during the test: the patient will need to remove the gown, but will be covered with sheets and sterile drapes. Tell him that he'll lie supine on a table during the test. The nurse will attach EKG electrodes, apply a blood pressure cuff, and start an I.V. line. After injecting a local anesthetic, the doctor will make a cutdown incision or a percutaneous needle puncture in an antecubital, femoral, jugular, or subclavian vein. Warn the patient that he may feel pressure. Next, the doctor will insert and advance a catheter

TEACHING PATIENTS ABOUT
RESPIRATORY TESTS *(continued)*

TEST AND PURPOSE	TEACHING POINTS
Pulmonary angiography *(continued)*	through the vein to the right side of the heart and the pulmonary artery, where he measures pressures and withdraws blood samples. Inform the patient that a radiopaque dye will be injected into the catheter. Warn him that he may experience a flushed feeling, nausea, or a salty taste for a few minutes after the dye's injected. X-ray films will be taken as the dye circulates through the pulmonary vessels. When the test is completed, the catheter will be withdrawn and a pressure dressing will be applied to the insertion site. Instruct the patient to tell the doctor if he experiences dyspnea, palpitations, chest pain, persistent nausea, paresthesias, or wheezing during the test. • Describe what will happen after the test: the patient's vital signs will be monitored during the first hour or two, and the catheter insertion site will be checked. If a femoral or antecubital vein was used, the patient may need to restrict activity in the affected limb for 4 to 6 hours. Instruct him to report wheezing, palpitations, chest pain, itching, nausea, vomiting, irritability, or euphoria after the test. Also tell him to report redness, swelling, or bleeding at the insertion site.

Pulmonary function tests
• To determine the cause of dyspnea
• To evaluate disability for legal or insurance purposes
• To determine whether a functional abnormality is obstructive or restrictive
• To estimate the degree of pulmonary dysfunction in obstructive and restrictive diseases
• To evaluate the effectiveness of therapy, such as use of bronchodilators or steroids
	• Explain to the patient that these tests evaluate his pulmonary function. Tell him who will perform the test, and where and when it will be done.
	• Describe the pretest restrictions: the patient mustn't smoke for 4 hours before the test and must avoid eating a large meal or drinking a large amount of fluid before the test.
	• Describe the preparation for the test: the patient should put on loose, comfortable clothing. If he wears dentures, advise him to keep them in to help form a tight seal around the mouthpiece. Just before the test, instruct him to void.
	• Explain what will happen during the test: he'll sit upright and need to wear a noseclip. Or he may sit in a small airtight box called a body plethysmograph. Then he won't need a noseclip. Warn him that he may experience claustrophobia. Assure him that he won't suffocate and that he can communicate with the technician through the window in the box.
	  Tell him that he'll be asked to breathe a certain way for each test; for example, to inhale deeply and exhale completely, or to inhale quickly. Explain that he may receive an aerosolized bronchodilator and may then repeat one or two tests to evaluate the drug's effectiveness. An arterial puncture may also be performed during the test for ABG analysis.
	  Emphasize that the test will proceed quickly if the patient follows directions, tries hard, and keeps a tight seal around the mouthpiece or tube to ensure accurate results.
	  Tell the patient that he may experience dyspnea and fatigue during the test but will be allowed to rest periodically. Instruct him to inform the technician if he experiences dizziness, chest pain, palpitations, nausea, severe dyspnea, or wheezing. He should also report swelling or bleeding from the arterial puncture site and any paresthesias or pain in the affected limb.

(continued)

**TEACHING PATIENTS ABOUT
RESPIRATORY TESTS** *(continued)*

TEST AND PURPOSE	TEACHING POINTS
Thoracentesis (pleural fluid aspiration) • To obtain a specimen of pleural fluid for analysis • To relieve lung compression caused by pleural fluid, blood, or air • To obtain a lung tissue biopsy specimen	• Explain to the patient that this test provides samples of tissue or fluid from around the lungs to help diagnose his respiratory disorder. It may also be done therapeutically to relieve respiratory distress. Tell him who will perform the test, and where and when it will be done. • Describe the preparation for the test: the patient will need to don a hospital gown. After his vital signs are taken, the area around the needle insertion site will be shaved. • Explain what will happen during the test: the patient will be comfortably positioned—either sitting with his arms on pillows or an overbed table or lying partially on his side in bed. The doctor will clean the needle insertion site with a cold antiseptic solution, then inject a local anesthetic. Warn the patient that he may feel a burning sensation as the doctor injects the anesthetic. After the patient's skin is numb, the doctor will insert the needle. Warn the patient that he will feel pressure during needle insertion and withdrawal. Instruct him to remain still during the test, to avoid the risk of lung injury. Encourage him to relax and breathe normally during the test, and warn him not to cough, breathe deeply, or move. Tell him to notify the doctor if he experiences dyspnea, palpitations, wheezing, dizziness, weakness, or diaphoresis; these may indicate respiratory distress. After withdrawing the needle, the doctor will apply slight pressure and then an adhesive bandage. • Describe what will happen after the test: the patient's vital signs will be monitored frequently for the first few hours. Instruct him to report any fluid or blood leakage from the needle insertion site as well as signs of respiratory distress. Explain that a chest X-ray will be taken to detect any post-test complications.
Ventilation scan • To assess general and regional lung ventilation • To help diagnose respiratory disorders, such as pulmonary embolism and chronic obstructive pulmonary disease	• Explain to the patient that this test evaluates lung ventilation during respiration. Tell him who will perform the test, where and when it will be done, and that it takes about 30 minutes. • Describe the pretest restrictions: the patient must avoid eating a large meal, drinking a large volume of fluids, and smoking for 3 hours before the test. He may continue to take his medications, unless the doctor orders otherwise. • Before the test, have the patient remove all jewelry and metal objects. • Explain what will happen during the test: the patient will be asked to sit down and to breathe a radioactive gas through a mouthpiece or a tightly fitted face mask. A nuclear scanner will monitor the gas distribution in the lungs. Tell the patient that he'll be instructed to breathe deeply, hold his breath, breathe out, and then breathe normally. Instruct him to remain still when he's asked to hold his breath. Assure him that the amount of radioactive gas used is minimal and that it's mixed with air. Tell him to report any dyspnea or wheezing during the test.

SURGERY

Thoracotomy—the surgical incision of the chest wall—may be performed to diagnose a respiratory disorder or to treat its complications. For example, the doctor may perform a thoracotomy for open lung biopsy to diagnose lung cancer or pulmonary fibrosis. Or, he may perform this surgery to suture ruptured blebs or bullae associated with emphysema or pulmonary fibrosis, or to drain an empyema or repair a bronchopleural fistula associated with chronic bronchitis.

Before thoracotomy, you'll need to teach the patient about the surgery and outline postoperative care measures.

Explain thoracotomy
Begin by telling the patient why the doctor has scheduled the thoracotomy. Then, point out where he'll make the incision—posterolateral, anterolateral, anterior, lateral, or mediastinal. Next, teach the patient about possible complications—most notably, atelectasis and acute respiratory failure. Explain how chronic respiratory disease limits cardiopulmonary reserve and increases his risk of complications. Tell him that treatment measures will aim to minimize atelectasis and to promptly reverse it. Note that significant atelectasis could prolong his need for intubation and mechanical ventilation as well as lead to pneumonia, sepsis, and acute respiratory failure.

Outline postoperative care
To encourage cooperation, discuss these measures with the patient.
• *Endotracheal intubation.* Tell the patient he'll remain intubated for 4 to 6 hours after surgery, or perhaps overnight, to support his breathing and/or to clear mucus from his lungs. Warn

him that the endotracheal tube may be uncomfortable and that he won't be able to talk while it's in place. Instruct him not to try to remove the tube, since this can cause larnygeal injury.

Explain that his mucus will be suctioned through the tube, possibly causing brief dyspnea and coughing. Assure him that he'll receive extra breaths with an Ambu bag or on the respirator after suctioning.
• *Chest tube placement.* Unless the patient's scheduled for a pneumonectomy, tell him he'll have a chest tube in place after surgery, to drain blood and fluid and to help expand his lung. Note that the chest tube drainage system will be attached to suction, which makes a bubbling noise. Warn the patient that the chest tube will cause discomfort.
• *Positioning.* Prepare the patient for frequent position changes after surgery. Usually, he'll be repositioned at least once an hour immediately after surgery and then every 2 hours for the first day after surgery.
• *Bronchial hygiene.* Emphasize the importance of coughing and deep-breathing exercises after surgery. Show the patient how to splint his incision.

Also teach him segmental breathing exercises, using biofeedback. Have the patient place his hand over the anticipated incision site and apply moderate pressure. Then, tell him to relax and concentrate on getting air to the lung segment underneath his hand. Have him practice pursed-lip breathing until he can expand this segment with minimal effort.
• *Pain control.* Tell the patient that he'll receive analgesics postoperatively, but the dosage won't be strong enough to fully relieve pain. Explain that analgesics depress respiration and interfere with bronchial hygiene.
• *Activity.* Tell the patient that as soon as his vital signs are stable, he'll be assisted with dangling, sitting, and ambulation. Teach him ankle circles and leg- and arm-raising exercises to do while he's in bed.

TEACHING PATIENTS ABOUT RESPIRATORY DRUGS

DRUG	ADVERSE REACTIONS	INTERACTIONS*
Anticoagulants		
heparin (Liquaemin, Lipo-Hepin)	*Reportable:* bleeding gums, signs of internal bleeding (bloody urine, tarry stools, hemoptysis, vomiting blood), unusually heavy bleeding from menses or cuts and wounds, easy bruising, epistaxis	• Instruct the patient not to take aspirin, other salicylates, and nonsteroidal anti-inflammatory drugs, such as ibuprofen, to avoid increased risk of bleeding. • Tell the patient that foods and beverages don't influence the safety or effectiveness of heparin.
warfarin (Coumadin, Panwarfin)	*Reportable:* bleeding gums, signs of internal bleeding (bloody urine, tarry stools, hemoptysis, vomiting blood), unusually heavy bleeding from menses or cuts and wounds, dark blue toes, easy bruising, chills, prolonged diarrhea, epistaxis, fatigue, fever, sore throat *Other:* diarrhea, ecchymoses, slight hair loss, nausea	• Instruct the patient to avoid aspirin, regular use of acetaminophen, and high doses of vitamins A and E; he may take an occasional dose of ibuprofen with his doctor's permission. • Tell him to limit his alcohol consumption to 1 or 2 drinks per day. • Because vitamin K counteracts warfarin, stress the need to maintain a consistent intake of vitamin K and of fats, which enhance vitamin K absorption. Explain that this is necessary to precisely adjust his warfarin dosage.
Antihistamines		
azatadine (Optimine) **brompheniramine** (Dimetane) **chlorpheniramine** (Chlor-Trimeton, Teldrin) **clemastine** (Tavist) **dexchlorpheniramine** (Polaramine)	*Reportable:* unusual bleeding or bruising, severe drowsiness, severe dry mouth or throat, unusual fatigue or weakness, fever, hallucinations, sore throat *Other:* anorexia; blurred vision; thickened bronchial secretions; mild drowsiness; mild dry nose, mouth, or throat; insomnia; irritability; tremors	• Tell the patient that foods and nonalcoholic beverages don't influence the safety or effectiveness of these antihistamines. • Advise against taking these drugs with alcohol to avoid increased CNS depression. • Inform him that many over-the-counter cough and cold medicines contain antihistamines or alcohol. These may increase CNS depression and should be avoided if possible.
terfenadine (Seldane)	*Reportable:* sweating; visual disturbances; wheezing; yellowing of the skin, mucous membranes, and sclera *Other:* dizziness, mild drowsiness, dry mouth and throat, nausea	• Tell the patient that foods, beverages, and over-the-counter drugs don't influence the safety or effectiveness of terfenadine.

*Interactions include foods, alcohol, and over-the-counter drugs.

TEACHING POINTS

• Explain to the patient that this drug helps treat or prevent pulmonary emboli.
• Teach him how to properly administer an injection to prepare for self-care at home.
• Urge the patient to comply with regular checkups to monitor the drug's effectiveness.

• Advise against contact sports to avoid injuries. Also, tell him to use a soft toothbrush and to shave with an electric razor instead of a straight razor.
• Suggest that he wear a Medic Alert bracelet to identify himself as a heparin user.

• Explain to the patient that this drug helps treat or prevent pulmonary emboli.
• Tell him to make up a missed dose within 8 hours. He must not double-dose.
• Inform the patient that he'll need frequent blood tests to monitor the drug's effects.
• Suggest that he wear a Medic Alert bracelet to identify himself as a warfarin user.
• Teach him measures to reduce the risk of

bleeding, such as placing a nonslip mat in the bathtub, shaving with an electric razor, using a soft toothbrush, and wearing gloves for yard work.
• Warn the female patient of childbearing age to avoid becoming pregnant. Warfarin can adversely affect fetal development or cause placental bleeding.

• Explain to the patient that antihistamines help control symptoms associated with allergy, the common cold, or sinusitis.
• Inform him that antihistamines may cause drowsiness so he must be extremely cautious when using tools, walking up and down stairs, and driving a motor vehicle.
• Advise the patient to take the drug with food or milk to avoid gastric upset.
• Suggest that he chew sugarless gum, ice chips, or hard candy to help relieve mouth

and throat dryness. Tell him to drink extra fluids to help thin bronchial secretions.
• Since long-term use of antihistamines can cause blood dyscrasias, emphasize that the patient must comply with scheduled blood tests.
• Tell the patient that antihistamines interfere with the skin-test response in a desensitization program for allergy. Therefore, the doctor may temporarily discontinue the drug.

• Explain to the patient that this drug should help control symptoms associated with allergy, the common cold, or sinusitis.
• Tell him that this drug usually causes less drowsiness than other antihistamines.

• Advise the patient to take the drug with food or milk to avoid gastric upset.
• Suggest that he chew sugarless gum, ice chips, or hard candy to help relieve mouth and throat dryness.

(continued)

TEACHING PATIENTS ABOUT
RESPIRATORY DRUGS *(continued)*

DRUG	ADVERSE REACTIONS	INTERACTIONS*
Corticosteroids		
Inhalable and intranasal **beclomethasone** (Beclovent Oral Inhaler, Beconase Nasal Inhaler, Vancenase Nasal Inhaler, Vanceril Inhaler) **dexamethasone** (Decadron Phosphate Respihaler) **flunisolide** (AeroBid Inhaler, Nasalide) **triamcinolone** (Azmacort)	*Reportable:* bleeding from or ulceration of nasal passages, chest tightness, confusion, depression, dizziness, dyspnea, fainting, fatigue, fever, gastric distress, insomnia, itching, mouth and throat lesions, weakness, wheezing *Other:* increased appetite, burning of the nose, dry mouth and throat, hoarseness, altered taste perception	• Tell the patient that foods, beverages, and over-the-counter drugs don't influence the safety or effectiveness of these corticosteroids.
Oral systemic **prednisone** (Orasone)	*Reportable:* abdominal pain, acne, back or rib pain, bloody or tarry stools, easy bruising, unusual fatigue, fever, hypertension, leg swelling, menstrual irregularity, extreme personality changes, purple striae, sore throat, vomiting, weakness, significant weight gain, wounds that won't heal *Other:* unusual appetite, diaphoresis, dizziness, euphoria or feeling of well-being, headache, indigestion, insomnia, mild mood swings, mild nausea, nervousness, restlessness, slight weight gain	• Advise against taking this drug with alcohol to avoid GI ulceration. • Also, instruct him not to take over-the-counter drugs containing aspirin, unless the doctor specifically recommends them. Aspirin may increase the risk of GI ulceration. • Tell the patient to avoid over-the-counter drugs and foods that contain sodium to reduce the risk of fluid retention.
Expectorants and antitussives		
codeine	*Reportable:* confusion, dizziness, respiratory difficulty, sedation *Other:* constipation, drowsiness, dry mouth, nausea	• Tell patient that foods, nonalcoholic beverages, and over-the-counter drugs don't influence the safety or effectiveness of codeine. • Advise against taking this drug with alcohol to avoid increased CNS depression.

*Interactions include foods, alcohol, and over-the-counter drugs.

TEACHING POINTS

• Explain to the patient that the prescribed drug should reduce the frequency and severity of his airway spasms and dyspnea. As appropriate, tell him that the doctor has prescribed an inhalable dosage for his asthma or an intranasal dosage for his rhinitis.
• Warn him that the inhalable dosage won't relieve airway spasm immediately; he mustn't increase the prescribed dose in response. Tell him to call his doctor immediately if he experiences wheezing, chest tightness, or dyspnea after taking the prescribed dose.
• Emphasize that the patient must strictly follow his doctor's orders when initiating, terminating, or tapering the use of oral steroids in conjunction with inhalable steroids to avoid acute adrenal insufficiency. Sudden withdrawal of oral steroids may be fatal.
• If the patient is taking or has recently discontinued taking systemic corticosteroids, explain the need for additional steroids when coping with stress. He should call his doctor for instructions during stressful periods.
• Advise the patient to rinse his mouth and gargle with water after inhalation to remove drug deposits from his mouth and pharynx.
• If the patient is taking inhalation bronchodilators, instruct him to take the bronchodilator before the steroid. That way, the bronchodilator can fully dilate his airways, thereby improving deposition of the steroid. Since both drugs contain fluorocarbon propellants, tell the patient to wait 5 minutes between treatments to avoid potential toxicity.
• Remind the patient that it may take up to a month before he notices improvement from the steroid therapy.
• Warn the patient that inhalation cartridges are flammable and should not be used or stored near heat.

• Explain to the patient that this drug should help relieve symptoms of asthma or other respiratory inflammation.
• Emphasize that the patient must strictly follow his doctor's orders when initiating, terminating, or tapering the use of prednisone in conjunction with inhalable steroids to avoid acute adrenal insufficiency. Sudden withdrawal of prednisone may be fatal.
• If the patient's on long-term (greater than 2 weeks) or high-dose (greater than 40 mg daily) prednisone, teach him the signs of early adrenal insufficiency: fatigue, weakness, joint pain, fever, anorexia, nausea, dyspnea, dizziness, fainting, and weight loss.
• Also warn the patient on long-term therapy about cushingoid effects, such as acne, moon face, hirsutism, buffalo hump, truncal obesity with thinning of the limbs, and high blood pressure.
• Because this drug affects protein metabolism and water retention, instruct the patient to eat a salt-restricted diet high in protein and potassium.
• Advise him to take this drug with food to reduce gastric irritation.
• Instruct the patient on long-term therapy to wear a Medic Alert bracelet.
• Explain the need for additional steroids when coping with stress. Tell him to call his doctor for instructions during stressful times.
• Remind the patient that it may take up to a month before he notices improvement in his condition.

• Explain to the patient that this drug should help control his nonproductive cough. Advise him to consult his doctor if his cough becomes productive.
• Warn the patient that prolonged use of codeine can lead to drug tolerance and dependence.
• Because this drug can impair mental and physical function, advise the patient to use caution when operating a motor vehicle or heavy machinery, or using tools.
• Suggest that he chew sugarless gum, ice chips, or hard candy to relieve mouth and throat dryness.

(continued)

TEACHING PATIENTS ABOUT
RESPIRATORY DRUGS (continued)

DRUG	ADVERSE REACTIONS	INTERACTIONS*
Expectorants and antitussives (continued)		
dextromethorphan (Benylin DM, Comtrex, Coricidin Cough Syrup, DM Cough, Novahistine DMX, NyQuil, Robitussin-DM, Triaminicol, Vicks Children's Cough Syrup)	*Reportable:* unusual excitement, insomnia, irritability, nervousness *Other:* dizziness, drowsiness, gastric upset	• Tell the patient that foods, non-alcoholic beverages, and over-the-counter drugs don't influence the safety or effectiveness of dextromethorphan. • Advise against taking this drug with alcohol to avoid increased CNS depression.
guaifenesin (Coricidin Cough Syrup, Novahistine DMX, Robitussin, Triaminic, Vicks Children's Cough Syrup)	*Reportable:* nausea, vomiting *Other:* diarrhea, drowsiness, mild gastric upset	• Tell the patient that foods, beverages, and over-the-counter drugs don't influence the safety or effectiveness of guaifenesin.
Mast cell stabilizer		
cromolyn sodium (Intal [inhaler], Intal Capsules for use with Spinhaler, Intal Nebulizer Solution, Nasalcrom Nasal Solution)	*Reportable:* signs of anaphylaxis (such as angioedema, chest tightness, urticaria, increased wheezing), epistaxis, severe headache, nausea, painful urination, vomiting *Other:* cough, mild headache, nasal burning, nasal congestion, sneezing, bad taste	• Tell the patient that foods, beverages, and over-the-counter drugs don't influence the safety or effectiveness of cromolyn sodium.

*Interactions include foods, alcohol, and over-the-counter drugs.

TEACHING POINTS

• Explain to the patient that this drug should help control his cough. Since dextromethorphan is usually given in combination with antihistamines, sympathomimetics, or other drugs, emphasize that the patient must check with his doctor or pharmacist before taking any other cough or cold formulas.

• Instruct patient not to drive a car, operate heavy machinery, or use tools if the drug makes him drowsy.
• Suggest that he chew sugarless gum, ice chips, or hard candy to relieve mouth dryness.

• Explain to the patient that this drug should loosen mucous secretions in his lungs.
• If not contraindicated, also encourage him to drink as much water as possible to help thin his mucus.

• Advise the patient to check with his doctor before taking any expectorant, since most products that contain guaifenesin also contain other drugs, such as antihistamines and decongestants.

• When the doctor prescribes oral inhalable cromolyn sodium, explain to the patient that this drug helps prevent airway spasm and wheezing associated with asthma. Emphasize that it doesn't reverse acute airway spasm; the patient shouldn't increase the dosage to treat acute airway spasm.
• When the doctor prescribes intranasal cromolyn sodium, explain to the patient that this drug helps prevent or treat allergic rhinitis.
• Remind the patient that it may take up to a month before he notices improvement from the drug therapy.
• If the patient is also taking an inhaled bronchodilator, advise him to take the bronchodilator before the cromolyn sodium. That way,

the bronchodilator can dilate his airways, thereby improving deposition of the cromolyn sodium.
• Warn the patient that asthmatic symptoms may recur if he reduces the prescribed dosage or discontinues the drug. Tell him to notify his doctor if he experiences airway spasm and wheezing after taking an inhalable dose.
• Instruct the patient to store this drug in a tightly closed container away from moisture and light.
• Suggest that he rinse his mouth after taking the drug to minimize taste.
• Before administering the nasal solution, tell the patient to clear his nasal passage. During drug administration, he should inhale through his nose.

(continued)

**TEACHING PATIENTS ABOUT
RESPIRATORY DRUGS** *(continued)*

DRUG	ADVERSE REACTIONS	INTERACTIONS*
Methylxanthines		
aminophylline (Aminophyllin, Phyllo-contin, Somophyllin) **oxtriphylline** (Choledyl) **theophylline** (Bronkodyl, Elixophyllin, Theo-Dur, Theolair, Theospan-SR, Theostat)	*Reportable:* anorexia, diarrhea, dizziness, flushing, headache, insomnia, irritability, light-headedness, nausea, palpitations, pulse rate or rhythm changes, restlessness, seizures, tachypnea, tremulousness, vomiting *Other:* mild dyspepsia, bitter taste	• Tell the patient not to take over-the-counter drugs containing CNS stimulants, such as ephedrine or epinephrine, to avoid increased CNS stimulation. • Advise him that beverages containing xanthines, such as coffee and tea, can magnify the drug's effects. • Because cigarette smoking increases drug metabolism, tell the patient not to abruptly stop smoking during therapy to avoid drug toxicity. • Instruct him to take this drug on an empty stomach or 1 hour before or 3 hours after meals for best absorption.
Sympathomimetics		
albuterol (Proventil, Ventolin) **bitolterol** (Tornalate) **epinephrine** (Medihaler-Epi, Primatene Mist) **epinephrine, racemic** (microNefrin, Vaponefrin) **isoetharine** (Bronkometer, Bronkosol) **isoproterenol** (Isuprel, Medihaler-Iso) **metaproterenol** (Alupent, Metaprel) **terbutaline** (Brethine, Bricanyl)	*Reportable:* chest pain, diaphoresis, dizziness, dyspnea, flushing, headache, pallor, pounding heartbeat, vomiting *Other:* anxiety, fear, heartburn, insomnia, nausea, nervousness, palpitations, restlessness, mild tachycardia, bad taste, tremors, throat irritation	• Tell the patient not to take over-the-counter drugs containing CNS stimulants, such as ephedrine and epinephrine, to avoid increased adverse reactions and drug toxicity. • Tell patient that foods, beverages, and *most* other over-the-counter drugs don't influence the safety or effectiveness of sympathomimetics.

*Interactions include foods, alcohol, and over-the-counter drugs.

TEACHING POINTS

• Explain to the patient that this drug should control his wheezing and prevent airway spasm. Emphasize that he must take the drug exactly as ordered, even if he feels fine.
• Instruct him to notify the doctor if he comes down with the flu or develops a high fever; these may influence the drug's effectiveness.
• Teach the patient how to take his pulse. Advise him to take his pulse daily, and to notify his doctor if his pulse rhythm changes or pulse rate decreases or increases 20 beats or more per minute.
• If the patient experiences mild dyspepsia, advise him to take the drug with food.
• Inform the patient that it may take some time to regulate the drug so that it works without causing adverse reactions.

• Explain to the patient that this drug should reverse or control wheezing and airway spasm.
• Tell the patient to notify his doctor if he gets minimal or no relief from the prescribed dosage of the drug.
• Warn him that increasing the prescribed dosage can cause serious complications such as severe wheezing, stroke, myocardial infarction, and perhaps even death. Also advise against taking the prescribed dosage more frequently than ordered. Excessive use can cause respiratory distress or reduce the drug's effectiveness. Tell the patient to immediately stop using the drug and notify his doctor if he develops any symptoms of serious complications.
• Instruct the patient not to take more than one sympathomimetic at a time. He should wait at least 4 hours between dosages of separate drugs.
• Teach the patient how to use an inhaler (See *Using an Oral Inhaler,* page 170). Instruct him to clean the mouthpiece daily by running it under warm water or immersing it in alcohol. This will prevent clogging and also sanitize the mouthpiece.
• Advise the patient to discard the inhalation solution if it turns brown or contains a precipitate. Tell him to store the drug in its original container and to refrigerate it, if the label directs.
• Tell the patient to rinse his mouth with water or gargle after using an oral inhaler to minimize the bitter taste.

8

Gastrointestinal System

Gastrointestinal System

Introduction

Because gastrointestinal (GI) disorders occur so commonly, you'll need to understand them thoroughly to provide effective teaching. Your teaching topics, after all, can address simple alterations in bowel function, such as constipation, or life-threatening disorders, such as cirrhosis.

Despite their high incidence, however, GI problems are rarely discussed, which only contributes to poor understanding about their diagnosis, causes, and treatment. Patients commonly ignore their symptoms (often until surgery is necessary), or they attempt to gain relief through self-medication and questionable dietary practices.

Although a clear need exists for dispensing accurate, complete information about GI disorders, many factors interfere with the teaching-learning process. For example, the patient may feel too embarrassed to discuss his bowel habits or reluctant to admit such conditions as alcoholism, which can lead to chronic pancreatitis. The patient may also feel resistant to necessary life-style changes, or he may become unwilling to comply with therapy once his symptoms, such as pain from ulcers, subside.

What the patient needs to know
Despite these obstacles, the patient needs information in many areas. For such disorders as irritable bowel syndrome, management begins with finding the cause. But because of the vague nature of GI complaints and the lack of definitive diagnostic tests, the patient may undergo a number of procedures—many uncomfortable and embarrassing—to evaluate his problem.

Then, successful management often requires significant alterations in the patient's life-style. Your teaching usually takes three directions: dietary modification, such as a low-fat, high-protein diet for chronic pancreatitis and the importance of frequent small meals in hiatal hernia; medication administration, such as anticholinergics and antispasmodics for inflammatory bowel disease; and other measures that improve GI function, such as managing stress and eliminating smoking and alcohol.

If surgery (usually a last resort) becomes necessary, the patient will require instruction in preoperative dietary restrictions and bowel cleansing. He may also need to learn postoperative self-care measures, such as ostomy management.

Although the patient with a GI disorder generally finds these changes demanding, your sensitive teaching can help persuade him that he can master the skills necessary to control his condition.

DISORDERS

Chronic Pancreatitis

The prognosis for chronic pancreatitis is good if the patient complies with his treatment plan—and poor if he doesn't. Yet compliance may be difficult, requiring that the patient—commonly an alcoholic male between the ages of 45 and 60—change years of poor health habits and alcohol abuse. Compliance may also be difficult because family and social support often deteriorates in alcoholism. Your teaching, though, may help the patient begin to accept and control his problems.

You may need to teach the patient slowly and in short sessions because alcoholism can lead to cognitive deficits and slowed comprehension. You'll need to help him understand the relationship between his disorder and alcoholism. You'll also need to prepare him for tests to confirm the disorder or detect complications. And you'll need to teach about treatments—proper diet to reduce gastric secretion and drugs to relieve symptoms and prevent complications—that may allow him to control his disease.

Describe the disorder
Tell the patient that recurring episodes of inflammation progressively damage the pancreas. Explain that the pancreas normally secretes digestive enzymes. But in chronic pancreatitis, the duct through which these enzymes leave the pancreas becomes blocked. The enzymes back up into the pancreas and eventually begin to destroy pancreatic tissue.

Point out the cause of chronic pancreatitis—alcoholism or, less commonly, gallbladder disease, metabolic disorders, trauma, peptic ulcer, or drugs (such as diuretics, steroids, aspirin, or anticholinergics).

Point out possible complications
Stress that failure to comply with treatment may lead to pseudocysts, diabetes, GI bleeding, peptic ulcer, and steatorrhea.

Pseudocysts, containing fluid and amylase, form when digestive juices break through the normal pancreatic ducts, and diabetes results from islet cell damage in the pancreas. Variceal bleeding may result from portal or splenic vein thrombosis. And as gastric acidity increases in chronic pancreatitis, peptic ulcer may develop. Another common complication, steatorrhea, occurs with impaired fat digestion in the pancreas and with relapse from a low-fat diet.

Teach about tests
Prepare the patient for diagnostic tests to confirm chronic pancreatitis and de-

CHECKLIST

TEACHING TOPICS IN CHRONIC PANCREATITIS

☐ An explanation of the cause of chronic pancreatitis

☐ Complications, such as diabetes and GI bleeding, and their warning signs

☐ Preparation for diagnostic tests, including ERCP, biopsy, ultrasonography, and collection of stool specimens

☐ Dietary measures to decrease the demand for pancreatic enzymes

☐ Drug therapy to reduce gastric acidity, replace pancreatic enzymes, relieve pain, and control hyperglycemia

☐ Preparation for surgery, if necessary

☐ Measures to relieve symptoms and prevent complications, such as cessation of smoking and avoiding infection

☐ Availability of support groups

tect complications. These tests include biopsy to confirm pathology of pancreatic cells; endoscopic retrograde cholangiopancreatography (ERCP) to visualize the pancreatic ducts; and ultrasonography to determine the size of the pancreas. (See *Teaching Patients about Gastrointestinal Tests*, pages 233 to 240, for additional information on these studies.)

Teach the patient how to collect a stool sample. Then, tell him to maintain a fat-restricted diet for 2 to 3 days, and then to collect stool specimens for 3 days.

Teach about treatments

• *Diet.* Explain that diet therapy aims to reduce gastric secretion. Usually, the doctor prescribes a bland, low-fat, high-carbohydrate, high-protein diet to decrease the demand for pancreatic enzymes. Instruct the patient to avoid rich, fatty foods, which will aggravate his symptoms. Also discourage carbonated beverages, caffeine, and fruit juice; they increase gastric secretion.

Encourage the patient to eat small, frequent meals, thereby minimizing the secretion of pancreatic enzymes. Emphasize the importance of eliminating alcohol entirely. If diabetes is a problem, help the patient incorporate the necessary dietary restrictions. If he's malnourished or underweight, explore what foods he likes, so he can increase calories while maintaining his diet.

• *Medication.* Inform the patient that drug treatment relieves symptoms and prevents complications. Prescribed drugs may include antacids, cholinergics, and cimetidine to decrease gastric acidity; pancreatin or pancrelipase to replace pancreatic enzymes; narcotics to relieve pain; and insulin or oral hypoglycemic agents to control hyperglycemia. (See *Teaching Patients about Gastrointestinal Drugs*, pages 244 to 253.)

• *Surgery.* Prepare the patient for surgery, if necessary, to treat the complications of chronic pancreatitis. If the patient has an abscess, tell him it will

---

DANGER SIGNS IN CHRONIC PANCREATITIS

In chronic pancreatitis, the accumulation of corrosive enzymes in the pancreas may lead to life-threatening complications. Instruct the patient to contact the doctor if he experiences any of the following signs and symptoms of diabetes, GI bleeding, peptic ulcer, pseudocyst, or steatorrhea:

Diabetes
• Frequent urination
• Increased hunger
• Increased thirst
• Weakness
• Weight loss

GI bleeding
• Black, tarry stools
• Bloody stools
• Bloody or coffee-ground vomitus
• Dizziness upon standing
• Fatigue
• Pallor
• Weakness

Peptic ulcer
• Gnawing stomach pain
• Heartburn
• Indigestion

Pseudocyst
• Anorexia
• Epigastric pain radiating to the back
• Fever
• Nausea
• Vomiting

Steatorrhea
• Foul-smelling, frothy stools

---

be lanced and drained. If he has gallbladder disease, inform him that a cholecystectomy may be performed.

In sphincter spasm or hypertrophy, explain that a choledochojejunostomy restores free flow of bile into the jejunum by anastomosing the common bile duct to the jejunum. A sphincterotomy enlarges the pancreatic sphincter, which has been narrowed by fibrosis, and a vagotomy may relax the sphincter and decrease pancreatic secretion. If pain is severe, a splanchnic resection controls pain, but doesn't alter or prevent attacks.

• **Other care measures.** Advise the patient to reduce his risk of infection by avoiding contact with persons who are ill, obtaining adequate rest, and adhering to his treatment regimen. Tell him to contact his doctor immediately if he becomes ill.

Teach the patient the warning signs of the most common complications: pseudocyst, diabetes, gastrointestinal bleeding, peptic ulcer, and steatorrhea. (See *Danger Signs in Chronic Pancreatitis*, page 207.) Instruct him and his family to routinely examine stools for steatorrhea and for blood. If diabetes or peptic ulcer disease develops, teach the patient what he needs to know about the disorder.

Discourage smoking, as it alters pancreatic secretions that neutralize gastric acid in the duodenum. If appropriate, encourage the patient to seek help from Alcoholics Anonymous.

Cirrhosis

The progression of this life-threatening disorder can be stopped or slowed only by strict compliance with treatment. However, compliance is unlikely if the patient denies his illness and its precipitating factor—alcoholism. Your first teaching goal may well be to establish a trusting relationship with the patient and to encourage him to express his concerns. Only then can you successfully begin the necessary teaching about a high-protein diet, use of antacids, life-style changes, and possibly surgery.

Your teaching should also involve the family, whose relationship with the patient may be strained by his alcoholism. You'll need to pinpoint the family member who's most appropriate for supportive teaching—someone who can be counted on to help the patient adhere to his treatment regimen.

Describe the disorder

Inform the patient that cirrhosis is a chronic disorder involving irreversible damage to liver cells. Explain that the healthy liver plays a major role in carbohydrate, protein, fat, and steroid metabolism; vitamin storage; blood coagulation; and detoxification. Impairment of these functions results in such problems as nutritional deficiencies, increased susceptibility to infection, and increased potential for bleeding. Emphasize that once major symptoms occur, cirrhosis can't be cured; in fact, three quarters of the liver can be damaged without causing overt symptoms. Inform the patient that although the liver has remarkable powers of regeneration if he abstains from alcohol and follows his treatment plan, new tissue doesn't function as effectively. However, with proper treatment, he may experience long-term remission of symptoms.

Explain the cause of cirrhosis to the patient—alcoholism and drug abuse being the most common. Other predisposing factors include viral hepatitis, heart disease, gallbladder disease, and exposure to certain environmental pollutants and chemicals.

Point out possible complications

Emphasize that the patient can prevent or relieve complications by strict compliance with treatment. Stress that noncompliance with diet and medication therapy may hasten portal hypertension and hepatic encephalopathy—signaling progressive liver cell damage.

In portal hypertension, explain that impaired venous outflow from the liver elevates pressure in the portal system. This promotes the formation of collateral vessels to shunt blood from the higher-pressure portal system to the vena cava. Unfortunately, these new vessels are fragile and susceptible to the development of varices. If these varices rupture, massive hemorrhage may occur, requiring emergency treatment. (See *Esophageal Varices: A Deadly*

Complication, page 210.)

In hepatic encephalopathy, inform the patient that the liver can't convert ammonia (the end product of protein breakdown) to urea; consequently, serum ammonia levels rise. Extremely toxic to the brain, elevated ammonia levels produce neurologic changes. Warn the patient that untreated hepatic encephalopathy can ultimately lead to coma and death.

Explain that ascites, a less acute but still ominous complication, results from pathological changes in the failing liver. Uncontrolled ascites can compromise respiratory and renal function.

Teach about tests

Prepare the patient for scheduled diagnostic tests, such as liver scanning and biopsy, to confirm or evaluate cirrhosis. Serum, urine, and stool samples may also be collected to test liver function.(See *Teaching Patients about Gastrointestinal Tests*, pages 233 to 240.)

Teach about treatments

• *Diet.* Because cirrhosis is associated, in part, with nutritional deficiencies, emphasize the importance of following dietary instructions to achieve remission of symptoms. Tell the patient that his diet will depend on the severity of the disease. If he has uncomplicated cirrhosis, tell him that the doctor may prescribe a diet high in calories, carbohydrates, and protein to promote liver regeneration and provide energy for muscle repair and rebuilding. If he has elevated levels of serum ammonia, he'll follow a low-protein diet to minimize the risk of developing uremia. Instruct him to take supplemental vitamins as ordered—A, B complex, D, and K—to compensate for the liver's inability to store them, and vitamin B_{12}, folic acid, and thiamine to correct anemia.

Advise the patient to avoid fats if they cause indigestion or diarrhea. Also advise him to restrict sodium to prevent or reduce ascites. Above all, stress abstention from alcohol.

CHECKLIST

TEACHING TOPICS IN CIRRHOSIS

☐ An explanation of how cirrhosis causes irreversible damage to liver cells

☐ Complications of cirrhosis and their warning signs

☐ Preparation for diagnostic tests, including liver scanning and biopsy, and serum, urine, and stool studies, to confirm or evaluate cirrhosis

☐ Dietary measures and elimination of alcohol

☐ Importance of taking medication as prescribed, because of the liver's impaired ability to detoxify substances

☐ Preparation for portal-systemic shunting, if necessary

☐ Measures to reduce the risk of bleeding and infection

☐ Availability of support groups

If anorexia's a problem, reinforce the importance of an adequate diet for liver cell regeneration. Advise small, frequent meals, liberal snacking, favorite foods (if allowed), scrupulous mouth care (especially before meals to encourage adequate intake), and an attractive setting, to make eating more appealing.

• *Medication.* Instruct the patient to take medications carefully since the liver's ability to detoxify all substances is impaired. Inform the patient that antiemetics may be prescribed for nausea, diuretics for edema, steroids for reducing inflammation, and antacids for reducing the risk of GI bleeding. (See *Teaching Patients about Gastrointestinal Drugs*, pages 244 to 253, for more information on these medications.)

• *Surgery.* If necessary, prepare the patient for portal-systemic shunting to relieve portal hypertension and prevent hemorrhage. Explain that surgery diverts blood flow from the portal vein into another vein that empties directly

ESOPHAGEAL VARICES: A DEADLY COMPLICATION

Esophageal varices are often the first sign of portal hypertension. Normally, blood from the digestive tract and spleen flows through the portal vein and hepatic artery into the liver. This blood then drains into the hepatic veins and flows to the inferior vena cava.

In cirrhosis, hepatic fibrosis compresses the hepatic veins, impeding outflow and increasing portal pressure. Eventually, rising portal pressure causes blood to back up in the spleen and establishes collateral circulation between the portal and caval systems via the left gastric and short gastric esophageal veins. However, these thin-walled vessels accommodate the high-pressure portal circulation poorly: they become dilated and develop varices that easily rupture and leak large amounts of blood into the upper GI tract.

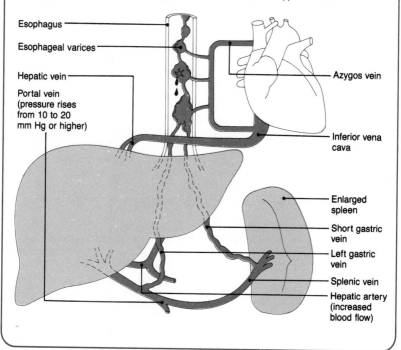

into the vena cava. Inform him that preoperative preparation may take 4 to 6 weeks. He'll require rest, a nutritious diet, supplemental vitamins, and adequate protein to relieve ascites and improve liver function. Explain that he'll receive neomycin for 1 week before surgery to cleanse the bowel.

Tell the patient what to expect after surgery. He'll return to the intensive care unit. (If possible, arrange for a visit before surgery.) Mention that he'll have several tubes and drains in place. For example, he'll have a nasogastric tube for 5 to 6 days to prevent distention by draining the GI tract and a drain (or chest tube) at the incision site for 2 to 3 days to remove accumulated fluid. He'll be connected to a cardiac monitor and also have several hemodynamic monitoring lines—pulmonary artery, arterial, and central venous pressure catheters. Assure him that monitoring of his vital signs is a normal procedure.

Inform the patient that usually he'll resume eating in 5 to 6 days, beginning with clear liquids and gradually progressing to solid foods. If he's not allowed to eat for more than a week, assure him that he'll receive adequate nourishment through I.V. hyperalimentation.

Pulmonary complications commonly occur after portal-systemic shunting because the surgical area lies close to the diaphragm. To help prevent them, instruct the patient to turn in bed, to cough and deep-breathe at least once every hour, and to use incentive spirometry. Advise him to ask for medication if moving and coughing cause pain. Show him how to splint his incision to minimize pain.

Tell the patient what to expect during the 6-to-8-week recovery period. Assure him that it's normal to feel tired. Explain that the doctor may prescribe a low-protein, low-sodium diet and vitamin supplements. Emphasize the importance of adequate rest to reduce the risk of bleeding and infection. Reinforce the need for strict adherence to the prescribed discharge regimen by pointing out common complications— encephalopathy, GI bleeding, and ascites. Instruct the patient to call the doctor if he experiences any symptoms of these complications. Advise him and his family to watch for neurologic alterations, such as confusion, irritability, or lethargy. These symptoms may occur as shunting prevents conversion of ammonia to urea by diverting blood past the portal circulation and into the systemic venous circulation.

• *Other care measures.* Because impaired hepatic production of prothrombin may cause a bleeding tendency, explain the warning signs of bleeding—weakness, hemoptysis, and blood in the stools and urine. Teach the patient to reduce this risk by avoiding aspirin, bruising, and straining during defecation. He should also avoid blowing his nose, sneezing, or coughing vigorously. Also suggest that he use an electric razor and a soft toothbrush.

Teach the patient to reduce his risk of infection by avoiding contact with persons who are ill, obtaining adequate rest, and maintaining his treatment regimen. Urge him to contact the doctor right away if he becomes ill.

Encourage the patient to seek counseling for alcohol or drug dependency, if appropriate.

Diverticular Disease

In diverticular disease, you'll need to adapt your teaching to the learning needs of the elderly and the obese. This most prevalent of colon disorders most commonly affects men and women over age 45 and occurs in 30% of the population over age 60. Half of those affected are obese.

For the elderly, your teaching should consider the possibility of visual and hearing loss and slower processing of information. If your patient's obese, you'll need to consider that his self-image and coping mechanisms may be poor and may detract from your teaching efforts.

You'll also need to consider that your teaching about diet, medication, lifestyle changes, and possibly colon resection may affect each patient differently, because of the age range involved. If individualized, your teaching can help the patient prevent the life-threatening complications secondary to this disease.

Describe the disorder

Tell the patient that in diverticular disease the intestinal mucosa pushes through the surrounding muscle, forming bulging pouches (diverticula). Explain that muscle layers of the colon have natural weak points where the marginal artery penetrates the colon wall. Thus, increased pressure in the colon's lumen may force the intestines to protrude into these weakened areas. Muscle weakness may be associated with aging, chronic constipation, or obesity.

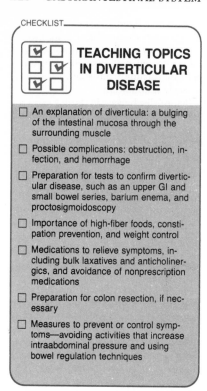

CHECKLIST

TEACHING TOPICS IN DIVERTICULAR DISEASE

☐ An explanation of diverticula: a bulging of the intestinal mucosa through the surrounding muscle

☐ Possible complications: obstruction, infection, and hemorrhage

☐ Preparation for tests to confirm diverticular disease, such as an upper GI and small bowel series, barium enema, and proctosigmoidoscopy

☐ Importance of high-fiber foods, constipation prevention, and weight control

☐ Medications to relieve symptoms, including bulk laxatives and anticholinergics, and avoidance of nonprescription medications

☐ Preparation for colon resection, if necessary

☐ Measures to prevent or control symptoms—avoiding activities that increase intraabdominal pressure and using bowel regulation techniques

Teach the patient about diverticulitis—inflammation of the diverticula, occurring anywhere along the GI tract, but most commonly in the descending and sigmoid colon.

Explain that episodes of pain may be related to inflammation or to the segmented action of the colon. Segmentation normally slows fecal movement, allowing water absorption and electrolyte exchange. However, this slowing action may cause pain from functional obstruction by fecal material. Inform the patient that symptoms of diverticulitis may also include rectal bleeding, abdominal pain, alternating constipation and diarrhea, gas, and a low-grade fever.

Point out possible complications

Inform the patient that diverticulitis may be acute or chronic. Caution him not to let decreased symptoms lull him into noncompliance with his medical regimen. If he fails to follow a proper diet and medication regimen, he risks the potentially fatal complications of obstruction, infection, and hemorrhage. Explain that obstruction occurs when fibrosis and adhesions narrow the gastrointestinal lumen. Infection results from rupture of the diverticulum, and hemorrhage occurs when ulceration is present.

Teach about tests

Prepare the patient for diagnostic tests to confirm diverticular disease. Inform him that an upper GI series detects diverticula of the esophagus and upper bowel, and a barium enema and proctosigmoidoscopy confirm or rule out diverticula of the lower bowel. Mention that these tests aren't performed during an acute attack since therapy aims to rest the colon and allow the inflammation to subside. (See *Teaching Patients about Gastrointestinal Tests*, pages 233 to 240.)

Teach about treatments

• *Diet.* If the patient has mild symptomatic diverticulitis, recommend a high-fiber diet. But tell him to avoid foods containing indigestible roughage, such as celery and corn, and to use bran to prevent constipation. Explain that he can also add bulk to his stools by eating fruits and vegetables with a high fiber content (seedless grapes, fresh peaches, carrots, and lettuce). Tell him to avoid extremely hot or cold foods and fluids, as they cause gas. Also tell him to avoid alcohol, because it irritates the bowel.

If the patient's overweight, stress the need for weight reduction; excess weight aggravates symptoms. Explore ways to help him maintain a calorie-restricted diet, such as reading labels for caloric content and using a calorie counter. Suggest that the patient contact a support group, if appropriate.

• *Medication.* Advise the patient to consult the doctor before trying to control constipation or diarrhea with nonprescription drugs. He should avoid enemas and nonprescription laxatives. The doctor may prescribe a bulk laxative to increase fecal size and consistency and an anticholinergic to reduce gastrointestinal spasms and hypermotility. (See *Teaching Patients about Gastrointestinal Drugs*, pages 244 to 253, for more information on these medications.)

• *Surgery.* If diverticular disease doesn't respond to dietary changes and drugs or if complications, such as hemorrhage or obstruction, develop, the patient may require colon resection. Inform him that resection involves excising the diseased or obstructed segments of the colon and rejoining the healthy segments. As a result, the patient may have a colostomy (temporary or permanent). Encourage him and his family to ask questions.

Describe the preparation for surgery. He'll be given vitamins C and K to build up a reserve; a low-residue diet for 4 to 5 days; a full liquid diet (such as applesauce, soups) for the next 48 hours; and a clear liquid diet (tea, bouillon) the evening before surgery. Also tell him to expect enemas and laxatives daily for 2 to 3 days before surgery. Inform him that he'll receive antiinflammatory and antibiotic medications rectally, and on the morning of the surgery, he'll have a nasogastric tube inserted.

Tell the patient what to expect after surgery: a nasogastric tube for several days to prevent distention by draining the GI tract, and a drain at the incision site for 2 to 3 days to remove any accumulated fluid. If the patient has a colostomy, describe the type—permanent or temporary. Explain that he'll return from surgery with a stoma and ostomy equipment. (See Chapter 18 for additional teaching points.) Inform him that he may not eat for several days, then he'll start with clear liquids and gradually advance to solid foods. If he's not allowed to eat for over a week, he'll receive I.V. hyperalimentation. Reinforce your preoperative teaching for the prevention of complications due to surgery. Show the patient how to minimize abdominal pain by splinting his incision, and tell him how to relieve gas pain by turning from side to side and by early ambulation.

Before discharge (in 1 to 2 weeks), advise him to avoid exertion or heavy lifting for several months. He'll probably be able to resume normal activities in 2 to 4 weeks. Outline discharge medication instructions: purpose, dosage, special considerations, and side effects. Also instruct the patient to continue the therapeutic measures followed before surgery: avoiding activities that increase intraabdominal pressure, promoting good bowel habits, and stopping smoking.

• *Other care measures.* Advise the patient to avoid activities that raise intraabdominal pressure. These include straining during defecation, bending, lifting, stooping, coughing, vomiting, and wearing constrictive clothing. To avoid constipation and colon irritation, explore strategies for bowel regulation. Recommend moderate exercise, a high-fiber diet, natural laxatives, and plenty of fluids. Tell the patient to set aside ample time for a bowel movement at the same time each day. Discourage smoking, as it irritates the gastric mucosa.

Emphasize the importance of notifying the doctor immediately if the patient experiences any signs of the following life-threatening complications: obstruction (lower abdominal cramping, distention, constipation), infection (fever, malaise, and fatigue), or hemorrhage (blood in the stool; black, tarry stools; or coffee-ground vomitus).

Hiatal Hernia

Even in its mildest form, hiatal hernia can disrupt the patient's life, forcing him to cope with recurring malaise and persistent dysphagia. To control his condition, your teaching will need to emphasize the direct relationship between the patient's symptoms and his meals, activities, and medications. He'll need to integrate the necessary restrictions into his life-style.

However, because the patient is usually over age 50 and has developed lifelong habits, he may resist your instructions. By helping him understand the need and the methods for preventing extended contact between stomach contents and the esophagus, you can help him reduce the number of painful episodes he experiences.

Describe the disorder

Inform the patient that a hiatal hernia results from a weakening or enlargement of the diaphragm opening that encircles the distal esophagus. This defect allows part of the stomach to protrude into the chest cavity when intraabdominal pressure rises, for example, with coughing or bending from the waist.

Explain to the patient that with these pressure changes, stomach contents and secretions push upward into the esophagus, causing gas or heartburn. (See *What Happens in Hiatal Hernia.*) This reflux of secretions can also erode the lining of the esophagus. Inform the patient that muscle weakening, causing insufficient closure of the opening, may result from congenital weakness, abdominal or chest injury, or a loss of muscle tone from aging, pregnancy, or obesity.

Point out possible complications

Stress that proper treatment may reduce the chances of complications. If the patient neglects his treatment, he risks developing esophagitis, gastritis, and aspiration pneumonia, as well as continued episodes of mild-to-severe pain. Explain that these complications result from the chemical effects of stomach contents on the esophagus or lungs.

Teach about tests

Prepare the patient for diagnostic tests to confirm hiatal hernia—barium swallow, endoscopy, and esophageal manometry. If he has esophagitis, prepare him for an acid perfusion test to evaluate gastric reflux. (See *Teaching Patients about Gastrointestinal Tests*, pages 233 to 240, for more information about these tests.)

Teach about treatments

• *Diet.* Teach the patient to modify the timing, size, and content of his meals to decrease the amount of acid secreted for digestion. Advise him to eat 4 to 6 small meals each day. This scheduling of meals prevents the stomach from becoming totally empty, thereby avoiding the acidic condition. A small meal prevents a large outpouring of digestive secretions and reduces stomach bulk, thus relieving symptoms resulting from displacement of other organs. To decrease his nighttime distress, instruct the patient to eat a small evening meal at least 3 hours before bedtime. Suggest

CHECKLIST

TEACHING TOPICS IN HIATAL HERNIA

☐ An explanation of hiatal hernia as muscle weakness of the diaphragm opening that encircles the distal esophagus and stomach

☐ Possible complications: esophagitis, gastritis, and aspiration pneumonia

☐ Preparation for tests to confirm hiatal hernia, such as barium swallow, endoscopy, and esophageal manometry

☐ Preoperative instruction for hernia repair, if necessary

☐ Meal scheduling, size, and contents

☐ Use of antacids, cholinergics, and other drugs to relieve symptoms and prevent complications

☐ Positioning, cessation of smoking, and avoidance of activities that increase intraabdominal pressure

WHAT HAPPENS IN HIATAL HERNIA

Hiatal hernia includes two classic types: sliding hernia and rolling or paraesophageal hernia.

In *sliding* hernia (which accounts for over 90% of adult hernias), the stomach cardia slips upward into the chest cavity, displacing organs and causing esophageal spasm when the patient lies down or when activities, such as bending or sneezing, increase intraabdominal pressure. The lower esophageal sphincter also moves into the chest, impairing its ability to prevent reflux of stomach contents into the esophagus. When the patient stands or intraabdominal pressure subsides, the cardia usually slides back into the abdominal cavity.

In *rolling* hernia, the stomach sphincter remains below the diaphragm, and the fundus rolls up beside the esophagus when intraabdominal pressure rises or the patient lies down.

Symptoms of hiatal hernia (occurring in about 50% of patients with the disorder) are severe and may cause complications. The most common is heartburn from gastric reflux. Other symptoms include belching and bloating due to increased swallowing from attempts to remove the acid from the esophagus. Reflux may cause aspiration pneumonia.

Other possible symptoms include pain, shortness of breath, and tachycardia, which result from rising intrathoracic pressure when a part of the stomach slides into the thoracic cavity. Accompanying esophageal spasm may cause severe pain radiating to the back, shoulder, or arm.

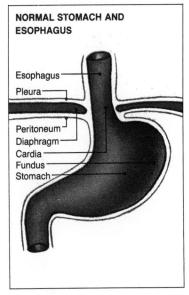

NORMAL STOMACH AND ESOPHAGUS

Esophagus
Pleura
Peritoneum
Diaphragm
Cardia
Fundus
Stomach

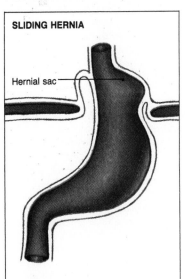

SLIDING HERNIA

Hernial sac

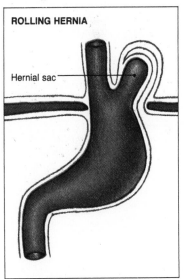

ROLLING HERNIA

Hernial sac

eating slowly to avoid a large outpouring of gastric secretions.

Instruct the patient to avoid beverages that may intensify his symptoms—fruit juice, caffeinated coffee or tea, alcohol, and carbonated beverages. He should also eliminate raw fruits, highly seasoned foods, and foods high in fat or carbohydrates. (Explain that he may have a greater desire for spicy foods because the aging process decreases the number of viable tastebuds.) Also, advise him to avoid extremely hot or cold foods and fluids, because they cause gas.

To prevent reflux, tell the patient to eat sitting up and not to lie down after meals. Also recommend drinking water after eating to cleanse the esophagus. If the patient's overweight, suggest a weight-loss program; excess weight increases intraabdominal pressure. Also suggest he use a calorie counter and read food labels. To promote compliance, emphasize the positive aspects of diet, rather than its restrictions.

• *Medication.* Educate the patient about the relationship between complications, which can be life-threatening, and the specific action of each medication. Explain that antacids neutralize the acid of gastric secretions, thereby relieving the symptoms of reflux. Cholinergics increase esophageal sphincter pressure, and antiemetics prevent vomiting, which can increase intraabdominal pressure. (See *Teaching Patients about Gastrointestinal Drugs*, pages 244 to 253, for more information.)

Give the patient tips to promote compliance: Tell him that antacids taste better cold, and, if needed, he should keep chewable antacids handy. Inform him that he'll take medications for a hiatal hernia indefinitely, even after surgical repair.

• *Surgery.* Inform the patient that surgery restores the stomach to its normal position, reducing the hernia. It also strengthens the lower esophageal sphincter. Tell him to expect laxatives and enemas the evening before surgery to cleanse the bowel and prevent postoperative complications.

Inform the patient that after surgery he'll have a nasogastric tube for 2 or 3 days to prevent gas by draining the GI tract. If the abdominal approach is used, he'll have a drain at the incision site to remove accumulated fluid for 1 or 2 days. If the thoracic approach is used, he'll have chest tubes. Explain that his intake may be limited to fluids for the first 24 hours. Then, he'll gradually resume his diet, starting on clear liquids and advancing to solid foods. Tell him to expect smaller, more frequent meals because the surgery reduces the storage capacity of the stomach. He may be asked to keep a record of his intake and output to evaluate the return of proper bowel function.

Stress the patient's susceptibility to pulmonary complications and his role in prevention. He should expect prophylactic antibiotics for 5 to 10 days. Assure him that he'll receive medication if he experiences pain with coughing and movement. Show him how to minimize abdominal pain by splinting his incision.

Explain that after surgery he may experience bloating. To relieve gas pain, instruct him in turning from side to side in bed, and advise early ambulation. Inform him that he'll be discharged about 1 week after surgery and will probably resume his normal activities in 2 to 4 weeks. Warn him to avoid exertion or heavy lifting for several months.

Explain that postoperative complications, such as a gastric fistula, are rare but do occur. Advise the patient to notify the doctor immediately if he experiences difficulty swallowing or reflux. If he's overweight, stress the need for weight reduction to prevent complications and recurrence of the hernia.

• *Other care measures.* Advise the patient to restrict activities that increase intraabdominal pressure—strenuous exercise, bending, coughing, and wearing constrictive clothing, such as a tight girdle or pantyhose. Also recommend methods to avoid straining with bowel movements, such as modifying his diet to include natural laxatives (high-fiber foods, citrus fruits) and, if prescribed, taking laxatives or stool softeners.

To relieve symptoms of heartburn, advise the patient to elevate his head with 2 or 3 pillows or to place 8- to 10-inch blocks under the head of his bed. Also suggest sleeping on his right side. Discourage smoking, because it alters pancreatic secretions that neutralize gastric acid in the duodenum.

Emphasize the warning symptoms of complications. Instruct the patient to contact the doctor immediately if he has symptoms of esophagitis, such as difficulty swallowing, chest pain, and bloody sputum; symptoms of gastritis, such as abdominal pain, belching, and nausea and vomiting; or symptoms of aspiration pneumonia, such as fever, difficulty breathing, rapid respirations, and pain with inspiration.

Inflammatory Bowel Disease

Teaching the patient with inflammatory bowel disease—either ulcerative colitis or Crohn's disease—requires understanding his psychological status as well as his physical problems. Typically, this patient is between the ages of 20 and 40 and involved in establishing a family and a career. Yet the pain and fatigue from bouts of this disorder leave him physically and psychologically debilitated. Also, recovery time is lengthy and rest imperative, possibly causing financial and child-care concerns.

To surmount this disorder, the patient must comply with dietary changes to rest the bowel, medication to manage pain and provide psychological rest, and life-style changes to relieve symptoms and possibly to cope with an ileostomy. But interruption of daily activities and the need to alter his goals may make him impatient with your teaching.

Despite these obstacles, your teaching can help the patient understand his disorder. In doing so, he may become less anxious and more willing to assume responsibility for managing symptoms and avoiding complications.

Describe the disorder

Inform the patient that inflammatory bowel disease involves chronic inflammation of the lining of the GI tract. Explain that this slowly progressive disease has two forms: ulcerative colitis and Crohn's disease.

Tell the patient with *ulcerative colitis* that this disease causes inflammation and destruction of the mucosa and inner muscle layer of the large intestine. Scar tissue replaces damaged areas and may eventually narrow the colon. Causes may include infection, destructive enzymes, allergic reactions, and psychological factors.

If appropriate, explain that remitting disease is the most common and the mildest form of ulcerative colitis. It involves the rectum or the rectosigmoid juncture. Attacks last 4 to 12 weeks and are interspersed with asymptomatic periods.

If the patient has chronic ulcerative colitis, explain that persistent inflammation affects parts of the colon above the rectum. Eventually, narrowing of the colon may necessitate surgery to prevent further progression.

If the patient's symptoms begin abruptly, he may have acute colitis. Explain that extensive symptoms—nausea, vomiting, and severe diarrhea—usually indicate involvement of the entire colon.

Inform the patient with *Crohn's disease* that it involves progressive inflammation and ulceration of all the layers of the bowel. It spreads from one bowel segment to another to involve every part

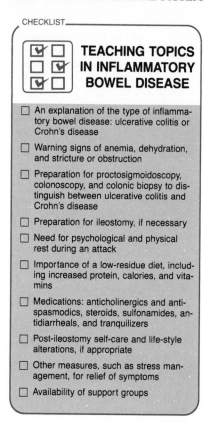

CHECKLIST

☑☐ ☐☑ ☑☐ **TEACHING TOPICS IN INFLAMMATORY BOWEL DISEASE**

☐ An explanation of the type of inflammatory bowel disease: ulcerative colitis or Crohn's disease

☐ Warning signs of anemia, dehydration, and stricture or obstruction

☐ Preparation for proctosigmoidoscopy, colonoscopy, and colonic biopsy to distinguish between ulcerative colitis and Crohn's disease

☐ Preparation for ileostomy, if necessary

☐ Need for psychological and physical rest during an attack

☐ Importance of a low-residue diet, including increased protein, calories, and vitamins

☐ Medications: anticholinergics and antispasmodics, steroids, sulfonamides, antidiarrheals, and tranquilizers

☐ Post-ileostomy self-care and life-style alterations, if appropriate

☐ Other measures, such as stress management, for relief of symptoms

☐ Availability of support groups

of the GI tract, which in later stages becomes thick and narrowed. Possible causes include allergies, lymphatic obstruction, and infection. Inform him that early features of Crohn's disease may be mild and nonspecific, but the disease may progress to acute inflammatory symptoms that mimic appendicitis (lower right quadrant pain, stomach cramps, tenderness, flatulence, nausea, fever, and diarrhea). However, chronic symptoms, including persistent diarrhea, lower right quadrant pain, fever, steatorrhea, and marked weight loss, are more typical in this disease.

Point out possible complications

Emphasize to the patient that failure to follow his diet can trigger the inflammatory process, leading to complications such as dehydration, malnutrition, and infection. Vomiting and diarrhea may cause the loss of body fluids and electrolytes, and the rapid movement of food through the intestines may cause deficiencies of fat, iron, calcium, and vitamins A, B_{12}, C, D, E, and K. Point out that symptoms may recur unless he controls emotional stress and follows his medication regimen.

Teach about tests

Prepare the patient for diagnostic tests, such as proctosigmoidoscopy, colonoscopy, and biopsy of the colon, to distinguish between ulcerative colitis and Crohn's disease. (See *Teaching Patients about Gastrointestinal Tests*, pages 233 to 240.) Also prepare him for serum, urine, and stool sample collections to detect pathological changes. For stool collection, instruct the patient to avoid red meats, poultry, fish, turnips, and horseradish for 48 hours before the collection period and throughout it. Also, as ordered, instruct him to stop taking medications for the same duration.

Teach about treatments

• *Activity.* Explain that physical and psychological rest are important treatment goals. To decrease intestinal motility during an attack, advise the patient to reduce physical activity. If his attack is mild, suggest that he get extra rest during the day. If he has a fever, toxemia, frequent bowel movements, bleeding, or pain, advise him to stay in bed and to use a bedside commode. If he's hospitalized with severe diarrhea, urge him to use the signal light whenever he needs help in going to the bathroom. If he can use the bathroom unassisted, instruct him to record the number of stools, noting their consistency, color, and the presence of bleeding.

If the patient's had a relapse, advise him to try to lead a normal life, including adequate rest and moderate activity to promote good bowel function and reduce anxiety.

• *Diet.* Explain that diet therapy allows the bowel to heal by decreasing its activity while providing the calories and nutrition necessary for healing. Stress the importance of following his diet to achieve remission and prevent complications. Make sure he understands his prescribed diet—high in protein, calories, and vitamins. Advise him to avoid foods that irritate his intestines or that require excessive intestinal activity, such as milk products, spicy or fried high-residue foods, raw vegetables and fruits, and whole-grain cereals. Explain that he'll be taking supplemental vitamins to compensate for the bowel's inability to absorb them. Discourage carbonated, caffeinated, and alcoholic beverages, as they increase intestinal activity. Also discourage extremely hot or cold food and fluids, because they cause gas.

Advise eating small, frequent meals. If anorexia's a problem, reinforce the importance of an adequate diet to promote healing. Suggest snacking, favorite foods if permitted, good mouth care (to enhance taste), and a pleasant atmosphere while eating.

• *Medication.* Inform the patient that he'll take several prescribed medications to relieve symptoms and prevent complications: anticholinergics and antispasmodics to decrease muscle spasm and pain; steroids to reduce inflammation; sulfonamides and antidiarrheals to control diarrhea; and antianxiety drugs to provide physical and emotional rest. (See *Teaching Patients about Gastrointestinal Drugs*, pages 244 to 253.)

• *Surgery and procedures.* If conservative treatments aren't successful or if the patient develops complications, such as obstruction, abscess, or fistula, prepare him for surgery to remove the diseased segment of the colon. Such surgery may eliminate his symptoms. Explain that the type of surgery depends on the location and extent of inflammation; colostomy and ileostomy are the most common operations. (See Chapter 18 for teaching points if the patient's having a colostomy.)

If the patient's scheduled for an ileostomy, explain that he may be unable to absorb vitamin B_{12} afterward, depending on the amount of bowel removed. If he's having the ileocecal valve removed, he can expect increased intestinal motility and altered protein and fat absorption.

Inform the patient that preoperative preparation extends over 3 to 4 days. He'll have cleansing laxatives and enemas and antibiotics to decrease the chance of infection after surgery. Tell him that his stoma site will be selected and marked. (Assure him that his preference for stoma location will be considered.) Describe the stoma, show him an ostomy pouch, and, if appropriate, ask him to wear it for several days to ensure proper fit. Also ask a representative of the United Ostomy Association to visit with the patient, thereby helping him get used to the idea of an ileostomy.

Inform the patient that he'll return from surgery with a pouch covering his stoma. The nurse will initially perform stoma care, changing the pouch as necessary, and gradually the patient will learn to do this for himself. Also describe the color and consistency of the drainage. Explain that it will change as his diet changes.

Tell him that he'll have a nasogastric tube in place for several days to prevent distention by draining the GI tract. Also explain that he won't eat for several days after surgery, but once he resumes his diet, he'll begin with clear liquids and gradually include solid foods. If eating's not permitted for more than a week, he'll have I.V. hyperalimentation.

To prevent pulmonary complications, instruct the patient to turn in bed, to cough and deep-breathe at least once every hour, and to use incentive spirometry. Assure him that he'll receive medication if movement and coughing cause pain. He'll also receive medication before ostomy appliance changes, for discomfort resulting from manipulation near the incision. To

EMPTYING AN OSTOMY POUCH

Dear Patient:

You'll empty your ostomy pouch when it's about one-third full. To prepare for the procedure, place a cup of warm water within reach.

1

Sit on the toilet with the ostomy pouch hanging between your legs. You can also sit on a chair next to the toilet, but be sure the pouch opening is in the toilet.

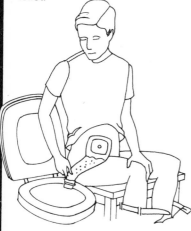

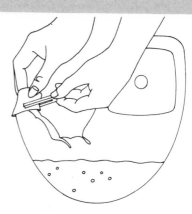

Then point the pouch's unclamped opening into the toilet.

To prevent splashing, place some toilet paper on the surface of the water, or flush the toilet as you lower the pouch opening into the bowl.

3

Then slide your thumb and index finger down the outside of the pouch, squeezing all the contents into the toilet.

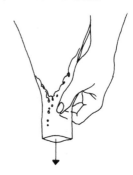

2

Now you're ready to empty your pouch. To do this, turn up the bottom of the pouch and remove the closure clamp, as shown at the top of the next column.

4

Next, use toilet paper to clean any remaining drainage from around and inside the pouch opening.

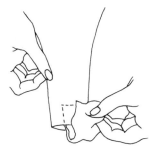

6

Now direct the pouch opening into the toilet. Let the pouch drain thoroughly. If you use a pouch deodorant, place it in the pouch, following the manufacturer's directions. Using toilet paper, clean and dry the outside of the pouch. Finally, refasten the pouch with a closure clamp. You can also refasten it with a rubber band, as shown below.

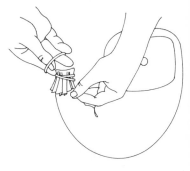

5

Hold the pouch opening upright and pour the cup of water into the pouch.

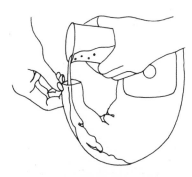

Swish the water around to remove any remaining drainage. As you work, avoid wetting your stoma or the pouch adhesive—doing so could break the seal.

REMOVING AN OSTOMY POUCH

Dear Patient:

When you remove your ostomy pouch, be sure you clean the area around the stoma at the same time. Here's the way to do both:

1

Gather gauze pads and, if needed, adhesive solvent and an eyedropper. (Note: Some adhesive solvents come in pre-saturated sponges or aerosol sprays and don't need to be applied with an eyedropper.) Also gather karaya gum or powder (if needed), a towel, and scissors.

2

Stand upright with the pouch exposed. Hold the skin taut around the stoma, as you gently peel back the top of the adhesive square (faceplate). Continue peeling downward to remove the faceplate.

3

If you have trouble removing the faceplate, don't use force. Instead, try loosening the adhesive that attaches the faceplate to your skin. If you've applied skin cement as an adhesive, use solvent to loosen it. To do this, fill an eyedropper with solvent and loosen each edge of the faceplate with a drop or two of solvent, or apply a presaturated sponge, an aerosol spray, or a gauze pad moistened with solvent to the faceplate. Wait a few seconds, and then try to remove the faceplate. Set the soiled pouch aside to be cleaned.

4

Perform stoma care by first gently wiping the stoma with toilet tissue or a gauze pad to absorb any leakage.

5

Wash the area around the stoma with warm, soapy water, and dry the skin thoroughly. If your skin is irritated, apply karaya gum or powder.

6

Trim any long hairs around the stoma with scissors. Avoid using a razor; it may irritate your skin. Don't be alarmed if you notice slight bleeding. It can occur anytime the stoma rubs against something rough, such as terry cloth.

minimize abdominal pain, show him how to splint his surgical site.

Include a family member in discharge teaching because common illnesses, such as viral infections, can have a devastating effect on the patient with inflammatory bowel disease. Also show the patient how to care for the skin around his stoma site to prevent skin breakdown and infection. Instruct him to contact the doctor if he observes redness, rash, or swelling, or if he experiences itching, warmth, pain, or unusual drainage. Teach him how to manage his ostomy equipment. (See *Emptying an Ostomy Pouch*, pages 220 and 221; *Removing an Ostomy Pouch*, page 222; and *Applying an Ostomy Pouch*, pages 224 and 225. If the patient's had a colostomy, see Chapter 18 for care instructions.)

Assure the patient that odor shouldn't be a problem if he cleans his pouch (if it's two-piece) or changes it (if it's one-piece) on a regular schedule. Suggest adding cranberry juice, buttermilk, or yogurt to his diet to help control odor. Also suggest a pouch deodorant. Instruct him to notify the doctor of any marked decrease in ostomy output or spurting or squirting of drainage from the stoma. This may signal stoma stricture and require medical intervention. Also tell him to report any unusually foul odor; it may indicate infection or may be only diet-related. To prevent gas from filling his pouch, advise him to avoid gas-producing foods, such as cabbage and broccoli. Also, he may want to use a pouch with a filter. Inform him that he may wear his pouch when taking a bath or shower, since water won't hurt his stoma.

If the patient's scheduled for a continent ileostomy, explain that it consists of an intraabdominal pouch surgically constructed from the terminal ileum. Solid waste collects in the nipple-valved pouch until the patient drains the pouch through the stoma with a catheter. Or he may have an an alternative procedure—the ileo-anal anastomosis. This involves dissection of the rectal area

from the submucosa and mucosa. The colon is removed, and the ileum sutured to the rectum via a straight anastomosis or by the creation of a J- or S-shaped reservoir pouch. With this procedure, the patient's able to move his bowels in a normal manner.

After a continent ileostomy, outline the procedure for emptying the pouch by inserting a lubricated #28 catheter through the stoma. Pouch capacity determines how often it should be drained. Because the pouch will stretch, it will hold only about 70 to 100 ml of fluid right after surgery. Six months later, it will hold about 600 ml and will need emptying only 3 or 4 times a day. Between intubations, instruct the patient to keep his stoma covered with a small gauze pad and to irrigate his pouch weekly—or more often if undigested food causes a drainage block. To prevent blocks, advise him to avoid fibrous foods, such as corn, nuts, lettuce, and celery.

Finally, answer the patient's questions about his life after surgery and suggest ways to ease his adjustment. (See *Questions Patients Ask about an Ostomy*, page 226.)

● *Other care measures.* Help the patient and his family identify causes of emotional tension, which can trigger inflammatory episodes. Suggest ways to eliminate or reduce the impact of stress. You may need to guide the patient in adjusting his work and home situations and establishing a realistic pattern of work and sleep. If necessary, encourage him to seek counseling for stress management.

Discourage smoking, because it contributes to altered bowel motility. If diarrhea's severe, teach the patient proper skin care. Because persistent diarrhea and vomiting may lead to serious metabolic complications, instruct him to report signs of dehydration (confusion, lethargy, dry skin and mucous membranes, dry mouth, muscle weakness, and decreased urine output). To reduce his risk of infection, advise him to avoid contact with per-

224

APPLYING AN OSTOMY POUCH

Dear Patient:

The nurse will show you how to apply the ostomy pouch. Then you can use this home care aid to help you remember the steps.

You can choose either a one-piece or a two-piece ostomy pouch. The one-piece pouch has an attached skin barrier, which creates a moisture-proof seal to prevent skin irritation around the stoma. With the two-piece pouch, you must apply a skin barrier separately.

Gathering the equipment

Assemble the equipment: a clean pouch, skin barrier (if applicable), stoma measuring guide, closure clamp or rubber band, and belt (optional).

Measuring your stoma

To ensure proper fit as your stoma shrinks while healing, you may need to measure your stoma, as shown here.

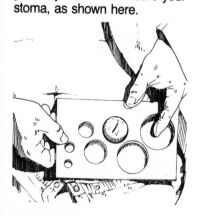

Then select a pouch with an opening that matches the size of your stoma.

Applying a one-piece pouch

1

Trace a circle the same size as your stoma onto the pouch's adhesive faceplate. Then fold the faceplate in half lengthwise and cut out the circle. (Or use a pouch with a precut opening of the right size.)

If desired, apply an additional skin barrier, such as karaya gum or powder, around the stoma to prevent skin breakdown.

2

Peel the paper backing away from the adhesive faceplate. Then center the pouch opening over your stoma, and press gently to secure the edges, as shown at the top of the next column. Also, if desired, attach the belt.

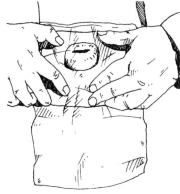

Your body temperature softens the wafer and molds it to the skin.

2

Now align the pouch flange with the wafer flange. Gently press along the circumference of the pouch flange, beginning at the bottom (as shown below), until it's secured to the

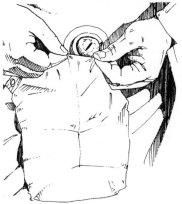

3

Now press air out of the pouch and attach a closure clamp at the bottom (or turn up the bottom of the pouch about 1½" (3.8 cm), fanfold across, and secure with a rubber band).

Applying a two-piece pouch with flanges

1

Fit a skin barrier wafer around the stoma and press gently.

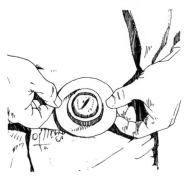

wafer flange. (The pouch will click into its secured position.) Also attach the belt, if desired.

3

Finally, press air out of the pouch and attach the closure clamp at the bottom (or turn up the bottom of the pouch about 1½", fanfold across, and secure with a rubber band).

QUESTIONS PATIENTS ASK ABOUT AN OSTOMY

Will I have to wear special clothes because I have an ostomy?

No, as long as you avoid putting pressure (as from a belt) directly over the stoma. Ostomy pouches lie flat against the body, so they're not detectable, even under snug-fitting clothing. But you shouldn't wear constrictive undergarments, such as long-line bras and girdles; they might injure the stoma. Instead, wear a lightweight stretch-type garment.

Must I eat special foods after my ostomy?

The doctor will probably first prescribe a low-residue diet that will rest the bowel so it can heal. Usually, you'll return to your regular diet within 4 to 6 weeks. But be sure to avoid gaseous foods, such as eggs, cabbage, and beer. Also stay away from foods that may cause constipation (such as celery, corn, popcorn, grapefruit, dried fruit, and seeds) and diarrhea (such as cabbage, beans, onions, cucumbers, and radishes).

Will my ostomy affect my sex life?

If your sex life was satisfying before surgery, it should remain so. Keep in mind that the stoma can't be injured by close physical contact. But before sexual intercourse, you may want to empty the pouch, or you may prefer to use a pouch cover.

If you've had surgery in the perineal area, you may expect some discomfort during sexual intercourse. That's normal until the wound heals. However, if you and your partner have difficulty adjusting sexually, you should consult a doctor to rule out a physical cause, and then, if necessary, contact a professional counselor to resolve psychological problems.

sons who are ill. Also advise traveling only in areas with proper sanitation.

Instruct the patient to notify the doctor if he experiences these warning symptoms of complications: fever, fatigue, weakness, or a rapid heart rate, along with abdominal cramping, vomiting, and acute diarrhea. Abdominal pain and cramping can signal progressive inflammatory bowel disease, indicating stricture or obstruction. Also instruct him to report symptoms of anemia: dizziness, fatigue, pallor, and muscle weakness.

If the patient has an ostomy, tell him to avoid laxatives, enteric-coated pills, and timed-release capsules, because they aren't absorbed and may obstruct the stoma. Urge him to contact the doctor if he acquires an infection, because diarrhea and vomiting can lead to life-threatening metabolic complications. Also arrange for follow-up by a health care professional. And emphasize the importance of wearing a Medic Alert bracelet or necklace at all times.

Advise the patient with inflammatory bowel disease to see the doctor regularly for checkups. Refer the patient with an ileostomy to the local chapter of the United Ostomy Association.

Irritable Bowel Syndrome

To teach the patient how to overcome this functional syndrome, you'll need to consider his emotional state—typically anxious and depressed—and the syndrome's prime trigger factor—stress. Often characterized as tense, rigid, and dependent, the patient commonly experiences irritable bowel syndrome as a reaction to stress. Consequently, he may have trouble changing ingrained responses in order to relieve the syndrome's symptoms. You'll need to adapt your teaching methods to his personality traits and enlist his cooperation before you can teach him ways to reduce stress and make the necessary life-style changes.

The patient may also be confused and frustrated by the diagnosis, finding it difficult to trust in treatment if symptoms have no organic cause and treatment doesn't produce a cure. You'll need to emphasize the positive, urging him to follow the treatment regimen so he can control his condition—and not let it control him.

Describe the disorder

Inform the patient that irritable bowel syndrome (also called spastic or irritable colon) is marked by chronic, excessive spasms of the large intestine. Although the GI tract has a normal structure, its function is impaired.

Explain that an overactive intestinal muscle is generally associated with psychological stress. Such stress may stimulate the autonomic nervous system and its innervation of the bowel, causing uncoordinated motor activity and slowed or accelerated movement of bowel contents. This produces abdominal pain, along with constipation or diarrhea or both. Physical factors, including seasoned, cold, or laxative foods, roughage, fruits, and alcohol, may also trigger or aggravate symptoms.

Point out possible complications

Tell the patient that he'll probably experience recurring bouts of irritable bowel syndrome with abdominal pain, constipation, and diarrhea if he doesn't follow the prescribed supportive treatment. Also mention that his general health will deteriorate with each bout.

Teach about tests

Explain that tests can't specifically diagnose irritable bowel syndrome, but they can rule out other disorders. A barium enema detects the syndrome's excessive intestinal spasms, and a proctosigmoidoscopy detects and eval-

---

CHECKLIST

TEACHING TOPICS IN IRRITABLE BOWEL SYNDROME

- ☐ Explanation of the disorder and its causative factors

- ☐ Preparation for tests, such as barium enema and proctosigmoidoscopy, to rule out other disorders

- ☐ Dietary measures to prevent pain, constipation, and diarrhea

- ☐ Medication administration: anticholinergics and tranquilizers

- ☐ Other care measures: stress management, cessation of smoking, and development of a regular bowel routine

---

uates inflammation and abnormalities. (See *Teaching Patients about Gastrointestinal Tests*, pages 233 to 240.) If the patient's scheduled for stool specimen collection to check for blood, bacteria, and parasites, instruct him to maintain a high-fiber diet and to avoid red meats, poultry, fish, turnips, and horseradish for 48 hours before the collection period and during it. As ordered, instruct the patient to stop taking medications for the same duration.

Teach about treatments

• *Diet.* Emphasize the importance of carefully following dietary instructions to prevent or relieve symptoms of irritable bowel syndrome. Instruct the patient to avoid fluids that will cause him pain, including carbonated and caffeinated beverages, fruit juice, and alcohol. Also instruct him to avoid foods that cause gas, especially extremely hot or cold foods or fluids. Advise him to eat slowly and carefully to prevent swallowing air and bloating. If his prescribed high-fiber diet contains unprocessed bran, explain that it adds essential soft bulk to his stools. If he's bothered by constipation, advise him to drink 8 to 10 glasses of fluid daily to regulate the consistency of his stools.

To promote compliance, emphasize the positive effects of the prescribed diet—a decrease in the patient's pain and diarrhea.

• *Medication.* Inform the patient that drugs are prescribed to relieve symptoms: anticholinergics to reduce intestinal hypermotility and mild tranquilizers or sedatives to relieve anxiety. (See *Teaching Patients about Gastrointestinal Drugs*, pages 244 to 253, for more information.) Advise him to consult the doctor before treating constipation or diarrhea with over-the-counter medications; most of them irritate the bowel.

• *Other care measures.* Teach the patient that effective treatment of irritable bowel syndrome may require lifestyle alterations that emphasize control of emotional tension. Be sure to help him set priorities by pinpointing the activities he enjoys, scheduling more time for rest and relaxation, and, if possible, shifting some of his responsibilities to other family members. If appropriate, encourage the patient to seek professional counseling for stress management.

Remind the patient that regular physical exercise helps eliminate anxiety and promotes good bowel function. Discourage smoking, because it contributes to altered bowel motility. Also help him establish a regular bowel routine.

Because irritable bowel syndrome is associated with a higher-than-normal incidence of diverticulitis and colon cancer, encourage regular physical examinations. For patients over 40, emphasize the need for an annual proctosigmoidoscopy and rectal examination.

Ulcer Disease

Although ulcer disease can lead to life-threatening complications, patient compliance with the prescribed regimen usually means a more favorable outcome. Compliance largely depends on the patient's understanding—and your teaching—of his responsibility for managing the disease.

One obstacle to successful teaching, though, may be the pain that's characteristic of ulcer disease. Its presence may delay your teaching; its absence may lessen the patient's motivation to learn and to complete his therapy. As a result, you'll need to help the patient understand the relationship between episodic pain and the need to follow his medication regimen to obtain relief and ensure complete healing. And because there's no guarantee that the ulcer won't recur, you'll need to emphasize to the patient the importance of controlling emotional stress and modifying his living, working, and eating habits. Your teaching must also stress the possibility of life-threatening complications. And because ulcer disease may be hereditary, you'll need to teach the patient's family to recognize its symptoms and contributing factors.

Describe the disorder

Inform the patient that an ulcer is an erosion of the lining of the GI tract caused by contact with strong gastric secretions (pepsin or hydrochloric acid). If the erosion penetrates the lining of the GI tract, it may invade the underlying blood vessels.

If the patient has a *duodenal* ulcer, inform him that lesions usually occur near the pylorus of the stomach. Explain that because his stomach secretes excess hydrochloric acid and also empties food more rapidly than normal, only part of the acid load is used on the food. This reduces the food's buffering effect and dumps the excess acid in the duodenum, where it erodes the GI tract lining.

If the patient has a *gastric* ulcer, explain that it results from destruction of the protective mechanisms that shield the lining of the GI tract. Consequently, this lining shows decreased resistance to gastric secretions, particularly pepsin. Mention that heredity, trauma, hormones, drugs, and psychological factors all contribute to development of a gastric ulcer.

Point out possible complications

Explain that the chances for life-threatening hemorrhage and perforation are greatly reduced if the patient adheres strictly to the treatment regimen. While slow hemorrhage from erosion of the gastric mucosa may go unnoticed, life-threatening hemorrhage can result from erosion of a major blood vessel. Also explain that after perforation of the ulcerated wall, gastroduodenal contents that leak into the peritoneum may lead to peritonitis, hemorrhage, and septic or hypovolemic shock. Also point out that failure to complete drug therapy may increase the chance of recurrence.

Teach about tests

Prepare the patient for diagnostic tests to confirm or evaluate ulcer disease. Such tests include upper GI endoscopy, upper GI series, and possibly a gastric acid stimulation test. (See *Teaching Patients about Gastrointestinal Tests*, pages 233 to 240.)

Teach about treatments

Teach the patient that treatment aims to help the stomach rest through dietary changes, medications, and physical and emotional relaxation.

• *Diet.* Inform the patient that small hourly feedings may relieve his symptoms by reducing the extent of distention, thereby reducing digestive juice secretion and gastric motility.

During the acute phase of his disease, make sure the patient understands his prescribed diet. If the doctor orders the Sippy diet, inform the patient that he'll have small amounts of milk and antacids alternately every 30 minutes. Gradually, he'll add frequent, small feedings of bland foods, such as cooked cereals, toast, and soft-boiled eggs. He won't be able to eat high-fiber

---

CHECKLIST

TEACHING TOPICS IN ULCER DISEASE

- [ ] An explanation of the type of ulcer disease: duodenal or gastric
- [ ] Warning signs of hemorrhage, obstruction, and perforation
- [ ] Preparation for diagnostic tests, such as upper GI endoscopy and upper GI series, to confirm and evaluate ulcer disease
- [ ] Dietary modifications to neutralize acid and reduce gastric motility and secretions
- [ ] Medications to relieve symptoms: antacids, anticholinergics, and tranquilizers
- [ ] If necessary, preparation for surgery, such as gastroenterostomy and vagotomy
- [ ] Other measures: adequate rest, stress management, and cessation of smoking

---

foods, such as cabbage, and irritating foods, such as soups and gravies. If constipation develops, the doctor will prescribe laxatives. Reassure the patient that eventually he'll resume a normal diet, but usually he'll remain on the restricted diet until a follow-up X-ray demonstrates ulcer healing. If the dietary regimen requires changes in cooking methods, be sure to include the family in your teaching.

After the acute phase, advise the patient to avoid large meals and high-fiber, gas-forming, and spicy foods that cause him pain. He should also eliminate fruit juices and carbonated, caffeinated, and alcoholic beverages, as they increase gastric secretion. Stress that *when* he eats is more important than *what* he eats, as any food acts as a neutralizing agent; he should avoid complete stomach emptying.

• *Medication.* Stress that symptoms usually disappear before the ulcer heals completely. Therefore, it's essential for the patient to complete his therapy (usually at least 8 weeks) to prevent symptoms from returning.

The doctor may prescribe antacids to reduce gastric acidity, histamine (H_2) receptor antagonists to reduce gastric secretion, anticholinergics to reduce gastric activity, and antianxiety drugs to promote rest and relaxation. (See *Teaching Patients about Gastrointestinal Drugs*, pages 244 to 253.)

Teach the patient to read the labels of nonprescription medications for the presence of aspirin (acetylsalicylic acid). Explain that aspirin injures the GI lining and increases its vulnerability to acid. Tell him to use alternative analgesics, such as acetaminophen.

• *Surgery.* Inform the patient that surgery may be necessary if conservative treatments fail or if complications develop. Explain the type of surgery to the patient.

Gastroenterostomy (removal of a part of the stomach) permits partial neutralization of gastric acid. However, because it doesn't decrease the secretory capacity of the stomach, it's often accompanied by a *vagotomy*. This partial severing of the vagus nerve prevents vagal impulses from reaching the stomach, thus reducing the stomach's motor activity. A *truncal vagotomy* completely severs both vagus nerves, sharply reducing stomach activity but also causing impaired emptying and diarrhea. A *superselective vagotomy*, denervating only the parietal mass cells of the stomach, prevents these problems.

A partial gastrectomy called *Billroth I* involves gastroduodenostomy (anastomosis between the stomach and the duodenum) following removal of the distal one third to one half of the stomach. A *Billroth II*, also a partial gastrectomy, involves gastrojejunostomy (anastomosis between the stomach and the jejunum) following removal of the distal segment of the stomach and antrum. Both Billroth procedures reduce gastric secretion and help restore gastric emptying. However, their possible complications include steatorrhea, dumping syndrome, weight loss, vomiting, and anemia. These complications tend to occur more commonly after the Billroth II procedure.

Pyloroplasty enlarges the pyloric sphincter, allowing reflux from the duodenum, which facilitates neutralization but doesn't inhibit gastric secretion. If combined with a vagotomy, pyloroplasty decreases gastric secretion and motility.

If the patient will be undergoing emergency surgery, inform him that preparation will include X-rays and immunohematologic studies. Explain the procedures for relieving the patient's pain and life-threatening symptoms—nasogastric suctioning, iced saline irrigations to stop bleeding, and medication.

If the patient will be undergoing planned surgery, inform him that he'll have cleansing laxatives and enemas the evening before and a nasogastric (NG) tube inserted on the morning of surgery. Explain that both measures prevent complications during surgery.

Tell the patient that the NG tube will prevent distention by draining the GI tract until his bowels begin to function in 2 to 3 days. Also inform him that he'll have a drain at the incision site for 1 or 2 days after surgery to remove any accumulated fluid, and he may be fed through a gastrostomy tube. He'll probably resume eating several days after surgery, beginning with clear liquids and gradually advancing to solid foods. If he's not allowed to eat for more than a week, he'll receive nourishment through I.V. hyperalimentation.

Explain to the patient and his family that coughing and deep breathing will be painful because of the incision, but that they're imperative to prevent postsurgical complications. (See Chapter 5 for teaching points.) Be sure the patient understands the splinting technique for coughing. Tell him that he'll go home in 1 to 2 weeks and that he'll probably resume normal activities 2 to 4 weeks later. Remind him to continue avoiding poorly tolerated foods, to follow stress

UNDERSTANDING THE DUMPING SYNDROME

If the patient's had a gastric resection with removal of the pylorus, he may develop dumping syndrome about 2 weeks after surgery. This syndrome usually occurs during meals and lasts about 1 hour. Its signs and symptoms include abdominal cramps, diaphoresis, diarrhea, palpitations, syncope, tachycardia, and weakness.

What causes dumping syndrome? After a gastric resection, food and fluid, which the stomach can no longer store, enter the small intestine in large quantities and at an abnormally fast rate. In an attempt to accommodate this sudden onrush, large amounts of fluid are drawn from the vascular system into the bowel lumen. As a result, the jejunum distends with food and fluid, and intestinal peristalsis and motility increase. This produces intestinal symptoms.

To minimize or prevent dumping syndrome, teach the patient to:
• Eat 4 to 6 small meals a day.
• Maintain a normal intake of foods containing fat and protein; they leave the stomach more slowly and attract less fluid into the intestine.
• Avoid foods with concentrated carbohydrates; they tend to attract more fluid into the intestine.
• Avoid drinking fluids with meals to decrease the fluid in the intestine.
• Avoid very hot or cold foods and fluids.
• Lie down for 1 hour after eating.
• Take anticholinergics and antispasmodics to slow intestinal motility, if ordered.

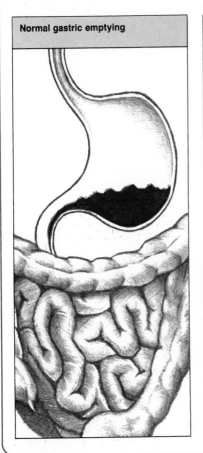

Normal gastric emptying

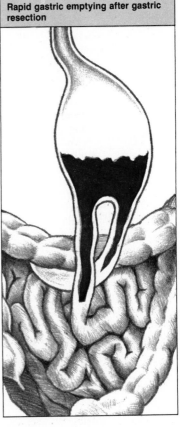

Rapid gastric emptying after gastric resection

DANGER SIGNS IN ULCER DISEASE

Although complications occur most commonly when the patient doesn't adhere strictly to his treatment regimen, they can still occur even with compliance. Instruct the patient and his family to call the doctor immediately if the patient experiences warning signs of life-threatening hemorrhage, intestinal obstruction, or perforation.

Intestinal obstruction

- A foul taste in the mouth and a coated tongue
- Abdominal fullness or distention worsening after meals and at night
- Nausea and vomiting of foul-smelling gastric contents
- Anorexia
- Weight loss

Hemorrhage

- Rapid, shallow breathing
- Bloody or coffee-ground vomitus
- Chills
- Sweating
- Dizziness upon standing
- Restlessness
- Bloody stools
- Black, tarry stools

Perforation

- Rapid, shallow breathing
- Facial flushing
- Fever
- Dizziness
- Sweating
- Abdominal rigidity
- Severe, diffuse abdominal pain that's decreased by bending at the waist or bringing the knees to the chest

management techniques, and to abstain from smoking (see *Other care measures*). If appropriate, describe the signs and symptoms of dumping syndrome and teach the patient to minimize or prevent this problem by properly managing his diet. (See *Understanding the Dumping Syndrome*, page 231.)

• *Other care measures.* Teach about necessary life-style changes, bearing in mind that the patient with ulcer disease may be assertive and independent, and changes may be difficult for him to accept. Inform him that emotional tension can precipitate an ulcer attack and prolong healing. Advise him and his family to identify stressors and explore ways to eliminate them or reduce their impact. Guide him in adjusting his work and home schedules to establish a realistic pattern of work and sleep. Recommend that the patient plan

short rest periods throughout the day. Also recommend appropriate relaxation activities, such as moderate exercise—but suggest that he eliminate the competition that can produce stress. For example, suggest playing tennis without keeping score. What relaxing hobbies and games does he like? Is he a reader? If the patient anticipates problems controlling stress, encourage him to seek counseling for stress management.

Discourage the patient from smoking, because it alters pancreatic secretions that neutralize gastric acid in the duodenum.

Instruct the patient to notify the doctor immediately if he has any signs of life-threatening complications—hemorrhage, obstruction, or perforation. (See *Danger Signs in Ulcer Disease.*) Remind the patient to visit the doctor regularly.

TEACHING PATIENTS ABOUT GASTROINTESTINAL TESTS

TEST AND PURPOSE	TEACHING POINTS
Acid perfusion test (Bernstein test) • To evaluate gastric reflux that causes esophagitis and heartburn • To distinguish chest pain caused by esophagitis from that caused by cardiac disorders	• Explain to the patient that this test helps determine the cause of chest pain. Tell him who will perform the test and where, and that it takes about 1 hour. • Instruct the patient to restrict antacids (if ordered) for 24 hours, food for 12 hours, and fluids and smoking for 8 hours before the test. • Explain what happens during the test: a flexible tube will be passed through the patient's nose into his esophagus. Assure him that the tube will be lubricated to ease its passage; however, he may feel some discomfort and may cough or gag as the tube is advanced. Tell the patient that the tube may feel cool as liquid flows through it and enters his esophagus. Instruct him to report immediately any pain or burning during the infusion. • Inform the patient that after the test he may have a sore throat, and that he'll resume his normal diet and medication as ordered.
Barium enema (lower gastrointestinal examination) • To aid diagnosis of disorders of the large intestine, such as inflammatory bowel disease • To detect diverticula, tumors, and polyps	• Explain to the patient that this test examines the large intestine through X-ray films taken after a barium enema, which clearly outlines the large intestine. Tell him who will perform the test and where, and that it takes 30 to 45 minutes. • Describe the preparation for the test: the patient must maintain a low-residue diet for 1 to 3 days and a clear liquid diet up to 24 hours before the test. About 1 hour before the test, he may have toast and black coffee or clear tea. He'll receive a laxative the afternoon before the test and up to three cleansing enemas the evening before or the morning of the test. The presence of food or fluid may prevent a clear outline of the intestine. Tell the patient that he'll wear a hospital gown. • Explain what happens during the test: the patient will be secured to a movable table. (Assure him that he'll be adequately draped.) Then, the doctor will take an X-ray of the bowel to make sure it's empty. If it is, the patient will lie on his left side and the doctor will insert a small, lubricated tube into his rectum. Instruct the patient to keep his anal sphincter tightly contracted against the tube, to hold it in position and help prevent barium leakage. Stress the importance of retaining the barium, as accurate test results depend on adequately coating the large intestine. (Assure him the barium is easy to retain because it's cool.) Once the tube's inserted, the barium slowly fills the bowel as X-ray films are taken. If air is also instilled through the tube, tell the patient the table may be tilted and he'll be assisted into various positions to aid filling. Inform him that he may experience cramping or the urge to move his bowels as the barium or air fills the large intestine. To ease the discomfort, instruct him to breathe slowly and deeply through his mouth. • Describe what happens after the test: the patient will expel

(continued)

**TEACHING PATIENTS ABOUT
GASTROINTESTINAL TESTS** (continued)

TEST AND PURPOSE	TEACHING POINTS
Barium enema (continued)	the barium into a bedpan or the toilet, and receive a laxative and an enema to clear the bowel of any remaining barium. Stress the importance of barium elimination, as retained barium may harden, causing intestinal obstruction or impaction. Tell the patient that barium will lightly color his stools for 24 to 72 hours after the test. Inform him that he may resume his diet and medications as ordered. Encourage fluid intake to prevent dehydration from the bowel preparation and test. Also, encourage rest, since the test is tiring.
Barium swallow (esophagography) • To help diagnose hiatal hernia, diverticula, and varices • To detect strictures, tumors, ulcers, or polyps in the pharynx and esophagus	• Explain to the patient that this test examines the pharynx and esophagus through X-ray films taken after a barium swallow, which clearly outlines these structures. Tell him who will perform the test and where, and that the test takes about 30 minutes. • Describe the preparation for the test: the patient must restrict antacids (if ordered) for 24 hours and food and fluids after midnight before the test. Tell the patient to remove jewelry, dentures, hairclips, and other objects that may obscure details on the X-ray films. Also tell him that he'll wear a hospital gown. • Explain what happens during the test: the patient will lie on an adjustable table and will be asked to swallow barium several times during the test. Explain that barium has a milkshake consistency and chalky taste, which may be unpleasant. First he'll swallow a thick mixture, then a thin one. If the doctor wants to accentuate small strictures or demonstrate dysphagia, the patient will swallow a special barium marshmallow (soft white bread soaked in barium). Tell the patient that as the barium outlines his pharynx and esophagus, the table will be adjusted so the doctor can take films from several angles. • Describe what happens after the test: the patient may resume his normal diet and medication as ordered, and will receive a laxative to help expel the barium. Stress the importance of barium elimination, as retained barium may harden, causing obstruction or impaction. The barium will lightly color his stools for 24 to 72 hours after the test.
Basal gastric secretion test • To evaluate epigastric pain	• Explain to the patient that this test measures the stomach's secretion of acid when he's fasting. Tell him who will perform the test and where, and that the test takes about 1½ hours. • Instruct him to withhold antacids, anticholinergics, cholinergics, cimetidine, reserpine, adrenergic blockers, or adrenocorticosteroids, as ordered, for 24 hours before the test. Tell him to restrict food for 12 hours and fluids and smoking for 8 hours before the test. • Explain what happens during the test: the patient will have a flexible tube passed through his nose into his stomach. Assure him that the tube will be lubricated to ease its passage; however, he may feel some discomfort and may cough or gag as the tube is advanced. Then the patient will lie in various positions as his stomach contents are suc-

TEACHING PATIENTS ABOUT
GASTROINTESTINAL TESTS *(continued)*

TEST AND PURPOSE	TEACHING POINTS
Basal gastric secretion test *(continued)*	tioned through the tube for analysis. Assure him that this won't hurt. • Inform the patient that after the test he may have a sore throat. Also tell him that he may resume his normal diet and, as ordered, his medications.
Cholangiography (percutaneous and postoperative) • To determine the cause of upper abdominal pain that persists after cholecystectomy • To evaluate jaundice • To determine the location, extent, and often the cause of mechanical obstruction	• Explain to the patient that this radiographic test examines the biliary ducts after injection of a contrast medium. Tell him who will perform the test and where, and that the test takes about 30 minutes. • Describe the preparation for the test: the patient must restrict food and fluids for 8 hours before the test, but should continue any drug regimen as ordered. Inform him that he'll be awake during the test, which may be uncomfortable, and that he'll receive medication to help him relax. • Explain what happens during the test: the doctor will drape and cleanse an area on the patient's abdomen, then inject a local anesthetic to minimize the discomfort of the test. Warn the patient that the injection will sting briefly. Instruct him to hold his breath, next, as the contrast medium is injected into the liver. (In postoperative cholangiography, the dye is injected through a T tube inserted into the common bile duct after surgery.) Warn him that this injection may cause a sensation of pressure and right upper back discomfort. Tell the patient to report immediately any side effects: nausea, vomiting, dizziness, headache, or urticaria. Instruct the patient to lie still, relax, breathe normally, and remain quiet as X-ray films are taken of the biliary ducts. • Describe what happens after the test: the patient's vital signs will be checked frequently for several hours, and he must remain in bed on his right side for at least 6 hours. Tell him that he may resume his normal diet after the test.
Computed tomography (CT) scan of the biliary tract, liver, or pancreas • To detect abnormalities of the biliary tract, liver, or pancreas, such as tumors, abscesses, cysts, and hematomas • To detect or evaluate pancreatitis • To determine the cause of jaundice	• Explain to the patient that this test examines the biliary tract, liver, or pancreas through computerized X-rays. Tell him who will perform the test and where, that the test is painless, and that it takes about 1½ hours. • Instruct him to restrict food and fluids after midnight before the test, but to continue any drug regimen as ordered. • Explain what happens during the test: the patient will lie on a table while X-rays are taken. Tell him to lie still, relax, breathe normally, and remain quiet, because movement will blur the X-ray picture and prolong the test. If the doctor is using an I.V. contrast medium, inform the patient that he may experience discomfort from the needle puncture and a localized feeling of warmth on injection. Tell the patient to report immediately any side effects: nausea, vomiting, dizziness, headache, or urticaria. Assure him that reactions are rare. • Inform the patient that he may resume his normal diet after the test.

(continued)

TEACHING PATIENTS ABOUT
GASTROINTESTINAL TESTS *(continued)*

TEST AND PURPOSE	TEACHING POINTS

Endoscopic retrograde cholangiopancreatography (ERCP)
• To help determine the cause of jaundice
• To evaluate tumors and inflammation of the pancreas, gallbladder, or liver
• To locate obstructions in the pancreatic duct and hepatobiliary tree
	• Explain to the patient that this test examines the liver, gallbladder, and pancreas through X-ray films. Inform him that these films are obtained with a flexible tube passed through the mouth into the intestine. Tell him who will perform the test and where, and that the test takes 30 to 60 minutes.
	• Describe the preparation for the test: the patient must restrict food and fluids after midnight before the test, but should continue any drug regimen as ordered. Tell the patient that he'll wear a hospital gown, and that he should urinate before the test, as ERCP may cause urinary retention.
	• Explain what happens during the test: the patient will lie on an X-ray table as a nurse takes his vital signs and inserts an I.V. line into his hand or arm to administer medication during the test. Inform the patient that he'll be awake during the test. Explain that although the test is uncomfortable, he'll receive a sedative to help him relax.
	   Before insertion of the tube, the patient's throat will be sprayed with a local anesthetic. Advise him that the spray tastes unpleasant and will make his mouth and throat feel swollen and numb, causing difficulty in swallowing. Instruct him to let the saliva drain from the side of his mouth. Tell him that he'll have a mouthguard to protect his teeth from the tube. Assure him that he'll have no difficulty breathing.
	   After insertion of the tube, the patient will receive an anticholinergic or glucagon I.V. to relax the small intestine. Tell him to report immediately any side effects: dry mouth, thirst, tachycardia, or blurred vision (from the anticholinergic); nausea, vomiting, urticaria, or flushing (from glucagon). Once the small intestine relaxes, the patient will be asked to assume various positions to advance the tube to the pancreas and hepatobiliary tree. He may experience warmth or flushing with injection of the contrast medium.
	• Describe what happens after the test: the patient's vital signs will be checked frequently for several hours. He'll be allowed to eat when his gag reflex returns, usually in about 1 hour. He may have a sore throat for several days.

Esophageal manometry • To detect achalasia, esophageal spasm, and esophageal scleroderma	• Explain to the patient that this test evaluates the function of the sphincter between the esophagus and stomach and the function of the esophagus. Tell him who will perform the test and where, and that the test takes about 45 minutes. • Instruct the patient to restrict smoking and alcohol for 24 hours and food and fluids for 4 hours before the test. Also tell him to stop taking cholinergics or anticholinergics, as ordered, for 24 hours before the test. • Explain what happens during the test: the doctor will measure the pressure of the patient's lower esophageal sphincter and esophagus with a small pressure transducer attached to a catheter. The patient will swallow the catheter, which may cause coughing or gagging. Once the catheter is in the esophagus, he'll sip water to stimulate esophageal peristalsis.

TEACHING PATIENTS ABOUT
GASTROINTESTINAL TESTS *(continued)*

TEST AND PURPOSE	TEACHING POINTS
Esophageal manometry *(continued)*	• Inform the patient that he may have a sore throat after the test. Also tell him that he may resume his normal diet and medication as ordered.
Gastric acid stimulation test • To aid diagnosis of duodenal ulcer, Zollinger-Ellison syndrome, pernicious anemia, and gastric carcinoma	• Explain to the patient that this test determines if the stomach is secreting acid properly. Tell him who will perform the test and where, and that the test takes about 1 hour. • Instruct the patient to stop taking antacids, anticholinergics, cholinergics, cimetidine, reserpine, adrenergic blockers, or adrenocorticosteroids, as ordered, 24 hours before the test. Tell him to restrict food, fluids, and smoking after midnight before the test. • Explain what happens during the test: a flexible tube will be passed through the patient's nose into his stomach. The tube is lubricated to ease its passage; however, he may feel some discomfort and may cough or gag as the tube is advanced. Then he'll receive a subcutaneous injection of a medication (pentagastrin) to stimulate acid secretion in his stomach. Tell the patient to report at once any side effects: abdominal pain, nausea, vomiting, flushing, dizziness, faintness, or numbness of the extremities. Next, the doctor will obtain several samples of stomach contents for analysis. • Inform the patient that he may have a sore throat after the test. Also tell him that he may resume his normal diet and medication as ordered.
Liver/spleen scanning • To detect abnormalities of the liver and spleen, such as tumors, cysts, and abscesses • To help diagnose diseases of the liver, such as cirrhosis and hepatitis • To assess the liver and spleen after abdominal trauma	• Explain to the patient that this test examines the liver and spleen through pictures taken with a special scanner or camera. Tell him who will perform the test and where, that the test is painless, and that it takes about 1 hour. • Explain what happens during the test: the patient will receive an injection of a radioactive substance (technetium sulfide—99m) through an I.V. line in his hand or arm to allow better visualization of the liver and spleen. Tell him to report immediately any side effects: flushing, fever, light-headedness, or difficulty breathing. Assure him that the injection contains only trace amounts of radioactivity and rarely produces side effects. If the test uses a rectilinear scanner, he'll hear a soft, irregular clicking noise as it moves across his abdomen. If the test uses a gamma camera, he'll feel the camera lightly touch his abdomen. Instruct him to lie still, relax, and breathe normally. He may be asked to hold his breath briefly, to ensure good-quality pictures.
Lower gastrointestinal (GI) endoscopy (colonoscopy, proctosigmoidoscopy) • To aid diagnosis of inflammatory and ulcerative bowel disease • To locate the origin of lower GI bleeding	• Explain to the patient that this test allows examination of the lower GI tract, using a flexible tube inserted into the rectum. Tell him who will perform the test and where, and that it takes about 30 minutes. • Describe the preparation for the test: the patient must maintain a clear liquid diet for up to 48 hours before the test, and, as ordered, fast the morning of the test. However, he should continue any drug regimen, as ordered. Inform the patient that he'll receive a laxative the afternoon before the

(continued)

TEACHING PATIENTS ABOUT
GASTROINTESTINAL TESTS *(continued)*

TEST AND PURPOSE	TEACHING POINTS
Lower gastrointestinal (GI) endoscopy *(continued)* • To detect abnormalities of the lower GI tract, such as tumors, polyps, hemorrhoids, and abscesses	test. Dietary restrictions and bowel preparation are essential to clear the lower GI tract for a better view. • Explain what happens during the test: the patient will lie on an X-ray table as a nurse takes his vital signs and inserts an I.V. line into his hand or arm to administer medication. He'll be awake, and although the test is uncomfortable, he'll be given a sedative to help him relax. The doctor will insert a flexible tube into the patient's rectum. Tell the patient that he may feel some lower abdominal discomfort and the urge to move his bowels as the tube is advanced. To control the urge to defecate and ease the discomfort, instruct him to breathe deeply and slowly through his mouth. Explain that air may be introduced into the bowel through the tube. If he feels the urge to expel some air, tell him not to try to control it. Also tell him that he may hear and feel a suction machine removing any liquid that may obscure the doctor's view, but it won't cause any discomfort. • Describe what happens after the test: the patient's vital signs will be checked frequently for 8 hours. He can eat after recovering from the sedative, in about 1 hour. If air was introduced into the bowel, he may pass large amounts of flatus. Instruct him to report any blood in his stool.
Oral cholecystography • To detect abnormalities of the gallbladder, such as gallstones, tumors, and inflammation	• Explain to the patient that this test examines the gallbladder through X-ray films taken after ingestion of a contrast medium. Tell him who will perform the test and where. Also tell him that the test is painless and takes about 30 to 45 minutes (or longer if a fat stimulus is to be given followed by another series of films). • Describe the preparation for the test: if ordered, the patient eats a meal containing fat at noon the day before the test and a fat-free meal that evening. After the evening meal, he can have only water, but should continue any drug regimen as ordered. He's given a cleansing enema, and 2 to 3 hours before the test he's asked to swallow six tablets, one at a time, at 5-minute intervals. The enema and tablets help outline the gallbladder on the X-ray film. Tell him to report immediately any side effects of the tablets: diarrhea, nausea, vomiting, abdominal cramps, or dysuria. • Inform the patient that during the test he'll lie on an X-ray table while films are taken of his emptying gallbladder and the patency of the common duct. • Describe what happens after the test: if test results are normal, he'll resume his usual diet. If another cholecystogram is necessary, he'll stay on a low-fat diet. If test results indicate a problem, he'll receive a special diet.
Percutaneous liver biopsy • To help diagnose cirrhosis, metastatic disease, and granulomatous infection	• Explain to the patient that this test diagnoses liver disorders through examination of liver tissue. Inform him that the doctor obtains a small specimen by inserting a needle. Tell him who will perform the test and where, and that the test takes about 15 minutes. • Instruct the patient to restrict food and fluids for at least 4 hours before the test.

TEACHING PATIENTS ABOUT
GASTROINTESTINAL TESTS *(continued)*

TEST AND PURPOSE	TEACHING POINTS
Percutaneous liver biopsy *(continued)*	• Explain what happens during the test: inform the patient that he'll be awake during the test. Although the test is uncomfortable, assure him that he'll receive medication to help him relax. Explain that the doctor will drape and cleanse an area on his abdomen and will inject a local anesthetic, which may sting and cause brief discomfort. Then, the patient will be asked to hold his breath and lie still as the doctor inserts the biopsy needle into the liver. Inform the patient that the needle may cause a sensation of pressure and some discomfort in his right upper back. Assure him that the needle will remain in his liver only about 1 second. • Describe what happens after the test: the patient's vital signs will be checked frequently for several hours. He must remain in bed on his right side for 2 hours and maintain bed rest for 24 hours. He may experience pain for several hours. Also tell him that he may resume his normal diet.
Ultrasonography of the gallbladder, biliary system, liver, spleen, or pancreas • To help diagnose disorders of the gallbladder and biliary system (such as cholelithiasis and cholecystitis), the liver (such as cirrhosis and hepatitis), and the pancreas	• Explain that this test examines body structures by means of sound waves. Tell him who will perform the test and where, and that the test takes about 15 to 30 minutes. • Instruct the patient to restrict food and fluids for 8 to 12 hours before the test. If he's having ultrasonography of his gallbladder and biliary system, instruct him to eat a fat-free meal the evening before the test before beginning his fast. • Explain what happens during the test: the patient will lie on a table in a slightly darkened room, and he'll feel the transducer moving across his abdomen. Assure him it won't be uncomfortable. Instruct him to lie still, relax, breathe normally, and remain quiet. Explain that any movement will distort the picture and prolong the test. He may also be asked to hold his breath or inhale deeply. If he's having ultrasonography of the gallbladder, he may receive an injection of a drug (sincalide) to stimulate gallbladder contraction. Tell the patient to report immediately any side effects: abdominal cramping, nausea, dizziness, sweating, or flushing. • After the test, the patient may resume his normal diet.
Upper gastrointestinal (GI) endoscopy (esophagogastroduodenoscopy) • To identify abnormalities of the esophagus, stomach, and small intestine, such as esophagitis, inflammatory bowel disease, Mallory-Weiss syndrome, lesions, tumors, gastritis, and polyps	• Explain that this test examines the esophagus, stomach, and the first part of the small intestine (duodenum), using a flexible tube inserted into the intestine through the mouth. Tell him who will perform the test and where, and that it takes about 30 minutes. • Describe the preparation for the test: the patient must restrict food and fluids for at least 6 hours before the test, but should continue any drug regimen as ordered. If the test is an emergency procedure, inform the patient that he'll have his stomach contents suctioned to permit better visualization. • Explain what happens during the test: the patient will lie on an X-ray table as a nurse takes his vital signs and inserts an I.V. line into his hand or arm to administer medication during

(continued)

**TEACHING PATIENTS ABOUT
GASTROINTESTINAL TESTS** (continued)

TEST AND PURPOSE	TEACHING POINTS
Upper gastrointestinal (GI) endoscopy (continued)	the test. Inform the patient that he'll be awake during the test. Explain that while the test is uncomfortable, he'll receive a sedative to help him relax. Before insertion of the tube, the patient's throat will be sprayed with a local anesthetic. Advise him that the spray tastes unpleasant and will make his mouth feel swollen and numb, causing difficulty in swallowing. Instruct him to let the saliva drain from the side of his mouth. Tell him that he'll have a mouthguard to protect his teeth from the tube. Assure him that he'll have no difficulty breathing. As the tube is inserted and advanced, he can expect pressure in the abdomen and some fullness or bloating as air is introduced to inflate the stomach for a better view. • Describe what happens after the test: the patient's vital signs will be checked frequently for 8 hours and he can resume eating when his gag reflex returns—usually in about 1 hour. He may have a sore throat for several days.
Upper gastrointestinal and small bowel series • To help diagnose hiatal hernia, diverticula, varices, regional enteritis, and malabsorption syndrome • To detect strictures, ulcers, or polyps in the esophagus, stomach, and small intestine	• Explain to the patient that this test examines the esophagus, stomach, and small intestine through X-ray films taken after swallowing barium, which clearly outlines the structures. Tell him who will perform the test and where. Inform him that the test requires several films to be taken up to 1 hour apart, so the test may take up to 6 hours. Advise him to bring an activity to help pass the time. • Describe the preparation for the test: the patient must maintain a low-residue diet for 2 to 3 days and must restrict food, fluids, and smoking after midnight before the test. As ordered, tell him to stop taking medications for up to 24 hours before the test. He'll receive a laxative the afternoon before the test and up to three cleansing enemas the evening before or the morning of the test. Explain that the presence of food or fluid may obscure details of the structures being studied. Tell the patient that he'll wear a hospital gown. • Explain what happens during the test: the patient will lie on a movable table and will be asked to swallow small amounts of barium several times during the test. Describe barium's milkshake consistency and chalky taste. Inform him that the doctor may compress his abdomen to ensure proper coating of the stomach and intestinal walls with barium. Also explain that the table will be adjusted to various positions so the doctor can take films from several angles. • Describe what happens after the test: the patient may resume his normal diet and medication as ordered. Tell him he'll receive a laxative or enema to help expel barium. Stress the importance of barium elimination, as retained barium may harden, causing intestinal obstruction or impaction. Explain that barium will lightly color his stools for 24 to 72 hours after the test.

SURGERY

Before you prepare the patient for GI surgery, consider his response to the scheduled procedure. For example, he may act restless and ask questions about pain, bleeding, or the unknown, signaling apprehension. Or he may, in fact, be looking forward to surgery if it promises an end to the daily disruptions of a disorder such as ulcerative colitis.

If the patient's scheduled for an ostomy, examine your own feelings about the surgery, too. Your hesitant response or facial expression can quickly convey negative feelings to the patient.

Begin your teaching by informing the patient of the purpose for his surgery. For example, tell him that an appendectomy is the only effective treatment for appendicitis. Bowel resection treats diverticulitis if perforation, obstruction, fistula formation, or hemorrhage occurs. Cholecystectomy treats gallbladder disease, and colostomy or ileostomy controls symptoms or manages complications of Crohn's disease and ulcerative colitis. Explain that partial or total gastrectomy resolves perforation or hemorrhage in ulcer disease; hemorrhoidectomy is indicated when hemorrhoids cause significant bleeding or severe discomfort; herniorrhaphy repairs a hernia; and portal-systemic shunting may be necessary to treat or prevent life-threatening esophageal varices in cirrhosis.

Continue your teaching by explaining what happens before and after surgery, including any special dietary or bowel preparation and the need for tubes and drains. Also demonstrate self-care procedures, and explain medications and dietary and activity restrictions.

Emphasize several general teaching points. Mention to the patient that the location of his incision and his decreased ability to move will place him at risk for pulmonary complications. Consequently, he must turn in bed and cough and deep-breathe at least once every hour. Also explain how to use incentive spirometry. To minimize abdominal pain when he moves or coughs, teach him to splint his incision. Encourage early ambulation to help relieve postoperative gas and prevent other complications. Tell him to ask for pain medication if he needs it.

This chapter's *Disorders* section contains specific teaching points for some types of gastrointestinal surgery; others are covered below.

Appendectomy

Your teaching will be brief, as prompt removal of the appendix is necessary to prevent complications, such as gangrene or perforation (if they haven't already occurred).

Begin by assuring the patient that removal of the appendix eliminates symptoms, but causes no change in body function. Explain that before surgery, he'll receive prophylactic antibiotics and I.V. fluids to maintain his blood pressure during surgery, and he'll have a nasogastric (NG) tube inserted. He'll be given a sedative and then a general anesthetic. After surgery, he can expect a dressing over his abdominal incision. If the surgery's complicated by gangrene or perforation, he'll have several drains at the incision site for 3 to 5 days.

Assure him that he'll recover rapidly from an uncomplicated appendectomy. He'll be up and walking, and following removal of the NG tube the day after surgery, he can have fluids and gradually resume his diet. Tell him that he'll go home on the third postoperative day and will return to his normal activity level in 2 to 4 weeks. If he's had complicated surgery, explain that he won't be allowed to eat right away, and he'll remain in bed for several days and will be discharged in 1 to 2 weeks.

Cholecystectomy

Explain that cholecystectomy, or gallbladder removal, is necessary when other measures fail to relieve symptoms of gallbladder disease. Assure the patient that his body can adjust; although the gallbladder's removed and the cystic duct's closed, the remaining ducts stay patent.

Tell the patient to restrict his diet to clear liquids for 24 hours before surgery and to fast after midnight. He'll have cleansing laxatives and enemas the evening before surgery and, to prevent postoperative complications, he'll have an NG tube inserted.

Inform the patient that after surgery the NG tube will be removed in 1 or 2 days, and he'll advance gradually from clear liquids to a low-fat diet. He can expect a drain at the incision site for 3 to 5 days to remove any accumulated fluid and bile, and a T tube in the common bile duct for 7 to 10 days to remove any retained stones. Or he may go home with the tube in place. He'll be ambulatory the day after surgery.

Tell the patient that he can go home in 1 to 2 weeks and resume normal activities in 4 to 6 weeks. Although he'll usually follow his regular diet, warn him that fatty, rich foods may cause discomfort at first, until his body adjusts to the lack of a gallbladder.

If he's returning home with a T tube, teach him to empty it (see *How to Empty the T-tube Drainage Bag*, page 243), change the dressing, and provide good skin care around the insertion site. Finally, point out possible complications, such as an obstructed T tube. Tell him to notify the doctor immediately if he observes little or no drainage and experiences abdominal tenderness, nausea, vomiting, and clay-colored stools. Warn him that his T tube may become dislodged if pulled.

Hemorrhoidectomy

Explain that a hemorrhoidectomy is necessary when other measures fail to relieve rectal bleeding and pain. Inform the patient that he'll have an enema to cleanse the bowel, a sedative to help him relax, and typically a local anesthetic.

Before discharge, which is usually the same day as surgery, teach the patient measures to relieve discomfort and promote healing, such as a sitz bath 3 or 4 times a day and after each bowel movement. Also teach him good perianal care: wiping gently with soft, white toilet paper (the dye in colored paper may be irritating), cleansing with mild soap and water, applying zinc oxide, and covering the area with a sanitary napkin. Stress the importance of good bowel habits to prevent recurrence. Recommend a high-fiber diet, 8 to 10 glasses of water daily, and avoidance of strong laxatives and straining during defecation. He shouldn't sit on the toilet too long, as this position promotes development of hemorrhoids. Caution against using stool softeners and laxatives right after surgery; a firm stool is necessary to dilate the anal canal and prevent strictures from scar tissue.

Herniorrhaphy

Explain to the patient that herniorrhaphy returns the protruding intestine to the abdominal cavity and repairs the abdominal wall defect in an inguinal hernia. He'll receive a cleansing enema before surgery, a sedative, and a spinal or general anesthetic. He'll have no tubes or drains unless surgery has been complicated by a strangulated or incarcerated hernia, but he can expect a dressing over his incision.

Assure him that recovery is usually rapid. He may go home the same day, and may resume normal activities in 2 to 4 weeks. Suggest using ice bags to relieve scrotal pain and swelling after inguinal hernia repair.

Recovery from a strangulated or incarcerated hernia will take longer. Inform the patient that he may have an NG tube for several days before he's allowed to eat or get out of bed. He'll go home in 1 to 2 weeks and will return to normal activities in 4 to 6 weeks.

HOW TO EMPTY THE T-TUBE DRAINAGE BAG

Dear Patient:

Empty your drainage bag at about the same time each day, or when it's two-thirds full. First, place a large measuring container within reach.

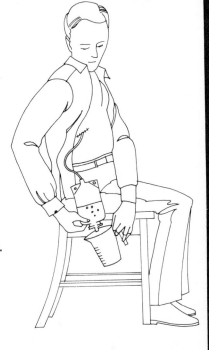

1

Sit on a chair and remove the Velcro belt that secures the drainage bag and connecting tubing to your abdomen. Uncoil the tubing, and position the spout at the bottom of the drainage bag over the measuring container, as shown at right. Don't place too much tension on the connecting tubing—you may dislodge the T tube.

2

Now, to empty the drainage bag, release the clamp on the drainage spout, so the bile flows freely into the measuring container. When the bag is empty, clean the drainage spout, using toilet paper. Close the clamp so the drainage bag is sealed.

3

Gently coil the connecting tubing. Then position the drainage bag and tubing *below* the wound site, and secure with the Velcro belt. *Never* place the drainage bag and connecting tubing higher than the wound site—that would allow bile to flow back up into the common bile duct.

4

Finally, note the amount, color, and odor of drainage. Report significant increases or decreases in the amount of drainage and any color or odor changes. These may signal complications, such as T-tube obstruction or infection.

TEACHING PATIENTS ABOUT GASTROINTESTINAL DRUGS

DRUG	ADVERSE REACTIONS	INTERACTIONS*
Antacids		
Calcium-containing antacids (Dicarbosil, Titralac, Tums)	*Reportable:* abdominal cramps, anorexia, constipation, dysuria, frequent urination, joint pain, mood or mental status changes, muscle pain, muscle twitching, nausea, nervousness, restlessness, vomiting, weakness *Other:* belching, chalky taste, confusion, mild constipation	• Tell the patient to take antacids 1 to 3 hours after meals and at bedtime. • Instruct him to space doses of iron preparations and these antacids as far apart as possible to prevent decreased iron absorption.
Magnesium-containing antacids (Maalox, Mylanta, Riopan)	*Reportable:* anorexia, dizziness, dysuria, headache, irregular heart rate, mood changes, muscle weakness *Other:* diarrhea, nausea, stomach cramps, vomiting, white specks in stools	• Tell the patient to take antacids 1 to 3 hours after meals and at bedtime. • Advise him not to take antacids within 2 hours of taking other medications. • Instruct him to space doses of iron preparations and antacids as far apart as possible to prevent decreased iron absorption.
Anticholinergics		
atropine	*Reportable:* blurred vision, confusion, dizziness, dyspnea, eye pain, flushing, rash, seizures, tachycardia, unusual tiredness or weakness *Other:* constipation; decreased sweating; drowsiness; dry mouth, nose, and throat; dysuria; headache; nausea; photophobia; vomiting	• Advise the patient to separate doses of atropine from doses of antacids and of kaolin- or pectin-containing antidiarrheals, to prevent decreased effectiveness of atropine. • Instruct him to take this drug 30 minutes to 1 hour before meals, as ordered. • Tell him to avoid alcohol and CNS depressants (increased adverse reactions possible).
methantheline bromide (Banthine) **propantheline bromide** (Probanthine)	*Reportable:* constipation, difficult urination, eye pain, rash, tachycardia *Other:* confusion, decreased sweating, dizziness, drowsiness, dry mouth, fatigue, headache, nausea, photophobia, vomiting	• Instruct the patient to take this drug 30 minutes to 1 hour before meals, as ordered. • Advise him that antacids and kaolin- or pectin-containing antidiarrheals may decrease these drugs' effectiveness. He should separate doses by 1 hour. • Instruct the patient to avoid alcohol and CNS depressants (increased adverse reactions possible).

*Interactions include food, alcohol, and over-the-counter drugs.

TEACHING POINTS

• Explain to the patient that this drug helps relieve heartburn or acid stomach.
• Instruct him to chew the tablet well before swallowing and to follow the dose with a full glass of water.
• Caution him about acid rebound if he takes this drug constantly for more than 2 weeks. Explain the dangers of self-medication, and advise him to consult his doctor before making any changes in his medication regimen.
• If the patient misses a dose, tell him to take the missed dose as soon as possible, then resume his schedule. He must never double dose.
• If constipation's a problem, the doctor may prescribe an alternate antacid, combination therapy, or a stool softener.

• Explain to the patient that this drug helps relieve heartburn and acid stomach.
• Instruct him to chew the tablet well before swallowing and to follow the dose with a full glass of water.
• Instruct the patient to shake the liquid form of this drug well before taking. Suggest mixing the tablet and liquid forms with fluids or food if preferred.
• If the patient misses a dose, instruct him to take the missed dose as soon as possible, then resume his schedule. He must never double dose.
• Warn the patient about the dangers of self-medication. Advise him to consult his doctor before making any changes in his medication regimen.
• If he experiences diarrhea, tell him that the doctor may prescribe an alternate antacid, combination therapy, or a stool softener.

• Explain to the patient that this drug helps relieve cramps or spasms of the intestines, stomach, and bladder. Explain that it's used in combination with other drugs to treat ulcer disease, and may also prevent nausea, vomiting, and motion sickness.
• If the patient misses a dose, instruct him to take the missed dose as soon as possible. If it's almost time for his next dose, he should skip the missed dose and resume his schedule. He must never double dose.
• Inform the patient that this drug often reduces sweating, allowing body temperature to rise. To prevent heat stroke, caution him to avoid becoming overheated during exercise or hot weather.
• Explain that this drug may make his eyes more sensitive to light. Suggest wearing sunglasses.
• Advise the patient to be sure his vision is clear before driving or performing other activities that require clear vision.
• Suggest that he chew sugarless gum or ice chips to relieve mouth dryness.

• Explain to the patient that this drug helps relieve stomach cramps, spasms, and acid stomach.
• If the patient misses a dose, instruct him to skip the missed dose and resume his schedule. He must never double dose.
• If this drug makes him feel drowsy, caution him to avoid driving, operating machinery, or performing other activities that require alertness.
• Explain that this drug may make his eyes more sensitive to light. Suggest wearing sunglasses.
• Inform the patient that this drug often reduces sweating, allowing body temperature to rise. To prevent heat stroke, caution him to avoid becoming overheated during exercise or hot weather.
• Suggest that he chew sugarless gum or ice chips to relieve mouth dryness.

(continued)

TEACHING PATIENTS ABOUT
GASTROINTESTINAL DRUGS *(continued)*

DRUG	ADVERSE REACTIONS	INTERACTIONS*
Antidiarrheals		
diphenoxylate and atropine (Lomotil)	*Reportable:* anorexia, bloating, constipation, nausea, shortness of breath, stomach pain, tachycardia, vomiting *Other:* blurred vision, depression, dizziness, drowsiness, dry mouth, dysuria, fever, headache, rash	• Tell the patient to avoid alcohol and cold, allergy, and sleep medications (increased adverse reactions possible). • Inform him that food and nonalcoholic beverages don't influence the safety or effectiveness of this drug.
kaolin and pectin (Kaopectate)	*Reportable:* none *Other:* mild constipation	• Inform the patient that food, beverages, and OTC drugs don't influence the safety or effectiveness of kaolin and pectin. • Advise him to separate doses of this drug and prescription drugs, since interactions occur commonly.
loperamide (Imodium)	*Reportable:* none *Other:* anorexia, bloating, constipation, dizziness, drowsiness, dry mouth, fever, nausea, rash, stomach cramps, vomiting	• Tell the patient that food, beverages, and OTC drugs don't influence the safety or effectiveness of loperamide.
paregoric	*Reportable:* abdominal pain, anorexia, constipation, depression, hypertension, nausea, rash, vomiting *Other:* dizziness, drowsiness, dysuria, increased sweating, oliguria	• Tell the patient to avoid alcohol and cold, allergy, and sleep medications (increased adverse reactions possible). • Inform him that food and nonalcoholic beverages don't influence the safety or effectiveness of this drug.
Antiemetics		
dimenhydrinate (Dramamine)	*Reportable:* fainting, fever, hallucinations, seizures, shortness of breath, sore throat, tachycardia, unusual bleeding or bruising, unusual tiredness *Other:* abdominal cramps; anorexia; blurred vision; diaphoresis; drowsiness; dry mouth, nose, and throat; dysuria; headache; nervousness	• Tell the patient taking this drug to avoid alcohol and cold, allergy, and sleep medications (increased adverse reactions possible). • Inform him that food and nonalcoholic beverages don't influence the safety or effectiveness of this drug.

*Interactions include food, alcohol, and over-the-counter drugs.

TEACHING POINTS

• Explain to the patient that this drug controls severe diarrhea by relaxing the intestinal muscles.
• If the patient misses a dose and still has diarrhea, instruct him to take the missed dose as soon as possible. Tell him to take any remaining doses for that day at evenly spaced intervals. If he misses a dose and his diarrhea has stopped, tell him to skip the missed dose and to take the next dose on schedule.
• Advise him to contact the doctor if he experiences any of the following after discontinuing the drug: muscle cramps, nausea, vomiting, shivering or trembling, stomach cramps, or increased sweating.

• Explain to the patient that this drug helps control diarrhea.
• Instruct him to shake the liquid well before taking.
• Advise the patient to check with the doctor if diarrhea doesn't stop within 1 to 2 days or if he develops a fever, as this may indicate infection.
• Instruct him to take this drug after a loose bowel movement. He doesn't need a regular dosage schedule, but tell him to check with the doctor for intervals between doses.

• Explain to the patient that this drug helps control severe diarrhea.
• If the patient misses a dose, instruct him to skip the missed dose and to take the next dose on schedule. He must never double dose.
• If this drug makes him feel drowsy, caution him to avoid driving, operating machinery, or performing other activities that require alertness.
• Suggest that he chew sugarless gum or ice chips to relieve mouth dryness.

• Explain to the patient that this drug helps control severe diarrhea.
• Instruct him to take the drug as directed, or it may become habit-forming.
• If the patient misses a dose, instruct him to take the missed dose as soon as possible. However, if it's almost time for his next dose, he should skip the missed dose and resume his regular schedule. He must never double dose.
• If this drug makes him feel drowsy, caution him to avoid driving, operating machinery, or performing other activities that require alertness.
• To minimize dizziness, advise him to rise slowly from a sitting or a lying position.

• Explain to the patient that this drug helps prevent motion sickness, nausea, vomiting, and dizziness.
• Instruct the patient to take tablets with food or with water or milk to decrease stomach irritation. Tell him not to chew tablets.
• If he's using the suppository form, provide instructions.
• For motion sickness, advise taking the drug at least 30 minutes and, for best results, 1 to 2 hours before travel.
• If the patient misses a dose, instruct him to take the missed dose as soon as possible. However, if it's almost time for the next dose, tell him to skip the missed dose and resume his regular schedule. He must never double dose.
• If this drug makes him feel drowsy, caution him to avoid driving, operating machinery, or performing other activities that require alertness.
• Advise the patient to let his doctor know he's taking this drug, because it may mask the symptoms of several disorders.

(continued)

TEACHING PATIENTS ABOUT
GASTROINTESTINAL DRUGS *(continued)*

DRUG	ADVERSE REACTIONS	INTERACTIONS*
Antiemetics *(continued)*		
metoclopramide hydrochloride (Reglan)	*Reportable:* confusion, muscle spasms, severe drowsiness, shuffling, tics, trembling hands *Other:* changes in menstruation, constipation, depression, diarrhea, dizziness, drowsiness, dry mouth, headache, insomnia, rash, unusual tiredness or weakness	• Tell the patient to avoid alcohol and cold, allergy, and sleep medications (increased adverse reactions possible). • For best absorption, advise him to take this drug 30 minutes before meals.
prochlorperazine (Compazine)	*Reportable:* diaphoresis, difficulty breathing, irregular pulse, loss of balance, orthostatic hypotension, seizures, shaking of fingers and hands, shuffling walk, tachycardia, trembling, unusual tiredness *Other:* constipation, decreased sweating, dizziness, drowsiness, dry mouth, nasal congestion, photosensitivity	• Tell the patient to avoid alcohol and cold, allergy and sleep medications (increased adverse reactions possible). • Instruct him to separate doses of this drug and antacids or antidiarrheals, such as kaolin-pectin, by 2 hours if possible. • Inform him that food and nonalcoholic beverages don't influence the safety or effectiveness of this drug.
scopolamine transdermal disc (Transderm Scop)	*Reportable:* none *Other:* constipation; dilated pupils; disorientation; dizziness; drowsiness; dry mouth, nose, and throat; fatigue; urinary retention	• Advise the patient to avoid alcohol and cold, allergy, and sleep medications as they cause increased drowsiness and CNS depression. However, these discs usually cause less CNS depression than oral and parenteral drugs.
trimethobenzamide (Tigan)	*Reportable:* back pain, jaundice, seizures, shakiness or tremors, unusual tiredness *Other:* blurred vision, diarrhea, dizziness, drowsiness, headache, muscle cramps	• Tell the patient to avoid alcohol and cold, allergy, and sleep medications (increased adverse reactions possible). • Tell him that food and nonalcoholic beverages don't affect this drug's safety or effectiveness.
Anti-inflammatory drugs		
sulfasalazine (Azulfidine)	*Reportable:* aching joints and muscles, dizziness, fever, headache, hematuria, itching, jaundice, low back pain, photosensitivity, rash, unusual bruising or bleeding *Other:* anorexia, GI upset, urine discoloration	• Inform the patient that food, beverages, and OTC drugs don't influence the safety or effectiveness of sulfasalazine.

*Interactions include food, alcohol, and over-the-counter drugs.

TEACHING POINTS

• Explain that this drug helps prevent nausea and vomiting.
• If the patient misses a dose, instruct him to take the missed dose as soon as possible. However, if it's almost time for his next dose, tell him to skip the missed dose and resume his regular schedule. He must never double dose.
• If this drug makes him feel drowsy, caution him to avoid driving, operating machinery, or performing other activities that require alertness.

• Explain to the patient that this drug relieves nausea and vomiting and may make him feel more relaxed and less anxious.
• Instruct him to mix the liquid form with water, milk, soft drinks, coffee, tea, tomato or fruit juices, or puddings. He should add the drug just before taking it.
• Caution him never to chew, break, or crush extended-release tablets. This destroys the coating and releases the full dose at once. To decrease stomach irritation, he should take tablets with food or a full glass of water.
• Inform him that this drug increases sensitivity to ultraviolet rays. Advise him to protect his skin from the sun's direct rays.
• Inform him that this drug often reduces sweating, allowing body temperature to rise. To prevent heat stroke, caution him to avoid overheating during exercise or hot weather.
• If this drug makes him feel drowsy, he shouldn't drive, operate machinery, or perform other activities that require alertness.
• To minimize dizziness, advise him to rise slowly from a sitting or a lying position.

• Explain that this drug helps prevent nausea and vomiting associated with motion sickness.
• Teach the patient how to apply the disc. If the disc becomes displaced, tell him to replace it on another site behind the ear.
• For best results, advise him to apply the disc the night before a trip. However, effects are still achieved when disc is applied 2 or 3 hours before experiencing motion.
• Instruct him to wash his hands thoroughly after handling the disc to remove any residual drug. Also, he should avoid touching his eyes before washing his hands.

• Explain to the patient that this drug helps prevent or relieve nausea and vomiting.
• For the suppository form, provide instructions; for the intramuscular injection form, demonstrate the correct technique.
• If this drug makes him drowsy, caution him to avoid driving, operating machinery, or performing other activities that require alertness.
• If the patient who regularly uses the medication misses a dose, instruct him to take the missed dose as soon as possible. However, if it's almost time for his next dose, tell him to skip the missed dose and resume his schedule. He must never double dose.

• Explain that this drug relieves inflammation of the colon in inflammatory bowel disease.
• Instruct the patient to take this drug with food to prevent stomach upset.
• Tell him not to chew, break, or crush tablets, as this may cause gastric irritation.
• Tell him to examine stools for the presence of intact enteric-coated tablets. If this occurs, conventional tablets will be prescribed.
• If he misses a dose, tell him to take it as soon as possible. If it's almost time for his next dose, tell him to skip the missed dose and resume his schedule. He must not double dose.
• Warn the patient that this drug may turn urine and skin a harmless orange-yellow.
• Advise him to protect his skin from the sun's direct rays, because this drug increases sensitivity to ultraviolet rays.

(continued)

TEACHING PATIENTS ABOUT
GASTROINTESTINAL DRUGS *(continued)*

DRUG	ADVERSE REACTIONS	INTERACTIONS*
Antilipemics		
cholestyramine (Questran) **colestipol** (Colestid)	*Reportable:* melena, nausea, severe constipation, unusual weight loss, vomiting *Other:* heartburn, indigestion, rash	• Inform the patient that food, beverages, and OTC drugs don't influence the safety or effectiveness of these drugs.
Digestants (pancreatic enzymes)		
pancreatin (Viokase) **pancrelipase** (Cotazym, Pancrease)	*Reportable:* diarrhea, hematuria, joint pain, nausea, stomach cramps, stomach pain, swelling of feet	• Inform the patient that food, beverages, and OTC drugs don't influence the safety or effectiveness of these drugs.
Histamine (H₂) receptor antagonists		
cimetidine (Tagamet) **ranitidine** (Zantac)	*Reportable:* confusion, unusual bleeding or bruising, unusual tiredness or weakness *Other:* diarrhea, decreased sexual ability, dizziness, gynecomastia, headache, muscle cramps or pain, rash	• Instruct the patient to take these drugs with or immediately after meals. Food delays absorption and prolongs drug effect. • Advise the patient to separate doses of these drugs and antacids by 1 hour (decreased absorption possible).
Laxatives		
Bulk-forming laxatives **methylcellulose** (Cologel) **psyllium** (Metamucil)	*Reportable:* breathing difficulty, diarrhea, itching, rash, swallowing difficulty, vomiting *Other:* nausea	• Inform the patient that food, beverages, and OTC drugs don't influence the safety or effectiveness of these drugs.
Emollient laxatives **docusate salts** (Colace, Surfak)	*Reportable:* rash *Other:* mild abdominal cramps, nausea, throat irritation (with liquid form)	• Inform the patient that food, beverages, and OTC drugs don't influence the safety or effectiveness of these drugs. • Avoid mineral oil while taking these drugs (increased mineral oil absorption and toxicity possible).

*Interactions include food, alcohol, and over-the-counter drugs.

TEACHING POINTS

• Explain to the patient that this drug helps remove excess bile salts from the body and relieves the itching that they cause.
• Instruct him to dissolve this drug in 2 to 6 ounces of preferred liquid. Caution him never to take this drug in its dry form; it irritates mucous membranes and may cause esophageal obstruction.

• If the patient's overweight, this drug will be less effective. Encourage him to consult his doctor about weight reduction.
• If the patient misses a dose, instruct him to take the missed dose as soon as possible. But if it's almost time for his next dose, tell him to skip the missed dose and resume his schedule. He must never double dose.

• Explain that this drug aids digestion when the pancreas isn't working properly.
• Tell him to follow the doctor's instructions regarding taking this drug with meals.
• Caution him never to chew, break, or crush the tablet form, because this destroys the

coating and may cause GI irritation. However, he may open the capsule form and gently mix the contents with soft foods.
• Tell him not to inhale the powder, which may result in a stuffy nose, shortness of breath, wheezing, and chest tightness.

• Explain to the patient that this drug relieves symptoms of ulcers by decreasing acid production by the stomach.
• Inform the patient that smoking interferes with the effect of this drug. Advise him to stop smoking. If abstinence is not possible, discourage smoking after taking the evening dose to prevent interference with drug control

of nocturnal gastric acid secretion.
• If the patient misses a dose, instruct him to take the missed dose as soon as possible. However, if it's almost time for his next dose, tell him to skip the missed dose and resume his regular schedule. He must never double dose.

• Explain to the patient that this drug helps relieve constipation or create a formed stool. Advise him to contact the doctor if he hasn't had a bowel movement after he's taken the medication for the prescribed time. Caution against overuse of laxatives.
• Instruct the patient to take tablets with a full glass of water and not to chew them. This prevents swelling of the medication in the

esophagus, which may cause obstruction.
• Instruct him to mix the powder form with a full glass of water, milk, fruit juice, or other liquid, and to drink it immediately.
• Advise him to drink 8 glasses of water a day to help prevent impaction.
• Inform him that the drug may work in 12 hours, but its effects may be delayed up to 3 days.

• Explain to the patient that this drug helps prevent constipation and hard stools. Tell him to take the drug for the prescribed time only.
• Advise him to contact the doctor if stools don't become softer in 1 to 3 days after taking the drug. Caution against overuse of laxatives.
• Advise him to drink 6 to 8 full glasses of

fluid a day while taking this drug, to help soften stools.
• Inform him that the liquid form has a bitter taste. To improve the flavor, suggest taking it in a glass of milk or fruit juice.
• Tell the patient to expect results in 1 to 2 days after the first dose; however, results may take up to 3 to 5 days.

(continued)

TEACHING PATIENTS ABOUT
GASTROINTESTINAL DRUGS *(continued)*

DRUG	ADVERSE REACTIONS	INTERACTIONS*
Laxatives *(continued)*		
Hyperosmotic laxatives **citrate of magnesia** (Magnesium Citrate)	*Reportable:* confusion, dizziness, irregular heart rate, unusual tiredness or weakness *Other:* abdominal cramps, diarrhea	• For best results, advise the patient to take this drug 1 hour before or 3 hours after meals. • Inform him that beverages and OTC drugs don't influence the safety or effectiveness of citrate of magnesia.
Lubricant laxatives **mineral oil** (Agoral Plain, Kondremul Plain)	*Reportable:* abdominal pain, nausea, vomiting *Other:* irritation of tissues around rectal area	• Inform the patient that mineral oil may reduce the absorption of fat-soluble vitamins A,D,E, and K. He should take them 2 hours apart. • Tell him not to take mineral oil within 2 hours of meals, to prevent decreased absorption of vitamins and other nutrients. • Tell him to avoid taking docusate salts when using mineral oil (increased absorption and toxicity of mineral oil possible).
Stimulant laxatives **bisacodyl** (Dulcolax) **cascara sagrada** **castor oil** **danthron** (Modane) **phenolphthalein** (Ex-Lax) **senna** (Senokot)	*Reportable:* burning on urination, confusion, headache, irregular heart rate, irritability, mood or mental status changes, muscle spasm, rash *Other:* belching, diarrhea, nausea, stomach cramps, urine discoloration	• For best results, tell the patient to take these drugs 1 hour before or 3 hours after meals. • Inform him that beverages and OTC medications don't influence the safety or effectiveness of these drugs (except bisacodyl). • Instruct the patient not to take bisacodyl with milk.
Miscellaneous		
simethicone (Mylicon)	None significant	• Inform the patient that food, beverages, and OTC drugs don't influence the safety or effectiveness of this drug.
sucralfate (Carafate)	*Reportable:* none *Other:* backache, constipation, diarrhea, dizziness, drowsiness, dry mouth, light-headedness, indigestion, nausea, rash, stomach cramps	• Instruct the patient to separate doses of this drug and antacids by 1 hour, to prevent decreased effectiveness of sucralfate. • Inform him that this drug may reduce absorption of fat-soluble vitamins A, D, E, and K. He should take them separately. • For best results, tell him to take the drug 1 hour before meals.

*Interactions include food, alcohol, and over-the-counter drugs.

TEACHING POINTS

• Explain to the patient that this drug helps relieve constipation. It may also be used to help cleanse the bowel before diagnostic studies or surgery.
• Advise him to contact the doctor if he doesn't have a bowel movement after he's taken the drug for the prescribed time. Caution against overuse of laxatives.
• Tell him to mix the drug with a full glass of water or fruit juice to improve the taste.
• Tell the patient that the drug works in about 2 to 6 hours; he should time his dose for convenience.

• Explain to the patient that this drug helps prevent constipation and hard stools. Advise him to contact the doctor if he doesn't have a bowel movement after he's taken the medication for the prescribed time. Caution against overuse of laxatives.
• Instruct him to take the drug with a full glass of water or fruit juice.
• Advise him to drink at least 6 to 8 full glasses of water a day while taking this drug, to help soften stools.
• Inform the patient that the drug works in about 6 to 8 hours. It's usually taken at bedtime.
• Warn the patient that this drug may cause leaking of oil from the rectum when taken for a long time. Suggest wearing a sanitary pad.

• Explain that this drug helps prevent or relieve constipation. It may also be used to help cleanse the bowel before diagnostic studies or surgery.
• Tell him to contact the doctor if he doesn't have a bowel movement after he's taken the drug for the prescribed time. Caution against laxative overuse.
• If he's taking the suppository form, provide instructions.
• Caution him never to chew, break, or crush bisacodyl tablets, as this destroys the coating and may cause gastric irritation.
• Inform the patient that these drugs begin to act in about 6 to 12 hours (except castor oil, which works in 2 to 6 hours, and bisacodyl suppositories, in about 10 minutes to 2 hours). He should schedule doses for convenience.
• Advise the patient to drink 6 to 8 full glasses of fluid a day while taking this drug, to help soften stools.
• Warn him that cascara sagrada, danthron, phenolphthalein, and senna may turn his urine a harmless pinkish-red or violet.

• Explain to the patient that this drug helps relieve gas in the stomach and intestines.
• For best results, instruct him to take the drug after meals and at bedtime, as ordered.
• If he's taking the tablet form, instruct him to chew tablets thoroughly.

• Explain to the patient that this drug helps relieve symptoms of ulcers and promotes healing.
• Instruct him to take the drug with a full glass of water.
• If the patient misses a dose, instruct him to take the missed dose as soon as possible. However, if it's almost time for his next dose, tell him to skip the missed dose and resume his regular schedule. He must never double dose.

9

Nervous System

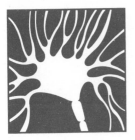

Nervous System

Introduction

Teaching a patient with neurologic dysfunction certainly poses a challenge to your teaching skills. Often it centers on teaching alternative methods of performing routine tasks to compensate for temporary or permanent neurologic deficits. And it often involves teaching the patient's family, because so many neurologic disorders cause progressive degeneration. You'll need the family to reinforce your teaching so the patient can maintain his independence for as long as possible. You can also teach them methods of coping with the demands the patient's disorder places on their lives.

Teaching varying age-groups
You'll need to tailor your teaching to suit different age-groups. For example, seizure disorders can strike children, the middle-aged, or the elderly; usually, multiple sclerosis (MS) occurs in young adults; and other degenerative diseases, such as Parkinson's and Alzheimer's, typically afflict the middle-aged or elderly.

Addressing widespread effects
Your teaching will need to address the widespread effects of neurologic disorders. In amyotrophic lateral sclerosis, MS, and cerebrovascular accident, physical deficits can prevent the patient from carrying out even routine daily activities, such as bathing, dressing, and eating. In some of these disorders, too, speech impairments hinder communication, emotional lability prevents productive activity, and cognitive deficits cause short attention and retention spans.

Dealing with long-term disability
In progressive neurologic disorders, perhaps your biggest challenge involves teaching the patient to function as independently as possible. One obstacle to teaching is the remissions and exacerbations that characterize many of these disorders. However, you can point out that failure to follow the prescribed treatment regimen may lead to increased and intensified symptoms. If the patient has mobility problems, explain that noncompliance with medication and exercise can lead to physical injury, immobility, and further complications, such as decubitus ulcers and pneumonia.

Another obstacle to your teaching may be the patient's emotional state. You'll need to evaluate his emotional response to his disorder, allowing him to express his grief for the loss of his former capabilities and encouraging him to discuss his problems. Your accepting attitude will make him more receptive to your teaching.

DISORDERS

Alzheimer's Disease

In this degenerative dementia, your primary teaching goal consists of preparing the patient and his family to meet the growing demands of progressive illness. You'll need to teach them about the inexorable course of the disease and the necessary measures they'll need to take to relieve its physical, emotional, and social strains. For example, you'll need to teach the family how to balance the sometimes conflicting needs of encouraging the patient's activity and independence while ensuring his safety.

Describe the disorder

Explain that the cause of Alzheimer's disease isn't known, but that several factors have been implicated: a deficiency in the brain's neurotransmitter substances, viruses, genetic predisposition, and environmental toxins. Also explain that the disease progressively affects the patient's ability to learn, remember, communicate, and act. In its early stages, the patient or his family may notice memory loss or personality changes. As the disease progresses, the patient's symptoms worsen: he becomes disoriented, emotionally labile, and unable to speak, write, or perform coordinated movements.

Tell the patient and his family that the disease progresses at an unpredictable rate.

Point out possible complications

Reinforce the need for precautions as the disease progresses to prevent the patient from injuring himself from his own violent behavior, wandering, or unsupervised activity. Also, explain that insufficient exercise and activity may lead to immobility and its complications, such as pneumonia and other infections. Mention that malnutrition and dehydration may also occur if the patient forgets or refuses to eat.

Teach about tests

Because no tests directly detect Alzheimer's disease, prepare the patient for studies that rule out other diseases. These studies may include a computed tomography (CT) scan, electroencephalography, positron emission tomography, and cerebrospinal fluid analysis. Also prepare the patient and his family for neuropsychological tests, which evaluate intellectual and emotional function. (See *Teaching Patients about Neurologic Tests*, pages 293 to 299, for additional information.)

Teach about treatments

• *Activity.* Explain that adequate exercise and activity during the day maintain mobility and promote a normal day and night routine. Encourage the family to find physical activities, such as dancing or light housework, that satisfy and occupy the patient.
• *Diet.* Stress the importance of a well-balanced diet with adequate fiber. If the patient is hyperactive, advise the family to increase his caloric intake with between-meal supplements. But tell them to avoid stimulants, such as coffee, tea, carbonated cola beverages, and chocolate.

Tell the family to limit the number of foods on the patient's plate, so he won't have to make decisions. If the patient has coordination difficulties, advise the family to cut his food and to provide finger foods, such as fruit and sandwiches. Suggest using plates with rim guards, built-up utensils, and cups with lids and spouts.

If the patient develops dysphagia, tell the family to serve semisoft foods. Suggest freezing liquids to a slush or mixing them with other foods. If the patient can't swallow or has no interest in food, nasogastric or gastrostomy tube feedings may be necessary; instruct the family accordingly.

If the patient puts almost anything in his mouth, whether it's food or not, tell the family to keep preferred foods readily available.

● *Medication.* Explain that no medications are currently available to treat Alzheimer's disease, but that several are being studied. Tell the family to check with the doctor before giving the patient a sedative; drug action may be reversed (due to slowed metabolism) in Alzheimer's disease, making the patient wakeful and restless. To control behavioral changes, the doctor may prescribe an antipsychotic, such as haloperidol, and antidepressants.

If the patient has trouble swallowing, tell the family to crush pills and mix them with a semisoft food or give them through the feeding tube.

● *Other care measures.* Encourage the family to provide the patient with as much independence as possible while ensuring his—and others'—safety. (See *Caring for a Person with Alzheimer's Disease*, page 258.) To combat the patient's confusion, emphasize maintaining a routine in *all* his activities. If the patient panics or becomes belligerent, advise the family to remain calm and to try distracting him.

Recommend dividing the patient's daily tasks into short, simple steps and then guiding him through them. Tell the family to use activities that stimulate or calm him appropriately. Suggest repetitive tasks, such as sanding wood and listening to music. Also, advise the family to avoid overstimulating the patient before bedtime and to limit fluids about 3 to 4 hours before bedtime, so the patient won't need to get up to urinate. If he develops irregular sleep patterns and wanders at night, he may harm himself and others. If necessary, tell the family to lock doors and windows, barricade stairways, and use night-lights. If the patient's confused about his surroundings, tell the family to use pictures to guide him. For ex-

CHECKLIST

TEACHING TOPICS IN ALZHEIMER'S DISEASE

☐ An explanation of the progressive course and worsening symptoms of the disease

☐ The role of diagnostic and neuropsychological tests

☐ The importance of establishing a daily routine for the patient

☐ The need for activity and exercise to maintain mobility

☐ Dietary adjustments for patients with restlessness, dysphagia, or coordination problems

☐ Techniques for managing confusion and preventing violent behavior

☐ Safety measures and assistive devices

☐ Drugs to help control the patient's behavior

☐ Referral to local and national organizations for information and support

ample, they can place a picture of a commode on the bathroom door and a picture of a bed on his bedroom door.

Teach the family about home safety measures, such as storing medication out of the patient's reach and removing throw rugs. If necessary, remind them to remove handles and buttons from appliances.

If the patient has coordination difficulties, suggest using Velcro strips instead of buttons and loafers or shoes with elastic shoelaces.

Teach the family about special equipment, such as a geriatric chair, that may protect the patient and make caring for him easier. Stress that the patient can't control his activities, although he may sometimes respond appropriately. And, if the patient no longer recognizes his family, urge them to still include him in their activities. Refer them to a local Alzheimer's support group and to the Alzheimer's Disease and Related Disorders Association for more information.

CARING FOR A PERSON WITH ALZHEIMER'S DISEASE

Dear Caregiver:

Caring for a person with Alzheimer's disease requires lots of patience and understanding. It also requires adapting his surroundings to control and protect him. You can use the following guidelines to help you provide a safe, stress-free environment for a person with Alzheimer's disease.

Safety tips

Survey the person's home for any potential safety hazards. Place objects that could cause injury—for example, knives and scissors—in a safe place. Also, use unbreakable plates, cups, and glasses, and check the temperature of the person's food before serving it to prevent burns. Lower the temperature on the water heater, too.

Install safety rails where needed—near the bathtub and toilet and on stairways. Remove throw rugs, toys, and other objects that might clutter the floor and stairways. Move furniture to the sides of rooms, and use padding to keep area rugs from sliding. If necessary, install high gates on stairways, and lock windows and doors. Also, have the person wear an identification necklace or bracelet. Be sure the family's address and phone number and the person's disorder appear clearly on it.

Tips for reducing stress

The person in your care will function better if you establish a daily routine for him. Do this by first listing his usual activities, including hygiene, scheduled medications, rest periods, hobbies, recreational walks, and housework or yard work. Then develop a schedule—and be sure to stick to it. Also, limit the number of people who interact with the person to one at a time.

After a break in the person's routine or when he's overtired, you can expect him to be more confused or even violent. To deal with him, use a calm voice and gentle physical contact, such as stroking or massage, to soothe him. If necessary, slowly move him to a less stimulating area.

Amyotrophic Lateral Sclerosis

Your teaching in this progressive, incurable disorder will be tailored to the stage of the patient's illness, focusing on supportive measures that the patient and his family can learn to help them deal with his worsening fatigue and muscle weakness. Early on, you'll need to stress the importance of exercise in maintaining strength in unaffected muscles. Later, you may need to teach the family how to give an intermittent feeding or how to ventilate and suction the patient.

To ensure the patient's safety and comfort, you'll need to teach the family about modifying the home environment. You'll also need to teach them how to handle the patient's drooling and dysphagia while providing good nutrition and ensuring that he receives his medications. When the disorder progresses to cause a loss of speech, you'll need to help the patient and his family establish an alternate means of communication.

Describe the disorder
Explain to the patient that amyotrophic lateral sclerosis (ALS) involves degeneration of the neurons that govern muscle movement. The disorder progressively affects more and more neurons, but at an unpredictable rate. Tell the patient to expect muscle weakness and spasms and progressive loss of muscle control. Also tell him that ALS usually doesn't affect mental status, eyelid movement, sensation, or bowel and bladder control.

Point out possible complications
Emphasize the importance of following supportive measures to forestall complications from severe muscle weakness or paralysis. If the patient neglects exercise and movement, explain that resulting immobility can lead to decubitus formation, respiratory infection, and life-threatening respiratory insufficiency.

Teach about tests
Teach the patient about scheduled diagnostic tests, such as electromyography and nerve conduction studies, to help distinguish ALS from muscle disorders. Additional tests, such as a CT scan, myelography, electroencephalography, and cerebrospinal fluid analysis, may be performed to rule out other disorders. (See *Teaching Patients about Neurologic Tests*, pages 293 to 299, for additional teaching points.)

Teach about treatments
• *Activity.* Encourage the patient to perform exercises that maintain the strength of unaffected muscles. Stress the importance of taking rest periods during exercise. Inform him and his family about splints, braces, and walk-

---

CHECKLIST

TEACHING TOPICS IN A.L.S.

☐ Explanation of how motor neuron degeneration affects muscles and motor function

☐ Preparation for electromyography, nerve conduction studies, and other tests to help distinguish ALS from other disorders

☐ The importance of exercise in maintaining strength in unaffected muscles

☐ Dietary changes, such as use of semisoft foods

☐ Techniques for nasogastric and gastrostomy tube feedings, if needed

☐ Palliative medications

☐ Techniques for respiratory support

☐ Alternate communication techniques

☐ Availability of information from the Muscular Dystrophy Association

HOW TO GIVE AN INTERMITTENT FEEDING

Dear Caregiver:

Because the person in your care can't chew foods or swallow liquids or even his own saliva, the doctor has placed a feeding tube in his stomach. This tube provides a direct route for delivering liquid feedings to the stomach. A *nasogastric feeding tube* goes through the person's nose and throat to his stomach. Another type of feeding tube, a *gastrostomy tube,* leads directly into his stomach from the abdomen, where it's sewn in place by the doctor. Whichever tube a person has, feeding him through it can provide adequate nutrition and prevent choking.

Use the following instructions to give a nasogastric or gastrostomy tube feeding.

Preparing for a feeding
Before you feed the person, gather the equipment, prepare the formula, and position him correctly. Follow this procedure:

1
First, gather the feeding formula; measuring, mixing, and pouring devices; a bulb or piston syringe; and warm water.

2
If the formula's in the refrigerator, take it out and let it warm to room temperature. (Formulas come premixed or in a powder or liquid to be mixed with water. The doctor will tell you which type of formula to use and how to feed it to the person.) Or warm the formula by placing the container in a basin of tepid water. *Note*: Never warm the formula over direct heat. Follow the manufacturer's directions for storing and reusing.

If the formula isn't premixed, measure and mix it as directed, for one feeding only.

3
Raise the person's head to *at least* a 30-degree angle (higher, if his condition permits), using pillows or a backrest. Always

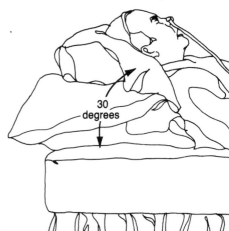

30 degrees

keep his head elevated at least 30 degrees during feeding.

Checking tube placement

Never begin a tube feeding if either of these tests is unsuccessful:

1

Draw fluid into the syringe. To do this, first remove the feeding tube's cap or plug. If you're using a bulb syringe, gently squeeze and hold the bulb. Attach the syringe to the end of the feeding tube and release the bulb. If you're using a piston syringe, pull back on the barrel. This should draw some gastric juices—yellow-green fluid— through the tube.

If you can't withdraw any fluid, the tube may be pressed against the stomach wall or curled in the stomach. Have the person move or turn. Then try again to draw up some fluid. If you're still unsuccessful, call the doctor.

If you're able to draw fluid into the syringe, squeeze the bulb or push in the barrel of the piston syringe to return the fluid to the stomach.

2

Next, listen with a stethoscope. If the person has a nasogastric tube, pay special attention to this step to ensure that the tube is correctly positioned in the stomach and hasn't drifted into the lungs. Place one end of a stethoscope in your ears, and place the other end over the person's stomach. Reattach the syringe to the feeding tube, and either squeeze the bulb or

(continued)

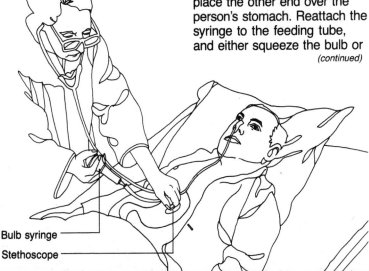

Bulb syringe
Stethoscope

HOW TO GIVE AN INTERMITTENT FEEDING *(continued)*

push in the barrel to inject a small amount of air into the tube. If you hear a gurgling sound, this means that air is entering the stomach and that the tube is clear. Now clamp the tube and remove the syringe. If you don't hear a gurgling sound, call the doctor.

Setting up and monitoring the feeding

After you've checked tube placement, gather a feeding bag, tubing, clamp, and an I.V. pole or hook. Now give the feeding this way:

1

Attach one end of the tubing to the feeding bag. Then clamp the tubing shut. Pour in the prescribed amount of formula, and hang the bag from the I.V. pole or hook. Unclamp the tubing, and slowly run the formula through it to remove all air bubbles. Then reclamp the tubing. Now attach the other end of the tubing to the person's nasogastric or gastrostomy tube. (You may need a connector.)

Set the bag at the correct height to get the flow rate the doctor prescribes. Unclamp the tubing to start the flow.

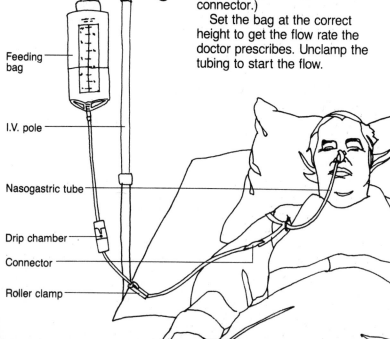

Feeding bag

I.V. pole

Nasogastric tube

Drip chamber

Connector

Roller clamp

2

Write down what time the flow began and when it's scheduled to end. Always give a tube feeding as slowly as the doctor orders. If you give it too quickly, the person may get diarrhea.

3

During the feeding, check the feeding bag and tubing to make sure the flow of formula doesn't stop or change. Squeeze the feeding bag every now and then to prevent clogging or settling.

Ending the feeding

After you've fed the person the prescribed amount of formula for the correct length of time, you're ready to end the feeding. Here's how:

1

First, clamp the feeding bag, and disconnect it from the person's nasogastric or gastros-

tomy tube. Then pour 2 ounces of water into the bulb or piston syringe that's attached to the feeding tube. Allow the water to flush the feeding tube. This clears away any leftover formula that could stick to and clog the tube.

Once you've disconnected the feeding bag from the feeding tube, clamp the tube shut. If the person has a nasogastric tube, replace the cap or plug and tape or pin the tube to the person's clothing until the next feeding. If he has a gastrostomy tube, apply the dressing, as directed. If the person complains of nausea, leave the feeding tube unclamped and uncovered until the feeling passes.

2

Keep the person in a sitting position for about 30 minutes to help prevent him from vomiting or inhaling any leftover formula. If he's uncomfortable sitting, help him lie on his side. Prop his head up with pillows, or partially elevate the head of the bed.

If the feeding bag is reusable, wash it with warm water, dry it, and store it.

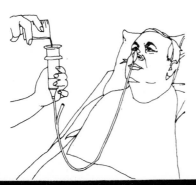

ers to help maintain mobility as long as possible.

If the patient with ALS is immobile, teach the family proper positioning techniques and passive range-of-motion exercises.

• *Diet.* If the patient has difficulty swallowing, tell him he may tolerate semisoft foods better than solid ones. But recommend that he avoid foods that stick in his mouth, such as peanut butter. Instruct the patient to avoid liquids or drink them cautiously. If appropriate, tell the family to freeze liquids to a slush or to mix them with other foods. If the patient drools, suggest avoiding foods and fluids (such as milk) that increase salivation. If he eats slowly, recommend using a warming tray to prevent foods from becoming cold.

Instruct the patient to always sit upright for meals and to tilt his head slightly forward to prevent choking. If he has a weak grip, recommend using built-up utensils, a plate guard, and a plate stabilized with a rubber soap holder. When swallowing eventually becomes impossible, teach the family to use gastrostomy or nasogastric tube feedings to ensure adequate nutrition and to prevent aspiration. (See *How to Give an Intermittent Feeding*, pages 260 to 263.)

Reinforce the need for adequate fluids and dietary fiber, since the patient may be prone to urinary stasis and constipation.

• *Medication.* Explain that medications help relieve the patient's symptoms. Neostigmine may be prescribed to minimize muscle weakness, and muscle relaxants may be given to relieve spasticity. If the patient has dysphagia, tell him to crush pills and mix them with a semisoft food to ease swallowing. If the patient is receiving gastrostomy or nasogastric tube feedings, tell the family to use a liquid form of medication, if one's available. Tell them to crush pills, mix them with water, and push them through the feeding tube with a syringe.

If necessary, teach the family how to insert suppositories and give the patient enemas.

• *Other care measures.* Advise the patient to avoid crowds and people with infections. Instruct him to report signs and symptoms of an infection (such as fever, headache, malaise) to the doctor.

Teach the patient how to perform deep-breathing and coughing exercises. If necessary, teach the family suctioning techniques. Ultimately, the patient may choose to be placed on mechanical ventilation. If he makes such a decision, you'll need to teach the family how to use mechanical ventilation and suction through a tracheostomy tube. Suggest that the family obtain a hospital bed to make caring for the patient easier and a foam rubber mattress to increase patient comfort and prevent skin breakdown and decubitus formation.

Instruct the patient to speak slowly and pronounce each word as communication becomes increasingly difficult. To help the patient conserve energy, suggest that he use a communication board, a magic slate, or an electric typewriter. In time, the patient and his family may have to use a code, such as eye blinking, or an electronic communication device. If the patient can't call for attention, tell the family to check on him frequently and to keep a squeeze toy or buzzer at his fingertips, if he has the strength to use it.

Instruct the family to watch for signs of depression (such signs include disinterest in surroundings, decreased appetite, or altered sleep and rest habits)—a common problem in ALS. Remind them that the patient is alert, oriented, and capable of feeling pain. Explain the need for maintaining a pleasant environment, with frequent contact with people, a radio, TV, and clock.

Refer the patient and his family to the Muscular Dystrophy Association for additional information about ALS and for the location of the nearest support group.

Cerebrovascular Accident

The most common cause of neurologic deficits, a cerebrovascular accident (CVA) poses difficult but not insurmountable teaching challenges. First of all, you'll need to teach the patient about his disorder and, perhaps, the need for surgery. Then, you'll need to teach him how to compensate for any temporary or permanent neurologic deficits. At times, the patient may feel depressed about his condition and the prospects of a lengthy rehabilitation. But you'll need to provide support and convince him of the benefits of rehabilitation and of avoiding CVA's risk factors.

Describe the disorder

Explain the patient's type of CVA. In an *ischemic CVA*, vascular narrowing or occlusion by a blood clot, plaque, or a clump of bacteria reduces cerebral perfusion. In a *hemorrhagic CVA*, arterial rupture causes bleeding into brain tissue. (If cerebral blood flow is only temporarily interrupted, a transient ischemic attack [TIA] results.)

Explain that brain cells in the area of disrupted perfusion no longer receive oxygen and glucose and therefore stop functioning. The resultant neurologic deficit can be specific or widespread, depending on the affected area of the brain. (See *Understanding Sites and Signs of Neurologic Deficits*, pages 266 and 267.) Tell the patient that the deficits may be temporary if brain cells were only injured or permanent if the cells were destroyed.

Point out possible complications

Explain that a temporary deficit may become permanent without the patient's active participation in his rehabilitation program, including range-of-motion exercises and speech and language therapy. Point out that immobility increases the risk of infection. Also point out that the patient may have another CVA if he fails to address risk factors.

Teach about tests

Prepare the patient for a CT scan and, possibly, for cerebral angiography to locate the infarct or hemorrhage. Other diagnostic tests, including digital subtraction angiography, positron emission tomography, and cerebral blood flow studies, may be performed, if available. (See *Teaching Patients about Neurologic Tests*, pages 293 to 299, for additional teaching points.) Blood tests may also be performed to evaluate clotting.

Teach about treatments

• *Activity.* Stress the importance of following the prescribed exercise program. Teach the patient to perform

CHECKLIST

TEACHING TOPICS IN C.V.A.

☐ An explanation of the type of CVA: ischemic or hemorrhagic

☐ Preparation for diagnostic tests, such as a CT scan and cerebral angiography

☐ If necessary, an explanation of the type of surgery: craniotomy, carotid endarterectomy, or extracranial/intracranial bypass

☐ The importance of rehabilitation in minimizing neurologic deficits

☐ A balanced program of activity and rest

☐ Dietary adjustments, such as semisoft foods for dysphagia

☐ Assistive devices

☐ Communication tips for the patient and his family

☐ Home safety tips

☐ Risk factors in CVA

☐ Sources of additional information and support

UNDERSTANDING SITES AND SIGNS
OF NEUROLOGIC DEFICITS

A cerebrovascular accident (CVA) can leave one patient with a mild hand weakness and another with complete unilateral paralysis. In both patients, the loss of function reflects damage to the area of the brain normally perfused by the occluded or ruptured artery. But the damage doesn't stop there. The resulting hypoxia and ischemia produce edema that affects distal parts of the brain, causing further neurologic deficits.

Most CVAs occur in the anterior cerebral circulation. These include middle cerebral artery syndrome, internal carotid syndrome, and anterior cerebral artery syndrome. However, CVAs of the posterior circulation,

deriving from the vertebral arteries, have a higher mortality. These include vertebral/basilar artery syndrome and posterior cerebral artery syndrome. The illustrations here show arterial circulation and the brain sites that control various body functions.

Middle cerebral artery syndrome
The most common deficits include motor or sensory deficits or both (contralateral to the lesion's hemisphere), aphasia, homonymous hemianopsia, neglect of paralyzed side (with nondominant hemisphere involvement), apraxia, agnosia, and paralysis of conjugate gaze.

SITES OF CEREBRAL FUNCTION

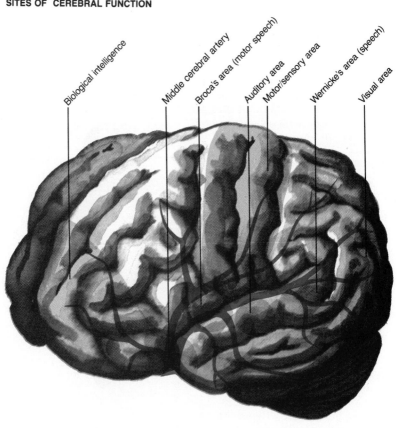

Biological intelligence — Middle cerebral artery — Broca's area (motor speech) — Auditory area — Motor/sensory area — Wernicke's area (speech) — Visual area

Anterior cerebral artery syndrome
This least common syndrome produces motor or sensory deficits or both, urinary incontinence, flat emotional affect, and gait apraxia.

Internal carotid syndrome
Similar to the middle cerebral artery syndrome, this syndrome causes motor or sensory deficits or both contralateral to the lesion, altered level of consciousness, neglect, and apraxia. It also causes homonymous hemianopsia, ipsilateral blindness, and aphasia.

Vertebral/basilar artery syndrome
Impaired vertebrobasilar circulation causes motor or sensory deficits or both on the same side of the body as the lesion, on both sides, or in all extremities; nystagmus; vertigo with nausea and vomiting; diplopia and lateral and vertical gaze palsies; visual field deficits; ataxia; dysphagia; dysarthria; and coma.

Posterior cerebral artery syndrome
This syndrome results in visual field deficits, blindness (if bilateral involvement), and sensory loss on one side.

MAIN CEREBRAL ARTERIES

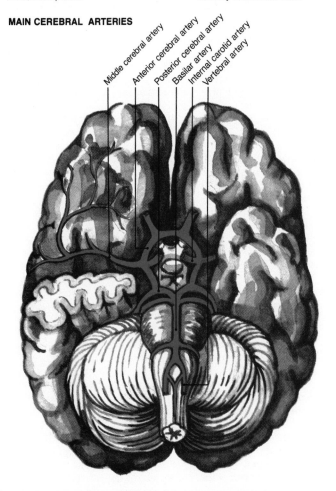

active range-of-motion exercises for the affected limb, or teach a family member to perform passive range-of-motion exercises. Advise frequently interrupting exercise with rest periods. Reinforce the importance of wearing slings, splints, or other prescribed devices to prevent complications.

• *Diet.* If the patient is obese or has elevated serum levels of cholesterol, lipoproteins, or triglycerides, you may need to explain a weight-reduction diet or one low in saturated fats. If he has dysphagia or one-sided facial weakness, tell him to eat semisoft foods and to chew on the unaffected side of his mouth.

Instruct the patient to sit upright when eating and to tilt his head slightly forward. Recommend preparing solid foods in a blender and freezing liquids to a slush or mixing them with other foods. If the patient has partial arm paralysis, advise him to use feeding aids, such as specially adapted plates with rims and built-up utensils. (See *Using Self-Help Aids.*)

• *Medication.* Instruct the patient about the schedule, dosage, and side effects of prescribed medications, such as anticoagulants, antiplatelet drugs (aspirin, dipyridamole), and antidepressants. Also, review foods and over-the-counter products that interact with these medications. (See *Teaching Patients about Neurologic Drugs*, pages 304 to 311.)

• *Surgery.* Depending on the cause and extent of the CVA, the patient may undergo a craniotomy (to remove a hematoma), endarterectomy (to remove atherosclerotic plaques), or extracranial/intracranial bypass (to circumvent an artery that's blocked completely by occlusion or stenosis).

If you're preparing the patient for a *craniotomy*, tell him that his head will be shaved and scrubbed and that he'll be given a general anesthetic. Explain that the surgeon will make an incision in his scalp and then will open the skull over the damaged area. (The size of the opening varies from a small hole, which

later fills with new bone, to a larger open flap, which is later replaced).

Tell the patient that after surgery his head will be bandaged. If he'll be having a supratentorial craniotomy, mention that the head of his bed will be elevated about 30 degrees. Or, if he'll be having an infratentorial craniotomy, mention that he'll lie flat in bed. Tell him he can turn from side to side, but caution him to avoid coughing, which may increase intracranial pressure. Instruct him to ask for medication if he experiences a headache after surgery.

After the patient recovers from surgery for a CVA, tell him that the surgeon will remove the sutures within 7 days. Also, mention that he'll be given a cap to wear after removal of the bandages. Before discharge, tell the patient he may wash his hair but should gently pat the incision area until dry. Advise the patient against scrubbing or rubbing the incision area.

If you're preparing the patient for a carotid *endarterectomy*, tell him that the skin on his neck will be thoroughly cleansed and shaved. If he'll be receiving a cervical block anesthetic, tell him he'll be awake during surgery. If not, tell him he'll receive a general anesthetic. Mention that dressings will be placed over the incision after surgery and that he may experience numbness and tightness in the incision area, a transient numbness in his earlobe, and a lump in his throat. Explain to the patient that these effects of swelling should resolve in a few days.

Tell the patient that he'll be able to resume his usual daily activities the day after surgery, barring complications. Mention that the doctor will remove any sutures before the patient's discharged from the hospital.

If you're preparing the patient for an *extracranial/intracranial bypass*, tell him that part of his head will be shaved and scrubbed and that he'll receive a general anesthetic. Explain that the surgeon will make an incision in the scalp above the ear to dissect and divide an artery. He'll then make an

USING SELF-HELP AIDS

Dear Patient:

Self-help aids help you conserve time and energy. The examples shown here are just a few of the many aids available.

Plate guard

To keep food from sliding off your plate, clip a guard onto the plate's edge. The guard also acts as a barrier, so you can push food against it to help get food onto a spoon or fork. To keep the plate itself from sliding, place a rubber disk (such as a soap holder with suction cups) or a damp paper towel or cloth under the plate.

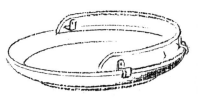

Utensils with built-up handles

You can build up a handle by wrapping a piece of cloth around it and securing it with adhesive tape. Or insert the utensil into a plastic foam curler or a bicycle grip. If the bicycle grip is too long, cut off the end. Fill the inside with lightweight clay, and insert the utensil.

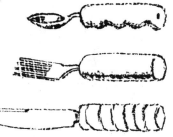

Special cups and glasses

If your hands are unsteady, you may find it easier to drink from a cup with a large handle. Or drink from a cup with a lip and a lid to help decrease spills. You can also use unbreakable plastic glasses and stretch terry-cloth coasters over glasses so they're easier to grasp.

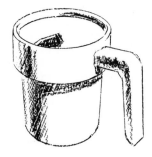

opening in the skull and splice one end of the dissected artery to an artery on the surface of the brain.

Inform the patient that after surgery for an extracranial/intracranial bypass he'll have a bulky dressing over the incision; he may also have a mild headache, caused by swelling in the surgical area. Warn the patient to avoid putting pressure on the surgical site even though he can resume most activities the day after surgery. And tell him to avoid lying on the affected side. If he wears eyeglasses, suggest that he remove the temple piece that extends over the surgical site.

Advise the patient that swelling normally occurs after surgery. Before discharge, instruct him to avoid wearing hats that exert pressure above the ear, thus causing damage to the suture line.

• **Other care measures.** If the patient has a *speech deficit*, recommend alternate methods of communicating, such as writing or using a picture board. Review his prescribed speech and language therapy and reinforce the importance of continuing it. Instruct the family to speak slowly to the patient in normal tones. Also recommend that they use gestures to clarify their message if the patient has receptive aphasia.

Also instruct the family to give the patient short, simple directions, cues, and lists. Warn them that the patient may overestimate his abilities, claiming he's capable of carrying out tasks, such as driving a car, that he's incapable of doing. Explain the importance of carefully monitoring the patient's abilities without frustrating his efforts for independence. Tell them to allow the patient to try most activities—short of those that could injure him or others or could cause excessive frustration or fatigue.

Mention to the family that the patient may be *emotionally labile*, crying or laughing at seemingly inappropriate times. Explain that he can't control these reactions.

Instruct the family to provide a safe environment for the patient who's had a CVA. Recommend installing grab bars near the toilet and bathtub, removing throw rugs, and securing carpets—or removing them entirely if the patient uses a walker or wheelchair. Also, instruct them to lower the water heater's temperature if the patient has sensory losses.

To prevent confusing the patient who has *difficulty generalizing*, tell the family to establish a routine and to minimize changes. For example, a patient who has learned to feed himself at home may have difficulty eating in a restaurant. One solution: take his utensils to the restaurant rather than risk his social withdrawal.

If the patient has a *one-sided deficit*, encourage him to bathe and dress the affected side first. Suggest calling attention to that side with a watch or a ring.

If the patient has *homonymous hemianopsia*, tell him to scan his environment by carefully looking from side to side.

To help prevent another CVA, you'll need to teach the patient about correcting any risk factors. For example, if the patient smokes, refer him to a stop-smoking program. As appropriate, tell him to maintain his ideal weight; to follow his prescribed diet, exercises, and stress-reduction program; and to check with the doctor before taking any nonprescription drugs. If the patient's a woman of childbearing age, tell her to avoid using oral contraceptives.

Encourage the patient and his family to contact a local support group and to obtain additional information from the local branch of the American Heart Association, the National Institute for Neurological and Communicative Disorders and Stroke, or the National Easter Seal Society for Crippled Children and Adults. In addition, advise the patient to obtain a medical identification bracelet or necklace if he's taking anticoagulants or antiplatelet drugs.

Multiple Sclerosis

As in other progressive degenerative disorders, multiple sclerosis (MS) requires complex teaching to help the patient adjust to its physical, emotional, and psychosocial effects. MS is a major cause of chronic disability in young adults and may progress rapidly, disabling the patient in the prime of life or even causing death within months of its onset. However, 70% of patients with MS lead active, productive lives with prolonged remissions.

Notorious for its spontaneous remissions and exacerbations, MS manifests itself in intermittent episodes that can be mild or severe. Because of this, the patient needs to know what factors can precipitate an exacerbation, how to care for himself during exacerbations (and remissions), and how to cope with any residual neurologic deficits, such as sensory alterations. He'll also need to learn what types of diet and exercise are compatible with his disorder and the importance of following his prescribed medication regimen. In addition, the patient will need information about sexual and childbearing concerns. (See *Questions Patients Ask about MS*, page 272.)

Describe the disorder
Explain that MS is thought to result from a viral infection, an autoimmune process, or both. It involves the destruction of myelin, a fatty substance covering the axons in the brain and spinal cord. As the disorder progresses, the myelin sheath is eventually destroyed, preventing the axon from transmitting impulses, thus causing a neurologic deficit. If destruction includes the axon or if the myelin fails to regenerate itself, scar tissue forms, causing a permanent (residual) deficit.

Inform the patient that his symptoms may come and go in no predictable pattern and that a deficit may appear during an exacerbation and recede during a remission, or it may be permanent. Explain to the patient that the type of deficit—motor, sensory, intellectual, or emotional—will depend on which part of the brain or spinal cord is involved.

Point out possible complications
Tell the patient that failure to follow his prescribed medication regimen and observe measures that compensate for deficits may lead to physical injury from falls, urinary tract infections, sensory alterations, and visual disturbances. Also, reinforce the importance of avoiding or minimizing factors that can trigger an exacerbation.

___ CHECKLIST

TEACHING TOPICS IN MULTIPLE SCLEROSIS

- [ ] Explanation of the effects of demyelination on sensory and motor function
- [ ] Preparation for tests, such as a CT scan, cerebrospinal fluid analysis, and evoked potential studies, to rule out other disorders
- [ ] Administration of drugs to relieve symptoms
- [ ] Preparation for stereotaxic thalamotomy, if ordered
- [ ] Balancing activity and rest
- [ ] Energy conservation
- [ ] Measures for minimizing neurologic deficits
- [ ] Dietary adjustments (such as semisolid foods) and proper elimination
- [ ] Bladder/bowel retraining to correct incontinence
- [ ] Self-catheterization technique or Credé's maneuver to correct urinary retention
- [ ] Precipitating factors for exacerbations
- [ ] Referral for financial and sexual counseling
- [ ] Sources of additional information and support

Teach about tests

Explain that no specific test can diagnose MS but that various tests can help distinguish it from other neurologic disorders. Prepare the patient for these diagnostic tests, including a CT scan, cerebrospinal fluid analysis, and evoked potential studies—visual, auditory, somatosensory, or all three. (See *Teaching Patients about Neurologic Tests*, pages 293 to 299, for further teaching points.)

Teach about treatments

• *Activity.* Stress the importance of frequent rest periods. (A great deal of energy is required to transmit nerve impulses past damaged myelin.) Tell the patient to plan activities after rest periods. If he holds a job, tell him to stagger rest periods throughout his working hours whenever possible.

Also, teach the patient about the importance of moderate exercise. Exercise helps decrease calcium loss from bones, prevents formation of calculi, maintains muscle strength and joint mobility, and promotes circulation. Advise him to perform stretching exercises to help decrease spasticity. Advise him to stagger exercise periods, too.

If the patient is immobile, teach the family proper turning techniques and passive range-of-motion exercises.

• *Diet.* Tell the patient he needs a nutritious, well-balanced diet to maintain his ideal weight and prevent constipation. Adequate fluid intake, including warm liquids, prune juice, and coffee, and high-fiber foods help prevent constipation. To help prevent calculi and urinary tract infection, encourage about 2 to 3 quarts (about 2 to 3 liters) of fluid each day—including some cranberry or other acidic juice.

If the patient has dysphagia, advise him to eat semisolid foods. He can prepare solid foods in a blender and freeze liquids to a slush or mix them with other foods to make them easier to swallow. Also, tell him to sit upright while eating and to keep his head tilted slightly forward. To stimulate the swallow reflex, tell him to stroke *up* from the base of the throat to the chin.

Teach the family to prepare and administer nasogastric or gastrostomy tube feedings if swallowing is extremely difficult or the potential for as-

QUESTIONS PATIENTS ASK ABOUT M.S.

Can I still have sex now that I have MS?

Yes, it's possible for you to have as active a sex life as before, but you may need to make some modifications. For example, you may need to vary your position and increase foreplay, stroking, or massage to avoid muscle spasms anywhere in your body. Be sure you discuss these changes with your partner.

Will MS affect my desire for sex?

In general, no. But fatigue, depression, or the medications you're taking may temporarily affect your desire for sex. And in some people, certain conditions associated with MS can affect their desire for sex. For example, if you have scar tissue in the area of the brain responsible for the sex drive, you may experience an increased or decreased desire for sex.

Will I be able to have children?

MS doesn't affect your reproductive capabilities, but before deciding whether to have children, you'll need to consider carefully the physical and financial changes MS will make in your life. For example, you'll find that you tire more easily now that you have MS. And, in time, MS may require additional financial expenditures for health or assistive care.

piration is great. (See *How to Give an Intermittent Feeding*, pages 260 to 263.)

● *Medication.* Explain to the patient that during acute exacerbations, the doctor may prescribe corticosteroids to help alleviate symptoms. During a remission, he may prescribe antispasmodics, anticholinergics, laxatives, and antidepressants, as needed.

● *Procedures.* Prepare the patient for plasmapheresis, if scheduled. Explain that although its success rate varies in MS, plasmapheresis is occasionally used to temporarily decrease the severity of symptoms. This procedure removes blood from the body, separates its components to allow removal of causative antibodies, and then returns the components to the body. Explain that the procedure involves two puncture sites—one to remove the blood and another to replace it. After the procedure, pressure is applied to the puncture sites for 15 to 30 minutes. Tell the patient he'll need to rest for 3 to 4 hours. Then he can resume his normal routine and medication schedule.

● *Surgery.* If drug therapy is ineffective and stereotaxic thalamotomy is ordered to control the patient's intention tremors, prepare the patient for surgery. Tell him that his head will be shaved and cleansed and that he'll be given a local anesthetic. Also tell him that he'll have a metal frame attached to his head to help him hold his head still and to guide the surgeon. Explain that the surgeon will drill a burr hole in the skull and will create a surgical lesion in the thalamus on the side *opposite* the tremors. (Explain that the right side of his brain controls the left side of his body, and vice versa.) Tell the patient that during surgery he'll be asked to follow commands, such as raising an arm. Also explain that he'll experience some discomfort when the surgeon applies the head frame and that he may have a headache after surgery.

● *Other care measures.* Educate the patient about factors that precipitate exacerbations, including stress, fatigue, temperature extremes, infection, trauma, menstruation, and pregnancy. Teach stress-reduction techniques, and advise the patient to get adequate rest. (See *How to Conserve Your Energy*, page 277.) Advise him to avoid hot baths and showers, to stay indoors in unusually cold or hot weather, and to use an air conditioner when appropriate. If he lives in a warm climate, tell him to plan activities for the cooler part of the day and to avoid prolonged sun exposure. Tell him to treat all fevers and to report any illness to the doctor. Stress the need to avoid exposure to infections.

If *incoordination* interferes with the patient's mobility, teach him to walk with a wide-based gait, to use a weighted cane or walker, if necessary, and to make his home safe for walking.

If the patient has head tremors, suggest resting his head against a high-backed chair to give him some stability. Also, teach him how to apply any prescribed collars or braces. If he has hand tremors, teach him to use weighted utensils or wrist weights (1 to 2 lb [0.45 to 0.9 kg]) while feeding himself. Also suggest using a plate with suction cups on its base, a plate guard, and a weighted cup or a cup with a lid and lip. (See *Using Self-Help Aids*, page 269.) To steady his arms while working, suggest he support them on a tabletop or on chair arms. This conserves energy and decreases tremors.

Instruct the patient with *spasticity* to use a cold pack and to apply splints (at night). Also, tell him how to decrease spasticity in his legs before sexual activity.

If the patient has *dysarthria, a low-pitched voice,* or *slow, scanning speech,* reinforce the need to perform phonation exercises, if prescribed. And, if appropriate, explain the use of a communication board and voice amplifiers.

Tell the patient with *diplopia* to use an eye patch or a frosted lens over one eye, alternating the patch every 2 to 4 hours. Warn about a loss of depth perception if the patient has vision in only

FOR WOMEN: HOW TO CATHETERIZE YOURSELF

Dear Patient:

Follow these instructions to perform catheterization.

1

Gather the equipment: catheter, lubricant, basin, clean wash-cloth, soap and water, paper towels, and plastic bag. Then wash your hands thoroughly. During the procedure, be sure to touch only the catheter equipment to avoid spreading germs.

2

Separate the folds of your vulva with one hand, and, using the washcloth, thoroughly clean the area between your legs with warm water and mild soap. Use downward strokes (front to back) to avoid contaminating the area with fecal matter. Now, pat the area dry with a towel.

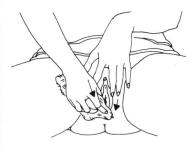

3

Open the lubricant and squeeze a generous amount onto a paper towel. Then roll the first 3″ of the catheter in it.

4

Spread the lips of the vulva with one hand, and, using the other hand, insert the catheter in an upward and backward di-rection about 3″ into the ure-thra. If you meet resistance, breathe deeply. As you inhale, advance the catheter, angling it upward slightly. Stop when urine begins to drain from it. Allow all urine to drain into the basin.

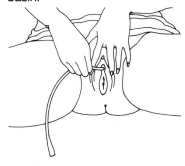

5

Pinch the catheter closed and slowly remove it. Wash it in warm, soapy water, rinse, and dry. Place it in a plastic bag for the next use. (After you've used the catheter a few times, boil it in water for 20 minutes to keep it germ-free.)

FOR MEN: HOW TO CATHETERIZE YOURSELF

Dear Patient:

Follow these instructions to perform catheterization.

1

Gather the equipment: catheter, lubricant, basin for collecting urine, clean washcloth, soap and water, paper towels, and plastic bag (optional). Then wash your hands thoroughly. During the procedure, touch only the catheter equipment to avoid spreading germs.

2

Wash your penis and the surrounding area with soap and water. Then pat dry.

3

Open the tube of lubricant and squeeze a generous amount onto a paper towel. Then roll the first 7″ to 10″ of the catheter in the lubricant.

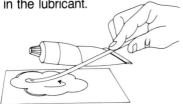

4

Put one end of the catheter in the basin or toilet. Hold your penis at a right angle to your body, grasp the catheter as you would a pencil, and slowly insert it into the urethra. If you meet resistance, breathe deeply. As you inhale, continue advancing the catheter 7″ to 10″ until urine begins to flow. Allow all urine to drain into the basin or toilet.

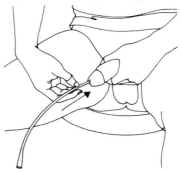

5

When the catheter stops draining, pinch it closed and slowly remove it. Empty the basin, then rinse and dry it. Wash the catheter in warm, soapy water, rinse it inside and out, and dry it with a clean towel. Place it in a plastic bag until the next use. (After you've used the catheter a few times, the doctor may tell you to boil it in water for 20 minutes to keep it germ-free.)

one eye. Suggest reading books with large print or listening to audiotaped publications. If the patient has corneal sensory loss, show him how to instill eye drops and use a clear eye shield.

If the patient has *sensory deficits*, stress caution near extremely hot or cold objects. Tell him to use a bath thermometer to test the temperature of his bathwater. Also tell him that he may perform activities better by observing his hand or foot movement.

The patient with MS may also experience *urinary deficits*—incontinence or retention. For either problem, he should drink 2 to 3 quarts (1.9 to 2.8 liters) of fluid each day but should restrict fluids about 2 hours before bedtime. If he's *incontinent*, help him reestablish a normal urinary pattern. First, advise him to keep a record of his fluid intake. (Remind him that such foods as ice cream and soup are sources of fluid.) Also tell him to record when he urinates in the toilet and when he has an episode of incontinence. After a few days, he'll know by checking his record when he's most likely to become incontinent (for example, after meals or during the night). Then tell the patient to set a schedule for urinating, starting every 2 hours and gradually extending the interval to 3 to 4 hours. (Does he have a watch or a clock within easy view to remind him?) Also stress the importance of staying near the bathroom. Encourage him to be patient if he still has episodes of incontinence. Suggest wearing incontinence briefs during bladder retraining. (Tell the family to avoid using plastic or rubber bed sheets because they promote skin breakdown.)

If *urinary retention* is a problem, explain to the patient the importance of completely emptying his bladder to prevent infection. Teach him to perform intermittent catheterization. (See *How to Catheterize Yourself*, on pages 274 and 275.) Also, recommend that the patient stimulate voiding by stroking the thighs and glans penis (or vulva), and by tapping the center of the abdomen below the navel about 10 to 15 times or until urination occurs. Eventually, the duration and intensity of tapping needed to produce emptying will decrease.

Credé's maneuver can also help empty the bladder. To perform this maneuver, the patient should tap the abdomen until he hears a dull sound, indicating a full bladder. Next, tell him to use the flat part of his fingertips to knead the bladder, progressively applying more pressure. (Caution him to avoid grinding his fingertips into his skin.) To ensure complete voiding, tell him to listen for a hollow sound, indicating an empty bladder.

For the patient with *constipation*, reinforce the need for a nutritious, well-balanced diet and physical activity. Describe a bowel retraining program—for example, using laxatives or suppositories at a prescribed time and then attempting to have a bowel movement about ½ hour after a meal (usually breakfast), when the gastrocolic reflex is the strongest. If the patient experiences *fecal incontinence*, explain that this usually results from illness, such as the flu, or from irritating substances, such as alcohol, spicy foods, or cigarettes, rather than from MS. Tell the patient to avoid irritating substances and hot liquids, to increase dietary fiber, and to wear incontinence briefs.

If the patient has a *hearing impairment*, tell him to always face the speaker (a hearing aid won't help). Refer him for instruction in lipreading (if available), unless visual disturbances are present. Also, tell him to look for motor vehicles before crossing a street (he shouldn't rely on sound.)

Suggest that the patient with *short-term memory loss* carry a pad and pencil so he can write down important information right away.

Refer the patient to appropriate sources for financial and sexual counseling. For further information about his disorder and support group services, refer him to the National Multiple Sclerosis Society.

HOW TO CONSERVE YOUR ENERGY

Dear Patient:

Your illness may cause you to tire easily, making it difficult to perform daily tasks. To avoid overexertion, remember to sit or lie down as soon as you feel tired. For other ways to help you conserve energy, follow these tips.

Sit down to do chores
When you're folding laundry, ironing, preparing food, or washing dishes, sit down whenever possible. (Also sit on a shower seat or stool when you're taking a shower.)

Use electrical equipment
Mixing a cake with an electric mixer takes less energy than stirring it by hand. Similarly, composing a letter on an electric typewriter or word processor takes less energy than writing one in longhand. Brushing your teeth with an electric toothbrush can also help.

Shop at home
Place orders by telephone, and use mail order and delivery services to avoid making trips to stores, the library, or the dry cleaner. When you do go shopping, park close to the store, using parking spaces marked for the handicapped.

More energy savers
Wear clothing that's easy to put on and take off, and make sure it's easy to fasten. Zippers and Velcro strips are easier than buttons. Also, eat frequent, small meals instead of three large ones if chewing tires you. (A warming tray is a good idea to keep food warm.)

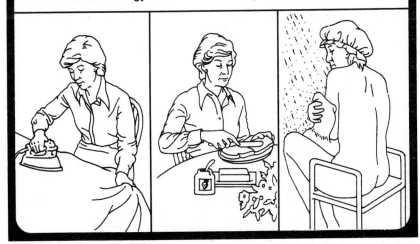

Myasthenia Gravis

In this disorder, your teaching focuses on helping the patient adjust to progressive fatigue and muscle weakness. This involves teaching him about the effects of his medication, the need to plan his activities around his medication schedule for maximum muscle strength, and the importance of lifelong compliance with medication therapy to alleviate symptoms.

You'll also need to teach the patient how to prevent or manage complications. For example, you'll need to teach him productive coughing to prevent pulmonary complications—a constant threat in a patient with weakened respiratory muscles. You'll also need to teach him and his family to recognize signs of myasthenic or cholinergic crisis.

Describe the disorder

Explain that myasthenia gravis is thought to be an autoimmune disorder that impairs transmission of nerve impulses.

Tell the patient that antibodies produced by his blood cells and thymus gland block and destroy the receptors that transmit the impulses required for muscle contraction. As a result, he experiences muscle weakness, causing him to work harder than usual to carry out an activity. Tell him he may experience periods during the day when fatigue and muscle weakness worsen. Also, mention that day-to-day fluctuations are common.

Point out possible complications

Emphasize the importance of following prescribed therapy by pointing out that severe respiratory difficulties may otherwise result. (See *Symptoms of Myasthenic Crisis.*) Respiratory distress can result from undermedication or overmedication.

Teach about tests

Prepare the patient for a Tensilon test or a neostigmine test, or both. But do *not* tell him the expected reaction because test results may be affected.

Other tests to confirm myasthenia gravis include electromyography, nerve conduction studies, X-rays, and a CT scan of the chest.

Blood tests, such as serum thyroxine, serum protein electrophoresis, erythrocyte sedimentation rate, and studies for antinuclear antibodies and acetylcholine receptor antibodies, may also help diagnose the disorder.

Occasionally, the doctor may order a test of vital capacity to measure the maximum amount of air the patient can exchange with each breath. Describe this test to the patient, and explain its purpose: to demonstrate the strength of his respiratory muscles.

CHECKLIST

☑☐ ☐☑ ☑☐ TEACHING TOPICS IN MYASTHENIA GRAVIS

☐ Explanation of the autoimmune process that impairs transmission of nerve impulses

☐ Warning symptoms of myasthenic crisis

☐ Preparation for tests that confirm myasthenia gravis, such as the Tensilon test, electromyography, and nerve conduction studies

☐ Antimyasthenic drugs and their administration

☐ Coordination of activities with drug administration schedule to take advantage of peak muscle strength

☐ Preparation for plasmapheresis or thymectomy, if necessary

☐ Dietary measures to compensate for muscle weakness

☐ Factors that increase symptoms and the risk of infection

☐ Sources of additional information and support

Teach about treatments

• *Activity.* Advise the patient to avoid repeated or prolonged activity that can cause muscle weakness and fatigue, and stress that rest periods are essential. Tell him to gauge his activities according to his level of tolerance—he should plan activities at times when his energy peaks, coinciding with administration of his medication.

Explain how he can conserve energy. For example, tell him to use a seat or a stool while taking a shower. If he's on bed rest, teach him to perform active

WARNING

SYMPTOMS OF MYASTHENIC CRISIS

A patient with myasthenia gravis may require immediate medical attention if he experiences sudden, severe muscle weakness that affects his breathing. Called a myasthenic or cholinergic crisis, this sudden worsening of the patient's condition may be associated with emotional stress, infection, surgery, trauma, or a medication overdose, commonly occurring within 1 hour after taking his medication. It can also occur if the patient forgets to take his medication.

Tell the family to call the doctor right away if the patient experiences any of these symptoms, especially within 1 hour after taking his medication:
• difficulty breathing, swallowing, or pronouncing words

• inability to cough
• increased salivation
• twitching around the mouth or eyes
• nausea and vomiting
• palpitations
• muscle spasms
• severe abdominal cramps
• severe weakness in any muscle
• cold, moist skin
• extreme restlessness
• confusion
• seizures
• fainting.

If the family is unable to awaken the patient, tell them to contact the doctor right away or take the patient to the hospital emergency department.

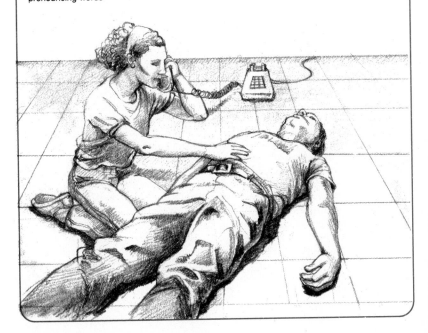

range-of-motion exercises to prevent the complications of immobility.

• *Diet.* If the patient experiences dysphagia and nasal regurgitation, advise him to eat semisoft foods (applesauce, mashed potatoes, solid foods prepared in a blender) and to freeze liquids to a slush or mix them with other foods. Eating semisoft foods will also conserve the energy he would need to chew foods. Tell him to avoid foods that stimulate saliva, such as milk, if he has dysphagia.

Explain that quinine (tonic water), excessive alcohol, and hot foods increase his weakness. (Eating warm rather than hot foods can help preserve his swallowing function, too.)

• *Medication.* Stress the importance of taking medications as scheduled to reduce the risk of relapse. Encourage him to premeasure doses. If the patient has a flexible medication schedule, instruct him to take a dose about 1 hour before meals and other important activities, such as exercise. If he's not taking sustained-release capsules for nighttime control, tell him to set his alarm so he can take the next scheduled dose.

Instruct the patient to check with the doctor before taking any nonprescription drugs; many of them interfere with antimyasthenic drugs. If he experiences respiratory distress or increased weakness, tell him to inform the doctor; he shouldn't attempt to adjust his medication dose or schedule on his own.

• *Procedures.* Plasmapheresis may be used if other treatments prove ineffective. Explain that this blood-cleansing procedure may help remove acetylcholine receptor antibodies, temporarily lessening the severity of his symptoms. Also explain that the procedure involves two puncture sites (arterial and venous or both venous). A technician removes blood from one site; then it's divided in a cell separator into plasma and other blood components. The plasma, which contains the antibodies, is discarded, and the other blood components are replaced via the second puncture site.

After the procedure, pressure is applied to the puncture sites for 15 to 30 minutes. Inform the patient that after resting for 3 to 4 hours, he can resume his routine activities and medication schedule.

• *Surgery.* If the patient has a thymoma, inform him that thymectomy may help control myasthenia gravis. Explain that his chest will be cleansed and shaved and that he'll be given a general anesthetic. If the incision is midsternal, he may have a chest tube after surgery to drain any accumulated blood; it will be removed in 1 to 2 days. If a transcervical approach is used, the patient will have a drain in place. Explain the possibility of intubation and mechanical ventilation. Tell him he'll receive his antimyasthenic medications I.V. or I.M. until he can again take them orally. Inform him that these medications are progressively withdrawn after surgery to assess his muscle strength. How soon he recovers depends on how soon he regains muscle strength and breathes without mechanical ventilation.

• *Other care measures.* If the patient has diplopia, tell him to use a frosted lens or an eye patch, alternating the patch every 2 to 4 hours.

Advise the patient to avoid activities or situations that worsen his condition. Common ones include very hot or cold weather, hot baths, and stress. Because the patient is vulnerable to respiratory infections and complications, tell him to avoid crowds and people with infections and to report any signs of infection to the doctor immediately.

Teach the patient how to cough productively, using his abdominal muscles. If necessary, instruct his family in suctioning techniques and airway insertion.

Also, tell the patient to keep the phone number for emergency assistance posted near his phone and to wear a medical identification bracelet or necklace. Be sure to refer him to the local chapter of the Myasthenia Gravis Foundation for more information.

Parkinson's Disease

Successful teaching in Parkinson's disease can help the patient effectively control the motor deficits that disrupt his coordination and movement and his ability to perform daily activities. To achieve success in teaching, you'll need to convince the patient of the importance of complying with a long-term drug regimen and various supportive treatments, such as a diet and exercise program, to stay active and independent. Tailored to his specific needs as his symptoms change, these treatments may allow him to maintain an optimum level of function.

Describe the disorder
Explain that this chronic, progressive disorder results from a deficiency of dopamine, a chemical that relays messages across the nerve pathways. This deficiency involves the area of the brain responsible for control of voluntary muscle movements and posture. As a result, most of the patient's symptoms relate to difficulty with posture and movement.

Inform the patient that the characteristic symptoms—tremors, slow movement (bradykinesia), and rigidity—may vary in severity from one patient to another. Also inform him that the disorder initially affects one side of the body but will eventually involve both sides. Tell him that tremors, beginning in the fingers, increase during stress or anxiety and decrease with purposeful movement and sleep.

Explain to the patient how bradykinesia changes his gait so that his body tilts forward while his arms remain at his sides (instead of swinging with walking). Mention that he may also notice muscle rigidity or a generalized stiffness when performing any activity. If the patient complains of other symptoms, such as oily skin, increased perspiration, insomnia, or mood changes,

explain that these are also part of the disease process. (See *Reviewing Clinical Features of Parkinson's Disease*, pages 282 and 283.)

Point out possible complications
To minimize or prevent complications, emphasize the importance of compliance with drug therapy and other supportive treatments. Noncompliance can lead to poorly controlled symptoms and injury. For example, postural and coordination difficulties may lead to falls if the patient's unable to quickly stop walking. Also, if he doesn't rise slowly from a sitting or recumbent position, orthostatic hypotension, a common symptom in Parkinson's disease, may lead to falls and injuries.

Failure to follow his exercise program may lead to decreased mobility and such complications as pneumonia, pulmonary emboli, and urinary tract infections. Does the patient perform his

---

CHECKLIST

TEACHING TOPICS IN PARKINSON'S DISEASE ☑☐ ☐☑ ☑☐

☐ An explanation of the progressive course of Parkinson's disease

☐ Preparation for tests, such as positron emission tomography (to rule out structural abnormalities) and cerebrospinal fluid analysis (to determine dopamine levels)

☐ Dietary modifications

☐ Exercise program and precautions

☐ Techniques for unlocking a position

☐ Medications, their effects, and their administration

☐ Stereotaxic thalamotomy, if appropriate

☐ Self-help aids for dressing and walking

☐ Measures for preventing orthostatic hypotension

☐ Modification of the home for safety

☐ Availability of information and support groups

REVIEWING CLINICAL FEATURES OF PARKINSON'S DISEASE

Signs and symptoms of Parkinson's disease reflect the degeneration of the basal ganglia, particularly the substantia nigra and corpus striatum. Progressive depletion of dopamine occurs in the areas of the brain that control voluntary muscle movement and posture.

Early unilateral features
Initially, the family may notice changes in the patient's posture, gait, facial expression, or speech. Early symptoms usually affect only one side of the body. A tremor in the arm, the most common symptom, usually occurs at rest. Also, the patient may lean slightly to one side. Other early symptoms include a blank facial expression and slight muscle rigidity that increases in resistance to passive muscle stretching. Muscle rigidity and tremor may also occur in the leg on the affected side, along with mild edema of the foot and ankle.

Later bilateral involvement
As symptoms of Parkinson's disease gradually spread from one side of the body to the other, the patient assumes a stooped posture. And he may complain of fatigue and weakness as bradykinesia progressively affects all his body movements. Gradually, his movements lose their spontaneity, becoming carefully executed. Eye blinking, arm swinging while walking, and expressive facial and hand gestures disappear. This

Early features

Loss of facial expression

Leaning to unaffected side

Arm in semiflexed position

Tremor

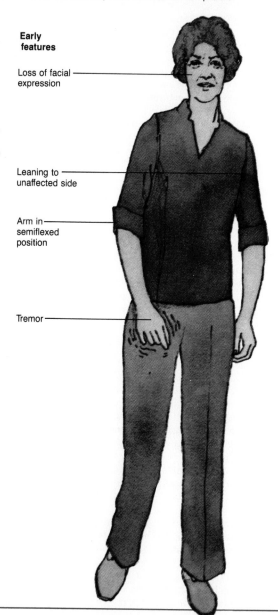

Later features

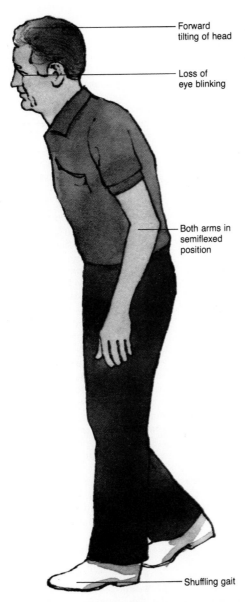

Forward tilting of head

Loss of eye blinking

Both arms in semiflexed position

Shuffling gait

loss of motor function may force the patient to stop working. Although he's still able to care for himself, he may become depressed and withdrawn, so you'll need to encourage the family to include him in their activities.

Gait problems and disability
The hallmarks of this stage include progressively pronounced gait disturbances. The patient walks more slowly in small, mincing steps and may unexpectedly find himself locked in a position, unable to move.

As his disability increases, the patient requires assistance for all activities of daily living. Tremors may not increase, but muscle rigidity and bradykinesia affect every aspect of his life, from rolling out of bed in the morning to eating.

Eventually motionless and unable to stand, the patient has little remaining voluntary motor function. Bradykinesia causes soft, monotonous speech, a masklike facial expression, and constant drooling. Neurogenic bladder and diminished thoracic excursion leave the patient susceptible to infection.

facial exercises? If not, dysphagia may occur, leading to weight loss and aspiration pneumonia.

Teach about tests

Although diagnosis of Parkinson's disease relies on clinical symptoms, you may need to prepare the patient for a CT scan or positron emission tomography to rule out structural abnormalities, such as tumors, and cerebrospinal fluid analysis and urinalysis to test for dopamine levels. (See *Teaching Patients about Neurologic Tests*, pages 293 to 299.)

Teach about treatments

• *Activity.* Stress the importance of moderate exercise to help improve mobility, decrease the risk of contractures, improve respiration and circulation, promote bowel function, lessen rigidity, and increase strength. Encourage the patient to perform range-of-motion exercises, if possible. (Passive exercises can be done, if necessary.) Tell him to exercise daily when movement is easiest—such as in the late morning or early afternoon, and soon after he takes his medication.

Review specific exercises with the patient, using pictures when helpful and providing a checklist so he can do them in order. (See *How to Do Stretching Exercises*, pages 286 and 287.) Caution him to avoid overexercise, though, because fatigue will interfere with his other daily activities. Instruct him to start his program slowly, gradually increasing his level of exercise. Enlist the family's assistance in encouraging daily exercise.

• *Diet.* Instruct the patient to avoid a high-protein diet because excess protein can affect the action of levodopa, an amino acid used to treat Parkinson's disease. But caution him against following a low-protein diet; this may cause nutritional imbalance. Also, tell him to avoid caffeine, which may worsen his symptoms. And because intestinal motility may decrease in Parkinson's disease, advise the patient to

drink adequate amounts of fluid and to eat more high-fiber foods if he's troubled by constipation.

If the patient has difficulty chewing or swallowing, recommend semisoft foods (applesauce, mashed potatoes, solid foods prepared in a blender) to help ensure adequate nutrition and minimize the risk of aspiration. Suggest freezing liquids to a slush or mixing them with other foods, such as cereals, to prevent choking. For the same reason, instruct the patient to sit up straight, move food to the back of his mouth, tilt his head slightly forward, and then swallow.

Remind the patient to keep a supply of napkins on hand to absorb excess saliva. If he has severe tremors, advise using an arm brace for steadiness. Suggest using flexible straws or cups with lid spouts (such as travel cups) to help make drinking easier. Also suggest using utensils with built-up handles to give him a better grip.

If the patient takes a long time to eat, advise eating small, frequent meals and keeping foods on a warming tray. If the patient's obese, instruct him in a weight-reduction diet. Explain that his weight affects his mobility and the absorption of his medications.

• *Medication.* Stress that the patient should never abruptly stop taking his medication because this may precipitate a parkinsonian crisis, intensifying his symptoms. Explain that as Parkinson's disease progresses, the doctor may increase the medication dosage. But caution the patient against increasing the dosage on his own, since toxicity could result.

Initially, the patient's medications may cause nausea and vomiting. Reassure him that these adverse reactions will disappear in a few months. Suggest taking medications after meals to decrease nausea.

If the patient has an intellectual impairment or memory difficulties, instruct him and his family to premeasure his medication doses for the day in separate containers, each marked with the scheduled administration time.

If the patient has difficulty swallowing, tell him to crush pills and open and mix the contents of capsules with a food that's easy to swallow, such as applesauce.

• **Surgery.** If medication fails to control the patient's tremors, stereotaxic thalamotomy may be used to relieve or eliminate them if they're unilateral. To prepare the patient for this surgery, tell him that his head will be shaved and cleansed and that a metal frame will be attached to his head to hold it still and to guide the surgeon.

Inform the patient that after he's given a local anesthetic, the surgeon will make a burr hole in his skull and create a surgical lesion in the thalamus on the side *opposite* the tremors. (Explain that the right side of the brain controls the left side of the body, and vice versa). This lesion will block the transmission of nerve impulses that cause the tremors.

Tell the patient that during surgery, he'll be asked questions to test his speech and memory, and he'll be asked to follow commands, such as raising an arm. Tell him that he'll experience some discomfort when the doctor applies the head frame and that he may have a headache after surgery.

• **Other care measures.** To provide support when sitting down and getting up, tell the patient to sit in chairs with arms. Also suggest tying a sheet to the foot of his bed to help pull himself to a sitting position. If he's experiencing orthostatic hypotension, instruct him to rise slowly from a lying or sitting position.

To help the patient maintain his balance and a forward momentum, teach him to walk with a wide-based gait and to swing his arms. If appropriate, show him how to use a weighted cane or a walker. Teach him how to unlock a position if he becomes fixed in it. Some common unlocking techniques include turning the head, opening the mouth, placing an arm behind the back or across the chest, tapping a leg with the hand, bending the knees slightly, or raising the toes. Warn him against losing his balance and falling while using some of these techniques.

To prevent falls, recommend removing throw rugs and unstable furniture and moving furniture against the walls to widen traffic paths. Also tell the patient to wear sturdy shoes with good support and traction.

Explain to the patient the importance of daily bathing because of increased skin oiliness and perspiration. Advise him to avoid oil-based soaps or lotions, and tell him to use an antiperspirant deodorant on his hands if he has sweaty palms.

If the patient experiences urinary urgency, tell him to remain near a bathroom or to keep a urinal nearby. Suggest having a raised toilet seat and grab bars installed if he has difficulty sitting and standing.

If dressing's a problem, advise the patient to wear clothing with zippers rather than buttons or to use Velcro strips. Loafer-style shoes solve the problem of tying and untying shoes.

If the patient has dysarthria, instruct him to take his time pronouncing each word. If his voice is too soft, tell him to breathe deeply before beginning each sentence. Tell him that reading aloud and singing can help his articulation and voice projection.

Instruct the family to be aware of any signs of depression in the patient, such as anorexia, insomnia, and disinterest in his surroundings. Tell them to encourage the patient's participation in family discussions, even though facial rigidity may cause him to look disinterested. Also urge the family to encourage the patient's independence and need to maintain social contacts.

Stress the importance of wearing a medical identification bracelet or necklace at all times. Also, refer the patient and his family to a local support group, the National Parkinson Foundation, or the United Parkinson Foundation for more information.

HOW TO DO STRETCHING EXERCISES

Dear Patient:

Your doctor has prescribed exercises to help you maintain flexibility and muscle strength. At first, do each exercise 1 to 5 times daily. Then, gradually increase to 10 to 20 times daily. If you're unable to do these exercises standing up, you can do most of them sitting down.

Facial muscle exercises

Raise your eyebrows and then lower and squeeze them together. Next, open your eyes wide; then close them tight. Now, wrinkle your nose. Follow this by opening your mouth wide in a big "O", then closing it tight. Move your jaw side to side. Finally, give a big smile; then purse your lips, as though trying to whistle. Repeat.

Neck exercises

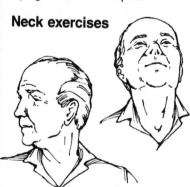

Begin by turning your head side to side. Next bend your head down and back. Repeat.

Shoulder exercises

Raise your shoulders to your ears as high as you can; then lower them. Repeat a few more times.

Arm and shoulder exercises

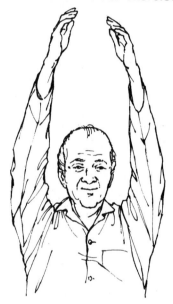

Raise your arms over your head; then swing them down, extending your arms behind your back. Repeat.

Trunk exercises
With your hands on your hips, twist your body side to side from the waist, keeping your hips and legs in place. Repeat this trunk exercise.

Hip and knee exercises

Knee exercises

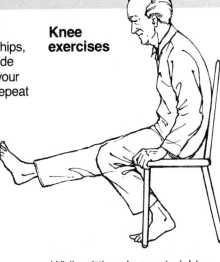

While sitting down, straighten your right knee and extend your right leg out in front of you. Then bend your right leg back under the chair as far as you can. (Keep your ankle flexed to avoid a muscle spasm.) Repeat with your left leg.

Perform this knee exercise several times.

Ankle and foot exercises
While sitting down, make circles with your right foot, first in one direction and then the other. Repeat with your left foot. Do this exercise a few more times.

Ankle and toe exercises
While sitting down, extend your leg and point your toes toward the floor; then point them up toward your nose. Try this several more times.

Holding on to a counter or a sturdy piece of furniture, raise your right knee toward your right shoulder; repeat with your left knee, raising it toward your left shoulder. Repeat these movements.

Seizures

In seizure disorders, the patient's ability to lead a productive life may hinge on your success in teaching him about his specific seizure-triggering factors and the importance of strict compliance with long-term drug therapy. You'll also need to explain that his drug therapy may change, depending on his symptoms and the rate at which he metabolizes the drug. What's more, you'll need to teach him about possible activity restrictions, precautions for an imminent seizure, preparation for diagnostic tests, and, if ordered, surgery.

Remember to include the family in your teaching, too, so they'll know how to help the patient during a seizure.

Describe the disorder

Explain to the patient that the cause of seizures can't always be identified. Tell him that seizures result from the rapid, uncontrolled discharge of central nervous system (CNS) neurons. Mention that the site of this cerebral hyperactivity determines the patient's signs and symptoms.

Explain the patient's type of seizure: focal, psychomotor, or generalized tonic-clonic. A *focal seizure* results from an irritable focus in the cerebral cortex, lasts about 30 seconds, and doesn't usually alter the patient's level of consciousness. A *psychomotor seizure* occurs when a focal seizure begins in the temporal lobe and causes confusion or some other change in the patient's level of consciousness. A *generalized tonic-clonic seizure* occurs when cerebral hyperactivity isn't confined to the original focus or to a localized area but extends to the entire brain.

Tell the patient that he may experience more than one type of seizure. Also tell him that during the initial phase of a seizure he may have noticed an aura—a sensory phenomenon, such as seeing stars or smelling roses—but that not everyone experiences auras.

Point out possible complications

Emphasize the need for strict adherence to the drug regimen to prevent overmedication or undermedication. Overmedication may cause increased side effects. In contrast, undermedication can increase the duration, frequency, and number of seizures. The result: an increased risk of injury.

Emphasize to the patient that he can seriously injure himself and others if he has a seizure while driving a car or operating machinery.

Teach about tests

Teach the patient about diagnostic tests, such as electroencephalography, a CT

CHECKLIST

TEACHING TOPICS IN SEIZURES

- ☐ Explanation of how the brain's abnormal electrical activity leads to seizures
- ☐ The patient's type of seizure: focal, psychomotor, or generalized tonic-clonic
- ☐ Preparation for diagnostic tests, such as electroencephalography and a CT scan, to help determine the seizure's cause
- ☐ Drugs and their administration, including the risks of overmedication and undermedication
- ☐ Trigger factors, including fatigue and hypoglycemia
- ☐ Importance of a normal diet to provide energy for normal neuron function
- ☐ Preparation for craniotomy, if necessary
- ☐ Measures, such as wearing a medical identification bracelet, to alert others to the patient's condition
- ☐ Precautions for an imminent seizure
- ☐ How the family or other caregivers should manage a seizure
- ☐ Sources of additional information and support

scan, or, occasionally, cerebrospinal fluid analysis, that may help identify the etiology of the seizures. If appropriate, explain any blood tests to check anticonvulsant drug levels and to detect any blood dyscrasias resulting from drug therapy. (See *Teaching Patients about Neurologic Tests*, pages 293 to 299, for further information.)

Teach about treatments

• *Diet.* Instruct the patient to eat regular meals and to check with the doctor before dieting. Maintaining adequate blood glucose levels provides the necessary energy for CNS neurons to work normally. Skipping meals or dieting may lead to decreased glucose levels (hypoglycemia). This can cause unstable neurons to malfunction, thus triggering a seizure. Teach the patient to recognize the symptoms of hypoglycemia, so he can eat a snack when needed.

• *Medication.* Make sure the patient understands that anticonvulsant drugs can't cure his seizures but will control them. Advise him to take his medication exactly as ordered—both undermedication and overmedication can cause seizures. Explain that the doctor will regulate drug dosage according to his blood levels, so the dosage may periodically change (for example, with age or illness). If illness prevents the patient from taking his medication, tell him to have a family member or other caregiver contact the doctor immediately. The doctor may decide to administer medication by another route.

Tell the patient what to do if he misses a dose, but caution him to avoid applying missed dose instructions for an anticonvulsant drug to any other drug he's taking, because instructions will vary according to each drug's mechanism of action. Stress that withdrawal seizures are possible if he abruptly stops taking his anticonvulsant drug.

Explain that he'll be taking medication as long as he needs it to control his seizures. Even if he doesn't have a seizure for years, he shouldn't stop taking it unless ordered by the doctor. The length of time he'll require an anticonvulsant drug (a few years or for life) depends on many factors, such as the cause of his seizures and his age.

• *Surgery.* Prepare the patient for a craniotomy, if ordered. Explain that

QUESTIONS PATIENTS ASK ABOUT SEIZURES

Will seizures interfere with my normal activities?

Once your seizures are under control, you'll be able to continue your normal activities—with some safety considerations. Avoid swimming alone and working at heights. (For example, don't climb a ladder to paint your house.) If you drive, contact your state's motor vehicle office. Most states prohibit you from driving a motor vehicle until you're seizure-free for a certain time period, usually 1 year.

What will happen if I have a seizure in a public place?

To ensure proper management of your seizure, you should always wear a medical identification bracelet or necklace stating that you have a seizure disorder. This will alert others to your condition. If you feel a seizure coming on, find a safe spot and lie down. (Of course, you should be aware of your trigger factors and avoid them, if possible.)

Will I lose my job?

You shouldn't lose your job because you have seizures. If you're honest with your employer about your disorder, you're protected by the equal opportunity laws. However, keep in mind that your exact job description may change, depending on the position's requirements and liability considerations.

HELPING A SEIZURE VICTIM

Dear Caregiver:

A person with a seizure disorder may have an attack at any time in any place. During a seizure, he may lose awareness of his surroundings. If this happens, follow these instructions:

During the seizure

1
Turn the person on his side.

2
Remove hard or sharp objects from the area, loosen restrictive clothing, such as a collar or a belt, and place something soft and flat under his head.

Never force anything into the person's mouth, especially your fingers. Ask onlookers to leave the area.

3
If you suspect the person has swallowed his own vomit, call a doctor immediately.

After the seizure

1
Allow the person to lie quietly. As he awakens, gently call him by name, and reorient him to his surroundings and to recent events.

2
If the person has an injury, such as a profusely bleeding tongue, take him to the doctor's office or to the hospital emergency department.

Also write an accurate description of the seizure as soon as possible. The doctor may request certain information, including the seizure's duration and the victim's activity immediately before, during, and after the seizure.

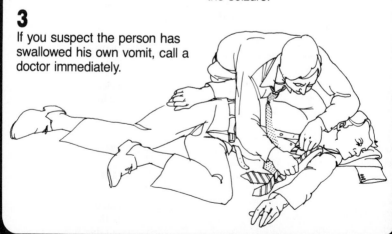

this surgery can remove a structure or lesion that can cause seizures, or it can sever a structure that allows abnormal electrical discharges to spread to other unstable neurons. Tell him that the success rate of craniotomy varies, but that this surgery may decrease the number and severity of seizures. Inform the patient that he may still require anticonvulsant drugs after surgery.

Advise the patient to wash his hair on the day before surgery, if possible. Tell him that a technician will shave his head at the incision site. (Reassure him that his hair will grow back and that the surgery won't affect his memory, his feelings, or his ability to think.) Explain to the patient that after he receives an anesthetic, the surgeon will open a part of the skull to expose the brain tissue. The size of the opening varies from a small burr hole to a larger open flap. The burr hole later fills in with bone growth; the large bone flaps are put back or replaced by synthetic material.

Inform the patient that after surgery he'll have a bandage over his head, and that the head of his bed will be elevated about 30 degrees (for a supratentorial craniotomy) or kept flat (for an infratentorial craniotomy). Caution him to avoid changing the bed's position; however, tell him that he can turn from side to side. Also tell him to avoid coughing, which could increase intracranial pressure. Remind him to ask for medication if he develops a headache.

Explain that the doctor will remove his skin sutures within 7 days and that he'll wear a cap to keep his head warm after removal of the bandages. (Tell him that the size of the scalp incision doesn't necessarily reflect the size of the skull opening.)

Before he's discharged from the hospital (usually 7 to 10 days after surgery), remind the patient to keep his head warm. Tell him he may wash his hair (but should avoid scrubbing around the incision), gently patting the incisional area dry. Instruct him to report any signs of infection (redness, warmth, drainage) or separation of the incision. Inform him that he can resume most routine activities, but that he'll require the doctor's permission to return to work or to engage in strenuous activities, such as running or contact sports.

• **Other care measures.** Help the patient identify factors that can trigger a seizure. These factors may include stressful situations and, in some seizure disorders, flashing lights on video games, computer screens, and sights and sounds associated with highway construction. Emphasize to the patient that seizures can be triggered even if he's taking his anticonvulsant medication as prescribed.

Encourage the patient to pursue his normal activities if possible, but remind him that fatigue can trigger seizures. For his own safety, warn him to avoid activities that require complete alertness until his seizures are under control. The same rule applies to operating any equipment that could cause an injury. If the patient has a driver's license, tell him to notify the Bureau of Motor Vehicles. (See *Questions Patients Ask about Seizures*, page 289.)

Make sure the patient's family knows what to do if a seizure occurs. (See *Helping a Seizure Victim.*) If the patient's a child, instruct the parents to notify day-care or school authorities of their child's condition.

Stress the importance of wearing a medical identification bracelet or necklace at all times. Also encourage the patient to contact the Epilepsy Foundation of America for additional information. Refer him to a local support group.

Vascular Headaches

In vascular headaches, your teaching can help the patient learn to manage pain and prevent disruption of his life.

For example, you'll need to teach him about the need to recognize and avoid factors that precipitate his headaches. You'll also need to reinforce the importance of taking his medications on time and adjusting his diet and activities appropriately.

Describe the disorder

Explain the patient's type of vascular headache: migraine (most common in women) or cluster (most common in men).

Migraine headaches have three phases. In the first phase, symptoms characteristically vary from patient to patient but may include an aura of visual, sensory, or motor disturbances. In the second, or vasoconstrictive, phase, the patient may experience ataxia, nausea and vomiting, and vertigo. Headache pain, often accompanied by nausea, occurs during the final phase (vasodilation).

Cluster headaches tend to occur at night and last about 1 hour. Usually, the patient experiences no warning symptoms, but he may notice dilation of the pupil on the same side as his headache. He may also experience increased tearing, nasal congestion, ptosis, and flushing. Explain that these headaches commonly occur in a series of closely spaced attacks. Also tell him that cluster headaches may have a genetic link.

Point out possible complications

To minimize persistent headaches, emphasize the importance of avoiding precipitating factors. Tell him that maximum relief hinges on compliance with his medication schedule, diet, and activity restrictions.

Teach about tests

Prepare the patient for a provocative histamine test to help diagnose the cause of his headache. Also prepare him for a computed tomography (CT) scan or electroencephalography to rule out other disorders, such as a lesion or infection. (See *Teaching Patients about Neurologic Tests*, pages 293 to 299.)

Teach about treatments

• *Diet.* Educate the patient about a low-tyramine diet. Tell him to avoid foods that contain tyramine, such as cheese, alcohol (especially red wines), liver, and yeast extracts. Also tell him to avoid or limit other foods, such as chocolate, that trigger attacks.

• *Medication.* Tell the patient with migraine headaches to take prescribed ergotamine with the onset of symptoms. If a headache develops, the patient may take prescribed analgesics. For the patient with cluster headaches, review the actions of his medications and the use of oxygen.

• *Other care measures.* Advise the patient to lie down in a dark, quiet room during an attack. Be sure to caution him to avoid bending over, coughing, and sneezing. Such activities increase intracranial pressure, thus increasing his pain. Also suggest that he apply an ice pack to his head to help decrease pain.

Review common precipitating factors in headaches, such as stress, hormonal changes, foods, lack of sleep, and barometric pressure changes. Instruct him to avoid these factors whenever possible.

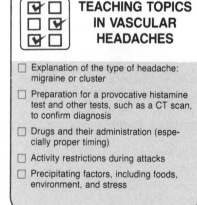

CHECKLIST

TEACHING TOPICS IN VASCULAR HEADACHES

☐ Explanation of the type of headache: migraine or cluster

☐ Preparation for a provocative histamine test and other tests, such as a CT scan, to confirm diagnosis

☐ Drugs and their administration (especially proper timing)

☐ Activity restrictions during attacks

☐ Precipitating factors, including foods, environment, and stress

TEACHING PATIENTS ABOUT NEUROLOGIC TESTS

TEST AND PURPOSE	TEACHING POINTS
Cerebral angiography (cerebral arteriography) • To detect disruption or displacement of the cerebral circulation by occlusion or hemorrhage	• Explain that angiography shows blood circulation in the patient's brain. Tell him who will perform the test and where. Also tell him that the test takes about 2 hours and that he may experience some discomfort from lying still that long. • Describe the preparation for the test. Instruct the patient to restrict food and fluids for 4 hours before the test. Tell him that just before the test he'll need to change into a hospital gown and to urinate. Mention that a technician will shave and cleanse the injection site—the carotid or the femoral artery—and may also immobilize the patient's head with tape or straps. If the carotid artery is used, inform the patient that he may have his face covered with a drape and his arms immobilized to maintain a sterile field. • Explain what happens during the test: as the patient lies on an X-ray table, the doctor will inject a local anesthetic and then insert a catheter. Next, during injection of the contrast medium, the patient may experience pressure, warmth, a transient headache, nausea, or a salty taste. Tell him to report any of these sensations to the doctor. Immediately after injection, he'll hear clacking sounds from the X-ray equipment. Explain that multiple injections of the contrast medium may be required to completely visualize the blood vessels. Instruct the patient to lie still throughout the test to avoid blurring the films. Also tell him to follow the doctor's instructions to move an arm or a leg. • Describe what happens after the test: tell the patient the catheter is removed, pressure is applied to the puncture site for about 15 minutes, a pressure dressing and an ice pack are applied, and his distal pulses are checked frequently. Instruct him to hold his head and neck (carotid approach) or leg (femoral approach) straight for 4 to 12 hours. Tell him he can resume his usual diet but should increase fluid intake for the rest of the day to help expel the contrast medium.
Cerebral blood flow (CBF) studies • To measure CBF • To detect abnormalities in cerebral perfusion • To evaluate the effectiveness of surgery, such as extracranial/intracranial bypass and cerebral aneurysm clipping	• Explain that CBF studies evaluate blood flow to the brain. Tell the patient who will perform the test and where, and that it takes about 30 minutes. Inform him that the test is painless and exposes him to less radiation than other radiologic studies, such as a chest X-ray. • Explain that he'll lie on a table during the test and have a frame placed around his head. For the inhalation technique, he'll breathe through a mask or mouthpiece (wearing noseclips) for 10 minutes as readings are taken. For the injection technique, he'll receive an I.V. injection and breathe through a mask or dome. • Tell the patient to lie still during the test. After it, he can immediately resume his usual activities.

(continued)

TEACHING PATIENTS ABOUT
NEUROLOGIC TESTS *(continued)*

TEST AND PURPOSE	TEACHING POINTS
Cerebrospinal fluid (CSF) analysis • To help detect infection, multiple sclerosis, or malignancy • To help detect obstruction of the subarachnoid space around the spinal cord • To inject medication or contrast medium into the central nervous system	• Explain that the test involves the removal and laboratory analysis of spinal fluid. Tell him who will perform the test and where, and that it takes about 15 minutes. Inform him that he'll feel some pressure during the procedure as the needle is inserted. • Describe the preparation for the test: *for a cisternal puncture,* instruct the patient to restrict food and fluids for 4 hours before the test, if ordered. Explain that he'll assume a sitting position with his chin resting on his chest, or he'll be positioned on his side at the edge of a bed, with a small pillow placed beneath his forward-bending head. After cleansing and possibly shaving the upper neck area, the doctor will inject a local anesthetic. *For a lumbar puncture,* tell the patient he'll be seated with his head bent toward his knees, or he'll lie on the edge of a bed or table, with his knees drawn up to his abdomen and his chin resting on his chest. After cleansing the lumbar area, the doctor will inject a local anesthetic. Tell the patient to report any tingling or sharp pain. • Explain what happens during the test: *in a cisternal puncture,* the patient should remain still as the doctor inserts a hollow needle into the midline of the vertebral column below the occipital bone. *In a lumbar puncture,* the doctor inserts a hollow needle into the subarachnoid space surrounding the spinal cord. Tell the patient to hold still to avoid dislodging the needle. Also tell him he may be asked to breathe deeply or to straighten his legs and that the doctor may apply pressure to the jugular veins. • Describe what happens after the test: *after a cisternal puncture,* the doctor removes the needle and applies an adhesive bandage. The patient briefly lies flat on his back while the puncture site seals. Then he can resume his usual activities. *After a lumbar puncture,* the doctor removes the needle and applies an adhesive bandage. The patient lies flat for 4 to 24 hours to prevent a headache. His head should be even with or below the level of his hips. Remind him that although he must not raise his head, he can turn from side to side. Also tell him to increase fluid intake for the rest of the day to help replenish CSF and to prevent a headache.

**TEACHING PATIENTS ABOUT
NEUROLOGIC TESTS** *(continued)*

TEST AND PURPOSE	TEACHING POINTS
Computed tomography (CT) scan (CAT scan) • To identify structural abnormalities, edema, and lesions, such as nonhemorrhagic infarction, hematomas, aneurysms, and tumors, in the brain and spinal cord	• Explain that this test produces X-rays of the brain or spinal tissue. Tell the patient who will do the test and where, and that it takes about 30 to 60 minutes. Tell him the test causes no discomfort, but he may feel chilled because the equipment requires a cool environment. • If the doctor will be using a contrast medium, tell the patient to restrict food and fluids for 4 hours before the test. • Explain what happens during the test: tell the patient that a technician will position him on an X-ray table and will place a strap across the part of the body to be scanned to restrict any movement. The table then slides into the circular opening of the scanner. If a contrast medium is ordered, the patient will receive it through an I.V. site; the infusion takes about 5 minutes. Instruct the patient to tell the technician immediately if it causes any discomfort, a feeling of warmth, or itching. (The technician can see and hear him from an adjacent room.) Then tell him he will hear noises from the scanner and may notice the machine revolving around him. • Describe what happens after the test: tell the patient he can immediately resume his usual activities and diet. Advise him to increase his fluid intake for the rest of the day to help expel the contrast medium.
Digital subtraction angiography (DSA) • To evaluate the patency of the cerebral vessels and to determine their position • To detect and evaluate lesions and vascular abnormalities	• Explain to the patient that DSA visualizes the blood vessels in his head and neck. Tell him who will perform the test and where, and that it will take about 30 to 45 minutes. Inform him that he may experience a feeling of warmth or a metallic taste upon injection of the contrast medium. • Instruct the patient to restrict solid food for 4 hours before the test. • Explain what happens during the test: the patient will be positioned on an X-ray table and an I.V. needle or catheter will be inserted. Caution him to lie still during the test. After the doctor injects a contrast medium, a series of X-rays are taken. Instruct the patient to tell the doctor immediately if he feels any discomfort or shortness of breath. • Describe what happens after the test: after the doctor removes the needle or catheter, the patient can resume his usual activities. Encourage him to increase his fluid intake for the rest of the day to help expel the contrast medium.

(continued)

TEACHING PATIENTS ABOUT
NEUROLOGIC TESTS *(continued)*

TEST AND PURPOSE	TEACHING POINTS
Electroencephalography (EEG) • To evaluate the brain's electrical activity in such disorders as seizures • To aid diagnosis of intra-cranial lesions, such as abscesses and tumors	• Explain to the patient that the EEG records the electrical activity of his brain. Assure him that the test is painless and that the electrodes won't give him an electric shock. Tell him who will perform the test and where, and that it takes about 45 minutes. • Depending on the type of EEG ordered (such as sleep, sleep deprivation, or photic stimulation), explain the necessary restrictions. Instruct the patient to wash his hair 1 to 2 days before the test to remove hair spray, cream, or oil. • Explain what happens during the test: the patient will be positioned comfortably in a reclining chair or on a bed. After lightly abrading the patient's skin to ensure good contact, a technician will apply paste and attach electrodes to the patient's head and neck. Tell the patient to remain still throughout the test. Review the activities that he may be asked to perform, such as breathing deeply and rapidly for 3 minutes (hyperventilating) or sleeping, depending on the type of EEG. • Describe what happens after the test: the technician will remove the electrodes. He'll also remove the paste, using acetone. (This may sting where the skin was scraped.) Tell the patient to wash his hair to remove residual paste; then he can resume his usual activities.
Electromyography (EMG) • To evaluate neuromus-cular disorders, such as myasthenia gravis	• Explain to the patient that this test measures the electrical activity of specific muscles. Tell him who will perform the test and where, and that it takes about 1 hour. • Explain what happens during the test: inform him that he'll be lying down or sitting up, depending on the muscle to be tested. A technician will cleanse the skin over the muscle. Tell the patient he may experience some discomfort as the doctor inserts a needle attached to an electrode into the muscle. Then the doctor will place another electrode, which delivers a mild electrical charge, on the patient's limb. This may also cause discomfort as each muscle is stimulated to test its response at rest and during voluntary contraction. Tell the patient he must remain still during the test, except when asked to contract or relax a muscle. Also explain that an amplifier may cause crackling noises whenever his muscle moves. • Tell the patient that the electrodes are removed after the test and that he can resume his usual activities.

**TEACHING PATIENTS ABOUT
NEUROLOGIC TESTS** (continued)

TEST AND PURPOSE	TEACHING POINTS
Evoked potential studies (evoked responses) • To measure the brain stem's electrical response to an external stimulus	• Explain to the patient that evoked potential studies measure his nervous system's electrical response to a visual, auditory, or sensory stimulus. Tell him who will perform the test and where. Also tell him that the test lasts about 1 hour and is painless. • Tell the patient to wash his hair 1 to 2 days before the test. • Describe what happens during the test: tell the patient he'll be positioned on a bed or table or in a reclining chair. Emphasize that he should lie still during the test. Mention that a technician will cleanse his scalp and apply paste and electrodes to his head and neck. Also tell him he may hear noises from the test equipment. Explain that he'll be asked to perform various activities, such as gazing at a checkerboard pattern or a strobe light, or listening with headphones to a series of clicks. Or he may have electrodes placed on an arm and leg, and be asked to respond to a tapping sensation. Tell the patient that the technician will remove the electrodes and paste after the test and that the patient can resume his normal activities. Tell him to wash his hair to remove residual paste.
Magnetic resonance imaging (MRI) (nuclear magnetic resonance scan) • To aid diagnosis of intracranial and spinal lesions	• Explain that this test evaluates the condition of the brain or spinal cord. Tell the patient that the test involves no radiation exposure but does involve exposure to a strong magnetic field. As a result, tell him to report any metal objects in his body (such as a pacemaker, aneurysm clips, a hip prosthesis, or bullet fragments) so the machine can be adjusted. • Tell the patient who will do the test and where. Also tell him that the test takes about 1 hour and causes no discomfort. • Explain what happens during the test: the patient will be positioned on a table that slides into a large cylinder housing the MRI magnets. Tell him that his head, chest, and arms will be restrained to help him remain still. Stress that lying still prevents blurring the images. Also explain that a technician can see and hear him from an adjacent room. Tell the patient he'll hear a loud knocking noise while the machine is running. If the noise bothers him, he may be given earplugs or pads for his ears. • Tell the patient he can resume his normal activities after the test.

(continued)

**TEACHING PATIENTS ABOUT
NEUROLOGIC TESTS** *(continued)*

TEST AND PURPOSE	TEACHING POINTS
Nerve conduction studies • To determine the velocity of impulses traveling along a nerve • To aid diagnosis of diseases that affect the peripheral nervous system, such as Guillain-Barré syndrome	• Explain to the patient that nerve conduction studies measure the speed at which electrical impulses travel along a nerve. Tell him who will do the test and where, and that it takes about 1 hour. Tell him he may experience discomfort during needle insertion and delivery of each stimulus. • Explain what happens during the test: the patient will lie on a bed or sit on a chair, depending on the nerve to be tested. The technician will cleanse the patient's limb and tape surface electrodes to the skin at the distal end of the nerve. The doctor will then insert the needle at various sites along the nerve route, and with each insertion will deliver a slight electrical charge. Tell the patient he must remain still during the test because movement may distort results, prolonging the test. • Tell the patient that the technician will remove the electrodes and needle after the test and that the patient can resume his usual activities.
Neuropsychological tests • To evaluate cognitive function • To help distinguish organic from psychiatric disorders	• Explain that a battery of neuropsychological tests evaluates simple to complex mental and verbal abilities. It also includes a personality inventory. Tell the patient who will administer the tests and where, and that the tests take about 1 to 2 hours. • Tell the patient that he may be asked to perform such activities as making calculations, solving problems, and answering questions about current events. • Tell the family that after the test, the patient with memory loss may show increased confusion and restlessness.
Oculoplethysmography (OPG) • To aid detection and evaluation of carotid occlusive disease	• Explain that OPG indirectly evaluates carotid blood flow. Tell the patient who will perform the test and where, and that it will take only a few minutes. • Describe the preparation for the test: tell the patient to remove any contact lenses. Also tell him he'll have anesthetic drops instilled in his eyes, which may cause burning. Explain that his head will be placed in a frame and that he'll have eyecups placed on his eyes (held in place with light suction) and photoelectric cells clipped to his earlobes. • Tell the patient to remain still and avoid blinking during the test. If he's also having ophthalmic artery pressure studies, mention that he'll briefly lose his vision when suction is applied to his eyes. • Tell the patient that the doctor will remove the eyecups and head frame after the test. Tell him not to rub his eyes or replace his contact lenses for at least 2 hours. Also tell him to blink and to protect his eyes until the effects of the anesthetic drops wear off.

**TEACHING PATIENTS ABOUT
NEUROLOGIC TESTS** (continued)

TEST AND PURPOSE	TEACHING POINTS
Positron emission tomography (PET) scan (positron emission trans-axial tomography) • To evaluate cerebral glucose metabolism • To evaluate cerebral perfusion • To aid diagnosis of tumors and disorders that alter cerebral metabolism, such as Alzheimer's disease, Parkinson's disease, multiple sclerosis, and cerebrovascular accident	• Explain that a PET scan evaluates brain cell function. Tell the patient who will perform the test and where. Also tell him that the test takes about 1 hour, is painless, and involves minimal radiation exposure. Mention that he'll lie on a moving table and that his head will be immobilized and placed inside a ring-shaped opening in the machine. • Explain what happens during the test: if the doctor uses the *inhalation method*, tell the patient he'll inhale a radioactive tracer through a mask. Tell him to breathe normally; he won't smell or taste anything odd. If the doctor uses the *I.V. method*, tell the patient he may feel a warm sensation during injection of the tracer. Tell him to notify the technician if he feels any discomfort. In both methods, tell the patient he'll have a dome-shaped hood placed over his head and face to prevent the *exhaled* tracer from circulating in the room. Stress the importance of lying still to avoid blurring the images. • If the I.V. method is used, explain that the doctor will remove the needle after the test and collect a blood sample. Tell the patient he can resume his normal activities.
Provocative histamine test • To evaluate the response of cerebral blood vessels to histamine	• Explain that this test helps diagnose vascular headaches. Tell the patient he'll receive one or two subcutaneous injections of histamine. He may resume his usual activities after the test.
Tensilon test (edrophonium test) • To aid diagnosis of myasthenia gravis	• Explain to the patient that this test helps evaluate muscle function. Tell him who will perform the test and where, that it takes about 15 to 30 minutes, and that he may feel discomfort upon needle insertion. Also tell him that the doctor will check his facial or peripheral muscle strength before the test. • Explain what happens during the test: the skin over the vein is cleansed. For multiple injections, the doctor inserts an I.V. cannula, injects Tensilon or a placebo, and checks the patient's muscle strength. Do *not* tell the patient about the placebo injection. (If the doctor injects a placebo, he next injects Tensilon and checks muscle strength.) After the cannula is removed, the patient can resume his usual activities.

SURGERY

More so than other surgeries, neurosurgery can threaten a patient's sense of self. After all, it invades the very seat of his thoughts, feelings, and sensations. In so doing, it can easily evoke fear and denial—two barriers you'll have to overcome before you can begin teaching. Only then will the patient be receptive to your teaching.

Once you're ready to begin teaching, explain the purpose of surgery. A carotid endarterectomy, for example, promotes cerebral circulation by revascularizing brain tissue. A craniotomy removes tumors and hematomas and allows insertion of shunts. A stereotaxic thalamotomy decreases tremors in Parkinson's disease and multiple sclerosis. In myasthenia gravis, thymectomy reduces circulating levels of the antibodies that block nerve impulse transmission necessary for muscle contraction. (See the entries in this chapter for more information.)

Continue your teaching by describing what happens before, during, and after surgery. On this and the following page, you'll find this information for carpal tunnel release, rhizotomy, spinal cord surgery, transsphenoidal hypophysectomy, and ventricular shunt. In the entries earlier in this chapter, you'll also find this information for carotid endarterectomy, craniotomy, and other surgeries.

Carpal tunnel release
Explain that this procedure relieves pressure on the median nerve in the patient's wrist and restores sensation and mobility to his hand. Tell him to restrict food and fluids after midnight on the day of surgery. Mention that he'll have his arm shaved and cleansed and a local anesthetic injected into his wrist

and hand. Inform him that he may have a feeling of pressure during surgery.

Tell him that after surgery he'll have a dressing wrapped around his hand and arm. To reduce swelling and discomfort, instruct him to elevate his hand above his elbow for at least 24 hours (using a sling when walking and pillows when lying down). Tell him to check his fingers for circulation, to gently open and close his hand every hour to prevent stiffness, and to take mild analgesics for pain. After 24 hours, the doctor will remove the dressing and place an adhesive bandage over the incision.

Instruct the patient to keep the incision site dry and to avoid lifting anything heavier than a thin magazine. Also have him avoid repetitive wrist movements (like typing).

Rhizotomy
Explain that after pain pathways are identified, a surgical rhizotomy severs and destroys the nerve roots to relieve pain. Alternatively, the nerve root can be injected with alcohol or destroyed with a needle to relieve pain. If it's successful, the patient will be free of leg pain but will have diminished or absent sensation in the affected area.

Tell the patient that he'll need to restrict food and fluids after midnight on the day of surgery and that he'll have the sacral area cleansed and shaved. After surgery, he can expect medication and neurologic and circulation checks. Explain that he'll lie on his abdomen and have a bulky dressing over the incision. Mention that his movement in bed will be limited to rolling no more than 30 degrees from his abdomen to either side. Instruct him in logroll turning—moving the whole spine as a unit without flexion.

Inform him that sutures will be removed in 7 to 10 days. Before discharge, remind him to use good body mechanics and not to lift anything heavier than 5 lb (2.3 kg) to avoid putting pressure on the suture line. Explain that he needs the doctor's permission to return to work or to engage in strenuous sports or other activities.

Spinal cord surgery

Explain that spinal surgery allows removal of a tumor, a hematoma, bone fragments, or a foreign body. If the patient's having high cervical spinal surgery, tell him to wash his hair the day before surgery and explain that the back of his neck may be shaved.

Explain that after surgery he'll be given medication, as needed, for pain. Review any activity restrictions, such as bed rest, and special beds. Remind him to cough, deep-breathe, and perform leg exercises (hip flexion may be limited). Explain how to logroll. Demonstrate correct spinal alignment, and caution the patient to avoid flexing or twisting his back.

Tell the patient when he can resume activities, and teach him the technique for getting into and out of bed. Instruct him to report any signs of infection to the doctor.

Transsphenoidal hypophysectomy

Tell the patient with a pituitary tumor that this procedure involves making an incision in the upper gum above the teeth, passing a surgical instrument through the sphenoidal sinus, and removing pituitary tissue. Instruct him to brush and floss his teeth before surgery to help prevent infection.

Explain that after surgery he'll have a nasal packing in place for 1 or 2 days and that this packing consists of antibiotic-soaked gauze. (He may also have a permanent packing near the pituitary that consists of tissue from his hip or thigh or synthetic dura.) He'll have a dressing on the donor site and a nasal sling or "moustache" dressing to absorb nasal drainage. The head of his bed will be elevated to reduce swelling, and he'll receive medication for headache. Instruct him to gently brush his teeth with a soft toothbrush or to use a water pick after surgery. Tell him to

deep-breathe but to avoid coughing, which can rupture the suture line. After removal of the nasal packing, instruct the patient not to cough, sneeze, blow his nose, or instill anything into his nose unless prescribed. Stress the importance of reporting excessive thirst or urination after removal of his indwelling catheter. (This may indicate delayed diabetes insipidus resulting from decreased pituitary hormone levels.)

If the patient's pituitary is partially removed, stress the importance of compliance with lifetime hormone replacement therapy to prevent life-threatening complications. Tell him to watch for signs of infection at the incision site and to avoid pressure changes, such as flying in an airplane, for 3 to 4 weeks after surgery.

Ventricular shunt

Explain that this procedure is similar to a craniotomy but involves insertion of a flexible tube into a ventricle to drain cerebrospinal fluid. The surgeon places one end of the shunt in a ventricle and the other end in a cavity large enough to absorb additional fluid, such as the abdominal cavity, a vessel leading to the heart, or a space at the back of the head. Placement in the back of the head is temporary; in the other areas, it's permanent. The shunt extends from the ventricle to the scalp, where it's tunneled under the skin to the appropriate cavity.

Explain to the patient that he can usually resume activities the day after shunt insertion and that he'll have a small dressing on his head and abdomen or chest. If the patient wears glasses, tell him to have the temple piece adjusted so it doesn't put pressure on the shunt.

Before the patient's discharged, review the procedure for pumping the shunt, if ordered. Tell the patient to report any signs of infection or shunt malfunction (for example, drowsiness, headache, restlessness, nausea, vomiting) to the doctor.

302

CARING FOR THE PERSON WITH A HALO BRACE

Dear Caregiver:

The doctor has placed the person you're caring for in a halo brace to stabilize his head and neck. The brace allows him mobility while keeping his head in the proper position. The guidelines below will help you care for the person during the early phases of his recovery.

Cleaning the pin sites

To prevent infection, clean the pin sites (where the screws secure the halo to the head) each day. Pour hydrogen peroxide over a cotton-tipped applicator and then use the applicator to clean the scalp around the pins.

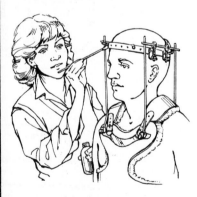

To prevent spreading any possible infection, begin at the pin insertion site, rotating the applicator while cleaning in a circular motion around the pin. Use a different applicator for each pin. Also, if an applicator becomes soiled, discard it and use another one to finish cleaning the pin site. *Never* pour more peroxide over a soiled applicator to rinse it.

While cleaning the pin sites, check the pins for stability. Does a pin feel loose? Is the skin puckered around it? If so, tell the person you're caring for to remain still. A loose pin may also make a clicking sound, which the person can hear. If you detect a loose pin, call the doctor immediately.

Also, check at each pin site for any signs of infection: unusual redness, tenderness, puffiness, or drainage. Ask the person in your care if he feels feverish or has a headache. Report any unusual findings to the doctor.

Cleaning under the vest

To clean the skin under the vest, first gather a basin of water, soap, a washcloth, and a towel. Then, ask the person to lie down (on his back or abdomen, as shown on the next page) and to support his head with a pillow so there's no pressure on the halo brace. (Place the pillow between the posts on the brace.) Remember, *never* loosen the vest while the per-

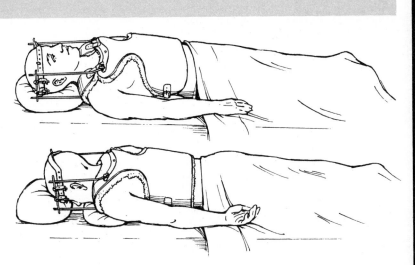

son's sitting up (even for comfort's sake; for example, after a large meal). This will remove the support necessary for his neck.

Now loosen *one* side of the vest at a time. Wash and thoroughly dry the area under the vest on that side and inspect it for redness, bruising, irritation, or any other signs of pressure. If you notice any of these signs, pad the area surrounding the pressure spot with sheepskin or a foam pad.

Refasten the opened side of the vest before opening the opposite side. Then repeat the procedure on the opposite side: wash, dry, and inspect the skin for signs of pressure.

If the vest lining gets wet, dry it with a hand-held hair dryer set on a low, warm temperature.

Moving about safely
Remember these safety rules:
• Tell the person to use a cane on steps and uneven terrain and to wear flat shoes to help maintain balance. The brace weighs 5 to 10 lb, so it will make him top-heavy. Also, make sure he has extra room when moving around. Never allow anyone to pull on the brace.
• Tell him to turn his entire body (not just his head) when looking to the side. He may attach mirrors to the brace to extend his field of vision. Tell him to avoid activities, such as driving, that require head turning.
• When he's getting into a car, check that the brace can fit under the car roof. Tell him to back himself in—buttocks first.

TEACHING PATIENTS ABOUT NEUROLOGIC DRUGS

DRUG	ADVERSE REACTIONS	INTERACTIONS*
Anticonvulsants		
carbamazepine (Tegretol)	*Reportable:* blurred vision, bradypnea, confusion, dark urine, depression, easy bruising or bleeding, edema of the legs or ankles, fever, hives, itching, jaundice, mouth ulcers, nightmares, nystagmus, palpitations, paresthesias, rash, sore throat, unusual tiredness or weakness, urinary retention *Other:* abdominal pain, aching muscles or joints, ataxia, constipation, diarrhea, diaphoresis, dizziness, drowsiness, dry mouth, glossitis, headache, nausea	• Tell the patient that foods, alcohol, and over-the-counter drugs don't influence the safety or effectiveness of carbamazepine.
ethotoin (Peganone) **mephenytoin** (Mesantoin) **phenytoin** (Dilantin, Novophenytoin)	*Reportable:* ataxia, blurred vision, confusion, easy bruising or bleeding, fever, gingival hyperplasia (with phenytoin), gingivitis (with ethotoin), hallucinations, jaundice, joint pain, lymphadenopathy, nystagmus, rash, seizures, severe abdominal pain, slurred speech, sore throat *Other:* constipation, diarrhea, drowsiness, headache, hirsutism, insomnia, mild dizziness, muscle twitching, nausea, urine discoloration, vomiting	• Tell the patient to avoid regular consumption of alcohol and large doses of salicylates. Tell him not to take vitamins containing folic acid without first consulting his doctor. • Advise him not to take antacids within 3 hours of taking his anticonvulsant. • Inform him that foods don't influence the safety or effectiveness of his anticonvulsant.
phenobarbital (Luminal, Nova-Pheno)	*Reportable:* ataxia, bradycardia, bradypnea, confusion, depression, easy bleeding or bruising, fever, hives, hyperexcitability, insomnia, jaundice, joint or muscle pain, rash, severe drowsiness or weakness, shortness of breath, slurred speech, sore throat *Other:* anxiety, dizziness, drowsiness, headache, irritability, nausea, nightmares, vomiting	• Tell the patient to avoid alcohol and hay fever, allergy, cold, and sleeping medications that contain central nervous system (CNS) depressants, such as antihistamines. • Also tell him that foods don't influence the safety or effectiveness of phenobarbital.

*Includes food, alcohol, and over-the-counter products.

TEACHING POINTS

• Explain to the patient that this drug helps control his seizures.
• If the patient misses a dose, tell him to take it as soon as he remembers unless it's almost time for the next dose. Tell him not to double-dose.
• Advise him to take the drug with food to reduce nausea. If he experiences a dry mouth, tell him to suck on ice chips or sugarless candy or to chew sugarless gum.
• Warn the patient to operate machinery cautiously and to avoid driving if he experiences dizziness, drowsiness, or ataxia.
• Because the patient may be sensitive to ultraviolet light, tell him to avoid using sunlamps and to wear a sunscreen and protective clothing in the sun.
• Stress the importance of keeping appointments for blood and eye tests.
• Tell the diabetic patient that this drug may affect urine glucose levels.
• Tell the patient that before any surgery, he should inform his doctor or dentist that he's taking this drug.

• Explain to the patient that this drug helps control his seizures.
• If he's taking one daily dose, tell him not to take it after his scheduled administration time. If he's taking several daily doses, tell him to take a missed dose as soon as he remembers.
• If he's using a liquid form, tell him to shake it *well* and to use a measuring spoon, not a household teaspoon. If he's taking the chewable form, tell him he *must* chew or crush the tablets.
• Tell the patient to take this drug with food if he develops nausea.
• Warn him to operate machinery cautiously and to avoid driving if he feels dizzy (more common with ethotoin and mephenytoin).
• Stress the importance of good oral hygiene and dental care to the patient taking phenytoin.
• Explain that these drugs may turn his urine pink or reddish brown.
• Warn the patient that changing brands or abruptly stopping the drug may cause withdrawal seizures.
• Stress the importance of keeping follow-up blood test and doctors' appointments.
• Tell the diabetic patient that this drug may affect his urine and blood glucose levels.
• Tell the patient that before any surgery, he should inform his doctor or dentist that he's taking this drug.

• Explain to the patient that this drug helps control his seizures.
• If he misses a dose, tell the patient to take it as soon as he remembers unless it's almost time for the next dose. He must never double-dose.
• Warn the patient not to crush, chew, or break extended-release capsules.
• Tell him to operate machinery cautiously and to avoid driving if he feels dizzy or drowsy.
• Warn the patient to take the drug as ordered to prevent possible dependence on it.
• Caution him never to abruptly stop the drug because withdrawal seizures could occur.
• Tell him that before any surgery, he should inform his doctor or dentist that he's taking this drug.

(continued)

TEACHING PATIENTS ABOUT NEUROLOGIC DRUGS *(continued)*

DRUG	ADVERSE REACTIONS	INTERACTIONS*
Anticonvulsants *(continued)*		
primidone (Mysoline, Sertan)	*Reportable:* ataxia, confusion, difficulty breathing, easy bruising or bleeding, facial edema, hives, itching, nervousness, rash, restlessness, sore throat, unusual tiredness, visual changes *Other:* anorexia, decreased libido, dizziness, drowsiness, headache, nausea, unsteadiness, vomiting	• Tell the patient to avoid alcohol and cold, hay fever, allergy, or sleeping medications containing CNS depressants, such as antihistamines. • Tell him that foods don't influence the safety or effectiveness of primidone.
valproic acid (Depakene)	*Reportable:* dark urine, depression, easy bruising or bleeding, jaundice, nausea, nightmares, rash, seizures, severe abdominal pain, visual changes, vomiting *Other:* constipation, diarrhea, dizziness, drowsiness, indigestion, mild abdominal pain, transient alopecia	• Tell the patient to avoid alcohol and hay fever, allergy, cold, or sleeping medications containing CNS depressants, such as antihistamines. • Tell him to avoid aspirin, which may increase the risk of bleeding and bruising, and to avoid taking the drug with milk.
Antimyasthenic drugs		
ambenonium (Mytelase) **neostigmine** (Prostigmin) **pyridostigmine** (Mestinon, Regonol)	*Reportable:* blurred or double vision, bradycardia, dyspnea, dysphagia, dizziness, fainting, increased weakness, tachycardia, twitching *Other:* abdominal cramps, diaphoresis, GI upset, salivation, urinary frequency	• Tell the patient to avoid drinking quinine and tonic water. • Tell the patient that foods, alcohol, and over-the-counter drugs don't influence the safety or effectiveness of these antimyasthenic drugs.
Antiparkinson drugs		
amantadine (Symmetrel)	*Reportable:* confusion, depression, edema, fainting, hallucinations, insomnia, nystagmus, shortness of breath, slurred speech, sore throat, urinary retention *Other:* anorexia, difficulty concentrating, dizziness, dry mouth, indigestion, irritability, lethargy, nightmares, orthostatic hypotension, rose-colored skin mottling	• Tell the patient to avoid alcohol (which may worsen dizziness and confusion) and decongestants that contain CNS stimulants (which may increase irritability). • Tell the patient that foods don't influence the safety or effectiveness of amantadine.

*Includes food, alcohol, and over-the-counter products.

TEACHING POINTS

- Explain to the patient that this drug will help control his seizures.
- If he misses a dose, tell him to take it only within 2 hours of the scheduled administration time. He must never double-dose.
- Tell the patient never to abruptly stop the drug, because seizures are possible.
- If the patient's taking the suspension form, tell him to shake the bottle *well* before pouring and to use a measuring spoon (not a household teaspoon).

- Tell the patient to take this drug with meals if he develops nausea.
- Tell the patient to operate machinery cautiously and to avoid driving if he feels dizzy, drowsy, or unsteady.
- Stress the need for follow-up blood tests and medical visits.
- Tell the patient that before any surgery, he should inform his doctor or dentist that he's taking this drug.

- Explain to the patient that this drug helps control his seizures.
- If the patient misses a dose, tell him to take it when he remembers. But if his next scheduled dose is within 6 hours, tell him not to take the missed dose. Never double-dose.
- Caution him never to stop the drug abruptly because withdrawal seizures may occur.
- Tell him never to chew the drug because it will irritate his mouth and throat.
- Tell the patient to take this drug with meals

(but not with milk) if he experiences GI distress.
- Tell him to operate machinery cautiously and to avoid driving if he feels drowsy.
- Stress the importance of follow-up blood tests and medical visits.
- Inform the diabetic patient that this drug may produce false urine ketone results.
- Tell the patient that before any surgery, he should inform his doctor or dentist that he's taking this drug.

- Explain to the patient that this drug improves his muscle strength.
- If the patient misses a dose, tell him to take it as soon as he remembers unless it's almost time for the next dose. He must never double-dose.

- Instruct him to take this drug with meals or milk if he experiences GI distress.
- Warn the patient to operate machinery cautiously and to avoid driving if he feels dizzy or has vision problems.

- Explain to the patient that this drug helps relieve symptoms of Parkinson's disease.
- If the patient misses a dose, tell him to take it when he remembers. But if his next scheduled dose is within 4 hours, tell him not to take the missed dose. Never double-dose.
- Tell him to schedule his last daily dose at least 3 hours before bedtime to help prevent insomnia.
- Warn the patient that abruptly stopping the drug could cause a parkinsonian crisis.

- If he experiences a dry mouth, tell him to suck on ice chips or sugarless candy or to chew sugarless gum.
- Warn him to operate machinery cautiously and to avoid driving if he feels dizzy or has blurred vision.
- To reduce the risk of orthostatic hypotension, tell him to rise slowly from a sitting or a lying position.
- Caution against overexertion when his symptoms subside.

(continued)

TEACHING PATIENTS ABOUT
NEUROLOGIC DRUGS (continued)

DRUG	ADVERSE REACTIONS	INTERACTIONS*
Antiparkinson drugs (continued)		
benztropine mesylate (Cogentin) **trihexyphenidyl** (Artane, Tremin)	*Reportable:* abdominal cramps, ataxia, confusion, eye pain, hallucinations, insomnia, muscle weakness, rash, shortness of breath, tachycardia *Other:* blurred vision, decreased sweating, dizziness, dry mouth, mild constipation, nausea, orthostatic hypotension, photosensitivity, sore mouth or tongue, vomiting	• Tell the patient to avoid alcohol and drugs that contain CNS depressants, such as antihistamines. Such drugs include cold and cough preparations and allergy and sleeping medications. • Instruct him to take antacids or antidiarrheals at least 1 hour before or after taking this drug. Antacids and antidiarrheals may decrease absorption of this drug. • Tell the patient that foods don't influence the safety or effectiveness of this drug.
bromocriptine mesylate (Parlodel)	*Reportable:* abdominal pain; melena; confusion; fainting; hallucinations; hematemesis; orthostatic hypotension; persistent constipation; twitching *Other:* anorexia, constipation, diarrhea, drowsiness, headache, leg cramps, nausea, stuffy nose, tingling fingers/toes when cold, vomiting	• Tell the patient that foods, alcohol, and over-the-counter drugs don't influence the safety or effectiveness of this drug.
levodopa (Dopar, Larodopa, Levopa) **levodopa-carbidopa** (Sinemet)	*Reportable:* depression, dysuria, frequent blinking, mouth ulcers, orthostatic hypotension, sore throat, tachycardia, tremors, twitching, vomiting, weakness *Other:* blurred vision, constipation, diarrhea, dry mouth, mild dizziness, mood changes, nausea, nightmares, urine discoloration	• Tell the patient to avoid vitamin preparations containing vitamin B_6 (with levodopa only); cough, cold, sinus, or allergy medications that contain sympathomimetics or CNS stimulants; and foods high in vitamin B_6 (with levodopa only), such as avocados, bacon, beans, beef liver, powdered milk, oatmeal, peas, pork, sweet potatoes, and tuna. • For best absorption, tell him to take this drug at least 1 hour before meals, if possible.

*Includes food, alcohol, and over-the-counter products.

TEACHING POINTS

- Explain to the patient that this drug improves muscle control and relieves muscle spasms.
- If he misses a dose, tell him to take it as soon as he remembers. But if his next scheduled dose is within 8 hours, tell him not to take the missed dose. He should never double-dose.
- Tell the patient to take this drug with or immediately after meals to help prevent GI distress.
- Warn him that abruptly stopping the drug could trigger a parkinsonian crisis.
- To minimize orthostatic hypotension, tell the patient to rise slowly from a sitting or a lying position.
- Warn the patient to operate machinery cautiously and to avoid driving if he feels dizzy or has blurred vision.
- Tell him that this drug may cause heat intolerance. As a result, he should avoid overexertion in warm temperatures.
- Also tell him that his eyes may be sensitive to sunlight; wearing sunglasses should help.
- If he experiences a dry mouth, tell him to suck on ice chips or sugarless candy or to chew sugarless gum.

- Explain to the patient that this drug helps relieve symptoms of Parkinson's disease.
- If he misses a dose, tell him to take it as soon as he remembers. But if his next scheduled dose is within 4 hours, tell him not to take the missed dose. He should never double-dose.
- Tell him to take this drug with or immediately after meals to reduce GI distress.
- To minimize orthostatic hypotension, advise the patient to rise slowly from a sitting or a lying position.
- Warn him to operate machinery cautiously and to avoid driving if he feels drowsy.

- Explain to the patient that this drug helps relieve symptoms of Parkinson's disease (tremors, stiffness, slow movements).
- If the patient misses a dose, tell him to take it as soon as he remembers. But if the next scheduled dose is within 2 hours, tell him not to take the missed dose. He must never double-dose.
- Warn him that he could trigger a parkinsonian crisis by abruptly stopping the drug.
- Tell the patient to take the drug with or immediately after meals if he experiences GI distress. If he experiences a dry mouth, tell him to suck on ice chips or sugarless candy or to chew sugarless gum.
- Warn him to operate machinery cautiously and to avoid driving if he feels dizzy or has blurred vision.
- Caution against overexertion when his symptoms subside.
- To reduce the risk of orthostatic hypotension, tell the patient to rise slowly from a sitting or lying position. Also tell him to avoid hot baths or showers if they cause dizziness.
- Explain that his urine may turn a harmless red or dark brown. Also tell him that bathroom cleaning products may turn dark if they come into contact with his urine.
- Warn the diabetic patient that this drug may interfere with urine glucose and ketone tests.
- Advise the patient that before any surgery, he should inform his doctor or dentist that he's taking this drug.

(continued)

**TEACHING PATIENTS ABOUT
NEUROLOGIC DRUGS** *(continued)*

DRUG	ADVERSE REACTIONS	INTERACTIONS*
Skeletal muscle relaxants		
baclofen (Lioresal) **dantrolene sodium** (Dantrium)	*Reportable:* bloody stools, bradycardia, chest pain, depression, fainting, fever, hematuria, insomnia, itching, jaundice, mouth sores, rash, seizures, severe diarrhea or constipation, shortness of breath, sore throat, tinnitus, urinary frequency *Other:* abdominal pain, ataxia, blurred vision, confusion, constipation, diarrhea, dizziness, drooling, drowsiness, dysuria, fatigue, headache, muscle aches, nausea, orthostatic hypotension, slurred speech, vomiting, weakness	• Tell the patient to avoid alcohol and cold, cough, allergy, or sleeping medications containing CNS depressants, such as antihistamines. • Also tell him to avoid diet pills and antacids. • Tell the patient that foods don't influence the safety or effectiveness of baclofen or dantrolene sodium.
Miscellaneous		
ergotamine tartrate (Ergomar, Ergostat, Wigrettes) **ergotamine tartrate and caffeine** (Cafergot, Cafetrate) **ergotamine tartrate, caffeine, belladonna alkaloids, and pentobarbital** (Cafergot P-B)	*Reportable:* abdominal pain; anxiety, bloating; bradycardia; confusion; dyspnea; edema of legs or feet; itching; mouth, throat, or lung infection (with Medihaler); pain in arms, legs, or lower back; paresthesias; red or violet blisters on hands or feet; tachycardia; visual changes; weakness *Other:* cough, diarrhea, drowsiness, dry mouth, itching, nausea, sore throat (Medihaler), vomiting	• Tell the patient that tobacco constricts his peripheral blood vessels and alcohol dilates his blood vessels, thereby aggravating his headache. • Tell the patient that foods and over-the-counter drugs don't influence the safety and effectiveness of this drug.
methysergide (Sansert)	*Reportable:* anorexia, bradycardia, chest pain, cold hands or feet, difficulty concentrating, dyspnea, dysuria, edema, feeling of dissociation, flank pain, hallucinations, leg cramps, low back pain, nightmares, paresthesias, severe dizziness, tachycardia, visual changes, weight loss *Other:* abdominal pain, anxiety, clumsiness, diarrhea, dizziness, drowsiness, insomnia, mild depression, nausea, vomiting, weight gain	• Tell the patient that tobacco constricts peripheral circulation. • Inform him that foods, alcohol, and over-the-counter drugs don't influence the safety or effectiveness of methysergide.

*Includes food, alcohol, and over-the-counter products.

TEACHING POINTS

• Explain to the patient that this drug helps relax his muscles and relieve spasticity and stiffness.
• If he misses a dose, tell him to take it as soon as he remembers. If it's almost time for the next dose, tell him not to take the missed dose. He should never double-dose.
• If he's taking the liquid form, tell him to use a measuring spoon and to *shake the bottle well.*
• Tell the patient to operate machinery cautiously and to avoid driving if he feels confused, weak, dizzy, or drowsy.
• To prevent dizziness, tell him to rise slowly from a sitting or lying position and to avoid hot baths or showers.
• Tell the diabetic patient that baclofen may elevate his glucose levels.
• If the patient's taking dantrolene sodium, tell him to avoid excessive exposure to sunlight.
• Tell the patient that before any surgery, he should inform his doctor or dentist that he's taking this drug.

• Explain to the patient that this drug helps constrict blood vessels during the vasodilation phase of a migraine headache.
• Tell him to take the prescribed dose at the first sign of a headache and to lie down in a dark, quiet room.
• If the patient's taking the sublingual form, tell him to let it dissolve completely under his tongue; otherwise, it will be ineffective.
• Warn him not to take more than the prescribed dose, because ergotism, cerebrovascular accident, and gangrene could result.
• If the patient has a dry mouth, tell him to suck on sugarless candy or to chew sugarless gum.
• Tell the patient that prolonged exposure to cold temperatures could worsen the side effects of the drug.
• Warn the patient that illness or infection could make him more sensitive to this drug.
• If the patient's taking Cafergot P-B, advise him not to operate machinery or drive until he's accustomed to the drug's effects.
• If he's using an inhaler, tell him that gargling after each dose may relieve his sore throat. Tell him to save his inhaler for refill.

• Explain to the patient that this drug helps prevent vascular headaches.
• If he misses a dose, tell him not to take it even if he remembers later. He must never double-dose or abruptly stop taking the drug.
• Tell the patient to take this drug with meals or milk if it upsets his stomach.
• Instruct him to operate machinery cautiously and to avoid driving if he feels dizzy or drowsy.
• Advise him to get up slowly from a sitting or lying position to prevent orthostatic hypotension.
• Warn him that exposure to cold temperatures worsens the drug's side effects.

10 Musculoskeletal System

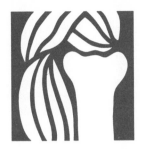

Musculoskeletal System

Introduction

The musculoskeletal system protects the body's organs, makes movement possible, stores calcium and other minerals, and serves as a site for hematopoiesis. Because of this system's wide-ranging effects, you'll find that certain teaching topics recur in many musculoskeletal disorders.

Most obviously, musculoskeletal disorders can limit the patient's mobility and thus threaten his sense of independence. Many of these disorders also follow a chronic course that's frequently marked by pain.

To promote mobility, you'll need to stress the importance of a balanced program of exercise and rest. Exercise maintains joint mobility and muscle strength, while rest prevents undue joint fatigue. For the patient with a musculoskeletal disorder, rest may involve using protective or assistive devices as well as modifying daily activities to avoid joint and muscle strain. As a result, you may need to teach him how to apply, use, and care for splints, braces, and other orthopedic devices, as appropriate. Keep in mind, though, that these devices can be baffling for the patient. He'll need your instruction—and encouragement—to use them properly.

Because many musculoskeletal disorders are chronic, much of your teaching will focus on home care. To perform home care successfully, the patient must first understand how even simple daily choices and activities—such as what he eats for dinner or how he sits in a chair to watch television—can make a difference. You'll need to emphasize to the patient the importance of a diet rich in calcium and vitamin D as well as the use of good posture and proper body mechanics at all times. These measures help keep bones strong and healthy. And they help prevent further musculoskeletal injury, especially to the back.

When pain also characterizes a musculoskeletal disorder, you'll face an even greater teaching challenge. Chronic pain can deplete the patient's emotional resources and tempt him to abuse his pain medication. To discourage this, your teaching must emphasize other pain-relief measures, such as heat or cold therapy, massage, and prescribed exercises, to minimize joint and muscle stiffness.

For some patients, surgery is necessary to correct joint deformity, strengthen unstable joints, replace joints, or repair traumatic injury. Among the surgical procedures you may be called on to teach about are arthroscopy, arthrodesis, debridement, joint replacement, laminectomy, osteotomy, closed or open reduction, and amputation.

DISORDERS

Congenital Hip Dysplasia

When teaching about congenital hip dysplasia (CHD), you'll be dealing with parents who are probably anxious and perplexed about their child's disorder. In all likelihood, their first questions will be "Why did this happen to our child?" and "What did we do (or not do) to cause it?" Besides explaining CHD and helping to assuage their feelings of guilt, your teaching must help them understand the importance of early treatment. In neonates, CHD can usually be corrected by conservative measures like splinting, while in older infants and children it may require surgery and a hip spica cast.

Many parents will be bewildered by the orthopedic devices and techniques, such as traction, used for treatment. You'll need to assure them that these devices aren't painful for the child, nor will they impede his growth and development. Because treatment for CHD usually takes 2 to 6 months to complete, you'll also need to address parental feelings about separation from their child and the psychological effects of hospitalization. This separation will probably motivate parents to learn about home care. After all, the sooner they can master skills like cast care, the sooner their child can return home. To ensure their confident and competent home care, your teaching must combine written instruction with return demonstration and must allow ample time for parents to ask questions.

Describe the disorder

Tell the parents that CHD is a common abnormality of the hip joint that's present at birth. Explain what type of hip dysplasia their baby has. In unstable hip dysplasia, the ligaments around the hip are lax, making the hip prone to dislocation. In subluxation, the head of the femur is partially displaced out of the acetabulum, whereas in frank dislocation, it's totally displaced. Most dislocations occur at birth or shortly thereafter; a few occur during fetal development.

Point out possible complications

Stress to the parents that the femur and acetabulum must fit together correctly for these bones to continue growing normally. Otherwise, the hip joint won't be able to move correctly. If CHD isn't treated, their child will develop an abnormal gait and restricted mobility of the hip joint. A unilateral dislocation will also shorten one of his legs, leading to scoliosis. Bony abnormalities of the femur and acetabulum may also develop, possibly causing painful degenerative joint disease later in life.

Teach about tests

Explain the clinical tests that the doctor may perform to detect CHD, including Ortolani's, Barlow's, and Trendelenburg's tests. Warn the parents that the

CHECKLIST

TEACHING TOPICS IN C.H.D.

☐ An explanation of the type of dysplasia: instability, subluxation, or dislocation

☐ Clinical tests to screen for CHD

☐ Importance of treatment to ensure a normal gait and to avoid degenerative joint disease later in life

☐ An explanation of selected treatment: external splinting, application of traction, surgery (open or closed reduction)

☐ Hip spica cast care, if needed

DEGREES OF DYSPLASIA

When teaching the parents of a child with congenital hip dysplasia (CHD), you'll need to clarify the extent of dysplasia. Begin by telling them that the head of the femur normally fits snugly into the acetabulum, allowing the hip to move properly. In CHD, flattening of the acetabulum prevents the head of the femur from rotating adequately. The hip may be unstable, subluxated (partially dislocated), or completely dislocated. Explain that the degree of dysplasia—and the child's age—will determine the doctor's treatment choice.

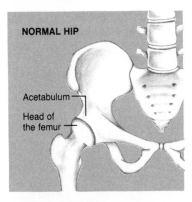

NORMAL HIP

Acetabulum

Head of the femur

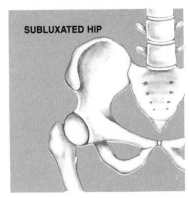

SUBLUXATED HIP

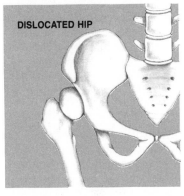

DISLOCATED HIP

child may fuss or cry since these tests cause some discomfort. Also prepare them for X-ray studies to evaluate the extent of dislocation and any bony abnormalities or soft-tissue contraction around the hip. Assure them that the small amount of radiation used in these studies won't harm their child. During treatment, inform them that follow-up X-rays will be taken at intervals to ensure that the hip is healing properly.

Teach about treatments
• *Procedures.* Typically, external splinting can correct CHD in neonates. Various devices are available, such as the Frejka splint and the Pavlik harness. Teach the parents how to apply

and remove the splint—with the doctor's approval—and review the schedule for wearing it. Usually, the doctor will allow them to do this when the hip's unstable but not dislocated. If the neonate has a harness, stress that parents mustn't remove it without the doctor's approval (see *Caring for Your Child's Pavlik Harness,* page 316).

If treatment isn't initiated until the infant is several months old, traction is usually necessary to correct soft-tissue contraction around the hip joint. Explain to the parents that traction pulls down on the femur, stretching the muscles and soft tissues around the hip. This will allow the femoral head to be reduced into the acetabulum. Traction

CARING FOR YOUR CHILD'S PAVLIK HARNESS

Dear Parent:

The doctor has applied a Pavlik harness to correct your baby's hip problem. Carefully follow these guidelines at home.

An important caution
Never remove the harness without the doctor's approval. He probably won't let you remove it for any reason, because removal may cause the baby's hip to dislocate again. However, if the hip is partially dislocated, he may let you remove the harness just for bathing.

Checking the harness
Several times a day, check the straps to see if they've loosened. You can tell by checking the black lines that the doctor

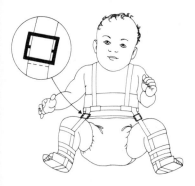

marked on the harness to show where the straps should pass through the buckles. Adjust as necessary.

If the harness becomes fully unbuckled, call the doctor.

Bathing your baby
Give your baby a daily sponge bath and check his skin, especially under the straps, for irritation. Also gently massage the skin with alcohol to stimulate circulation. Avoid using powder or lotion, which may become caked and irritate the skin.

Dressing and diapering your baby
With the doctor's approval, you can undo the shoulder straps to change your baby's shirt. Carefully adjusting these straps, as instructed, shouldn't affect the baby's hip position.

When changing your baby, fasten diaper ends *under* the straps so that the diaper doesn't pull on them. Use plastic pants with side snaps to keep the harness clean. Or choose disposable diapers with elastic legs.

Cleaning the harness
If the harness becomes soiled, simply sponge it clean with a mild soap. If your baby has a subluxated hip, the doctor may let you remove the harness to wash it. But he'll give you another for the baby to wear in the meantime.

CARING FOR YOUR CHILD'S HIP SPICA CAST

Dear Parent:

The doctor has immobilized your child's hip with a cast. To make sure the hip heals correctly, follow these instructions.

Check circulation and sensation

At least 3 times a day, check your child's circulation by pressing briefly on his large toenail. Release pressure when the skin under the nail turns white. If normal pink color doesn't return quickly, call the doctor. Also call him if the skin above or below the cast looks blue or mottled or if your child's toes feel cold and don't warm up when you cover them.

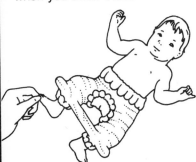

Several times a day, squeeze your child's toes. If he pulls away or seems in pain when you do this, call the doctor. Also call the doctor if your child seems unusually irritable or uncomfortable or keeps his feet and legs increasingly still.

Clean and check the skin

Every day, wash the skin along the cast's edges using water and mild soap. Be sure to first cover the edges with plastic wrap. Also clean the skin you can reach under the cast, but don't wet the cast itself. Finally, massage the skin under and along the cast's edges.

Don't let your child insert anything inside the cast. To relieve any itching, try using a hair dryer, set on "cool." Never apply lotion or powder.

Every day, inspect as far under the cast as possible, using a flashlight. Check for redness, bits of plaster, and rough edges. Petal any rough edges to avoid skin irritation. Call the doctor if you notice any object stuck in the cast, any change in the cast's fit, or a foul smell or fresh stain.

Keep cast dry and clean

If your child isn't toilet-trained, tuck a folded disposable diaper under the perineal edges of the cast. Fasten a second diaper around the cast to hold the first one in place. If your child is toilet-trained, insert plastic wrap into his cast when he's using a bedpan.

When the cast becomes dirty, clean it with a damp cloth and a powdered cleanser.

may be needed for several weeks or more, until X-rays show that the soft tissues have been stretched enough. If possible, teach the parents how to apply and maintain skin traction at home. Also teach them how to check neurovascular status. Have them keep the child's head and trunk elevated, when possible, to prevent pooling of secretions in the pharyngeal cavity, leading to otitis media.

If appropriate, explain to the parents of an older infant why he must remain hospitalized for skeletal traction.

• *Surgery.* To replace the head of the femur into the acetabulum, the doctor may perform closed or open reduction. Both require anesthesia and are performed in the operating room. Explain to the parents that open reduction involves an incision and is usually necessary when soft tissue lies between the head of the femur and the acetabulum. After reduction, the doctor may place the child in a series of spica casts so that the hip joint can remodel. As a result, you'll need to teach the parents the basics of cast care (see *Caring for Your Child's Hip Spica Cast*, page 317). Their most challenging task will be keeping the cast clean. If the child has been toilet-trained, instruct them to tuck plastic wrap around the cast's edges to prevent soiling. If the child hasn't been toilet-trained, teach them how to diaper around the cast or describe available devices, such as the split Bradford frame, that help prevent soiling. Inform the parents that the child may need to wear a splint at night after the cast is removed. If so, teach them to apply it correctly.

Herniated Nucleus Pulposus

In North America, low back pain rivals the common cold as one of the most prevalent health problems. And one of its causes, herniated nucleus pulposus (HNP), calls for your command of a wide range of teaching topics. For example, you'll need to convey the importance of strict activity restrictions and techniques for pain control—typically the first treatment measures selected. You'll also need to routinely emphasize proper body mechanics to help prevent further or recurrent back injury. Your teaching here can often spell the difference between successful home care and necessary hospitalization.

For some patients, though, HNP does demand hospitalization, forcing difficult career and life-style changes. You may need, for example, to teach the patient about surgery and about exercises and care measures during convalescence.

Describe the disorder
Explain to the patient that one of his intervertebral disks—the shock absorbers in his spine—has been injured, allowing the gelatinous center of the disk (nucleus pulposus) to push through its strong outer ring (anulus fibrosus). This compresses the nerve roots in his spine, causing pain and, possibly, sensory and motor loss.

Point out possible complications
Although symptoms occasionally abate spontaneously, HNP may cause persistent sciatica without treatment. It may also cause permanent motor or sensory loss, such as weakness in one or both legs, and bowel or bladder problems.

Teach about tests
Explain the procedures that the doctor may perform to confirm sciatica, a characteristic symptom of HNP. In the straight leg raise, the patient will lie supine on a table. The doctor will then support the patient's heel in his hand and lift the patient's leg, keeping the knee straight. Normally, a person can raise his leg 80 degrees before feeling pain. If the patient feels pain at a lesser

angle, the doctor will lower the leg slightly and dorsiflex the foot. If this too elicits pain, the patient has sciatica.

In the sitting root test, the patient must sit erect on the examination table with his legs dangling and his chin bent to his chest. The doctor will hold the patient's thigh against the table and then attempt to straighten the patient's leg. If the patient has sciatica, he'll feel pain before his leg is completely extended.

Next, prepare the patient for a battery of tests to confirm HNP. Usually, he'll be X-rayed first to screen for bony changes. Then he'll likely undergo myelography, which can accurately define the level of the herniated disk. Next, he'll usually have a computed tomography (CT) scan to evaluate any bone or soft-tissue involvement.

Teach about treatments

• *Activity*. For acute HNP, the doctor typically orders 2 weeks of bed rest at home. Explain to the patient that bed rest reduces pressure on his spine, which allows the herniated disk to subside. This, in turn, relieves pressure on the irritated nerve root, which decreases pain. Suggest that the patient use the semi-Fowler or side-lying position with his knees flexed; both help flatten the lower back and reduce tension on the spine. Recommend that he use a bedpan or a bedside commode, as ordered.

When the patient's acute pain eases, the physical therapist will start him on an exercise program to strengthen his back and abdominal muscles and to promote good posture. Reinforce the importance of following the prescribed exercise program. Include the family in your teaching to give the patient extra encouragement and support.

Also emphasize the use of proper body mechanics in daily activities. Advise the patient to avoid lifting heavy objects, like groceries, and bending at the waist. Suggest assistive devices, such as reachers. In some cases, the patient may have to make a more dra-

matic change in his life-style, such as a career move, to avoid aggravating his back problem.

• *Diet*. Explain to the patient that excess body weight aggravates the strain on his spine. If the doctor prescribes a weight-reduction diet, make sure the patient has a written copy. When teaching about meal planning, include other family members—especially the one who does most of the cooking. Consult the dietitian for additional help with meal planning.

• *Medication*. For acute HNP, the doctor may order narcotic analgesics and muscle relaxants to relieve pain and steroids to reduce inflammation. Because narcotic analgesics may cause constipation, he may also suggest concomitant use of an over-the-counter laxative. Teach the patient that a high-fiber diet with plenty of fresh fruits and vegetables and adequate fluid intake also help prevent constipation.

CHECKLIST

TEACHING TOPICS IN H.N.P.

☐ An explanation of the disorder, including how it causes back and leg pain

☐ Warning signs and symptoms of nerve root compression

☐ An explanation of procedures to confirm sciatica

☐ Preparation for X-rays, myelography, and possibly a CT scan

☐ Initial treatments, such as bed rest

☐ Back-strengthening exercises

☐ Importance of using proper body mechanics

☐ Medications and their administration

☐ Other pain-relief measures: heat or cold therapy, massage, TENS

☐ Chemonucleolysis, if performed

☐ Surgery (laminectomy or spinal fusion), if performed

☐ Postoperative exercises and wound care

STAGING HERNIATION

In herniated nucleus pulposus, the gelatinous center of an intervertebral disk (nucleus pulposus) pushes through the disk's outer fibrocartilaginous ring (anulus fibrosus). This process often occurs in stages, which determine the choice of treatment.

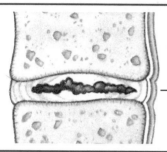

Degeneration
In this stage, certain areas of the spine may weaken from degeneration related to aging.

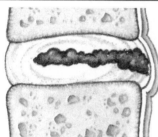

Protrusion
In this stage, the nucleus pulposus bulges at a weakened area.

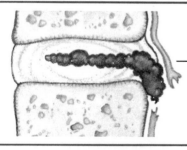

Extrusion
In this stage, the nucleus pushes through the ruptured anulus into the spinal canal.

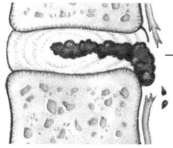

Sequestration
In this stage, fragments of the nucleus may escape into the spinal canal.

● **Procedures.** Teach the patient about adjunctive measures for pain relief: applying local heat or cold helps reduce muscle spasms, while use of pillows, a bed board, or a firm mattress helps ensure comfortable positioning. If the patient has decreased sensation, stress the importance of frequent skin checks during use of heat or cold therapy.

If the patient's hospitalized, traction may also enhance the effects of bed rest. Explain to the patient that traction involves the application of a pulling force to the body. In pelvic traction, a girdlelike device around the hips keeps the lower spine properly aligned to help ease back pain. Tell the patient how long he'll be in traction and how often he'll be allowed out of bed. Usually, the doctor orders traction for 2 weeks, with the patient allowed out of traction for 4 hours out of every 24 to take meals, use the bathroom, and perform other activities of daily living.

When these conservative measures combined fail to relieve pain, there's one alternative before surgery for some patients—chemonucleolysis. Explain that this procedure may be done in the X-ray department or operating room, under local or general anesthesia, and that it takes about 45 minutes. Tell the patient he'll receive an injection of the enzyme chymopapain. This enzyme shrinks the nucleus pulposus, thereby relieving pain. (Mention that current diagnostic tests can't always reveal how far the nucleus pulposus has pushed into the spinal canal. Sometimes, the enzyme can't reach this herniated tissue, especially if it's fragmented.) Most patients experience immediate pain relief. However, tell the patient that he may have to wait 3 to 6 weeks for total relief. After the procedure, inform the patient that he'll probably be on bed rest for 24 hours. Then reinforce the prescribed exercise program, outlined below under "Surgery." If necessary, teach him about measures to manage pain and muscle spasms, such as epidural steroid injections and use of transcutaneous electrical nerve stim-

QUESTIONS PATIENTS ASK ABOUT LEG PAIN

Why do I have so much leg pain if the problem is in my back?

Your leg pain occurs because the herniated disk is pressing on certain nerve roots in your spine. These nerve roots belong to the sciatic nerve, which courses along your hip, buttock, and leg. This explains why your shooting leg pain is commonly called sciatica.

How can the doctor tell for sure that something isn't wrong with my leg?

By ordering a myelogram. This diagnostic test can clearly show the herniated disk and where it's located. A myelogram can also rule out other back problems that might cause you to have the same symptoms.

Will my leg pain go away on its own?

Usually, bed rest will give the herniated disk time to subside, or slip back into its proper position. When this happens, there'll be no more pressure on the nerve roots and, best of all, no more leg pain.

ulation (TENS). Advise the patient that he should plan to be out of work for 2 to 8 weeks, depending on his occupation.

● **Surgery.** When conservative measures fail, you'll need to prepare the patient for surgery—most commonly, laminectomy—to relieve back pain. Explain that laminectomy involves the removal of a flat, bony section of the vertebra known as the lamina. Once the surgeon removes the lamina, he can remove the protruding fragments of the disk or the entire disk (diskectomy) to relieve nerve root compression.

CARING FOR YOUR BACK

Dear Patient:

To help manage your back pain, good posture is a must—whether you're sitting, standing, or lying down. Good posture strengthens the abdominal and buttock muscles that support your hard-working back. The guidelines here will teach you what good posture means as well as how to safely rest and exercise your back. In your daily activities, you'll also want to keep in mind the list of "do's and don'ts" to protect your back from further injury.

How to stand correctly
When you're standing correctly, you should be able to draw an imaginary line from your ear through the tip of your shoulder, middle of your hip, back of your knee, and front of your ankle. You won't be able to do this if you stand with your lower back arched, your upper back stooped, or your abdomen sagging forward.

To correct your posture, stand 1 foot away from a wall. Then lean back against the wall with your knees slightly bent. Tighten your abdominal and buttock muscles to tilt your pelvis back and flatten your lower back. Holding this position, inch up the wall until you're standing. This is the posture

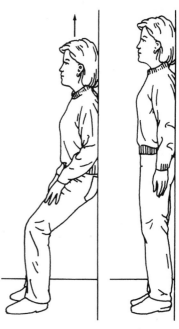

you should always assume when standing. As you walk away from the wall, try to maintain this posture. Periodically check yourself against the wall to see how you're doing.

How to sit correctly
If possible, choose a straight, hard chair to sit on. When sitting, you should avoid slumping down in the chair and thrusting your head and neck forward. Instead, you should sit with your neck and back in as straight a

line as possible, as shown in the illustration at right.

To relieve strain, sit well forward in the chair, tighten your abdominal muscles to flatten your back, and cross your knees. To correct swayback, use a footrest to bring your knees higher than your hips.

When you drive, position the seat close to the pedals to avoid emphasizing the curve in your lower back. Tighten the seat belt or use a hard backrest to flatten your lower back.

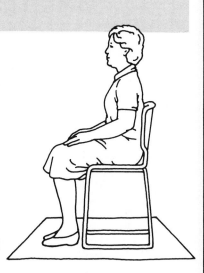

How to lie down correctly

A firm mattress is a must to achieve correct posture in bed. Either buy one or use a bed board or piece of plywood to support a soft mattress. Avoid using high pillows and sleeping flat on your back or on your stomach. These positions exaggerate swayback, and strain your neck and shoulders. In-

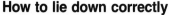

stead, lie on your side with your knees bent and a pillow between them to flatten your back. Use a flat pillow to support your neck, if you wish. Or you can sleep on your back if you support your knees with pillows. To read in bed, support your back with pillows.

(continued)

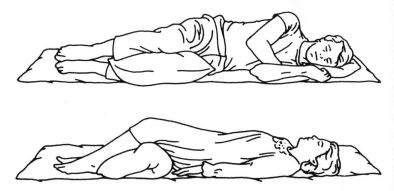

324

CARING FOR YOUR BACK *(continued)*

Exercising your back

To help improve your posture, you should exercise your back regularly while you're lying in bed or whenever you have a spare moment during the day. To exercise in bed, lie on your back with your knees bent and a pillow supporting your neck. Bring one knee up to your chest. Then lower it slowly without straightening your leg. Repeat with each leg 10 times. Next, bring both knees slowly up to your chest. Tighten your abdominal muscles and press your back flat against the bed. Hold this position for 20 seconds, then lower your knees slowly. Repeat five times. Finally, clasp both knees to your chest and gently rock back and forth (but not side to side).

During the day, periodically:
• rotate your shoulders, forward and backward.
• turn your head slowly from side to side.
• slowly touch your left ear to your left shoulder, and your right ear to your right shoulder.
• raise both shoulders, then lower them as far as possible.
• pull in and tighten your abdominal muscles, and count to 8 while holding your breath. Relax slowly. Gradually increase the count and practice breathing normally with your abdominal muscles tightened while you're sitting, standing, and walking.

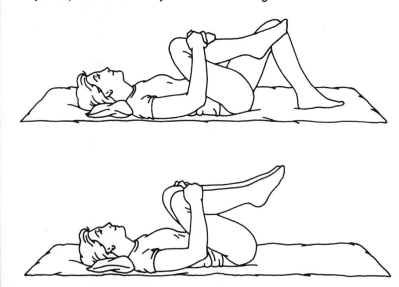

Resting your back

To relieve a tired or aching back, assume one of the positions shown here. Maintain the position for 5 to 25 minutes for the most benefit.

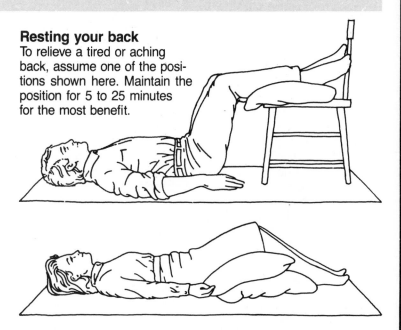

Some do's and don'ts

Do:
• keep your neck and back as straight as possible, whether you're standing, sitting, or lying in bed.
• cross your legs to rest your back during prolonged sitting.
• use a footrest to avoid tiring your back during prolonged standing.
• bend from the hips and knees, not from the waist.
• consult your doctor before doing any exercises for physical fitness.
• wear shoes with moderate heels. Avoid alternating between low and high heels.

• turn and face any object that you wish to lift.
• hold heavy objects close to your body.
• avoid rapid, jerky movements and suddenly overloading your back muscles.

Don't:
• carry unbalanced loads or anything heavier than you can manage with ease.
• lift a heavy object above your waist.
• try to move heavy furniture.
• sit on soft chairs or deep couches.
• strain to open windows or doors.

Occasionally, the surgeon may perform spinal fusion to enhance vertebral stability. Explain to the patient that this surgery involves placing bone chips from his iliac crest or a bone bank over the unstable area of his spine.

Emphasize that laminectomy and spinal fusion won't immediately relieve back pain and neurologic symptoms. That's because irritation and swelling from chronic nerve root compression will take some time to subside. In fact, the patient may temporarily have more back pain, stiffness, or muscle spasms after surgery. Assure him that analgesics and muscle relaxants will be available. If the doctor also orders a back brace or corset to support the spine, teach the patient to apply it.

After surgery, teach the patient to logroll when he gets in and out of bed, to prevent back strain and twisting.

When he's discharged (usually 6 to 10 days after surgery), make sure he understands the importance of resuming activity gradually. Have him start with a few short walks inside his home, then progress to longer walks outdoors. Advise him to rest between or during activities to avoid overdoing it. He'll probably prefer to lie down—rather than sit—to rest, since sitting places more stress on the spine. For the same reason, advise the patient to avoid long car trips at first. When sitting, he should prop his feet on a low stool to flex his hips and knees so that his knees are higher than his hips, which will keep his lower back flat against the back of a chair. When standing, he should alternately place one foot on a low stool to straighten his lower back and relieve strain. Also instruct him to wear supportive shoes with a moderate heel, to avoid bending over or lifting heavy objects, and to use a firm mattress or bed board. Tell the patient that he can resume sexual activity whenever he feels comfortable doing so. Suggest a side-lying or supine position to reduce back strain. Also, prepare the patient to do prescribed exercises—such as the pelvic tilt, leg lifts, and toe pointing—

when the doctor tells him to begin (usually about 2 months after surgery).

Besides teaching about postoperative activity, instruct the patient or his care giver about daily care of the posterior incision that the patient will have after surgery. Advise him to shower facing the stream of water and not to soak his wound in the bath until stitches have been removed (usually 1 to 2 weeks after surgery). Describe signs of infection—redness, swelling, increased pain or tenderness, fever exceeding 102° F. (38.9° C.), or changes in color or odor of drainage—that the patient should report to his doctor.

Osteoarthritis

Because chronic joint pain in osteoarthritis has no cure, your patient teaching must stress compliance with measures to help manage pain and maintain joint mobility. For pain relief, the patient can combine medication, heat or cold therapy, and massage. Most important, though, you'll need to emphasize how a balanced program of exercise and rest can help restore or maintain joint mobility and muscle strength and keep the patient as independent as possible. Incorporating such a program into his life-style may be difficult for the patient—especially if he has a set routine. But with your encouragement, he can learn to discipline himself and pace his daily activities to avoid overdoing it.

Occasionally, osteoarthritis requires surgery to correct deformity or to improve function by fusing or replacing a joint. After surgery, you'll need to teach the patient how to care for his brace or cast, and when and how to safely resume exercise.

Describe the disorder
Explain to the patient that osteoarthritis is a common degenerative disorder in which the smooth elastic

cartilage of his joints gradually wears down. The bones underneath this worn cartilage harden, and bony spurs develop around the joint, narrowing the joint space. During movement, the bones can rub together, resulting in inflammation, pain, and, possibly, loss of joint function.

Tell the patient what type of osteoarthritis he has, so he can begin to address the contributing cause. (See *Classifying Osteoarthritis*, page 328.) Be sure to point out that symptoms can vary greatly from one person to another. Similarly, a treatment may work well for one person but not for another. As a result, advise the patient to avoid comparing his condition to that of other osteoarthritic patients.

Point out possible complications
Tell the patient that if he fails to follow the prescribed exercise program, he may suffer permanent loss of function and deformity in the affected joint.

Teach about tests
Explain the tests that the doctor may order to confirm a diagnosis of osteoarthritis or to evaluate its underlying cause. Blood and urine tests can help rule out other forms of arthritis and detect metabolic disorders associated with secondary osteoarthritis. Other useful tests include joint aspiration, X-rays, tomography, and arthrography. (See *Teaching Patients about Musculoskeletal Tests*, pages 336 to 339, for more information on these tests.)

Teach about treatments
● *Activity*. Perhaps more than any other treatment measure, a balanced program of exercise and rest is critical to restore, maintain, and improve joint function and to keep the patient as independent as possible. Tell the patient that the health care team—you, the doctor, and the physical therapist—will help tailor a program to meet his needs. The amount and type of exercise will depend on the severity of his disease,

---

CHECKLIST

TEACHING TOPICS IN OSTEOARTHRITIS

- [ ] An explanation of the disease process: primary or secondary osteoarthritis
- [ ] Importance of exercise to prevent loss of joint function and deformity
- [ ] Range-of-motion, extension, flexion, and isometric exercises
- [ ] Use of protective and assistive devices to avoid joint fatigue
- [ ] Medications and their administration
- [ ] Surgery: debridement, osteotomy, arthrodesis, or joint replacement
- [ ] Postoperative exercises and activity restrictions, if appropriate
- [ ] Other pain-relief measures: heat or cold therapy, massage

---

the specific joints affected, and his lifestyle.

Explain to the patient that exercise maintains joint mobility and muscle strength while rest prevents undue joint fatigue. Tell him to perform range-of-motion (ROM) exercises daily, as instructed. Emphasize that his usual daily activities won't put his joints through full ROM.

Teach the patient to do extension and flexion exercises at least three times a day. (Many elderly people tend to hold themselves in a flexed position.) These exercises can easily be performed almost anywhere—for example, if the patient's sitting in a chair, he can periodically stretch his arms up and back.

To maintain muscle strength, show the patient how to do isometric exercises. These exercises place little stress on the joints and don't require many repetitions for maximum effect. Tell the patient to count to 6 out loud during each exercise to prevent holding his breath and to get the most benefit from the exercise.

Caution against excessive exercise,

CLASSIFYING OSTEOARTHRITIS

Osteoarthritis can be classified as *primary* or *secondary*. Primary (or idiopathic) osteoarthritis can't be linked to an underlying factor or disease. In contrast, secondary osteoarthritis has an identifiable cause. The list below outlines the forms of primary osteoarthritis and the causes of secondary osteoarthritis.

PRIMARY OSTEOARTHRITIS

- Primary generalized osteoarthritis
- Diffuse idiopathic skeletal hyperostosis
- Erosive inflammatory osteoarthritis

SECONDARY OSTEOARTHRITIS

- Acute or chronic trauma
- Multiple dysplasia
- Other inflammatory arthritic disorders, such as infectious, rheumatoid, or gouty arthritis and calcium pyrophosphate crystal deposition disease
- Old fractures
- Hemarthrosis associated with blood dyscrasias
- Neuropathic disorders, such as diabetic neuropathy
- Overuse of intraarticular corticosteroids
- Metabolic disorders, such as Wilson's disease, ochronosis, or acromegaly
- Avascular necrosis
- Chondrocalcinosis

which may worsen joint inflammation. Advise the patient to adjust his exercise program if he notices increased joint pain or swelling or decreased ROM or muscle strength. If joint pain or swelling worsens, the patient should reduce the repetitions of his exercises. However, if his ROM decreases, he should increase the repetitions. If these changes don't help or if new joints become symptomatic, advise the patient to call the doctor. Stress the importance of regular checkups to evaluate ROM and muscle strength.

Make sure the patient understands that rest doesn't mean bed rest. In fact, he should avoid prolonged immobility, which will only worsen joint pain and stiffness. Explain how recommended assistive or protective devices—such as reachers, splints and braces, or crutches, cane, or walker—can rest joints and avoid stressing them during daily activity. Teach the patient how to use any recommended devices, as necessary. Also teach him relaxation techniques to reduce stress.

- *Diet.* Because obesity places an added burden on the joints, advise the patient to follow a weight-reduction diet, if necessary.
- *Medication.* To treat osteoarthritis, the doctor will commonly prescribe aspirin and other salicylates and nonsteroidal anti-inflammatory drugs. (See *Teaching Patients about Musculoskeletal Drugs,* pages 344 to 349.) Taking these drugs for pain relief before exercise can help the patient adhere to his prescribed program.
- *Surgery.* Although not a cornerstone of treatment, surgery may be necessary to correct deformity or to avoid progression of osteoarthritis. Among the surgeries that a doctor may perform are debridement, osteotomy, arthrodesis, and partial or total joint replacement.

In *debridement,* the doctor smooths irregular joint surfaces and removes loose bodies and inflamed synovium. Tell the patient that this surgery's usually done in the early stages of osteoarthritis. After surgery, the affected joint

TIPS FOR BALANCING EXERCISE AND REST

Dear Patient:

The doctor wants you to exercise to keep your joints flexible and your muscles strong. But he doesn't want you to overdo it. Here are some tips to help you safely perform exercises and to protect your joints during your daily activities.

Exercising safely
- Dress comfortably.
- Use slow, smooth movements during exercise.
- Gradually build up repetitions.
- Exercise one side at a time.
- Expect mild discomfort when you exercise, but stop if you feel pain.
- Don't use weights during exercise, unless prescribed.
- Check with the doctor before exercising a swollen, hot, red, or painful joint. He may want you to rest the joint completely or to use it sparingly.
- Apply heat or cold before you exercise to reduce pain. Use trial and error to determine what works best for you. For heat therapy, try a heating pad or a hot water bottle. But remember, never apply heat for more than 30 minutes. Another option is to soak in a warm tub or to take a shower, which gently massages joints and muscles.

For cold therapy, try applying a double plastic bag filled with ice or directly massaging a joint with an ice cube. But remember, never apply cold for more than 20 minutes. Remove the plastic bag or ice when the area becomes numb.

Making the most of daily activities
- Set priorities to conserve your energy and to accomplish the most important things.
- Alternate light and heavy chores and rest frequently between chores. Use lightweight equipment or assistive devices.
- When performing activities, use your largest and strongest muscles first. For example, close the door with your arm instead of with your hand.
- If an activity causes pain with minimal effort, stop. If the pain continues or worsens, call the doctor.
- Be flexible. Explore new ways to perform tasks if a certain activity causes pain.
- Change positions often— alternate sitting, standing, and lying down—to help reduce strain on joints and muscles.
- Always maintain good posture. And be careful not to contribute to joint deformity. For example, rest your chin on your palm, not on the back of your hand, which forces fingers into a deformed position.

CARING FOR YOURSELF AFTER TOTAL HIP REPLACEMENT

Dear Patient:

Your new artificial hip is designed to eliminate pain and to help you get around better. But go easy at first. To avoid placing too much stress on it, follow these "do's and don'ts" for the next 3 months—or for as long as your doctor orders.

Do:

● sit only in chairs with arms that can support you when you're getting up. Then, when you do stand up, move to the edge of the chair. Place the affected leg in front of the unaffected one, which should be well under the chair; push up with your arms, not with your legs. Most of your weight will be on your arms and the unaffected leg.

● keep your affected leg facing forward, whether you're sitting, lying down, or walking.

● exercise regularly, as ordered. Stop exercising immediately if you feel severe hip pain.

● lie down and raise your legs if they swell after walking.

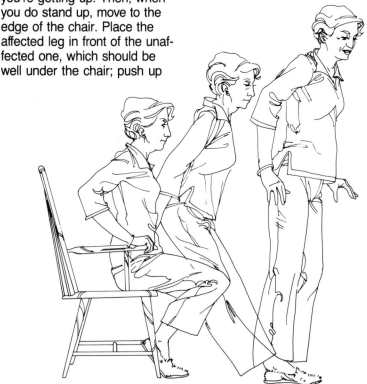

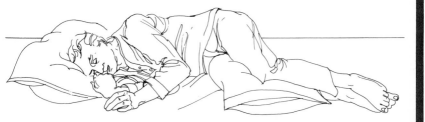

- place a pillow between your legs when lying on your side.
- wear your support stockings except when you're in bed at night.

Don't:
- lean far forward to stand up.
- sit on low chairs or couches.
- bend way over when picking up objects or tying your shoes.
- cross your legs or turn your hip or knee inward or outward.
- scrub your hip incision.
- take a tub bath.
- lift heavy items.
- have sexual intercourse until your doctor says you can.
- play tennis, run, jog, or do other strenuous activities.
- drive a car.

Call your doctor if you have:
- redness, swelling, or warmth around your incision
- drainage from your incision
- fever or chills
- severe hip pain the prescribed pain medication doesn't control
- sudden sharp pain and a clicking or popping sound in your joint
- leg shortening, with your foot turning outward
- loss of control over leg motion or complete loss of leg motion.

An important caution:
You'll need to take antibiotics just before and 2 days after any tooth extractions, dental procedures other than routine fillings, or any other surgery.

will be immobilized for a few days. Then the patient will need ROM exercises to restore joint mobility. Tell the patient to bear partial or full weight on the joint, as the doctor instructs.

To correct joint misalignment, explain that the doctor may perform *osteotomy*. Usually performed on the knee, this procedure involves cutting the bone to change the weight-bearing surfaces. Assure the patient that osteotomy usually relieves joint pain and improves joint mobility and stability. Describe the bulky dressing and knee immobilizer that he'll have to wear for 2 to 3 days after surgery until swelling subsides. After that, the doctor will apply a long leg cylinder cast.

In *arthrodesis* (or *fusion*), the doctor fuses a joint to relieve pain or provide support. Although typically performed on the cervical or lumbar spine, this surgery can also treat other joints. After surgery, the affected joint must be immobilized until it heals—usually in 3 to 6 months, as confirmed by X-rays. Accordingly, prepare the patient to wear a halo vest or cervical collar (for cervical vertebrae); a brace, body cast, or clam shell cast (for other spinal vertebrae); a hip spica cast; external fixation device; long leg cast; or a knee immobilizer. Instruct him how to apply and care for his devices.

When the patient has severe joint pain and disability, partial or total *joint replacement* may be the only option. Explain that the doctor will replace some or all of the joint with a plastic and/or metal prosthesis. This surgery can be done on all joints except the spine, with hip and knee replacements being the most common. It usually achieves pain relief and improved joint function. Stress the importance of starting an exercise program immediately to maintain joint mobility.

After a total knee replacement, the doctor will usually recommend continuous passive motion (CPM). Explain that this may involve use of a stationary, electrically controlled machine or a series of suspended pulleys and ropes.

Tell the patient that applying continuous ROM to the affected joint promotes healing. The degree of flexion will be increased gradually to reach full flexion. Inform him that he probably won't be allowed out of CPM for more than 4 hours a day for meals, bathroom visits, and other activities of daily living, and that his first time out of bed won't be until 2 to 3 days after surgery. When the patient's up, tell him that he'll have to wear a knee immobilizer. Teach him how to apply it.

After a total hip replacement, instruct the patient to keep his hips abducted and not to cross his legs, to avoid dislocating the prosthesis. When getting in and out of bed or a chair, he must avoid flexing his hips more than 90 degrees.

• *Other care measures.* Teach the patient other measures to relieve discomfort, including massage and heat or cold therapy. Heat and cold can temporarily relieve pain and increase joint ROM, making prescribed exercises easier to do. Heat can also help relieve morning stiffness. Advise the patient to experiment to discover what works best for him.

Emphasize safety measures and use of assistive devices to compensate for restricted mobility. Mention that aids are available for personal care, eating, driving, and walking, to name a few. Suggest that the patient consider adapting his home, if necessary. Refer him to the Arthritis Foundation for additional help.

Osteoporosis

Called the "silent disease," osteoporosis often goes undetected until the patient sustains a fracture and must be hospitalized. This makes your first opportunity for patient teaching more complicated than usual. You'll have to ensure that the fracture heals properly as well as help the patient understand how to avoid new fractures. Also, because osteoporosis has long been viewed as an inevitable part of aging, the patient may feel that there's little she can do to slow or prevent its occurrence. But your teaching can help her understand the importance of proper diet, vitamin and mineral supplements, and a regular exercise program in controlling osteoporosis. To help prevent new fractures, you'll need to emphasize use of proper body mechanics and close attention to safety during daily activities.

Describe the disorder

Explain to the patient that bone is continually being resorbed and formed throughout life and that between ages 30 and 35, the bones reach maturity. After this time, the rate of bone resorption exceeds that of bone formation, resulting in the gradual loss of bone mass known as osteoporosis. This bone loss makes the bones brittle and prone to fractures. Next, review with the patient the risk factors that can accelerate osteoporosis.

Explain the cause of the patient's osteoporosis, if known. There are two forms of osteoporosis—primary (divided into Type I and Type II) and secondary. Type I osteoporosis affects postmenopausal women and is linked with estrogen deficiency. Patients with this type are especially susceptible to vertebral and Colles' (distal radius) fractures. Type II osteoporosis affects men and women between the ages of 70 and 85 and is associated with persistent deficiency of calcium and vitamin D. Patients with this type are most susceptible to hip fractures.

Point out possible complications

Tell the patient that failure to observe safety measures and use proper body mechanics increases the risk of fractures. Explain that a fracture can result from minor trauma, such as a fall, or from a simple activity, such as getting up from a chair, bending over, or rais-

---

CHECKLIST

TEACHING TOPICS IN OSTEOPOROSIS

- [ ] An explanation of the disease process: Type I or Type II
- [ ] Risk factors for developing osteoporosis
- [ ] Importance of safety measures and proper body mechanics to prevent fractures
- [ ] Preparation for blood and urine studies, X-rays, and bone biopsy, if necessary
- [ ] Bone-strengthening exercises
- [ ] Importance of dietary calcium and sources of this mineral
- [ ] Vitamin and mineral supplements

---

ing a window. That's why the patient should report even minor falls to the doctor if pain, swelling, or stiffness continues.

Teach about tests

Explain the diagnostic tests that may be scheduled to confirm osteoporosis and differentiate Type I and Type II. Routine X-rays can show fractures and advanced bone loss. More sensitive radiologic tests, such as photodensitometry and single-photon absorptiometry, can detect bone loss as slight as 1% to 3%. Transiliac bone biopsy, the most valuable test, allows direct examination of osteoporotic changes in bone cells.

Prepare the patient for blood and urine studies, as appropriate. Typically, a blood sample will be drawn for blood urea nitrogen and serum calcium, phosphorus, triiodothyronine, and thyroxine levels and for serum protein electrophoresis. If the doctor orders serum alkaline phosphatase and creatinine tests, instruct the patient to fast before the sample's drawn. If he orders 24-hour urine collection for calcium, creatinine, and hydroxyproline levels, teach the patient how to collect the sample.

REVIEWING CALCIUM REGULATION

Thyroid hormone, vitamin D, and, to a lesser extent, calcitonin and adrenal steroids regulate blood levels of calcium by influencing the absorption and excretion of this mineral. They also regulate mobilization of calcium from bones and teeth, which together store over 98% of the body's calcium.

The body absorbs calcium from the gastrointestinal tract, provided sufficient vitamin D is present, and excretes it in the urine and feces. When calcium levels fall, parathyroid hormone and vitamin D enhance intestinal absorption of calcium, as illustrated here, and promote renal retention of calcium and mobilization of calcium from bones and teeth. When calcium levels rise, calcitonin—secreted by the thyroid gland—inhibits the release of calcium from bone and enhances renal excretion of calcium.

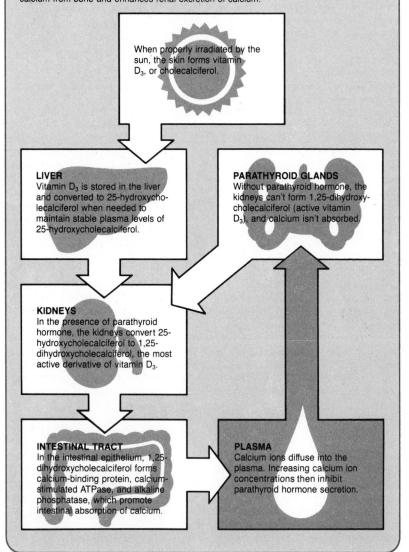

When properly irradiated by the sun, the skin forms vitamin D_3, or cholecalciferol.

LIVER
Vitamin D_3 is stored in the liver and converted to 25-hydroxycholecalciferol when needed to maintain stable plasma levels of 25-hydroxycholecalciferol.

PARATHYROID GLANDS
Without parathyroid hormone, the kidneys can't form 1,25-dihydroxycholecalciferol (active vitamin D_3), and calcium isn't absorbed.

KIDNEYS
In the presence of parathyroid hormone, the kidneys convert 25-hydroxycholecalciferol to 1,25-dihydroxycholecalciferol, the most active derivative of vitamin D_3.

INTESTINAL TRACT
In the intestinal epithelium, 1,25-dihydroxycholecalciferol forms calcium-binding protein, calcium-stimulated ATPase, and alkaline phosphatase, which promote intestinal absorption of calcium.

PLASMA
Calcium ions diffuse into the plasma. Increasing calcium ion concentrations then inhibit parathyroid hormone secretion.

Teach about treatments

• *Activity.* Describe the benefits of exercise: it increases the rate of bone formation; improves muscle strength, which increases bone density; and promotes circulation, which enhances intestinal absorption of nutrients—including calcium. Explain that exercises which put stress or weight on the bone help prevent or slow osteoporosis. Examples of such exercises include walking, jogging, and bicycling.

Instruct the patient to closely follow the prescribed exercise program.

• *Diet.* Explain that adequate daily intake of calcium can't replace lost bone, but it may slow or prevent further bone loss. Teach the patient about good sources of calcium: milk, cheese, ice cream, yogurt, tofu, dark green vegetables, sardines, and salmon. Emphasize that dietary calcium is absorbed better than artificial supplements. What's more, foods high in calcium are usually high in protein, vitamin D, phosphorus, and fiber—all of which affect bone formation.

Emphasize that the patient should adhere to the calcium intake requirements prescribed by the doctor. (These requirements vary, especially among premenopausal, pregnant, lactating, and postmenopausal women.) Caution against excess protein, coffee, and alcohol, which may increase bone loss.

Prepare the patient for a visit from the dietitian to discuss ways to meet prescribed calcium intake. For example, if the patient's watching her weight, the dietitian may recommend substituting skim milk and powdered milk for whole milk.

• *Medication.* Explain that the doctor may order calcium and vitamin D supplements to bolster the patient's dietary intake of these nutrients. An adjunctive therapy, fluoride supplements, may also promote bone formation. When the doctor orders estrogen to treat a menopausal or postmenopausal woman, stress the importance of frequent gynecologic visits to monitor for endometrial cancer.

OSTEOPOROSIS: RISK FACTOR PROFILE

Various factors can accelerate or predispose to the cortical bone loss that's characteristic in osteoporosis. These factors include:

• inadequate dietary calcium, vitamin D or C, or protein

• sex (women generally have less bone mass than men)

• family history of osteoporosis

• small bone structure or chronic underweight

• immobility or a sedentary life-style

• smoking or consumption of alcohol, which decreases calcium absorption and retention

• menopause (although the mechanism is unclear, decreased estrogen levels are linked with increased bone resorption)

• long-term use of certain drugs, such as steroids, antacids, diuretics, heparin, tetracycline, and anticonvulsants

• history of hyperthyroidism, gastrectomy, intestinal malabsorption, rheumatoid arthritis, or renal calculi.

• *Other care measures.* Since osteoporosis places the patient at risk for fractures, teach about potential safety hazards. To prevent falls, instruct the patient to remove throw rugs, to install handrails on stairs, to place a nonslip mat in the bathtub, and to avoid walking about in dimly lit rooms. Also caution against lifting heavy objects and bending deeply. Describe available assistive devices to make daily activities easier, such as a sock donner, shoe horn, long-handled sponge, or reacher. Advise the patient to wear well-fitted shoes with rubber heels to help cushion the spine during walking. If appropriate, suggest a cane or walker to maintain balance, reduce the risk of falls, and decrease lower back pain from weight bearing.

TEACHING PATIENTS ABOUT MUSCULOSKELETAL TESTS

TEST AND PURPOSE	TEACHING POINTS
Arthrography • To detect abnormalities of the menisci, cartilage, and ligaments of the knee • To detect shoulder abnormalities, such as a torn rotator cuff and anterior capsule derangement • To evaluate the need for surgery	• Explain to the patient that this radiographic test involves injecting air or a radiopaque contrast medium into the joint space. Tell him that it's performed by a doctor in the X-ray department and that it takes about 1 hour. • Explain what will happen during the test: after the patient's joint is anesthetized, the contrast medium will be injected. Warn the patient that he may experience a tingling sensation or pressure in the joint. X-rays will then be taken as the contrast medium fills the joint space. The patient will be asked to quickly assume various positions for these X-rays, then to remain as still as possible. If the knee is being studied, tell the patient that he may have to take a few steps. • Describe what will happen after the test: the patient may experience some swelling or discomfort or may hear crepitant noises in the joint. Advise him to apply ice to the joint to reduce swelling and to take a mild analgesic for pain. If symptoms persist more than 2 days, tell the patient to contact the doctor. Advise the patient to rest the joint for at least 12 hours after the test. If the doctor applies an elastic bandage after a knee arthrogram, tell the patient to keep the bandage in place for several days. Teach him how to rewrap it.
Arthroscopy • To detect and diagnose meniscal, patellar, condylar, extrasynovial, and synovial diseases • To monitor the progression of disease • To perform joint surgery or biopsy • To monitor the effectiveness of therapy	• Explain to the patient that this test allows direct examination of the inside of a joint and that it's a safe, convenient approach for surgery, if necessary. Tell the patient that arthroscopy is usually done in the operating room, under general or local anesthesia, by an orthopedic surgeon, and that it takes 30 to 60 minutes. • Describe the physical preparation for the test: the patient must not eat or drink after midnight before the test. Immediately before the test, he'll receive a sedative and have the area around the joint shaved. • Explain what will happen during the test: the patient may feel transient discomfort as the local anesthetic is injected (if applicable). The doctor will make a small incision and insert the arthroscope into the joint cavity. • Explain what will happen after the test: the patient will be allowed to walk as soon as he's fully awake. Tell him that he'll experience mild soreness and a slight grinding sensation in his knee for a day or two. Instruct him to notify the doctor if he feels severe or persistent pain or develops a fever with signs of local inflammation. Advise against excessive use of the joint for a few days after the test. Tell him that he may resume his normal diet, which was discontinued before the test.

TEACHING PATIENTS
ABOUT MUSCULOSKELETAL TESTS *(continued)*

TEST AND PURPOSE	TEACHING POINTS
Bone biopsy • To distinguish between benign and malignant bone tumors • To detect metastatic bone diseases and infection	• Explain to the patient that this test allows direct examination of a small sample of bone and that it takes 15 to 30 minutes (for needle biopsy) or 30 to 60 minutes (for open biopsy). Tell the patient who will perform the test and where, and whether he will receive a local or general anesthetic. • Describe pretest restrictions: if the patient will be receiving a general anesthetic, he mustn't eat or drink for 12 hours before the test. • If the patient will undergo needle biopsy with a local anesthetic, tell him he'll feel a sharp, sticking sensation as the local anesthetic is injected into the skin. The doctor will make a small incision, then insert the needle into the bone. Warn the patient that he'll feel pressure as the needle's advanced into the bone. • Explain what will happen after the test: the patient will experience some pain and tenderness for 1 to 3 days after a needle biopsy or for 2 to 6 days after an open biopsy. Advise him to call the doctor if pain or tenderness worsens, if drainage from the biopsy site increases, or if fever develops. Tell the patient that he can resume his normal activities after the test as soon as he's comfortable doing so. If he has undergone open biopsy, tell him the doctor will remove the stitches or sutures in 5 to 10 days.
Bone scan (bone scintigraphy) • To detect or rule out malignant bone lesions when radiographic findings are normal but cancer is confirmed or suspected • To detect occult bone trauma due to pathologic fractures • To monitor degenerative bone disorders • To detect infection	• Explain to the patient that this painless test can often detect bone abnormalities before conventional X-rays can. Tell him who will perform the test and where. • Tell the patient that fasting before the test isn't necessary. However, he should avoid eating a meal or drinking large amounts of fluids right before the test. • Explain what will happen during the test: after applying a tourniquet on the patient's arm, the doctor will inject a small dose of a radioactive isotope. Assure the patient that the isotope emits less radiation than a standard X-ray machine. Mention that there'll be a 2- to 3-hour waiting period after the isotope's injected. During this time, the patient will need to drink 4 to 6 glasses of fluid. Then he'll be asked to lie supine on a table within the scanner. The scanner will move slowly back and forth, recording images for about 1 hour. Instruct the patient to lie as still as possible during the test. Tell him that he may be asked to assume various positions on the table.

(continued)

TEACHING PATIENTS
ABOUT MUSCULOSKELETAL TESTS *(continued)*

TEST AND PURPOSE	TEACHING POINTS
Computed tomography (CT) scan (CAT scan, computerized axial tomography) • To aid diagnosis of bone tumors and other abnormalities	• Explain to the patient that this test helps detect bone abnormalities and that it takes 30 to 90 minutes. Tell him who will perform the test and where. • Describe the pretest restrictions: if he's scheduled to receive a contrast medium, the patient mustn't eat for 4 hours before the test. • Describe the physical preparation for the test: the patient will be asked to don a hospital gown and to remove all jewelry before the test. Instruct him to empty his bladder just before the test. • Explain what will happen during the test: the patient will be asked to lie on a table within the large tunnel-like scanner. Then, he may be given a contrast medium by mouth or by injection. During the test, the table he's lying on will move a small distance every few seconds. Tell him that the scanner will rotate around him and may make a clicking or buzzing noise. Instruct him to remain still during the test. Although he'll be alone in the room, assure the patient that he can communicate with the technician through an intercom system. • If the patient received a contrast medium, encourage him to drink plenty of fluids after the test.
Joint aspiration (arthrocentesis) • To aid in differential diagnosis of arthritis • To identify the cause of joint effusion • To relieve pain and distention resulting from accumulation of fluid within the joint • To administer local drug therapy (usually corticosteroids)	• Explain to the patient that this test removes a fluid sample from within the joint space for analysis. Tell him where the test will be done and that it takes about 10 minutes. • Explain what will happen during the test: the patient will be asked to assume a position and then remain still. After cleansing the skin over the joint, the doctor will insert the needle. After withdrawing the fluid, he'll apply a small bandage to the puncture site. • Explain what will happen after the test: ice or cold packs may be applied to the joint to reduce pain and swelling. If the doctor removed a large amount of fluid, tell the patient that he may need to wear an elastic bandage. Advise him not to use the joint excessively after the test to avoid joint pain, swelling, and stiffness. Instruct him to report any increased pain, tenderness, swelling, warmth, or redness as well as fever; these may signal infection.
Myelography • To detect spinal abnormalities, such as tumors, herniated intervertebral disks, fractures, and inflammation	• Explain to the patient that this test reveals obstructions in the spinal canal. Tell him that it's done in the X-ray department and that it takes about 1 hour. • Explain what will happen during the test: the patient will be positioned prone on a tilting X-ray table. After cleansing the skin on the patient's lower back with an antiseptic, the doctor will inject an anesthetic. Warn the patient that he may experience a stinging sensation. Next, the doctor will insert a needle between two vertebrae of the patient's spinal cord and will inject an oil- or water-based contrast medium. Warn the patient that he may feel a transient burning sensation during injection. He may also feel flushed and warm and may experience a headache, a salty taste, or nausea and vomiting. X-rays will be taken as the table is tilted

TEACHING PATIENTS
ABOUT MUSCULOSKELETAL TESTS *(continued)*

TEST AND PURPOSE	TEACHING POINTS
Myelography *(continued)*	vertically and then horizontally to allow the contrast medium to flow through the spinal canal. After completing the test, the doctor will withdraw the oil-based contrast medium or allow the water-based medium to be absorbed. He'll then apply a small dressing to the puncture site. • Describe what will happen after the test: if an oil-based medium was used, the patient must remain flat in bed for 6 to 8 hours and avoid abrupt movement. He must drink plenty of fluids and can resume his normal diet. If nausea prevents this, explain that he may receive I.V. fluids and an antiemetic. If a water-based medium was used, the patient must sit in a chair or lie with the head of the bed elevated for 6 to 8 hours, and then remain on bed rest for an additional 6 to 8 hours. He must drink plenty of fluids and can resume his normal diet, as tolerated. If he's on phenothiazine therapy, tell the patient that he must temporarily discontinue the drug, as ordered by the doctor. • Tell the patient to notify the doctor if he has a headache for more than 24 hours after the test or if he develops weakness, numbness, or tingling in his legs.
Photodensitometry • To measure cortical bone density as an aid in early diagnosis of osteoporosis	• Explain to the patient that this test can detect osteoporosis before it's apparent on conventional X-rays. Tell him that the test takes about 20 minutes. • Mention that during the test his hand will be positioned next to a small piece of aluminum alloy. As X-rays are taken, a computer will compare the density of the bone to that of the aluminum.
Photon absorptiometry (single) • To measure cortical bone density as an aid in early diagnosis of osteoporosis	• Explain to the patient that this painless test can accurately detect osteoporosis, even with bone loss as slight as 1% to 3%. Tell him that the test takes about 20 minutes. • Tell him that his arm will be positioned in a cradle and that X-rays will be taken of the radius—a bone in his forearm.
Photon absorptiometry (dual) • To measure trabecular bone density as an aid in early diagnosis of osteoporosis	• Explain to the patient that this painless test can detect osteoporosis before most other tests. Tell him that the test takes about 20 minutes. • Tell him that he'll be positioned on his back in a tunnel-like machine that will take X-rays of his lumbar spine.
Sinography • To determine whether a sinus tract communicates with bone as an aid in evaluating osteomyelitis • To differentiate osteomyelitis from a local abscess	• Explain to the patient that this test explores the course of his sinus tract. • Describe what will happen during the test: the doctor will insert a catheter into the sinus tract, then instill a contrast medium through the catheter. He'll take serial X-rays as the medium flows through the sinus tract. • After the test, tell the patient that the contrast medium will be absorbed into the bloodstream or by the dressing over the sinus tract.

SURGERY

For some patients with musculoskeletal disorders, surgery can offer a bright alternative to a life of chronic pain and disability. To treat degenerative joint changes in osteoarthritis, for example, the doctor may perform arthrodesis, debridement, osteotomy, or joint replacement. Surgery can also treat joint dislocation and musculoskeletal trauma. As a result, you'll need to be prepared to teach about closed or open reduction for congenital hip dysplasia and laminectomy or arthrodesis for herniated nucleus pulposus. (See these entries for specific information about the surgeries).

For other patients, such surgery as amputation may be palliative but may have a dramatic impact on self-image. In this section, you'll find out more about your teaching responsibilities in amputation as well as in closed and open reduction and in arthroscopy.

Surgical preparation

One of the first things to discuss before orthopedic surgery is the sterile shave and prep. Why? Because it's usually more extensive than that required for general surgery.

You'll also have to focus on helping the patient cope with altered mobility and body image.

Arthroscopy

During arthroscopy, the surgeon can visually examine and operate on internal joint structures through a fiber-optic scope. Explain the type of anesthetic—local or general—that the surgeon will use. If the patient will be receiving a general anesthetic, instruct him not to eat after midnight. Also tell him he may receive a sedative an hour before surgery. Mention that after sur-

gery he'll briefly have an I.V. line in place. Describe the dressing that he can expect over the site. After knee arthroscopy, review prescribed exercises and ambulation with a cane or crutches, as needed. Tell the patient to watch for signs of infection, effusion, or hemarthrosis—unusual drainage, redness, joint swelling, or a "mushy" feeling in the joint. Instruct him to call the doctor if pain, swelling, or stiffness persists for more than a week.

Closed reduction

Explain that this surgery involves external manipulation of fracture fragments or dislocated joints to restore their normal position and alignment. It may be done under local, regional, or general anesthesia. If the patient will be receiving general anesthesia, instruct him not to eat after midnight.

Tell him he'll receive a sedative before the surgery. If appropriate, explain how traction can reduce pain, relieve muscle spasms, and maintain alignment while he awaits surgery. Mention that he'll need to wear a bandage, sling, splint, or cast postoperatively to immobilize the fracture or dislocation. Before discharge, teach him how to apply (if appropriate) and care for the immobilization device. Tell him to regularly check his skin under and around the device for irritation and breakdown. Stress the importance of following prescribed exercises.

Open reduction and internal fixation

During open reduction, the doctor surgically restores the normal position and alignment of fracture fragments or dislocated joints. He then inserts internal fixation devices—such as pins, screws, wires, nails, rods, and plates—to maintain alignment until healing can occur. Because this procedure requires general anesthesia, instruct the patient not to eat after midnight. Note that he'll receive a sedative and antibiotics before going to the operating room. Describe the bulky dressing and surgical drain that he'll have in place for several days postoperatively. Tell him that he may need a cast or splint for support when the drain's removed and swelling subsides. Teach the patient how to apply (if appropriate) and care for the device. Tell him to regularly check his skin under and around the device, if possible, for irritation and breakdown. Also instruct the patient to watch for signs of incisional infection. Advise him to exercise and place weight on the affected joint only as the doctor instructs.

Amputation
Perhaps more than any other surgery, amputation can dramatically change a patient's life. As a result, you'll have to do considerable teaching both before and after surgery. Before surgery, reinforce the doctor's explanation of the procedure and clear up any misconceptions the patient may have. Support the patient as he comes to grips with the emotions surrounding loss of a limb.

Explain that after surgery the doctor will apply a cast or elastic wrap around the stump. This will help control swelling, minimize pain, and mold the stump so that it fits comfortably into a prosthesis. As appropriate, instruct the patient to report any drainage through the cast, warmth, tenderness, or a foul smell. Tell him that if the cast slips off as swelling subsides, he should immediately wrap the stump (see *How to Wrap Your Stump*, pages 342 and 343). Or show him how to slip on a custom-fitted elastic stump shrinker.

Emphasize that proper home care of his stump can speed healing. Tell the patient to carefully inspect his stump daily, using a mirror. Instruct him to call the doctor if the incision appears to be opening, looks red or swollen, feels warm, is painful to touch, or is seeping drainage. Teach him to clean the stump daily with mild soap and water, then rinse and dry it thoroughly.

Instruct the patient to rub the stump with alcohol daily to toughen the skin.

Have him avoid applying powder or lotion, which may soften or irritate the skin. Tell him to massage the stump *toward the suture line* to mobilize the scar and prevent its adherence to bone. Advise him to avoid exposing the skin around the stump to excessive perspiration, which can be irritating. He may need to change his elastic bandages or stump socks during the day to avoid this.

As stump muscles adjust to amputation, tell the patient he may have twitching and spasms, or phantom limb pain. Teach him to decrease these symptoms by using heat, massage, or gentle pressure. If his stump is sensitive to touch, tell him to rub it with a dry washcloth for 4 minutes three times a day.

Stress the importance of performing prescribed exercises to help minimize complications, maintain muscle strength and tone, prevent contractures, and promote independence. If appropriate, teach the patient triceps-strengthening exercises for crutch-walking, such as push-ups and flexion and extension of the arms using traction weights.

Also stress the importance of positioning to prevent contractures. If the patient's had a partial arm amputation, tell him to keep his elbow extended and shoulder abducted. If he's had a leg amputation, tell him not to prop his stump on a pillow to avoid hip flexion contracture. After a below-the-knee amputation, have him keep his knee extended to avoid hamstring contracture. After leg amputation, also advise him to lie prone for 4 hours each day to help stretch flexor muscles and to prevent hip flexion contracture. To prevent leg abduction, tell him to keep his legs close together.

To prepare the stump for a prosthesis, teach progressive resistance maneuvers. Begin by telling the patient to push his stump gently against a soft pillow. Have him progress to pushing it against a firm pillow, a padded chair, and, finally, a hard chair.

HOW TO WRAP YOUR STUMP

Dear Patient:

When wrapping your stump, follow these steps so that your bandage doesn't slip off.

1

Gather the supplies you'll need for wound and skin care. Also get two 3-inch elastic bandages, one 4-inch elastic bandage, and adhesive tape, safety pins, or clips. Now perform the routine wound and skin care the nurse taught you in the hospital.

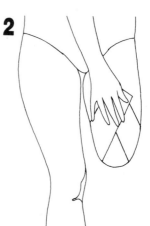

2

Make three turns back and forth to adequately cover the ends of your stump. Hold the bandage ends as shown.

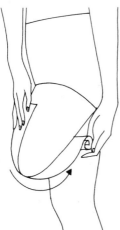

Hold the end of a 3-inch bandage at the top of your thigh. Bring the bandage's opposite end downward over your stump and to the back of your leg, as shown above.

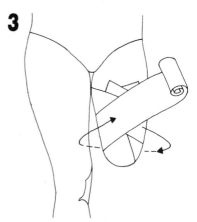

3

Using the other 3-inch bandage, make figure-eight turns around your leg to secure the first bandage.

4

Be sure to include the roll of flesh in your groin area. Use even pressure as you wrap the stump, keeping it narrow toward the end for a more comfortable fit in the prosthesis. Secure the bandage with clips, safety pins, or adhesive tape.

5

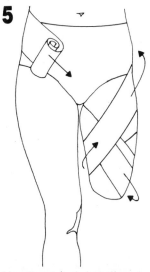

Use the 4-inch bandage to anchor the stump bandage around your waist.

6

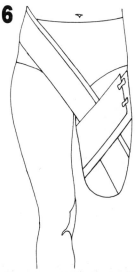

Secure the bandage with clips, safety pins, or adhesive tape. However, if you have a below-the-knee amputation, you won't need to do this. You can use your knee to anchor the bandage in place.

Check your stump bandage regularly. Rewrap it if it bunches at the end.

TEACHING PATIENTS ABOUT MUSCULOSKELETAL DRUGS

DRUG	ADVERSE REACTIONS	INTERACTIONS*
Aspirin and salicylates		
aspirin (Bayer Aspirin, Ecotrin, St. Joseph's Aspirin for Children) **aspirin and caffeine** (Anacin) **buffered aspirin** (Ascriptin, Bufferin) **choline and magnesium salicylates** (Trilisate) **magnesium salicylate** (Doan's Pills) **salsalate** (Disalcid) **sodium salicylate** (Pabalate)	*Reportable:* abdominal pain, unusually fast or deep breathing, bloody stools, bloody urine, chest tightness, confusion, severe diarrhea, severe drowsiness, uncontrollable flapping of the hands, hallucinations, hearing loss, severe nausea, seizures, unusual sweating, unusual thirst, tinnitus, visual disturbances, vomiting (especially bloody or resembling coffee grounds), wheezing *Other:* heartburn, indigestion	• Tell the patient to inform the doctor if he's taking acetaminophen, antacids, other aspirin or salicylate products, or cellulose-containing laxatives. • Advise against taking this drug with alcohol. • Tell the patient that foods and other beverages and over-the-counter (OTC) products don't influence the safety or effectiveness of this drug.
Nonsteroidal anti-inflammatory agents		
ibuprofen (Advil, Motrin, Nuprin) **indomethacin** (Indocin, Indocin SR) **meclofenamate** (Meclomen) **naproxen** (Anaprox, Naprosyn) **piroxicam** (Feldene) **sulindac** (Clinoril) **tolmetin** (Tolectin)	*Reportable:* unusual bleeding, bloody or tarry stools, bloody urine, bruises, fever, skin rash, sore throat, decreased urine output, wheezing, yellowing of skin and eyes *Other:* diarrhea, dizziness, drowsiness, heartburn, indigestion, nausea, vomiting	• Tell the patient not to take this drug with aspirin, acetaminophen, or alcohol. • Have him take the drug on an empty stomach 1 hour before meals or 3 hours after meals for best absorption.
Skeletal muscle relaxants		
carisoprodol (Rela, Soma)	*Reportable:* blurred or double vision; shortness of breath; fever; unusually fast, slow, or pounding heartbeat; hives; itching; skin rash; swollen lips, tongue, and face; wheezing *Other:* dizziness, drowsiness, hiccups, nausea, stomach cramps, vomiting	• Tell the patient to ask his pharmacist or doctor before taking over-the-counter CNS depressants, such as antihistamines or sleeping pills. • Advise against drinking alcohol. • Tell him that foods and other beverages and OTC products don't affect drug safety or action.

*Interactions include food, alcohol, and over-the-counter drugs.

TEACHING POINTS

• Explain to the patient that aspirin and other salicylates relieve pain and reduce fever.
• If the patient is taking this drug for arthritis, tell him that he may not experience relief from symptoms for several weeks.
• Advise parents against giving aspirin to children without the doctor's approval.
• If the drug doesn't relieve the patient's symptoms, tell him to call the doctor and not to adjust the dosage himself.
• If he's on a sodium-restricted diet, inform the patient that buffered aspirin, effervescent tablets, and sodium salicylate may contain a large amount of sodium.
• Tell the patient that he can chew, crush and dissolve, or swallow whole chewable aspirin tablets. To take effervescent tablets, he should dissolve them in water, immediately drink all of the water, then add more water to the glass and drink that also. He shouldn't crush aspirin, although his pharmacist may allow the aspirin to be gently broken. To take an aspirin suppository, he should moisten the suppository with water or lubricant, then insert it well up into the rectum.
• If the patient experiences gastric upset, instruct him to take this drug with food or a full glass of water.
• If the patient misses a dose, tell him to take it as soon as he remembers. But if it's almost time for the next dose, tell him to skip the missed dose. He shouldn't double-dose.
• Advise the patient to avoid aspirin and other salicylates for 5 days before any surgery or dental work to avoid increased bleeding.
• Inform him that the doctor may order biweekly serum tests until optimal blood levels of the drug are achieved.

• Explain to the patient that this drug should help relieve his arthritis, joint inflammation, or pain associated with sprains, strains, bursitis, tendinitis, or gout.
• If the patient misses a dose, tell him to take the dose as soon as he remembers. However, if it's almost time for the next dose, tell him to skip the missed dose; he shouldn't double-dose.
• If he experiences gastric upset, tell the patient to take the drug with meals or with an antacid.
• If this drug makes the patient drowsy, advise him not to drive or operate machinery.

• Explain to the patient that this drug relaxes certain muscles in his body and should help relieve pain caused by strains, sprains, and other injuries.
• If the patient misses a dose but remembers within an hour, advise him to take the missed dose. If he doesn't remember until later, he should skip the missed dose. He mustn't double-dose.
• Because this drug may cause dizziness or drowsiness, caution the patient to get out of bed and change positions slowly. Have him lie down whenever he feels dizzy. Warn against driving or operating machinery when he feels this way.

(continued)

TEACHING PATIENTS
ABOUT MUSCULOSKELETAL DRUGS *(continued)*

DRUG	ADVERSE REACTIONS	INTERACTIONS*
Skeletal muscle relaxants *(continued)*		
cyclobenzaprine (Flexeril)	*Reportable:* breathing difficulty, buzzing in ears, confusion, severe drowsiness, fainting, fever or decreased temperature, hallucinations, unusually fast or irregular heartbeat, hives, muscle stiffness, severe vomiting *Other:* dizziness, slight drowsiness, dry mouth	• Tell patient to check with his doctor before taking this drug with any over-the-counter CNS depressants, such as antihistamines or sleeping pills. • Advise him not to drink alcohol. • Tell him that foods and other beverages and OTC products don't influence the safety or effectiveness of cyclobenzaprine.
diazepam (Valium)	*Reportable:* confusion, severe drowsiness, hallucinations, hostility, insomnia, restlessness, slurred speech, staggering, severe weakness *Other:* constipation, transient drowsiness, dry mouth, nausea, vomiting, weakness	• Tell patient not to take this drug with alcohol or any over-the-counter CNS depressants, such as antihistamines or sleeping pills. • Tell him that foods and other beverages and OTC products don't influence the drug's safety or action.
methocarbamol (Robaxin)	*Reportable:* fever, hives, itching, skin rash *Other:* blurred vision, dizziness, drowsiness, headache, light-headedness, nausea, nervousness, unsteadiness, vomiting	• Tell the patient not to take this drug with other CNS depressants, such as antihistamines or sleeping pills, or with alcohol. • Tell him that foods and other beverages and OTC products don't influence the drug's safety or action.
Vitamins and minerals		
calcitonin (Calcimar)	*Reportable:* hives, skin rash *Other:* pain, redness, soreness, or swelling at the injection site; nausea; vomiting	• Tell the patient to inform the doctor if he's taking any other medication containing calcium or vitamin D. • Tell him that foods, alcohol, and other over-the-counter products don't influence the safety or effectiveness of calcitonin.
calcium carbonate (Caltrate 600, Os-Cal, Tums)	*Reportable:* abdominal pain, unusually slow breathing, severe constipation, dysuria, persistent headache, mood or mental changes, muscle pain or twitching, nausea, nervousness or restlessness, frequent urination, vomiting *Other:* anorexia, belching, chalky taste, flatulence	• Tell patient to avoid spinach, rhubarb, and whole grain cereals as they decrease drug absorption. • Advise him to avoid bisacodyl laxatives and salicylates and to space doses of iron preparations far apart from this drug. • Tell him to take this drug 1 to 2 hours after meals, and not at the same time as other oral medications.

*Interactions include food, alcohol, and over-the-counter drugs.

TEACHING POINTS

• Explain to the patient that this drug relaxes certain muscles in his body and should help relieve pain caused by strains, sprains, and other injuries.
• If the patient misses a dose but remembers within an hour, advise him to take the missed dose. If he doesn't remember until later, he should skip the missed dose. He mustn't double-dose.

• Because this drug may cause dizziness or drowsiness, caution the patient to get out of bed and change positions slowly. Have him lie down whenever he feels dizzy. Warn against driving or operating machinery when he feels this way.
• If the patient experiences dry mouth, tell him that sucking on ice chips or sugarless candy or chewing gum may provide relief.

• Explain to the patient that this drug relaxes certain muscles in his body and should relieve muscle spasms.
• Advise him to take the drug with food or a full glass of water. He should swallow capsules whole and not crush or chew them.
• If the patient misses a dose but remembers within an hour, advise him to take the missed dose. If he doesn't remember until later, he

should skip the missed dose. He mustn't double-dose.
• Instruct the patient not to drive or operate machinery when he's taking this drug.
• Inform him that diazepam may be habit-forming.

• Explain to the patient that this drug relaxes certain muscles in his body and should relieve muscle pain associated with strains, sprains, bursitis, or surgery.
• Tell the patient that this drug can be taken by mouth or injection. For easy swallowing, instruct him to crush the tablets and mix them with food or liquid.

• If the patient misses a dose, advise him to take it as soon as he remembers. But if it's almost time for the next dose, tell him to skip the missed dose. He mustn't double-dose.
• If the drug makes him drowsy, instruct the patient not to drive or operate machinery.

• Explain to the patient that this drug helps treat Paget's bone disease and osteoporosis.
• Show how to administer drug by injection.
• If the patient's on an every-other-day schedule and misses a dose, advise him to take the missed dose as soon as he remembers it. If he doesn't remember until the next day, he should take it then and go back to the every-other-day schedule.

If the patient's on a daily schedule, he should take a missed dose as soon as he remembers it. If he doesn't remember until the next day, he shouldn't double-dose.
If the patient receives injections twice a day, he should take a missed dose within 2 hours of its scheduled time; otherwise, he should skip that dose and continue with the regular schedule.

• Explain to the patient that this drug supplements his dietary intake of calcium and helps prevent or treat osteoporosis.

• Instruct him to take the drug in two divided doses or at one time, as the doctor orders.

(continued)

TEACHING PATIENTS
ABOUT MUSCULOSKELETAL DRUGS *(continued)*

DRUG	ADVERSE REACTIONS	INTERACTIONS*
Vitamins and minerals *(continued)*		
sodium fluoride (Fluoritab)	*Reportable:* abdominal pain, constipation, diarrhea, joint pain and stiffness, nausea, tarry or black stools, vomiting	• Instruct the patient to avoid aluminum-containing antacids. • Tell him that foods, alcohol, and other over-the-counter products don't influence the safety or effectiveness of sodium fluoride.
Vitamin D (Calciferol, Drisdol)	*Reportable:* anorexia, constipation, diarrhea, fatigue, headache, hypertension, irregular heartbeat, metallic taste, nausea or vomiting, seizures, severe stomach pain, unusual thirstiness, unusual weakness	• Tell the patient to avoid excessive use of aluminum-containing antacids and mineral oil. • Mention that foods, alcohol, and other beverages don't influence the safety or effectiveness of vitamin D.
Miscellaneous		
allopurinol (Lopurin, Zyloprim)	*Reportable:* chills, fever, hives, muscle aches and pains, nausea, skin rash, vomiting *Other:* diarrhea, drowsiness	• Tell the patient not to take vitamin C or any other urinary acidifier with this drug to avoid increasing the risk of renal calculi. • Instruct him not to take this drug with alcohol. • Tell him that foods and other beverages and over-the-counter products don't influence the safety or effectiveness of allopurinol.
colchicine	*Reportable:* abdominal pain, bloody urine, breathing difficulty, diarrhea, mood or mental changes, severe muscle weakness, nausea, vomiting *Other:* anorexia	• Instruct the patient not to use this drug with alcohol to avoid causing GI upset or decreasing the drug's effectiveness. • Tell him that foods and over-the-counter products don't influence the safety or effectiveness of colchicine.
probenecid (Benemid)	*Reportable:* low back pain, bloody urine, breathing difficulty, dysuria, edematous feet or lower legs, suddenly decreased urine output, severe vomiting, unusual weakness or fatigue *Other:* anorexia, dizziness, headache, nausea, mild vomiting	• Instruct the patient to avoid aspirin, salicylates, and alcohol since these may decrease this drug's effectiveness. • Tell him that foods and other beverages and over-the-counter products don't influence the safety and effectiveness of probenecid.

*Interactions include food, alcohol, and over-the-counter drugs.

TEACHING POINTS

• Explain to the patient that this drug helps treat osteoporosis and that it's usually prescribed with calcium and vitamin D supplements.
• If the patient misses a dose, advise him to take the missed dose as soon as he remembers. But if it's almost time for the next dose, he should skip the missed dose.
• Instruct the patient to chew or crush chewable tablets before swallowing them. He can add liquid doses to food or juice to make them more palatable.

• Explain to the patient that this drug supplements his dietary intake of vitamin D and helps treat osteoporosis and osteomalacia.
• Tell the patient to try to follow the prescribed administration schedule, but not to worry about missing a dose. Advise against taking large doses of vitamin D for an extended period without his doctor's approval.

• Explain to the patient that this drug helps treat gout or gouty arthritis by reducing the body's production of uric acid. Remind him that he must take the drug regularly to prevent gout attacks.
• If the drug makes him nauseated, advise him to take it after meals. Also encourage him to drink ten to twelve 8-oz glasses of fluid a day to help prevent renal calculi.
• If the patient's taking one dose a day, he should take a missed dose as soon as he remembers. However, if he doesn't remember until the next day, he should skip the missed dose.
   If the patient's taking more than one dose a day, he should take a missed dose as soon as he remembers. If that's close to the next scheduled dose, and the dose is one 100-mg tablet, then he should take two tablets. If the scheduled dose is two 100-mg tablets, then he should take three tablets for the next dose.

• Explain to the patient that this drug helps prevent or treat gout attacks. He may take it when he has an attack, or in regular small doses to prevent attacks.
• If the patient takes this drug to treat attacks, instruct him to start taking it at the first sign of an attack and then to discontinue it as soon as the pain subsides or if he develops nausea, vomiting, diarrhea, or abdominal pain. He should take only the prescribed dose and shouldn't take it more often than every 3 days.
• If the patient takes this drug regularly to prevent attacks, he should increase the dose, as instructed, at the first sign of an attack, then discontinue the larger dose as soon as the pain subsides or if he develops nausea, vomiting, diarrhea, or abdominal pain.

• Explain to the patient that this drug helps treat gout or gouty arthritis by removing extra uric acid from the body.
• Remind him that he must take the drug regularly to prevent gout attacks. These attacks should decrease in severity and frequency with continued therapy.
• When he first starts therapy, tell the patient to drink ten to twelve 8-oz glasses of fluid a day to make his urine less acidic.
• If the patient misses a dose, he should take that dose as soon as possible. However, if it's almost time for the next dose, he should skip the missed dose.
• To reduce GI upset, instruct the patient to take this drug with meals or an antacid.
• Inform the patient that this drug may cause a false-positive Clinitest for urine glucose.

11

Renal and Urologic System

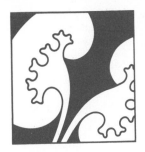

Renal and Urologic System

Introduction

Because of increasingly accurate diagnostic tests and growing numbers of elderly patients, you'll be devoting more time than ever before to teaching about renal and urologic disorders. And when you do, you'll be faced with special teaching challenges. Because the kidneys play such a critical role in maintaining homeostasis, their dysfunction or failure produces widespread systemic effects. That means you'll be called upon to demonstrate your command of all other body systems. You'll also have to tailor your teaching to meet varied learning needs.

What will determine the patient's learning needs? Among other factors, his chief complaint, or primary symptom. For the patient with renal calculi, this symptom may be the telltale excruciating pain of urinary tract obstruction. But in chronic renal failure, the patient may look and feel quite well, even though his kidneys have lost 75% of their normal function.

The diversity that characterizes symptoms of renal and urologic disorders also appears in their diagnosis and treatment. For example, to prepare the patient for a diagnostic workup, you may teach him how to collect a urine sample for routine urinalysis or what to expect in complex invasive tests, such as percutaneous renal biopsy or antegrade pyelography. To prepare him for treatment, you may explain revolutionary procedures, such as extracorporeal shock wave lithotripsy (ESWL) to shatter renal calculi. Or your focus may be renal transplantation, an increasingly common treatment for chronic renal failure. To prepare the patient for home care, you may need to discuss dramatic changes in his normal routine, such as performing continuous ambulatory peritoneal dialysis to treat chronic renal failure, as well as comparatively minor changes, such as drinking plenty of fluids to prevent recurrence of renal calculi.

Throughout your teaching, you'll need to keep in mind that many renal and urologic symptoms, tests, and treatments cause considerable emotional and physical stress. For example, the patient scheduled for nocturnal penile tumescence testing may feel discouraged and afraid of what the results may indicate about his impotence.

Also, you'll often need to explain renal and urologic physiology to promote the patient's understanding and compliance. For example, by explaining how the kidneys normally filter wastes from the blood, you can help him understand how dialysis works. Or by showing him a diagram of the urinary tract, you can help him understand how prostatic enlargement obstructs urine outflow.

DISORDERS

Acute Renal Failure

When teaching about acute renal failure (ARF), you'll be dealing with a patient who is typically troubled by the disorder's initial sign—sudden onset of oliguria or, rarely, anuria. Such a patient may also be frightened by the prospect of losing renal function or becoming dependent on dialysis. To allay the patient's fears, your teaching must

stress that early detection and aggressive therapy can usually reverse ARF and prevent it from progressing to chronic—and often fatal—renal failure. As always, the therapy's effectiveness will hinge on the patient's compliance.

To actively involve the patient in his care, you'll need to teach him how to monitor his fluid balance daily by taking his blood pressure, measuring his weight, and recording his intake and output.

Describe the disorder

Tell the patient that ARF is the sudden inability of the kidneys to remove waste materials from the blood and to maintain proper fluid and electrolyte balance. Inform him whether his ARF is classified as prerenal, intrarenal, or postrenal.

Prerenal failure results from conditions outside the kidneys that impair renal perfusion, such as congestive heart failure and other cardiovascular disorders, hypovolemia, and renovascular obstruction. *Intrarenal failure* results from disorders that damage the kidneys themselves, such as acute tubular necrosis. *Postrenal failure* results from bilateral obstruction of urinary outflow, for example, by renal calculi or ureteral constriction.

Explain which phase of ARF the patient is experiencing. In the *oliguric phase,* urine output usually drops to less than 500 ml/day. The patient may need to restrict his fluids during this phase, which typically lasts from 7 to 21 days. A longer oliguric phase may herald chronic renal failure. In the *diuretic phase,* the kidneys abruptly begin to produce larger volumes of urine—from 3 to 7 liters/day. Because of this, many patients assume that the diuretic phase indicates an improvement in renal function. For patients whose ARF is reversible, the diuretic phase often *does* indicate recovery. But for patients whose ARF is irreversible, you'll need to clear up any misconceptions by explaining that the oliguric

---

CHECKLIST

☑☐ TEACHING TOPICS
☐☑ IN ACUTE
☑☐ RENAL FAILURE

☐ An explanation of ARF, including its cause (prerenal, intrarenal, or postrenal) and phase (oliguric or diuretic)

☐ The importance of treatment to prevent complications, most notably chronic renal failure

☐ Signs and symptoms of uremia, hypervolemia, hypovolemia, and hyperkalemia

☐ Preparation for laboratory tests, such as arterial blood gas analysis, serum electrolytes, and urinalysis

☐ Preparation for kidney-ureter-bladder radiography, renal ultrasonography, or other scheduled imaging studies

☐ Dietary restrictions, such as avoidance or limited intake of potassium, sodium, and protein

☐ Instructions to restrict or increase fluids, as indicated

☐ Drugs and their administration

☐ An explanation of hemodialysis or peritoneal dialysis, if appropriate

☐ How to monitor fluid balance

and diuretic phases often form a recurrent cycle in the normal progression of ARF. Mention that the diuretic phase may last from several weeks or months to a year before returning to the oliguric phase.

Point out possible complications

Emphasize that compliance with therapy may help prevent serious complications, including uremia, hypervolemia, hypovolemia, and hyperkalemia. What's more, it may prevent or delay the development of chronic renal failure.

Explain that *uremia* is an accumulation of protein waste products in the blood. When these waste products reach toxic levels, such complications as uremic pericarditis and uremic pneumonitis may result. Instruct the patient to watch for and report signs and symptoms of uremia. These include nausea, vomiting, headache, decreased level of consciousness, dizziness, decreased visual acuity, urinous breath odor, and increased blood pressure.

Explain that *hypervolemia* is an abnormal increase in the volume of fluid circulating in the body. This excess fluid may accumulate in the patient's blood vessels or body tissues. Unchecked, hypervolemia can result in such serious complications as hypertension, congestive heart failure, and pulmonary edema. Teach the patient to watch for and report signs of hypervolemia, such as sudden weight gain, swelling of the hands and feet, and increased blood pressure. Instruct him to go to the hospital immediately if he experiences difficulty breathing or an inability to lie down flat; both of these warning signs suggest that hypervolemia has progressed to life-threatening congestive heart failure or pulmonary edema.

Explain that *hypovolemia* is an abnormal decrease in the volume of fluid circulating in the body. Mention that hypovolemia can progress to shock if

it's untreated. Teach the patient to watch for and report signs of hypovolemia—sudden weight loss, dry skin and mucous membranes, decreased urine output, muscle cramps, fatigue, dizziness, or decreased blood pressure.

Explain that *hyperkalemia* results when an excessive amount of potassium—an electrolyte that's normally excreted by the kidneys—accumulates in the blood. Mention that hyperkalemia can result in an irregular heart rate, leading to cardiac arrest and death. Instruct the patient to notify the doctor if he experiences weakness, malaise, nausea, diarrhea, or abdominal cramps—warning signs of hyperkalemia.

Teach about tests

Instruct the patient about the routine blood and urine tests the doctor will order to evaluate renal function. Blood tests may include a complete blood count (CBC); analyses of arterial blood gases (ABGs) and electrolytes; and measurement of serum protein, creatinine, and uric acid levels and of blood urea nitrogen (BUN) level. As appropriate, inform the patient who will perform the venipuncture and when. Or warn him that the arterial puncture required for ABG analysis may cause momentary pain. Mention that follow-up blood tests will be performed regularly during treatment to ensure that ARF is being managed properly. Teach the patient how to collect a clean-catch midstream urine specimen for urinalysis to help evaluate the kidneys' diluting and concentrating ability and to help determine the cause and degree of renal failure.

Also teach the patient about radiographic studies, such as kidney-ureter-bladder (KUB) radiography, computed tomography scan, renal ultrasonography, and retrograde ureteropyelography, to reveal abnormal kidney size or shape, fluid accumulation, or obstruction of urinary outflow. Renal angiography may also be performed to reveal obstruction or renal artery dysplasia.

If the results of laboratory and radiologic studies are inconclusive, you may need to prepare the patient for renal biopsy to evaluate renal failure. Biopsy may also be helpful when oliguria lasts longer than 4 to 6 weeks. (See *Teaching Patients about Renal and Urologic Tests*, pages 372 to 379.)

Teach about treatments

• *Activity.* Instruct the patient with severe ARF to limit his activity in order to conserve energy. If the doctor orders bed rest for the patient, stress the importance of early, progressive ambulation.

• *Diet.* Although diet alone can't treat ARF, it does play an important role in therapy. In collaboration with the doctor and the dietitian, teach the patient how to manage ARF by adjusting his diet.

Explain to the patient that a diet high in calories and low in protein, sodium, potassium, and phosphorus can prevent further renal damage, yet maintain nutritional balance. Inform him that his diet will depend on his renal function, so he must carefully follow the one prescribed by the doctor or dietitian. When teaching about meal planning, be sure to include other family members—especially the one who does most of the cooking.

Depending on the cause of his ARF, the patient may need to either restrict or increase his intake of fluids. If the patient must restrict fluids, suggest that he suck on ice chips to relieve thirst. (Remind him to include the ice chips as part of his total daily fluid intake.) Advise him to spread the amount of fluid allowed over the entire day and to accurately measure his urine output to avoid fluid overload. If the patient must increase fluids, explain that the doctor will order supplemental fluids for him to drink or to receive intravenously.

• *Medication.* Inform the patient that he may need to discontinue the medications he normally takes—particu-

larly if they're concentrated in the kidneys and excreted in the urine. Since ARF delays urine excretion, the patient has an increased risk of toxic drug reactions. Warn him, though, not to discontinue any medication without first checking with his doctor. (See *Teaching Patients about Renal and Urologic Drugs*, pages 382 to 385, for more information.)

If the patient's ARF results from a prerenal cause, inform him that he may be given diuretics to increase his urine output after adequate hydration has been achieved by replacing fluids.

• *Procedures.* If ARF fails to respond promptly to other treatment measures, you'll need to prepare the patient for dialysis. Explain the purpose of dialysis and discuss which type the patient will receive—hemodialysis or peritoneal dialysis. (See *Comparing Hemodialysis and Peritoneal Dialysis*.) Tell him what to expect during and after dialysis.

If the patient will be undergoing hemodialysis, explain that he'll first require surgery to create vascular access. Two small catheters will be placed into a vein and an artery near the vascular access—usually in the upper or lower arm or the upper thigh. His blood will leave his body through one of the catheters; circulate through a dialyzer, which removes waste products; and then return to his body through the other catheter. Reassure the patient that it's normal to feel tired for several hours after hemodialysis, as his body adjusts to the treatment.

If the patient will be undergoing peritoneal dialysis, explain that a catheter will be inserted in the peritoneal cavity through a small incision in his abdomen. A dialysate solution will then be instilled through the catheter into the peritoneal cavity, where it will remain long enough to allow excess fluid, electrolytes, and accumulated wastes to move through the peritoneal membrane into the dialysate. At the end of the prescribed dwelling time, the dialysate will be drained from the pa-

COMPARING HEMODIALYSIS AND PERITONEAL DIALYSIS

When the patient requires dialysis, you'll need to teach him how it works to encourage his compliance. The two types of dialysis—hemodialysis and peritoneal dialysis—share a common purpose: to remove toxic wastes from the blood when renal failure prevents the kidneys from carrying out this function. But each technique accomplishes this quite differently, as explained here.

Hemodialysis

In this technique, blood is pumped through an external dialyzing system. Within the dialyzer, blood flows between hollow fibers, plates, or coils of semipermeable material while a special dialysis solution is pumped around the other side under hydrostatic pressure. Because the blood contains toxic wastes and higher concentrations of hydrogen ions and other electrolytes, these solutes diffuse across the semipermeable material into the solution. Any solute that's more concentrated in the dialysis solution (glucose or bicarbonate) diffuses into the blood. Thus, hemodialysis removes excess water and toxins, reverses acidosis, and corrects electrolyte imbalance.

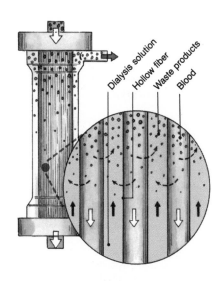

Peritoneal dialysis

In this technique, a hypertonic dialyzing solution is instilled through a catheter into the peritoneal cavity. By osmosis, water moves from the blood into the dialysis solution; by diffusion, excessive concentrations of toxins also move across the peritoneal membrane. After an appropriate dwelling time, the dialysis solution is drained, taking toxins with it.

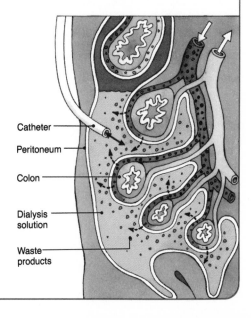

tient's peritoneal cavity, taking toxins with it.

Whether the patient's undergoing hemodialysis or peritoneal dialysis, tell him that he'll be awake and alert during the procedure. Instruct him to notify the dialysis nurse if he experiences faintness, dizziness, nausea, vomiting, or headache—possible indicators of overly rapid fluid loss.

• *Surgery.* If ARF results from a postrenal cause, treatment usually includes catheterization to drain urine from the bladder and either a surgical or nonsurgical procedure to free the obstruction. If the patient requires surgery, explain the procedure to him, including who will perform it and where, and how long it will take. For example, you may need to prepare him for removal of calculi from a ureter or renal pelvis. (See "Renal Calculi" in this chapter.)

• *Other care measures.* Prepare the patient for home care by teaching him how to monitor his fluid balance. To do this, he'll need to measure and record his daily weight, blood pressure, and intake and output.

Instruct the patient to weigh himself at the same time each day, using the same scale and wearing the same type of clothing. Tell him to notify the doctor if his weight increases or decreases by more than 5% of his total body weight from one day to the next. Explain the difference between weight gain from fluid accumulation and that from increased intake of calories.

Teach the patient the proper technique for taking accurate blood pressure readings. Stress that he should compare every blood pressure reading against his baseline reading. Tell him to notify the doctor if blood pressure exceeds 140/86 mm Hg or drops below 90/60 mm Hg.

Emphasize the importance of accurately recording daily intake and output of fluids. When the patient totals his fluid intake, remind him to include any food that's liquid at room temperature—for example, gelatin, custard, and ice cream.

Benign Prostatic Hyperplasia

Because benign prostatic hyperplasia (BPH) progresses slowly, a patient may not realize he has this disorder until his prostate enlarges enough to create such problems as a weak urinary stream or a frequent urge to urinate. Besides helping your patient recognize these and other warning signs of BPH, your teaching must stress the importance of prompt treatment and clearly explain its possible side effects, such as infertility.

Because BPH most commonly affects elderly men, your teaching may need to overcome age-related learning barriers, such as impaired vision, confusion, or physical limitations. These factors may also hinder compliance with at-home treatments, such as catheter care.

Describe the disorder

Tell the patient that BPH is a nonmalignant overgrowth of tissue in the prostate, a spherical gland that surrounds the urethra at the base of the bladder. As the gland becomes increasingly rigid, it compresses the urethra and may obstruct urine flow. Inform the patient that by the age of 70, most men have some degree of prostatic enlargement as a result of the aging process. Explain that the cause of BPH is unknown, but researchers suspect it's linked to a hormonal or metabolic change.

Point out possible complications

Using an anatomic drawing of the male renal and urologic system, explain that BPH may lead to serious complications if it remains untreated. For example, urine retention may result if the bladder muscles can't overcome the resistance to urine outflow caused by the rigid prostate. This, in turn, may cause bladder infection as pools of urine within the bladder become stagnant. And, if urine outflow is obstructed or blocked for a prolonged time, pressure within the bladder will increase and may precipitate life-threatening bladder rupture.

Teach about tests

Explain the procedures that the doctor will perform to evaluate BPH. Tell the patient that the doctor will observe him as he voids, to determine the size and force of his urine stream. Then he'll examine the prostate gland by inserting a gloved finger into the patient's rectum. He'll also evaluate the rectal sphincter, which indirectly reflects the state of bladder innervation. Reassure the patient that he'll be given complete privacy during these often embarrassing procedures.

Next, explain to the patient the variety of laboratory tests that the doctor will order to evaluate BPH. Inform him that blood samples will be collected to measure BUN, creatinine, and acid phosphatase levels. In addition, a urine sample will be obtained for urinalysis to check for infection. Also prepare him for catheterization to obtain a residual urine sample to assess urine retention and rule out the presence of stricture.

As ordered, prepare the patient for urodynamic studies; radiologic tests, such as intravenous pyelography (IVP); and endoscopic tests, such as cystoscopy. Inform him who will perform the tests and when, and advise him of any pretest restrictions. (See *Teaching Patients about Renal and Urologic Tests*, pages 372 to 379.)

Teach about treatments

• *Procedures.* Although surgery is the primary treatment for BPH, radiation therapy may be ordered instead of or before surgery to shrink the enlarged gland. Make sure the patient understands when and where he'll receive radiation therapy and who will administer it. Typically, he'll receive ther-

---

CHECKLIST

TEACHING TOPICS IN B.P.H.

- [ ] An explanation of nonmalignant tissue overgrowth in the prostate
- [ ] Signs and symptoms of BPH
- [ ] The importance of treatment to prevent complications, such as bladder infection or rupture
- [ ] Preparation for physical examination of the prostate and for blood tests, urinalysis, and invasive diagnostic tests
- [ ] An explanation of radiation therapy, if appropriate
- [ ] An explanation of open prostatectomy or transurethral resection of the prostate
- [ ] At-home catheter care, if appropriate
- [ ] Referral for sexual counseling, if appropriate, to deal with postoperative infertility or, rarely, impotence

---

apy daily for 4 to 6 weeks.

Reinforce the doctor's explanation of the procedure, and answer any questions the patient may have. Warn him that he may experience bladder spasms or rectal discomfort during therapy; however, these side effects usually abate after therapy. Also mention that he may be sensitive to sunlight during therapy and should avoid prolonged exposure to the sun.

• *Surgery.* The primary treatment for BPH, surgery aims to remove excess prostate tissue and thus relieve obstructed urine outflow. Explain which surgical procedure the patient requires—open prostatectomy or transurethral resection of the prostate (TUR). In open prostatectomy, the doctor makes an incision in the lower part of the abdomen and cuts away the excess tissue. In TUR, he passes a thin tube up the urethra to the prostate and slices away the excess tissue with an electric cutting loop at the tip of the tube. TUR takes less time to perform, requires a shorter hospital stay, and produces less postoperative pain than

BENIGN PROSTATIC HYPERPLASIA: REVIEWING PATHOPHYSIOLOGY

Before you teach patients about benign prostatic hyperplasia (BPH), review the illustrations here to clarify your understanding of the disorder.

Nearly every man has some degree of prostate enlargement by the age of 70. This doesn't necessarily cause problems, even if the prostate becomes quite large. Why? Because the size of the prostate matters less than its consistency, as the gland normally relaxes to allow urine flow. However, an increasingly rigid prostate, as in BPH, fails to relax adequately and thus constricts the urethra. If the bladder muscles aren't strong enough to force urine through the constricted urethra, urine flow diminishes, resulting in urine retention. Eventually, increased bladder pressure from urine retention may precipitate life-threatening bladder rupture.

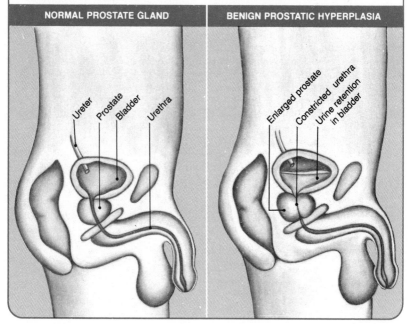

NORMAL PROSTATE GLAND	BENIGN PROSTATIC HYPERPLASIA

Labels (normal): Ureter, Prostate, Bladder, Urethra

Labels (BPH): Enlarged prostate, Constricted urethra, Urine retention in bladder

open prostatectomy. However, it's not feasible when the prostate is extremely enlarged or when the tissue overgrowth lies beyond the reach of the cutting loop.

Whether the patient's undergoing open prostatectomy or TUR, explain what will happen before, during, and after surgery. As ordered, instruct the patient to observe food and fluid restrictions before surgery. If appropriate, discuss how a full bowel preparation before open surgery helps prevent infection. Tell the patient that he'll be given a low-residue diet for 3 days, then high-calorie fluids for 24 hours before surgery. He'll also receive antibiotics—usually erythromycin 500 mg and neomycin 1 g every 4 hours for 24 hours before surgery. The night before surgery, he may be given enemas to cleanse fecal material from the bowel.

Inform the patient how long the surgery will take and how long he'll be hospitalized after surgery. Mention that he'll have a catheter in his bladder for several days after TUR. The catheter will be connected to a continuous irrigation machine to clear away blood

HOW TO CARE FOR YOUR CATHETER

Dear Patient:

Your catheter is a tube that will continually drain urine from your bladder, so you won't need to urinate. To care for your catheter, follow these guidelines.

Empty the drainage bag

How often? Usually, every 8 hours will do. First, unclamp the drainage tube and remove it from its sleeve, without touching its tip.

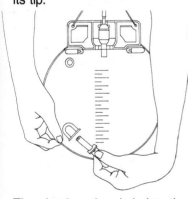

Then let the urine drain into the toilet or into a measuring container, if required. When the bag's completely empty, swab the end of the drainage tube with povidone-iodine solution.

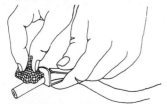

Reclamp the tube and reinsert it into the sleeve of the drainage bag.

To maintain good drainage from the catheter, frequently check the drainage tubing for kinks and loops. Never disconnect the catheter from the drainage tubing, for any reason. Also, keep the drainage bag below your bladder level, whether you're lying, sitting, or standing.

Care for your skin

Use soap and water to wash the area around your catheter twice each day. Also wash your rectal area twice each day and after each bowel movement. Periodically check the skin around the catheter for signs of irritation, such as redness, tenderness, or swelling.

Report problems early

Contact the doctor immediately if you have any problems, such as urine leakage around the catheter, pain and fullness in your abdomen, scanty urine flow, or blood in your urine. Above all, never pull on your catheter or try to remove it yourself.

from the bladder. Reassure him that it's normal to have blood in the urine for several days after surgery.

Reinforce prescribed limits on activity after surgery. Warn against lifting and strenuous exercise, since these may increase bleeding tendency. Also caution the patient to restrict sexual activity for several weeks after surgery, as his doctor orders.

Inform the patient that he may experience a sensation of heaviness in the pelvic region, urinary urgency, or bladder spasms, which can often be relieved with pain medication. Instruct him to take antibiotics, as prescribed, and tell him the indications for using gentle laxatives. Urge him to seek medical care immediately if he can't void or if fever develops.

• **Other care measures.** If the patient will be going home with an indwelling (Foley) catheter in place, teach him how to care for the catheter properly. (See *How to Care for Your Catheter*, page 359, for more information.) Tell him when to return to the hospital for the catheter's removal.

Rarely, a patient will experience temporary or permanent impotence after surgery. (See "Impotence" in this chapter.) More commonly, a patient may still be able to have an erection but will become sterile because his semen is expelled backwards into the bladder instead of being ejaculated. Reassure the patient that seminal fluid in the bladder does no harm; it's simply eliminated in the urine. If the patient has problems adjusting sexually, refer him and his sexual partner to a professional counselor.

Chronic Renal Failure

Thanks to dialysis and renal transplantation, patients with chronic renal failure (CRF) are surviving longer than ever before. That means you'll probably have more occasions to teach CRF patients and their families how to manage this life-threatening disorder. Above all, you'll need to convince them that complying with prescribed treatment really *can* improve the quality of life, despite the disorder's irreversible and progressive course. To promote compliance, you'll need to provide thorough teaching about dietary restrictions, drug regimens, and dialysis options. You'll also need to provide emotional support to help the patient cope with frequent hospitalizations and the prospect of his impending death.

Describe the disorder
Tell the patient that CRF results from extensive, irreversible damage to the nephrons—the structural and functional units of the kidney. Then explain what stage of CRF he's experiencing. In the first stage, *decreased renal reserve*, the kidneys respond to illness or injury with mildly to moderately decreased function. Typically, the patient is asymptomatic during this stage because of the renal system's compensatory mechanism. In the second stage, *renal insufficiency*, the kidneys are unable to concentrate urine, resulting in nocturia or polyuria. However, these and other symptoms are frequently mild, even though about 75% of renal tissue has been destroyed. Because the patient's renal reserve is so low during this stage, any stress—infection, dehydration, or other trauma—will further impair renal function. By the time the patient reaches the third stage, *end-stage renal disease (ESRD)*, 90% of renal tissue has been destroyed and oliguria is characteristic. In this stage, every body system demonstrates the effects of renal failure.

Point out possible complications
Stress that failure to comply with therapy hastens the onset of ESRD and thus shortens the patient's life. It may also

lead to complications, such as uremia, hypervolemia, hypovolemia, hyperkalemia, and calcification.

Explain that *uremia* is an accumulation of protein waste products in the blood. When these waste products reach toxic levels, such complications as uremic pericarditis and uremic pneumonitis may result. Teach the patient to watch for and report signs and symptoms of uremia, such as nausea, vomiting, headache, decreased level of consciousness, dizziness, decreased visual acuity, urinous breath odor, and increased blood pressure.

Explain that *hypervolemia* is an abnormal increase in the volume of fluid circulating in the body. This excess fluid may accumulate in the patient's blood vessels or body tissues. Unchecked, hypervolemia can result in such serious complications as hypertension, congestive heart failure, and pulmonary edema. Teach the patient to watch for and report signs of hypervolemia, such as sudden weight gain, swelling of the hands and feet, and increased blood pressure. Caution him to go to the hospital emergency department immediately if he experiences difficulty breathing or an inability to lie down flat—warning symptoms that hypervolemia may have progressed to life-threatening congestive heart failure or pulmonary edema.

Explain that *hypovolemia* is an abnormal decrease in the volume of fluid circulating in the body. Mention that hypovolemia can progress to shock if it's untreated. Teach the patient to watch for and report signs and symptoms of hypovolemia—sudden weight loss, dry skin and mucous membranes, decreased urine output, muscle cramps, fatigue, dizziness, or decreased blood pressure.

Explain that *hyperkalemia* results when an excessive amount of potassium—an electrolyte that's normally excreted by the kidneys—accumulates in the blood. Mention that hyperkalemia can result in an irregular heart rate, possibly leading to cardiac arrest.

TEACHING TOPICS IN CHRONIC RENAL FAILURE

CHECKLIST

- [ ] An explanation of nephron damage in CRF, including its stage of progression
- [ ] Importance of treatment to delay onset of end-stage renal disease and prevent complications, such as uremia
- [ ] Preparation for blood and urine tests and for other scheduled diagnostic studies, such as KUB radiography and renal ultrasonography
- [ ] Prescribed diet and fluid restrictions
- [ ] Drugs and their administration
- [ ] An explanation of hemodialysis or peritoneal dialysis
- [ ] Preparation for renal transplantation or nephrectomy, if indicated
- [ ] How to prevent peritonitis at home
- [ ] How to monitor fluid balance at home

Teach the patient to watch for and report signs and symptoms of hyperkalemia, such as weakness, malaise, nausea, diarrhea, muscle twitching, or abdominal cramps.

Explain that *calcification* results when calcium phosphate deposits accumulate in soft tissues throughout the body. Teach the patient to watch for and report signs and symptoms of calcification, such as itching, conjunctivitis, and bony enlargement around the joints in the hands.

Teach about tests

Prepare the patient for routine blood and urine tests that the doctor will order to evaluate renal function. Blood tests may include a CBC; analyses of ABGs and electrolytes; and measurement of serum protein, creatinine, and uric acid levels and of BUN level. Mention that follow-up blood tests will be performed regularly during treatment to ensure that CRF is being managed properly.

Teach the patient how to collect a

clean-catch midstream urine specimen for urinalysis to help evaluate the kidneys' diluting and concentrating capacity and to help determine the cause and stage of renal failure.

Also teach the patient about radiologic studies, such as KUB radiography and renal ultrasonography, to visualize the kidneys and lower urinary tract. In addition, prepare the patient for a chest X-ray to evaluate his heart and lungs and for an EKG to detect cardiac abnormalities that may indicate hyperkalemia. Mention that bone and skeleton X-rays will be performed to help detect calcification. Stress the importance of returning for follow-up X-rays.

If indicated, explain that renal biopsy helps identify progression of renal failure. Describe what will happen before, during, and after renal biopsy. (See *Teaching Patients about Renal and Urologic Tests,* pages 372 to 379.)

Teach about treatments

• *Activity.* Emphasize the need for regular exercise to maintain muscle strength and mobility, to help prevent bone demineralization, and to decrease protein breakdown. However, tell the patient to avoid contact sports, crowds, and persons with respiratory infections.

• *Diet.* In collaboration with the doctor and the dietitian, teach the patient how to manage CRF by adjusting his diet. Explain that a diet high in calories and low in protein, sodium, potassium, and phosphorus helps avoid taxing his kidneys. Inform the patient that his diet will depend on his renal function, so he must carefully follow the one prescribed by the doctor or dietitian. If he complains of nausea in the morning, have him wait 2 to 3 hours before eating and then eat small, frequent meals. When teaching about meal planning, include other family members—especially the one who does most of the cooking.

Encourage the patient to adhere to fluid restrictions. Suggest that he suck on ice chips or hard candies to relieve thirst. Advise him to spread the allowed amounts of protein, calories, and fluid over the entire day.

• *Medication.* Typically, patients with CRF require a variety of drugs to help control the disorder's effects and to relieve associated symptoms. For example, the patient may be given a beta-adrenergic inhibitor to help control hypertension and an antipruritic to relieve itching associated with dialysis. The patient may also benefit from supplemental vitamins and essential amino acids.

To promote the patient's compliance, discuss the purpose, side effects, and dosage instructions for each prescribed drug. (See *Teaching Patients about Renal and Urologic Drugs,* pages 382 to 385.) Also warn the patient about harmful drug interactions. Inform him that the doctor may order him to discontinue the medications he normally takes—particularly if they're concentrated in the kidneys and excreted in the urine. Since elimination of urine is delayed, a patient with CRF has a greater risk of toxic drug reactions than a person with normal renal function.

• *Procedures.* Explain the purpose of dialysis and discuss the advantages and disadvantages of the two types—hemodialysis and peritoneal dialysis. (See *Comparing Hemodialysis and Peritoneal Dialysis,* page 355.) If the patient will be undergoing hemodialysis, explain that he'll first require surgery to create an arteriovenous shunt or fistula for vascular access. Advise him of any preoperative restrictions, tell him who will perform the procedure and where, and mention that it takes from 1 to 2 hours. After surgery, explain that two small catheters will be placed into a vein and an artery near the vascular access—usually in the upper or lower arm or the upper thigh. His blood will leave his body through one of the catheters; circulate through a dialyzer, which removes waste products; and then return to his body through the other catheter. Tell the patient that he'll be awake and alert for each dialysis session. Instruct him to notify the nurse if he experiences faintness, dizziness, nausea, vomiting, or headache—possible signs and symptoms of overly rapid fluid loss. Reassure the patient that it's normal to feel tired for several hours after the hemodialysis session, as his body adjusts to the effects of treatment.

Teach the patient how to protect and care for the vascular access. Show him how to check its patency by palpating for a thrill or listening for a bruit. Instruct him to assess the access frequently for signs of blood clotting or infection. Advise him to go to the hospital's emergency department immediately if the skin near the access becomes hot, red, swollen, or painful. Suggest ways to protect the access—for example, by not covering it with tight clothing. In addition, if the patient has a shunt, instruct him to close off the tubing with a cannula clamp if the shunt becomes separated and then to go to the hospital's emergency department immediately. Advise him to carry extra cannula clamps at all times. If the patient has a fistula, teach him to apply pressure to the vascular access after dialysis.

If the patient will be using peritoneal dialysis, explain that a catheter will be inserted in the peritoneal cavity through a small incision in his abdomen. A dialysate solution will then be instilled through the catheter into the peritoneal cavity, where it will remain long enough to allow excess fluid, electrolytes, and accumulated wastes to move through the peritoneal membrane into the dialysate. At the end of the prescribed dwelling time, the dialysate will be drained from the peritoneal cavity, taking toxins with it.

Peritoneal dialysis may be performed manually, by an automatic cycler machine, or as continuous ambulatory peritoneal dialysis (CAPD). Regardless of which method your patient will be using, you must teach him how to prevent peritonitis.

(See *Tips for Preventing Peritonitis*, page 364.)

If the patient will be using manual dialysis, teach him or a family member to run the dialysate through the catheter into the peritoneal cavity, to allow the proper amount to infuse, to time the duration of the dwell, and to drain the dialysate from the peritoneal cavity. Explain that this process must be repeated for 6 to 8 hours a day, 5 to 6 days a week.

If the patient will be using a cycler machine, teach him or a family member how to connect the dialysate tubing, using sterile technique. Explain that the cycler machine will then automatically perform the rest of the procedure until it's disconnected from the peritoneal catheter.

Teach a patient who'll be using CAPD how to instill the dialysate solution into the peritoneal cavity from the plastic bag attached to the catheter. Mention that he can roll up the empty plastic bag, place it in a shirt pocket, and go about his normal routine until it's time to drain the solution 6 to 8 hours later. Demonstrate how to attach another bag of dialysate solution, using sterile technique. Also teach the patient how to observe the insertion site for signs of infection and how to clean the catheter. Instruct him to repeat this procedure as needed to ensure continuous dialysis 24 hours a day, 7 days a week.

• *Surgery.* If the patient's kidneys are infected, greatly enlarged, or causing uncontrollable hypertension, you may need to prepare him for renal transplantation or nephrectomy (see the "Surgery" section in this chapter for more information about nephrectomy). Begin teaching about renal transplantation by emphasizing that this surgery is a treatment, not a cure, for renal failure. Inform the patient whether he'll receive a donor kidney from a living relative or from a cadaver.

Before surgery, reinforce the doctor's explanation of the procedure. Mention that splenectomy may be performed during surgery to decrease lymphocyte

364

TIPS FOR PREVENTING PERITONITIS

Dear Patient:

Because you'll be using peritoneal dialysis at home, you must guard against peritonitis—an infection that occurs when harmful bacteria enter the dialysis system. Follow these tips to help prevent peritonitis.

Avoid contamination
• Wash your hands before opening the dialysis system, handling the dialysis solution, or changing the dressing over your catheter.
• Change the dressing over your catheter every day.
• Cover your mouth and nose with a surgical mask whenever you open the dialysis system—for example, to perform a solution exchange.
• Perform solution exchanges in a clean, dry room with the doors and windows closed; *do not* perform exchanges in the bathroom.
• Check dialysate drainage for cloudiness or particles—possible signs of infection.
• Don't use fresh dialysis solution that comes in a bag with excessive moisture on the outside: this could indicate a leak in the bag and, possibly, contamination of the solution.

• Take showers instead of baths to prevent bacteria from entering the dialysis system.

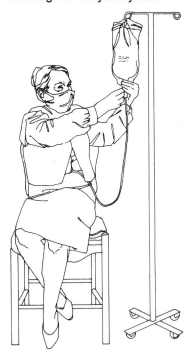

When to seek help
• Call your doctor immediately if the skin around the dialysis tubing becomes reddened, warm, or painful.
• Go to the hospital immediately if you detect signs of peritonitis, such as abdominal pain, cloudy dialysate drainage, fever, chills, nausea, vomiting, or diarrhea.

production. Also discuss possible complications with the patient and his family. Most important, explain how transplant rejection is detected—and treated.

Tell the patient who will perform the surgery and where, and that it takes about 3 to 4 hours. Inform him that he may be dialyzed immediately before surgery, to ensure optimal fluid, electrolyte, and acid-base balance and to reduce uremic toxins in the blood. Describe the midline incision that he should expect postoperatively. If the patient is very thin, he may feel a bulge next to the incision where the transplanted kidney has been placed.

Explain to the patient that he'll be monitored in an intensive care unit for several days after surgery. Prepare him for the placement of a catheter in his bladder to check hourly urine volumes. Mention that decreased urine output is a possible sign of transplant rejection. Explain that you'll also assess for other signs of rejection, such as fever, weight gain, and tenderness or redness at the incision site.

Before discharge, make sure the patient understands that renal transplantation doesn't guarantee a life free of medical problems and restrictions. Give him written information describing follow-up care and the required dietary and immunosuppressive drug regimens. Also teach him to watch for—and immediately report—signs of infection and transplant rejection. Note that recovery from the surgery usually takes 6 to 8 weeks. Emphasize, though, that medical follow-up must continue for the rest of the patient's life.

• **Other care measures.** Teach the patient the basics of good skin care to help prevent skin breakdown and infection. Also encourage frequent oral hygiene to reduce urinous breath odor. Recommend petrolatum or mineral oil to moisten cracked lips and mucous membranes. If the patient develops mouth sores, tell him to avoid spicy foods and to eat a soft, bland diet.

Prepare the patient to monitor his fluid balance after discharge. Teach him to measure and record his daily weight, blood pressure, and intake and output. Tell him to notify the doctor if his weight increases or decreases by more than 5% of his total body weight during 1 week or if his blood pressure exceeds 140/86 mm Hg or drops below 90/60 mm Hg.

Impotence

Few medical conditions have greater impact on a man's emotional well-being than impotence. By teaching your patient the facts about impotence and by stressing that effective treatment options exist, you can help him cope with this condition's often devastating effects. Begin by establishing a rapport with the patient to help him feel comfortable about discussing his sexuality. Remember, impotence can be both frightening and puzzling for your patient. To help relieve his confusion, take the time to carefully explain all the treatment options—such as penile im-

---

CHECKLIST

TEACHING TOPICS IN IMPOTENCE

☐ An explanation of the cause of impotence: psychological or physical

☐ The importance of treatment to prevent severe depression and psychosocial isolation

☐ Preparation for nocturnal penile tumescence monitoring, Doppler readings of penile blood pressure, and other diagnostic studies

☐ Discussion of treatment options, such as hormonal therapy, vasodilators, and penile implants

☐ Referral for psychiatric counseling, if appropriate

plants, drug therapy, and psychiatric counseling.

Describe the disorder

Describe impotence as the inability to sustain an erection sufficient for vaginal penetration. Explain that both psychological and physical factors can contribute to this problem. For example, such psychological factors as performance anxiety, depression, and marital conflict can trigger impotence. Underlying physical causes include hormonal imbalance, nerve damage, alcohol- or drug-induced dysfunction, or chronic disease, such as diabetes. Mention that it's sometimes difficult to determine impotence's exact cause.

Point out possible complications

Encourage the patient to comply with therapy by pointing out that impotence can foster loss of self-esteem and feelings of frustration, humiliation, and insecurity. When prolonged, it may set the stage for severe depression and, possibly, contemplation of suicide.

Teach about tests

Prepare the patient for evaluation of nocturnal penile tumescence to differentiate between organic and psychogenic impotence. (See *Teaching Patients about Renal and Urologic Tests,* pages 372 to 379.) As needed, also prepare him for blood tests to detect hormonal imbalance and for Doppler readings of penile blood pressure or penile arteriography to rule out vascular insufficiency. Other possible tests include voiding studies, nerve conduction tests, and psychological screening.

Teach about treatments

• *Medication.* Explain that many commonly used drugs—especially antihypertensives—can cause impotence that may be reversible if the drug is discontinued or the dosage reduced. However, caution the patient not to stop taking a drug or to change its dosage unless the doctor orders.

If the patient's impotence results from hormonal imbalance (such as insufficient testosterone or excessive prolactin levels), the doctor may order hormonal therapy. As ordered, teach the patient how to give himself testosterone injections or to take bromocriptine mesylate to reduce prolactin levels. (See *Teaching Patients about Renal and Urologic Drugs,* pages 382 to 385.)

If impotence results from nerve damage, such as spinal cord injury, the doctor may order papaverine hydrochloride or another vasodilator to dilate the penile arteries and induce erection. Teach the patient self-injection techniques and review dosage instructions to prevent side effects, such as priapism. Mention that erection should occur within 15 minutes and last for 1 to 2 hours. Tell the patient to notify the doctor if erection persists for 4 or more hours after drug injection.

• *Surgery.* If the patient's impotence can't be corrected with drugs or psychiatric counseling, the doctor may recommend surgery to insert a penile implant. When you teach about penile implants, try to include the patient's sexual partner in your session. Discuss the two basic types of penile implants—semirigid rods and inflatable cylinders. Make sure the patient knows that both types carry the risk of infection and initially cause discomfort. How long the discomfort lasts depends mostly on the degree of tissue trauma caused by surgery. Also tell him that he may need surgery again—particularly if he's getting an inflatable cylinder—to replace defective parts.

Tell the patient what to expect before, during, and after surgery. Inform him what type of anesthetic he'll receive—general or local—and advise him of any preoperative food or fluid restrictions. Describe the procedure for implanting the chosen device: to implant a semirigid rod, the doctor will make a small incision at the base of the patient's penis; to implant an inflatable cylinder, he'll make an incision in the patient's lower abdomen. Tell the patient who will perform the procedure and when, and how long it will last. During his recovery, tell him to wear loose-fitting underwear and clothing to avoid placing prolonged pressure on his penis. Have him notify the doctor if he develops a temperature of 101° F. (38.3° C.) or higher, if pain worsens, or if his penis becomes sore or drains pus. Also tell him to avoid sex for at least 6 weeks after surgery, to allow his incision to heal.

• *Other care measures.* Because the CNS-depressant effect of alcohol may cause or exacerbate impotence, caution the patient against drinking alcoholic beverages. If appropriate, encourage him to maintain follow-up appointments and treatment for underlying medical disorders.

Make sure the patient and his sexual partner understand that a diagnosis of impotence doesn't mean an end to sex or to sexual expression. As needed, refer them for counseling to overcome psychogenic impotence.

Renal Calculi

Since 90% of renal calculi are smaller than 5 mm in diameter, most of your patient teaching will involve explaining measures to promote their natural passage—most important, vigorous hydration and use of diuretics. However, for patients with larger calculi, your approach will differ significantly. Why? Because these sometimes excruciatingly painful calculi require medical removal to avoid urinary tract obstruction. Depending on the calculi's size and location, you'll need to prepare the patient for surgery or for a revolutionary noninvasive procedure—extracorporeal shock wave lithotripsy (ESWL). To prevent calculi from recurring, your teaching must then stress compliance with prescribed dietary restrictions and with drug therapy to adjust urine pH, if appropriate.

Describe the disorder

Tell the patient that renal calculi, or kidney stones, usually begin when tiny specks of material—normally dissolved and excreted in the urine—instead precipitate and remain in the urinary tract. As more material clings to these specks, they gradually develop into renal calculi. Explain that, although the exact cause of renal calculi is unknown, a variety of factors have been linked to their formation, including excessive dietary intake of calcium, immobility, altered urine pH, and infection.

Mention that small stones seldom cause problems, since they're easily carried into the ureter and passed in the urine. A larger stone, however, may cause excruciating pain if it enters the ureter. It may also obstruct urine outflow.

CHECKLIST

TEACHING TOPICS IN RENAL CALCULI

☐ An explanation of how calculi precipitate from urine, including factors that influence their formation

☐ The importance of treatment to prevent urinary tract obstruction, which may lead to kidney infection, hydronephrosis, and renal insufficiency

☐ Preparation for blood and urine tests to determine the cause and composition of calculi and for radiography or ultrasonography to pinpoint their location

☐ Importance of prescribed dietary restrictions and adequate hydration to prevent recurrence of calculi

☐ Drugs to adjust urine pH, if appropriate

☐ Preparation for surgery or extracorporeal shock wave lithotripsy, as indicated

☐ Home care of percutaneous nephrostomy tube, if appropriate

☐ How to strain urine for calculi and test urine pH

☐ Signs and symptoms of infection

Point out possible complications

Using an anatomic drawing of the renal and urologic system, explain how calculi too large for natural passage cause urinary tract obstruction. Point out that unless calculi are removed, urine trapped above the obstruction may set the stage for kidney infection. Eventually, the kidney's collecting system may also become abnormally dilated— holding up to several liters of urine— a condition known as hydronephrosis. If untreated, hydronephrosis may lead to renal insufficiency.

Teach about tests

Explain the blood and urine tests that the doctor may order to diagnose and evaluate renal calculi.

Inform the patient that blood will be drawn for a CBC and for determination of calcium, phosphorus, BUN, creatinine, glucose, uric acid, and electrolyte levels. Tell him who will perform the venipunctures and when. Explain that tests to measure serum calcium and phosphorus will be repeated on three different days to determine average levels; instruct the patient to fast for 8 hours before each test.

Teach the patient how to collect a clean-catch urine specimen for routine urinalysis and urine cultures to check for infection. If a 24-hour urine specimen is ordered—for example, to measure calcium, phosphorus, uric acid, creatinine, or magnesium levels—explain the collection technique.

Also prepare the patient for KUB radiography and intravenous pyelography or renal ultrasonography. (See *Teaching Patients about Renal and Urologic Tests*, pages 372 to 379.)

Teach about treatments

• *Diet.* In collaboration with the dietitian, teach the patient which foods to eliminate from his diet to prevent calculi from recurring. To avoid hypercalciuria, encourage him to eliminate carbonated soft drinks, cheeses, and other calcium- and phosphorus-rich foods from his diet. Stress the importance of accurately following the prescribed diet.

Also instruct the patient to drink at least 12 glasses of fluid a day. This will dilute his urine, making formation of calculi less likely. To prevent nocturnal dehydration, have him drink fluids before bedtime. Tell him to drink additional fluids when he gets up at night to urinate.

• *Medication.* Depending on the composition of the patient's renal calculi, the doctor may order drugs that adjust the urine pH to eradicate the calculi. For example, if the calculi are composed of phosphate, oxalate, or carbonate, he may order ascorbic acid to acidify the urine. If they're composed of uric acid, cystine, or urate, he may order sodium bicarbonate to alkalinize the urine. In addition, the doctor may order antibiotics to prevent infection, diuretics to increase urine output, and narcotic analgesics to relieve pain. Explain the rationale, dosage, and potential side effects of prescribed drugs, and inform the patient of any harmful interactions. (See *Teaching Patients about Renal and Urologic Drugs*, pages 382 to 385.)

• *Procedures.* A noninvasive procedure, ESWL provides an alternative to surgery for some patients with renal calculi. If your patient's scheduled for ESWL, describe the procedure to him. Explain that he'll receive a general or spinal anesthetic and then be lowered into a water bath. An electric spark generator will direct high-energy shock waves through the water at the affected kidney. These waves will shatter the calculi without damaging surrounding tissue. Afterward, the patient will be able to easily excrete the fine gravel-like remains of the calculi. Inform him that he may receive 500 to 1,500 shocks in 30 to 60 minutes; tell him not to be alarmed by the sound of the generator. Also assure him that he's in no danger of electric shock. After the procedure, tell the patient to increase his fluid intake to 8 to 10 glasses a day and to walk around as much as he can to promote passage of the calculi particles. Before he's discharged (usually the day after the procedure), make sure he understands the importance of straining his urine for stones after each voiding. Tell him when to return for follow-up tests to evaluate the procedure's effectiveness.

• *Surgery.* If the patient's calculi are too large to pass through the ureter, he may require surgery to remove them. Reinforce the doctor's explanation of the procedure, and answer any questions. Tell the patient what type of anesthetic he'll receive—local, spinal, or general—and advise him of any preoperative food and fluid restrictions or bowel preparation.

If the calculi are lodged in the ureter, the doctor may use a basketing instrument to remove them. Describe what will happen during surgery: the patient will be positioned on his back on a table, with his hips and knees flexed. The doctor will pass the basketing instrument through a cystoscope into the ureter, beyond the calculi. Then he'll open the basket to catch the calculi. After the calculi have been trapped, he'll remove the basketing instrument and the cystoscope. Inform the patient that he may have a catheter in place for 2 to 3 days after surgery to keep the ureter open.

When calculi are in the renal pelvis or upper ureter, you may need to prepare the patient for percutaneous nephrostomy. Explain that the doctor will insert a catheter and guide wire through a puncture wound in the patient's flank. Guided by fluoroscopy or ultrasonography, he'll move the catheter to the renal pelvis or upper ureter and inject a contrast medium to visualize the collecting system and to locate the calculi. Then he'll either grasp and remove the calculi or shatter them with ultrasound waves and flush away the fragments from the area. Tell the patient that he'll return from surgery with a urinary drainage tube in place. If the drainage tube is permanent, such as a nephrostomy tube, teach him how to care for it at home. (See *Caring for Your Nephrostomy Tube*, pages 370 and 371.) If the drainage tube is temporary, tell the patient that it will be removed 1 to 3 days after surgery, when X-rays reveal that the kidney is healing properly and no calculi remain. Inform the patient that he can return to work immediately if he has a sedentary job, or in 2 weeks if his job requires any lifting.

When renal calculi aren't accessible to the basketing instrument or to percutaneous nephrostomy, you may need to prepare the patient for pyelolithotomy or ureterolithotomy. Explain that he'll be positioned on his side and that the doctor will remove the calculi from the kidney (pyelolithotomy) or the ureter (ureterolithotomy) through an incision in his flank. Mention that he'll receive fluids through an I.V. line for 1 or 2 days after surgery. If a drainage tube will be inserted during surgery, tell the patient that it will be removed before he goes home. If the ureter will be opened during surgery, tell him that he'll have a catheter until the ureter heals (usually 4 to 6 days after surgery). Mention that full recovery will take 6 to 8 weeks.

Finally, if the calculi are embedded in one of the renal calyces (staghorn calculi), the doctor may order a nephrectomy. To relieve the patient's apprehension, emphasize that the body can adapt well to one kidney. (For more information, see the "Surgery" section in this chapter.)

• *Other care measures.* Instruct the patient to strain his urine after voiding and to save any solid material for analysis. Explain that knowing the composition of calculi will help the doctor pinpoint what's causing them to form. Also teach the patient how to test urine pH, if necessary.

Finally, tell the patient to watch for and report signs of infection, such as increased pain, inability to void, change in the color or odor of his urine, or fever exceeding 102° F. (38.9° C.).

CARING FOR YOUR NEPHROSTOMY TUBE

Dear Patient:

A nephrostomy tube allows urine to drain from your kidney into a collection bag attached to the free end of the tube with a length of tubing.

How to clean the tubing and collection bag

To help prevent infection, clean the tubing and collection bag daily. (Keep an extra bag and tubing available for use when you're cleaning the other set.)

1

Boil some water in a pot or kettle for 30 minutes. Set aside and allow to cool.

Meanwhile, disconnect the collection bag from the tubing and drain any urine from it. Then wash the bag and tubing with soap and water.

2

Fill the collection bag with disinfectant solution, and soak the tubing in the solution for 30 minutes. Remove the tubing with tweezers.

3

Rinse the tubing and the collection bag with the water that you've boiled and then cooled. Cover the upper end of the bag with sterile gauze. Then

place the bag and tubing on a hanger so they can air dry.

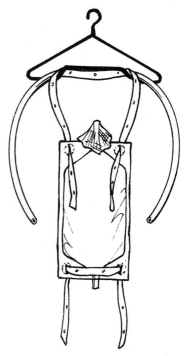

Next, cover the ends of the tubing with sterile gauze pads, and store in a covered container for future use.

How to change the dressing

To protect the skin around your nephrostomy tube, change the dressing daily, as your doctor orders.

1

Assemble the necessary equipment: sterile cotton-tipped applicator, hydrogen peroxide solution, sterile gauze pads, and adhesive tape.

2

Wash your hands. Then remove and discard the old dressing. Wash your hands again. Now, dip a cotton-tipped applicator into hydrogen peroxide solution, and carefully clean the skin around the tube.

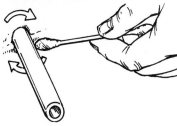

While you're waiting for the skin to dry, check around the tube for signs of infection, such as redness, swelling, or leakage.

3

Next, fold several sterile gauze pads in half and place them around the tube. Cover with an unfolded gauze pad.

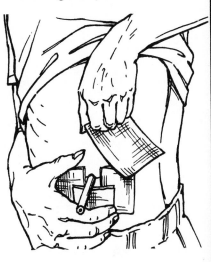

4

Apply adhesive tape to secure the gauze pads to your skin.

Some do's and don'ts

Keep in mind this list to ensure proper drainage and help prevent infection.

Do:
- Tape the tubing securely to your flank.
- Keep the collection bag below kidney level.
- Swab the tubing with an alcohol wipe before connecting or disconnecting it.
- Check the tubing for kinks.

Don't:
- Use your fingernails to disconnect the tubing.
- Touch the open ends of the tubing or bag with your fingers.

TEACHING PATIENTS ABOUT RENAL AND UROLOGIC TESTS

TEST AND PURPOSE	TEACHING POINTS
Antegrade pyelography • To evaluate obstruction of the upper collecting system by stricture, stone, clot, or tumor • To evaluate hydrone-phrosis revealed during excretory urography or ul-trasonography and to en-able placement of a percutaneous nephros-tomy tube • To evaluate the function of the upper collecting system after ureteral sur-gery or urinary diversion • To assess renal func-tional reserve before sur-gery	• Explain to the patient that this test allows radiographic ex-amination of the kidney. Tell him who will perform the test and where, and that it takes about 1 hour. • Explain what happens during the test: the patient will be positioned prone on an X-ray table and given a sedative to help him relax. Next, the skin over the kidney will be cleansed with an antiseptic solution and numbed with a local anesthetic. Then a needle will be inserted into the kidney to inject contrast medium. Explain that urine may also be col-lected from the kidney for testing and that a tube will be left in the kidney for drainage, if necessary. Warn him that he may feel mild discomfort as the local anesthetic is injected and transient burning and flushing from the contrast me-dium. Mention that the X-ray machine will make loud, clack-ing sounds as it exposes films of the kidney. • Describe what happens after the test: the patient's blood pressure, heart rate, and respirations will be monitored every 15 minutes for the first hour, every 30 minutes for the sec-ond hour, and every 2 hours for the next 24 hours. Also, his dressing will be checked for blood or urine leakage, and his fluid intake and urine output will be monitored for 24 hours. If a nephrostomy tube was inserted, note that it will be checked to be sure that it's patent and draining well. • Instruct the patient to report post-test chills, fever, and rapid pulse or respirations to the doctor immediately. Also tell him to report pain in the abdomen or flank or sudden on-set of chest pain or dyspnea.
Cystometry • To evaluate detrusor muscle function and tonic-ity • To help determine the cause of bladder dysfunc-tion	• Explain to the patient that this test evaluates bladder func-tion, especially as it relates to the urgency to void and the ability to suppress voiding. Tell him who will perform the test and where, and that it takes about 40 minutes. Ask him to urinate just before the test. • Explain what happens during the test: the patient will be placed in a supine position on an examining table, and a catheter will be passed into the bladder. As fluid is instilled into the bladder, he'll be asked to report his sensations, such as a strong urge to void, nausea, flushing, or a feeling of warmth. • Warn the patient that he may experience transient urinary burning or frequency after the test.

TEACHING PATIENTS ABOUT
RENAL AND UROLOGIC TESTS *(continued)*

TEST AND PURPOSE	TEACHING POINTS
Cystourethroscopy • To directly visualize the bladder wall, ureteral orifices, and urethra • To provide a channel for invasive procedures, such as biopsy, lesion resection, removal of calculi, or passage of a ureteral catheter to the renal pelvis	• Explain to the patient that this test permits visualization of the bladder and urethra. Tell him who will perform the test and where, and that it takes about 20 minutes. • If a general anesthetic has been ordered, inform the patient that he must fast for 8 hours before the test. • If a local anesthetic has been ordered, tell the patient that he may receive a sedative before the test to help him relax. • Describe what happens during the test: the patient will be positioned supine on an X-ray table, with his hips and knees flexed. His genitalia will be cleansed with an antiseptic solution, and he'll be draped. Then the doctor will administer a local anesthetic, if appropriate, and introduce the cystourethroscope through the urethra into the bladder. Next, he'll fill the bladder with irrigating solution and rotate the scope to inspect the entire surface of the bladder wall. If a local anesthetic was used, warn the patient that he may feel a burning sensation when the cystourethroscope is passed through the urethra. He may also feel an urgent need to urinate as the bladder is filled with irrigating solution. • Describe what happens after the test: the patient's blood pressure, heart rate, and respirations will be monitored every 15 minutes for the first hour after the test, then every hour until stable. Instruct him to drink plenty of fluids and to take the prescribed analgesics. However, he should avoid alcohol for 48 hours after the test. Reassure him that urinary burning and frequency will soon subside. Instruct him to take antibiotics, as ordered, to prevent bacterial infection. • Tell the patient to report flank or abdominal pain, chills, fever, or decreased urinary output to the doctor immediately. In addition, tell him to notify the doctor if he doesn't void within 8 hours after the test or if bright red blood continues to appear after three voidings.
Doppler ultrasonography • To assess penile arterial blood flow • To help diagnose penile vascular disease • To help differentiate between organic and psychogenic impotence	• Explain to the patient that this test evaluates the blood flow to his penis. Tell him who will perform the test and where, and that it takes about 10 minutes. • Explain what happens during the test: the technician will place a transducer against the patient's penis to assess its arterial blood flow. Next, a small blood pressure cuff will be placed around the base of the penis. Tell the patient that he may feel mild discomfort when the cuff is inflated to measure systolic penile blood pressure.

(continued)

TEACHING PATIENTS ABOUT
RENAL AND UROLOGIC TESTS *(continued)*

TEST AND PURPOSE	TEACHING POINTS
Excretory urography (intravenous pyelography) • To evaluate the structure and excretory function of the kidneys, ureters, and bladder • To support a differential diagnosis of renovascular hypertension	• Explain to the patient that this test evaluates the kidneys and urinary tract. Tell him who will perform the test and where, and that it takes about 1 hour. • Tell the patient to drink plenty of fluids and then to fast for 8 hours before the test. Inform him that he may receive a laxative or other bowel preparation before the test. • Explain what happens during the test: the patient will be placed in a supine position on an X-ray table. After injection of a contrast medium, X-rays will be taken at specific intervals. Mention that a belt may be placed around his hips to keep the contrast medium at a certain level. Also warn him that he may experience a transient burning sensation and metallic taste when the contrast medium is injected. Tell him to report these and any other sensations to the doctor. • Warn him that the X-ray machine will make loud, clacking sounds as it exposes films. • Instruct the patient to report symptoms of delayed reaction to the contrast medium.
External sphincter electromyography • To assess neuromuscular function of the external urinary sphincter • To assess the coordination of bladder and sphincter muscle activity	• Explain to the patient that this test evaluates how well his bladder and urinary sphincter muscles work together. Tell him who will perform the test and where, and that it takes about ½ to 1 hour. • Explain what happens during the test: if skin electrodes will be used, show the patient where they'll be placed. Tell him that a technician will first cleanse and possibly shave the areas before applying the electrodes. If needle electrodes will be used, also show the patient where they'll be placed. Tell him that he'll feel slight discomfort when the electrodes are inserted. Explain that the needles will be connected to wires leading to the recorder; assure the patient that there's no danger of electric shock. If an anal plug will be used, inform him that only the tip will be inserted into the rectum and that he may feel fullness or an urge to defecate. Reassure him that a bowel movement rarely occurs. • Advise the patient to drink 2 to 3 liters of fluids daily and to take warm sitz baths to ease post-test discomfort.
Lymphangiography • To detect metastatic infiltration in the lymph nodes	• Explain to the patient that this test permits evaluation of the lymphatic drainage system. Tell him who will perform the test and where, and that it takes about 1 hour. Mention that follow-up X-ray films will be taken within 48 hours of the test. • Explain what happens during the test: after the patient receives a local anesthetic, a catheter will be inserted into a vein in the foot and a contrast medium will be instilled. Warn him that he may experience mild discomfort as the local anesthetic is injected and transient burning and flushing from the contrast medium. • Inform the patient that he may have a bluish skin discoloration for several days after the test.

TEACHING PATIENTS ABOUT
RENAL AND UROLOGIC TESTS (continued)

TEST AND PURPOSE	TEACHING POINTS
Nephrotomography and renal computed tomography • To differentiate between a renal cyst and a solid tumor • To detect and evaluate renal pathology, such as tumor, obstruction, calculi, polycystic kidney disease, congenital anomalies, and abnormal fluid accumulation around the kidneys	• Explain to the patient that this test helps detect renal abnormalities by providing cross-sectional images of the kidney. In renal computed tomography, a computer translates these images for display on an oscilloscope screen. Tell him who will perform the test and where, and that it takes about 1 hour. • Instruct the patient to fast for 8 hours before the test, if he's scheduled to receive a contrast medium. If he has a history of hypersensitivity to iodine or iodine-containing foods, inform the patient that the doctor may forego administration of the contrast medium or may prescribe antiallergenic prophylaxis. • Describe what happens during the test: the patient will be positioned on an X-ray table, and he'll hear loud, clacking sounds as the scanner rotates around the body. Explain that he'll be asked to lie still to avoid distorting the X-ray films. After a series of films is taken, the patient may receive an injection of contrast medium. Warn him that he may experience transient flushing, headache, and metallic taste, as well as a burning or stinging sensation at the injection site. • If the patient received a contrast medium, tell him to report any post-test flushing, nausea, itching, or sneezing to the doctor.
Nocturnal penile tumescence • To differentiate between organic and psychogenic impotence	• Explain to the patient that this test determines whether or not he is able to have erections in his sleep. • Explain what happens during the test: before the patient goes to sleep, he must place a special Velcro band or a small circular wire around the base of his penis. If he's using the wire, he will then attach the leads to a recording device; assure the patient that there's no danger of electric shock. Tell him to carefully remove the device when he awakens and to return it to the doctor for evaluation.
Radionuclide renal imaging • To detect and assess functional and structural renal abnormalities (such as lesions), renovascular hypertension, and acute and chronic renal disease (such as glomerulonephritis) • To assess renal transplantation • To assess renal injury due to trauma or obstruction of the urinary tract	• Explain to the patient that this test permits evaluation of kidney structure, blood flow, and function. Tell him who will perform the test and where, and that it takes about 1½ hours. • Describe pretest preparations: pregnant women and young children may receive a super-saturated solution of potassium iodide 1 to 3 hours before the test to block thyroid uptake of iodine. • Explain what happens during the test: after the patient receives an injection of a radionuclide, several series of X-ray films will be taken of his bladder. Mention that he may experience transient flushing and nausea as the radionuclide's injected. However, emphasize that he'll receive only a small amount of radionuclide and that it's usually excreted within 24 hours. • Instruct the patient to flush the toilet immediately after each voiding for 24 hours after the test, as a radiation precaution.

(continued)

**TEACHING PATIENTS ABOUT
RENAL AND UROLOGIC TESTS** *(continued)*

TEST AND PURPOSE	TEACHING POINTS
Renal biopsy • To aid diagnosis of renal parenchymal disease • To monitor progressive renal disease and to assess effectiveness of treatment	• Explain to the patient that this test helps diagnose kidney disorders. Tell him who will perform the test and where, and that it takes about 15 minutes. Mention that the biopsy needle is in the kidney for only a few seconds. • Instruct him to restrict food and fluids for 8 hours before the test. Inform him that he'll receive a mild sedative before the test to help him relax. • Explain what happens during the biopsy: the patient will be placed in a prone position with a sandbag under his abdomen. After the biopsy site is numbed with a local anesthetic, he'll be asked to hold his breath as the biopsy needle is inserted through his back into the kidney. Warn him that he may experience a pinching pain as the needle's inserted. • Describe what happens after the test: pressure will be applied to the biopsy site to stop superficial bleeding; then a pressure dressing will be applied. Instruct the patient to lie flat on his back without moving for at least 12 hours to prevent bleeding. Tell him that his blood pressure, heart rate, and respirations will be closely monitored.
Renal or penile arteriography • To demonstrate the configuration of renal or penile vasculature • To determine the cause of renovascular hypertension, such as from stenosis, thrombotic occlusion, emboli, or aneurysms • To evaluate chronic renal disease or renal failure • To investigate renal masses and renal trauma • To detect complications following renal transplantation, such as a nonfunctioning shunt or rejection of the donor organ • To help differentiate between organic and psychogenic impotence	• Explain to the patient that this test permits visualization of vessels in the kidneys or penis. Tell him who will perform the test and where, and that it takes about 1 hour. • Describe pretest preparation: the patient must fast for 8 hours before the test. Tell him that he may receive a narcotic analgesic and a sedative before the test to help him relax. Instruct him to remove all metallic objects and to void just before the test. • Explain what happens during the test: the patient will be positioned supine on an X-ray table, and a peripheral I.V. infusion will be started. The skin over the arterial puncture site will be cleansed with antiseptic solution, and a local anesthetic will be injected. Then the femoral artery will be punctured and cannulated for instillation of a contrast medium. Warn the patient that he may experience transient discomfort (flushing, burning sensation, and nausea) as the contrast medium's injected. After this injection, a series of rapid-sequence X-ray films will be taken. Then the catheter will be removed, and pressure will be applied to the puncture site for 15 minutes to stop bleeding. • Describe what happens after the test: the patient will be kept flat in bed for 8 to 12 hours and nonambulatory for 24 hours after the test. His blood pressure, heart rate, and respirations will be monitored every 15 minutes for 1 hour; then every 30 minutes for 2 hours; then once every hour until they're stable. His popliteal and dorsalis pedis pulses will be monitored every 4 hours.

TEACHING PATIENTS ABOUT
RENAL AND UROLOGIC TESTS *(continued)*

TEST AND PURPOSE	TEACHING POINTS
Renal ultrasonography • To determine the size, shape, and position of the kidneys, their internal structures, and perirenal tissues • To evaluate and localize urinary obstruction and abnormal accumulation of fluid • To assess and diagnose complications following kidney transplantation	• Explain to the patient that this test helps detect abnormalities in the kidneys. Tell him who will perform the test and where, and that it takes about ½ hour. Reassure him that the test is safe and painless; in fact, it may feel like a back rub. • Explain what happens during the test: the patient will be placed in a prone position and the area to be scanned will be exposed. The technician will then apply ultrasound jelly and guide a transducer over this area. During the test, the patient may be asked to breathe deeply to assess kidney movement during respiration.
Renal venography • To detect renal vein thrombosis • To evaluate renal vein compression due to extrinsic tumors or retroperitoneal fibrosis • To assess renal tumors and detect invasion of the renal vein or inferior vena cava • To detect venous anomalies and defects • To differentiate renal agenesis from a small kidney • To collect renal venous blood samples for evaluation of renovascular hypertension	• Explain to the patient that this test permits radiographic study of the renal veins. Tell him who will perform the test and where, and that it takes about 1 hour. • If ordered, instruct him to fast for 4 hours before the test. • Explain what happens during the test: after the patient receives a sedative and a local anesthetic, a catheter will be inserted into a vein in the groin area for instillation of contrast medium. Warn him that he may feel mild discomfort as the local anesthetic is injected and transient burning and flushing from the contrast medium. Mention that the X-ray machine will make loud, clacking noises as it exposes the films. • Describe what happens after the test: the patient's blood pressure and pulse will be monitored closely and the puncture site will be checked for bleeding. Tell him to report chills, fever, rapid pulse or respirations, dyspnea, and chest, flank, or abdominal pain to the doctor immediately.
Residual urine test • To evaluate the bladder's ability to empty with voiding	• Explain to the patient that this test measures the amount of urine that remains in the bladder after urination. Tell him who will perform the test and where, and that it takes about 15 minutes. Ask the patient to void just before the test. • Explain what happens during the test: after the patient voids, a catheter will be inserted into the bladder. Mention that he may feel some discomfort as the catheter's inserted. The urine in his bladder will then be collected and measured.

(continued)

TEST AND PURPOSE	TEACHING POINTS
Retrograde cystography, ureteropyelography, or urethrography • To diagnose bladder rupture without urethral involvement, neurogenic bladder, recurrent urinary tract infections, reflux, diverticula, and tumors • To diagnose urethral strictures, laceration, diverticula, and congenital abnormalities • To examine the renal collecting system when excretory urography is contraindicated or inconclusive	• Explain to the patient that this test evaluates the structure and integrity of the bladder, renal collecting system, or urethra. Tell him who will perform the test and where, and that it takes about ½ to 1 hour. • Describe the pretest preparation: if a general anesthetic is ordered, tell the patient to fast for 8 hours before the test. However, before retrograde ureteropyelography, he must drink plenty of fluids to ensure adequate urine flow. • Explain what happens during the test: for retrograde urethrography and retrograde cystography, tell the patient that he'll be placed in a supine position on an X-ray table. A catheter will be inserted into the urethra (for urethrography) or the bladder (for cystography); then a contrast medium will be instilled through the catheter. He'll be asked to assume various positions while X-ray films are taken. For retrograde ureteropyelography, tell the patient that he'll be positioned on an X-ray table with his legs in stirrups and that a contrast medium will be injected through a urethral catheter. X-ray films will be taken while the catheter's in place and again after it's withdrawn. Warn the patient that he may experience some discomfort when the catheter is inserted and when the contrast medium is instilled through the catheter. Also mention that the X-ray machine will make loud, clacking sounds as it exposes the films. • Describe what happens after the test: after retrograde urethrography, instruct the patient to report flushing, nausea, itching, or sneezing to the doctor immediately. After retrograde cystography or ureteropyelography, tell him that his blood pressure, heart rate, and respirations will be monitored frequently until stable. His urine volume and color will also be monitored. Have the patient notify the doctor if blood continues to appear in his urine after the third voiding or if he develops chills, fever, or increased pulse or respiration rate.
Uroflometry • To evaluate lower urinary tract function • To demonstrate bladder outlet obstruction	• Explain to the patient that this test evaluates his pattern of urination. Tell him who will perform the test and where, and that it takes about 10 to 15 minutes. • Advise the patient not to urinate for several hours before the test and to increase his fluid intake so that he'll have a full bladder and a strong urge to void. • Explain what happens during the test: the male patient will be asked to void while standing; the female patient, while sitting. Tell the patient that he'll void into a special commode chair with a funnel that measures his urine flow rate and the amount of time he takes to void. Assure him that he'll have complete privacy during the test. To help ensure accurate results, instruct him to remain as still as possible while voiding.

TEACHING PATIENTS ABOUT
RENAL AND UROLOGIC TESTS *(continued)*

TEST AND PURPOSE	TEACHING POINTS
Voiding cystourethrography • To detect abnormalities of the bladder and urethra, such as vesicoureteral reflux, neurogenic bladder, prostatic hyperplasia, urethral strictures, or diverticula	• Explain to the patient that this test permits assessment of the bladder and the urethra. Tell him who will perform the test and where, and that it takes about 30 to 45 minutes. • Explain what happens during the test: the patient will be placed in a supine position, and a catheter will be inserted into his bladder. Then a contrast medium will be instilled through the catheter. Tell him that he may experience a feeling of fullness and an urge to void when the contrast medium is instilled. Explain that he'll be asked to assume various positions for X-ray films of his bladder and urethra. • Describe what happens after the test: the time, color, and amount of each voiding will be observed and recorded. The patient should drink plenty of fluids to reduce burning on urination and to flush out any residual contrast medium. Tell him to report chills or fever, since these may indicate urinary infection.
Whitaker test • To identify and evaluate renal obstruction	• Explain to the patient that this test evaluates kidney function. Tell him who will perform the test and where, and that it takes about 1 hour. • Describe the pretest restrictions: the patient mustn't eat or drink for at least 4 hours before the test. Instruct him to void just before the test. Also inform him that he may receive a mild sedative to help him relax. • Explain what happens during the test: the patient will be placed in a supine position on the X-ray table. A catheter will be placed in the bladder and then connected to a manometer for pressure readings. Warn the patient that he may feel some discomfort as the urethral catheter is inserted. Next, he'll receive an I.V. injection of contrast medium. Describe the transient burning and flushing he may experience as the contrast medium's injected. Then he'll be placed prone and X-rays will be taken to detect contrast medium in the kidney. Warn him that the X-ray machine will make loud, clacking sounds as the films are exposed. When they do so, the area over the kidney will be cleansed with an antiseptic solution and draped. A local anesthetic will be injected, and an incision will be made through the flank for cannulation of the kidney. Tell the patient that he'll be asked to hold his breath while the needle is inserted into the kidney. Then serial X-rays will be taken as contrast medium is perfused through the cannula while intrarenal pressure is measured. After the test is complete, the cannula will be removed and the wound dressed. • Describe what happens after the test: the patient must remain in the supine position for 12 hours after the test. His blood pressure, heart rate, and respirations will be monitored frequently for 24 hours, and the puncture site will be checked for bleeding or urine leakage. Assure him that colicky pain is transient and that he can request pain medication. Inform him that he may be given antibiotics for several days to prevent infection.

SURGERY

When teaching about surgery to treat renal and urologic disorders, you'll be challenged by the sheer number and diversity of current procedures. After all, surgery for these disorders may primarily involve the kidneys, the urinary tract, or the male genital tract. And such surgery may have a dramatic impact on the patient's life. For example, renal transplantation usually makes possible a relatively full and normal life for the patient with ESRD. In fact, it ranks as one of the most successful organ transplants. Surgery may also be the treatment of choice when renal calculi become lodged in the kidney or ureter or are too large for the patient to pass. Then the doctor may perform percutaneous nephrostomy, cystoscopy (to insert a basketing instrument), pyelolithotomy, ureterolithotomy, or nephrectomy (usually reserved for a staghorn calculus).

When conservative measures fail, surgery may also correct disorders of the male genital tract. For example, to relieve urinary obstruction in benign prostatic hyperplasia, the doctor may perform open prostatectomy or transurethral resection of the prostate. Or, he may use a penile implant to restore sexual function in physiologic impotence. (See the "Chronic Renal Failure," "Renal Calculi," "Benign Prostatic Hyperplasia," and "Impotence" entries for specific information about these surgeries.)

In this section, you'll discover your teaching responsibilities in nephrectomy, retroperitoneal lymphadenectomy, ureteral reimplantation, and urinary diversion. Part of what you'll teach to prepare the patient for surgery will be the same for these four procedures.

Surgical preparation

Inform the patient that he mustn't eat or drink for 8 hours before surgery. Explain that he also won't be allowed to eat or drink food or fluids for the first day after surgery, and that he'll be given I.V. fluids. After that, he can resume oral fluids—and later progress to solids—as long as he doesn't experience nausea or vomiting.

If appropriate, discuss how a full bowel preparation before surgery helps prevent infection. Tell the patient that he'll be given a low-residue diet for 3 days, then high-calorie fluids for 24 hours before surgery. He'll also receive antibiotics—usually erythromycin 500 mg and neomycin 1 g every 4 hours for 24 hours before surgery. Inform him that the night before surgery, he may also be given enemas to cleanse fecal material from the bowel.

Nephrectomy

Explain to the patient that nephrectomy is the removal of part or all of a kidney. Show him where the incision will be made—in the flank over the affected kidney. Tell him who will perform the surgery and where, and that it takes 2 to 3 hours.

Inform the patient that he'll have a catheter in his bladder after surgery to carefully monitor his urine volumes. Mention that he may also have a Penrose or Hemovac drain in place to remove fluid from the operative space, thereby preventing infection. Both the catheter and drain will be removed before the patient goes home. Tell him that full recovery takes 6 to 8 weeks.

Retroperitoneal lymphadenectomy

Discuss how this surgery helps stage testicular cancer. Tell the patient that the lymph nodes in the abdomen and pelvis will be removed and microscopically examined for the presence of cancer cells. Tell him who will perform the surgery and where, and that it takes 3 to 5 hours. Describe the incision that he should expect postoperatively.

After surgery, stress the importance of regular medical follow-up, including monthly examination of the remaining testicle. Depending on the outcome of surgery, you may need to prepare the patient for chemotherapy or radiation therapy.

Ureteral reimplantation

Explain to the patient that this surgery prevents urine from flowing back into the kidney and causing recurrent urinary tract infections. Tell him that one or both ureters will be detached from the bladder during surgery, then reattached to the bladder at new sites. Tell him who will perform the surgery and where, and that it takes 4 to 6 hours. Describe the midline incision that he should expect postoperatively.

Inform the patient that he'll have several tubes in place for a few days after surgery. Explain the purpose of each tube: a nasogastric tube to keep the bowel decompressed and prevent vomiting; an I.V. to maintain hydration; a catheter in the bladder to monitor urine volumes; and a ureteral stint to keep the ureter open until healing begins. Tell him that these tubes will be removed before he goes home. Assure him that he'll be able to void normally on his own. Teach him how to monitor his urine volumes at home and to watch for signs of infection. Mention that full recovery characteristically takes 6 to 8 weeks. Stress the importance of follow-up X-rays, as scheduled by the doctor.

Urinary diversion

Explain to the patient that this procedure provides an alternative route for urine excretion when the bladder has been removed or doesn't function. Describe the type of urinary diversion that he will have. In *ureterosigmoidostomy*, the ureters are attached to the sigmoid colon, allowing urine to flow into the colon and out of the rectum. Because the rectum maintains urinary control and acts as a reservoir for the urine, the patient needn't wear an external collection device. For an *ileal conduit*, the ureters are attached to a 6″ to 8″ segment of the ileum excised from the bowel. One end of the ileal segment is closed with sutures and the opposite end is brought through the abdominal wall to form a stoma. After this procedure is performed, the patient must use an external collection device. A new procedure, called a *continent ileal reservoir*, is similar to the ileal conduit, except that the bowel segment acts as a reservoir for the urine. The patient must catheterize himself periodically to empty the urine from the bowel segment. In a *cutaneous ureterostomy*, one or both ureters are brought through the abdominal wall to form a stoma or stomas. After this procedure is performed, the patient must use an external collection device.

Tell the patient who will perform the surgery and where, and that it takes 5 to 6 hours. Describe the midline incision that he should expect postoperatively. Also prepare him for a stoma, if appropriate. To do so, arrange for a visit with the enterostomal therapist. The therapist will mark the new stoma site, help explain the procedure, answer any questions, and show the patient the type of appliance he will need after surgery.

Explain to the patient that he'll have several tubes in place after surgery. For example, he'll have a nasogastric tube in place for 4 to 5 days to prevent the bowel from distending and damaging the suture line. He may have one or two catheters inserted into the stoma opening to drain urine and to provide splinting for the anastomosis. He may also have a temporary ileostomy bag placed over the stoma opening to collect the urine.

Before discharge, teach the patient how to care for his stoma, how to disinfect his equipment, and where to obtain supplies. Mention that full recovery will characteristically take 6 to 8 weeks. Review the signs and symptoms of infection, as well as any dietary and activity restrictions, if ordered by the doctor.

TEACHING PATIENTS ABOUT RENAL AND UROLOGIC DRUGS

DRUG	ADVERSE REACTIONS	INTERACTIONS*
Alpha-adrenergic blockers		
phenoxybenzamine hydrochloride (Dibenzyline) **phentolamine mesylate** (Regitine)	*Reportable:* fainting, persistent lethargy, unusually rapid heart rate, vomiting, weakness *Other:* dizziness, light-headedness, nausea, pinpoint pupils, postural hypotension, rapid heart rate, stomach pain, stuffy nose	• Tell the patient that foods, beverages, and over-the-counter products don't influence the safety or effectiveness of this alpha-adrenergic blocker.
Anticholinergics		
anisotropine methylbromide (Valpin) **belladonna alkaloids** (Atropine) **dicyclomine hydrochloride** (Bentyl) **glycopyrrolate** (Robinul) **propantheline bromide** (Pro-Banthine)	*Reportable:* difficult urination, eye pain, severe constipation, skin rash *Other:* blurred vision, decreased sweating, drowsiness, dry mouth and throat, mild constipation, rapid pulse	• Tell the patient to avoid over-the-counter products containing antihistamines. • If he's taking antacids and antidiarrhea drugs, tell him to take them at least 1 hour before or after he takes his anticholinergic, for best absorption. • Advise against taking this drug with alcohol. • Instruct the patient to take this drug ½ hour before meals.
Antispasmodics		
flavoxate hydrochloride (Urispas) **oxybutynin chloride** (Ditropan)	*Reportable:* confusion, difficult urination, eye pain, fever, skin rash, sore throat *Other:* blurred vision, constipation, decreased sweating, dizziness, drowsiness, dry mouth, impotence, nausea, rapid pulse	• Tell the patient that beverages and over-the-counter products don't influence the safety or effectiveness of this antispasmodic. • Have him take the drug on an empty stomach—1 hour before or 3 hours after meals—for best absorption.
imipramine hydrochloride (Tofranil)	*Reportable:* blurred vision, confusion or hallucinations, constipation, eye pain, fainting, irregular heart rate, urine retention *Other:* dizziness, drowsiness, dry mouth, fatigue, nausea, weakness	• Tell the patient to avoid taking this drug with systemic decongestants that contain sympathomimetics, such as epinephrine, and to use topical decongestants in moderation. • Advise against taking this drug with alcohol. • Tell him that food, nonalcoholic beverages, and other over-the-counter products don't influence this drug's safety or effectiveness.

*Interactions include food, alcohol, and over-the-counter drugs.

TEACHING POINTS

• Tell the patient that this drug should ease bladder contraction and improve voiding.
• Tell him that the drug's dosage will be increased gradually over a period of days until he obtains symptomatic relief without troublesome side effects. Note that mild side effects usually disappear after prolonged therapy.
• If the patient's being treated for hypertension, advise him that this drug will cause a further drop in his blood pressure.
• Because this drug may cause dizziness or light-headedness, caution the patient to rise slowly from a sitting or lying position.
• Warn a male patient that he may experience retrograde ejaculation.
• Advise the patient to stop taking the drug immediately if he experiences hypotension, fainting, vomiting, or lethargy. Tell him to lie down with his legs elevated until these symptoms subside. Have him call the doctor if symptoms are severe or don't improve within 24 hours.

• Explain to the patient that this drug inhibits bladder contraction and should increase his bladder capacity.
• Caution the patient not to drive or operate machinery while taking this drug.
• Because this drug can decrease sweating, tell him to avoid becoming overheated to prevent heatstroke. Inform the patient that hot baths may also make him feel faint or dizzy.
• Tell the patient to chew sugarless gum or ice chips to relieve dry mouth and throat.

• Explain to the patient that this drug inhibits bladder contraction and should relieve urinary discomfort and bladder spasm. Note that it delays the initial desire to void and may increase bladder capacity.
• Because this drug can decrease sweating, tell him to avoid becoming overheated to prevent heat stroke.
• Instruct the patient not to drive or operate machinery while taking this drug.
• If appropriate, warn a female patient that this drug can suppress lactation. Warn a male patient that it may cause impotence.
• Tell the patient to stop taking the drug immediately and to notify the doctor if he develops an allergic reaction.

• Explain to the patient that this drug should help control enuresis, particularly in children age 6 and older, or symptoms of urinary urgency and frequency. Note that prolonged use, however, may decrease drug effectiveness.
• Advise parents that children should take this drug 1 hour before bedtime. To lessen nausea, suggest that the child take the drug with food.
• Warn the patient not to stop taking the drug suddenly. He must taper the dosage gradually to prevent relapse of symptoms or development of withdrawal symptoms, such as headache and nausea.
• Because this drug can cause an irregular heart rate, inform the patient that he may need periodic EKGs.
• Instruct the patient not to drive or operate machinery while taking this drug.

(continued)

**TEACHING PATIENTS ABOUT
RENAL AND UROLOGIC DRUGS** (continued)

DRUG	ADVERSE REACTIONS	INTERACTIONS*
Carbonic anhydrase inhibitors		
acetazolamide (Ak-Zol, Diamox)	*Reportable:* confusion, hematuria, lower back pain, malaise, urinary difficulty *Other:* anorexia, diarrhea, drowsiness, gastric upset, metallic taste, tingling of extremities	• Tell the patient that foods, beverages, and over-the-counter products don't influence the safety or effectiveness of acetazolamide.
Cholinergics		
bethanechol chloride (Duvoid, Urecholine) **neostigmine methylsulfate** (Prostigmin)	*Reportable:* hypotension, shortness of breath, wheezing or tightness in the chest *Other:* abdominal cramps, dizziness, fainting, headache, nausea, excessive salivation, sweating and skin flushing, urinary frequency	• Tell the patient that foods, beverages, and over-the-counter products don't influence the safety or effectiveness of this cholinergic.
External sphincter relaxants		
baclofen (Lioresal)	*Reportable:* bloody urine, chest pain, fainting, itching, mood changes, skin rash, tinnitus *Other:* confusion, constipation, dizziness, drowsiness, dry mouth, nausea, urinary frequency, weakness	• Instruct the patient not to take this drug with other central nervous system depressants, such as antihistamines, or with alcohol. • Tell him that foods, nonalcoholic beverages, and other over-the-counter products don't influence the safety or effectiveness of baclofen.
dantrolene sodium (Dantrium)	*Reportable:* black or tarry stools, chest pain, dysuria, severe constipation, severe diarrhea, yellowing of eyes or skin *Other:* dizziness, drowsiness, mild constipation, mild diarrhea, muscle weakness, nausea, photosensitivity, unusual tiredness, vomiting	• Instruct the patient not to take this drug with alcohol or over-the-counter products that contain antihistamines. • Tell him that foods, nonalcoholic beverages, and other over-the-counter products don't influence the safety or effectiveness of dantrolene.
Miscellaneous		
phenazopyridine hydrochloride (Pyridium)	*Reportable:* bluish skin discoloration, yellowing of eyes or skin *Other:* dizziness, headache, indigestion, stomach cramps or pain, urine discoloration	• Tell the patient that foods, beverages, and over-the-counter products don't influence the safety or effectiveness of phenazopyridine.

*Interactions include food, alcohol, and over-the-counter drugs.

TEACHING POINTS

• Explain to the patient that this drug should promote urination and help prevent renal calculi by increasing urinary pH.
• If he experiences gastric upset, tell the patient to take this drug with food.
• Because this drug increases the amount and frequency of urination, advise him to take the last dose no later than 6 p.m., unless his doctor directs otherwise. Also tell him to check with his doctor before increasing his fluid intake.
• If ordered, encourage the patient to eat potassium-rich foods, such as bananas and citrus fruits and juices. Also note that he may require a potassium supplement.
• Teach the patient how to test his urine pH with nitrazine paper.

• Explain to the patient that this drug causes bladder contraction that should stimulate voiding.
• If he experiences nausea, tell him to take the drug 1 hour before or 2 hours after meals.
• Because this drug may cause dizziness, light-headedness, or fainting, advise him to rise slowly from a sitting or lying position.

• Explain to the patient that this drug helps treat uninhibited bladder contraction and promote adequate bladder emptying.
• Warn him not to stop taking this drug abruptly. He must gradually taper the dosage to avoid hallucinations and seizures.
• If this drug makes him dizzy or drowsy, tell the patient not to drive or operate machinery.

• Explain to the patient that this drug relaxes certain muscles in his body and should promote adequate emptying of the bladder.
• Inform him that because of the risk of hepatotoxicity, he'll need to undergo liver function tests while taking this drug.
• Because this drug may cause dizziness or drowsiness, caution the patient against driving or operating machinery.
• Instruct him to avoid overexposure to sunlight and to use a sunscreen to prevent sunburn.

• Tell the patient that this drug should relieve urinary burning, urgency, and frequency.
• Inform him that this drug colors the urine orange or red and can stain clothing.
• Tell him that this drug only relieves urinary tract discomfort. He should seek appropriate treatment for underlying causes of pain and not take this drug for more than 2 days.
• If he experiences gastric upset, instruct him to take the drug with food.

12

Obstetrics and Gynecology

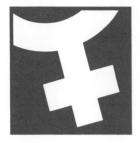

Obstetrics and Gynecology

Introduction

Nowadays, books, magazines, and the news media provide a wealth of information about women's health problems and needs. Yet, despite this explosion of interest and information, many women remain unsure about the basics of reproductive physiology—and may be too embarrassed to admit it. Some may not fully understand the reports they read about new treatments for age-old problems like menstrual discomfort or infertility. Others may persist in believing "old wives' tales" about menstruation, pregnancy, and menopause. Although women are becoming better informed about their health, they're still being exposed to misinformation from a variety of sources. And they may turn to you for clarification.

As a nurse, you're in an excellent position to help female patients understand the changes their bodies undergo throughout their reproductive years. In fact, you'll probably find yourself clearing up confusion and correcting misconceptions about a number of topics, from what causes disorders specific to women to how they're most effectively treated.

Of course, your teaching topics will vary with the patient's stage of life. For example, during the years when your patient is menstruating, your teaching may include a discussion of drug therapy to relieve dysmenorrhea or an ex-

planation of how laparoscopy can treat disorders like endometriosis. During pregnancy, you may teach a patient how to help ensure a healthy pregnancy and a normal delivery—or how to cope with a disorder such as pregnancy-induced hypertension. And during menopause, you may teach a patient about conjugated estrogen therapy to relieve symptoms associated with decreased estrogen production.

Keeping patients well-informed
Some of your most gratifying teaching experiences will involve informing patients about recent advances in obstetric and gynecologic care. Consider, for example, oral contraceptives. Thanks to lower levels of estrogen in current oral contraceptives, women who choose this form of birth control suffer fewer adverse reactions—such as thrombosis and high blood pressure—than women who took earlier types of oral contraceptives. However, the advent of triphasic oral contraceptives marks perhaps the final word in refining this drug therapy. These new drugs, which combine estrogen and progestogen in three different dosages administered during the menstrual cycle, more closely mimic a woman's natural hormonal fluctuations and thus produce maximum effectiveness with minimum side effects.

DISORDERS

Endometriosis

If you've taught patients about endometriosis, you're no doubt familiar with the anxiety, apprehension, and misconceptions surrounding this disorder. For example, a patient may justifiably fear that endometriosis will affect her ability to conceive. Or she may wrongly believe that endometriosis is a life-threatening disorder or a form of cancer. By clearly explaining the disorder, its possible complications, and the impact of treatment options on childbearing, you can clear up your patient's confusion and help her make informed decisions about her care.

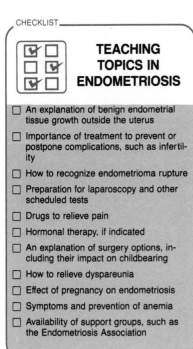

CHECKLIST

TEACHING TOPICS IN ENDOMETRIOSIS

☐ An explanation of benign endometrial tissue growth outside the uterus

☐ Importance of treatment to prevent or postpone complications, such as infertility

☐ How to recognize endometrioma rupture

☐ Preparation for laparoscopy and other scheduled tests

☐ Drugs to relieve pain

☐ Hormonal therapy, if indicated

☐ An explanation of surgery options, including their impact on childbearing

☐ How to relieve dyspareunia

☐ Effect of pregnancy on endometriosis

☐ Symptoms and prevention of anemia

☐ Availability of support groups, such as the Endometriosis Association

Describe the disorder

Using an anatomic drawing of the female reproductive system, explain that endometriosis is a benign growth of endometrial tissue outside the uterus. Such tissue is usually confined to the pelvic area, but it can appear anywhere in the body. Hormones secreted during the menstrual cycle influence this misplaced tissue, causing pain and bleeding during menstruation. As the tissue grows and spreads, it irritates and scars surrounding structures, leading to fibrosis, with adhesions and blood-filled cysts.

Explain to the patient that the cause of endometriosis is unknown but that it may be linked to retrograde tubal flow of menstrual discharge or to transformation of pelvic peritoneal tissue into endometrial tissue. Reassure the patient that endometriosis is not a life-threatening disorder.

Point out possible complications

Tell the patient that complying with prescribed treatment may help prevent or postpone complications, such as infertility and endometrioma (ovarian cyst) rupture. Instruct her to go to the hospital's emergency department immediately if she experiences sudden excruciating abdominal pain—the cardinal symptom of endometrioma rupture. Be sure to advise the patient to alert the doctor that she has endometriosis, to help prevent a possible misdiagnosis of acute appendicitis.

Mention that, rarely, an endometrial growth will become malignant. More often, patients with gross enlargement of one or both ovaries are found to have ovarian cancer unrelated to endometriosis.

Teach about tests

Describe the procedures that the doctor will perform to help detect endometriosis, such as pelvic examination and abdominal palpation. Also prepare the patient for laparoscopy to visualize the extent of tissue growth and confirm di-

QUESTIONS PATIENTS ASK ABOUT ENDOMETRIOSIS

Will endometriosis prevent me from conceiving?

That depends on how severe your endometriosis is and where the endometrial implants are located. Severe endometriosis that affects your ovaries or fallopian tubes might make conception difficult or impossible if it interferes with normal ovulation or fertilization. For example, extensive blood-filled cysts around the ovary may prevent the ovum from leaving the ovary. Or, adhesions in the fallopian tube, pelvic peritoneum, or cul-de-sac may obstruct the ovum's path from the ovary to the uterus.

How can treatment help me to conceive?

By shrinking the size of endometrial implants or suppressing their growth or by surgically removing implants that interfere with conception. To accomplish the first, the doctor will prescribe certain drugs for you that don't affect your ability to ovulate. If the doctor opts for surgery instead, he'll be sure to leave the uterus intact and preserve at least part of one ovary and its fallopian tube.

Should I try to conceive before my endometriosis gets worse?

Yes. In fact, you may find that the hormonal changes associated with pregnancy will cause endometriosis to improve or disappear.

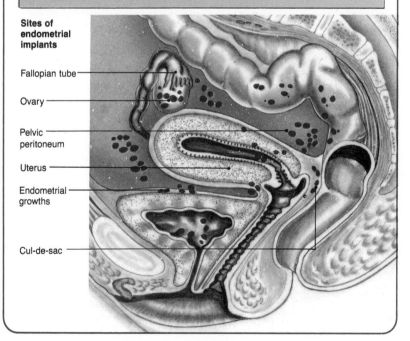

Sites of endometrial implants

Fallopian tube

Ovary

Pelvic peritoneum

Uterus

Endometrial growths

Cul-de-sac

agnosis. (See the "Surgery" section of this chapter for more information.) Explain that additional tests, such as barium enema, cystoscopy, or cul-de-sac aspiration, may also be ordered to establish sites of endometrial tissue growth.

Teach about treatments

• *Medication.* For minor pain, the doctor may order mild analgesics, such as aspirin or acetaminophen. For severe pain, he may order a prostaglandin inhibitor, such as ibuprofen. When pain isn't responsive to these drugs, the doctor may recommend hormonal therapy—for example, oral contraceptives to shrink endometrial tissue; testosterone to reduce pain without affecting ovulation; or the androgen danazol to suppress endometrial tissue growth. Review the dosage instructions with your patient, and inform her of any harmful side effects or interactions. (See *Teaching Patients about Obstetric and Gynecologic Drugs*, pages 396 to 399, for additional information.)

• *Surgery.* To treat severe pain, the doctor may perform presacral neurectomy. Make sure the patient understands that this procedure relieves pain but doesn't cure endometriosis. After surgery, teach the patient bowel or bladder retraining techniques, if needed. Also warn the patient that she may experience heavier menstrual periods after surgery because of vasodilation.

For a patient who has extensive endometriosis and doesn't want to bear children, the doctor may recommend total hysterectomy and bilateral salpingo-oophorectomy. Make sure the patient understands the extent of surgery planned, and explain that it will prevent recurrence of endometriosis. Inform the patient that she'll receive a general anesthetic, so she must fast from midnight before the surgery. Emphasize that performing prescribed exercises after surgery will speed recovery.

For a patient who wants to conceive,

the doctor may perform more conservative surgery, such as lysis of adhesions, resection of cysts, or uterine suspension. Reinforce the doctor's explanation of the recommended procedure and answer any questions the patient may have. Lysis of adhesions and excision of accessible implants may be performed during laparoscopy. (See the "Surgery" section of this chapter for more details.) More extensive or inaccessible implants and uterine suspension require laparotomy. Before surgery, tell the patient what type of anesthetic she'll receive—local or general—and advise her of preoperative food and fluid restrictions. Explain to the patient that after surgery, follow-up hormonal therapy—or pregnancy and its associated hormonal changes—may inhibit further ectopic endometrial growth.

• *Other care measures.* If appropriate, teach the patient measures to reduce dyspareunia. For example, suggest that she take an analgesic or apply a vaginal lubricant before sexual intercourse. Also suggest that she assume a superior or side-lying position to allow her greater control over the amount of pressure exerted during intercourse.

Since infertility is a possible complication of endometriosis, advise the patient who wants to have children not to postpone childbearing. Explain to the patient that pregnancy may also cause endometriosis and its symptoms to improve or disappear.

Teach the patient to notify the doctor if she experiences weakness or fatigue—possible signs of anemia related to heavier menstrual flow. Also stress the importance of eating iron-rich foods—such as mozzarella or American cheese, whole or enriched grains, milk, salmon, broccoli, liver, and clams—and getting adequate rest to help prevent anemia.

To help the patient cope with endometriosis, refer her to a support group, such as the Endometriosis Association.

Pregnancy-Induced Hypertension

Also called preeclampsia or eclampsia, pregnancy-induced hypertension (PIH) accounts for an estimated 30,000 still-births and neonatal deaths in the United States each year. That means when you teach about PIH, you'll be dealing with parents who are understandably concerned about their baby's survival. This concern frequently motivates a patient with mild PIH to learn how to monitor her condition at home. You'll need to teach the patient how to accurately measure her daily weight, blood pressure, and urine protein level. Your teaching here can help ensure a healthy pregnancy and a normal delivery.

A patient with severe PIH requires immediate hospitalization and, possibly, emergency delivery. If emergency delivery is necessary, you'll need to teach the patient and her partner about induced labor or cesarean section. And, if the baby's life can't be saved, you'll need to help them cope with stillbirth or neonatal death.

Describe the disorder

Inform the patient that PIH is a disorder of late pregnancy, in which the mother's blood pressure rises, her body retains excess fluid, and her urine contains excess protein. Explain that PIH causes spasms in the blood vessels that diminish cardiac output and decrease blood flow to all body organs—including the placenta, which provides the fetus with nutrients and oxygen. This may result in fetal malnutrition and growth retardation.

Tell the patient that the cause of PIH is unknown but that several theories link PIH to such varied factors as multiple pregnancies, hydatidiform mole, malnutrition, and metabolic or immunologic disorders.

CHECKLIST

TEACHING TOPICS IN P.I.H.

- [ ] An explanation of the classic signs of PIH and how the disorder compromises maternal and fetal blood flow
- [ ] Importance of treatment to preserve maternal and fetal health—and life
- [ ] How to collect urine for laboratory tests (a clean-catch midstream specimen and a 24-hour specimen)
- [ ] Preparation for amniocentesis and fetal monitoring, if appropriate
- [ ] Activity restrictions
- [ ] Importance of a nutritious, high-protein diet
- [ ] Drugs and their administration
- [ ] How to monitor PIH at home by measuring daily weight, blood pressure, and urine protein level
- [ ] Symptoms of worsening PIH
- [ ] Preparation for emergency delivery by induced labor or cesarean section, if indicated

Point out possible complications

Explain to the patient that uncontrolled PIH may lead to maternal heart failure, by increasing cardiac work load; renal failure, by decreasing renal perfusion; and seizures or cerebrovascular accident, by causing cerebral vasospasm. Inform her that continuously diminished blood flow to the placenta may lead to fetal or neonatal death.

Teach about tests

Prepare the patient for laboratory tests to measure urine protein and estriol levels and to determine creatinine clearance. As appropriate, teach her how to collect a clean-catch midstream urine specimen or a 24-hour specimen. For creatinine clearance, note who will perform the venipuncture and when.

Also prepare the patient for amniocentesis and fetal monitoring to evaluate fetal health and maturity. (See *Teaching Patients about Obstetric and Gynecologic Tests*, pages 393 to 394, for more information.)

Teach about treatments

• *Activity.* If the patient has mild PIH, the doctor may recommend bed rest at home. Tell the patient to lie quietly in a darkened room with as little stimulation as possible. Advise her to rest on her left side to increase blood flow to the fetus. Emphasize that she should get out of bed only to go to the bathroom. Explain that if her condition fails to improve within 3 or 4 days, she'll need to be admitted to the hospital to ensure proper rest and allow close observation.

• *Diet.* In collaboration with the dietitian, stress the importance of eating a well-balanced, nutritious diet that's high in protein. Be sure to determine what types of protein the patient prefers and can afford before recommending which foods she should include in her diet.

• *Medication.* Discuss prescribed drugs with the patient, including hydralazine and methyldopa to control her blood pressure; sodium phenobarbital to help her cope with prolonged bed rest and control convulsions; and diuretics, such as thiazides, furosemide, and ethacrynic acid, to increase her urine output. Review dosage instructions and warn the patient about any harmful side effects or interactions.

• *Procedures.* If appropriate, teach the patient how to monitor PIH at home by measuring and recording her daily weight, blood pressure, and urine protein level. Instruct her to weigh herself at the same time each day, using the same scale and wearing the same type of clothing. Tell the patient to notify the doctor if she gains more than 2½ lb per week after the 34th week of pregnancy.

Teach the patient how to take accurate blood pressure readings. Emphasize that she should compare each blood pressure reading against her baseline reading. Advise her to notify the doctor immediately if systolic pressure rises 30 mm Hg above baseline or diastolic pressure rises 15 mm Hg above baseline.

Explain how to measure protein in her urine. First, instruct the patient to collect a clean-catch midstream urine specimen—preferably in the morning, when urine is most concentrated and yields the most reliable information. Tell her to dip the reagent strip into the urine and to remove excess urine by tapping the strip against a clean surface or the edge of the container. Next, have her hold the strip in a horizontal position, place it close to the color block on the bottle, and carefully compare colors. Explain that the color block corresponds to levels of protein in the urine, and tell her to notify the doctor immediately if she detects protein levels of 300 mg/dl or more.

• *Surgery.* If the patient doesn't respond to conservative treatment or if PIH is severe, the doctor may attempt emergency delivery—either by inducing labor or by performing a cesarean section. Stress that delivery is necessary to preserve the health and possibly the life of the baby, the mother, or both. Reinforce the doctor's explanation of the procedure, and answer any questions the patient may have. Encourage parent-infant bonding as soon as practical after delivery.

Unfortunately, it's not always possible to save the baby's life through emergency delivery. Besides providing emotional support for the parents, you'll need to help them cope with stillbirth or neonatal death by describing the grieving process. (For additional information about the grieving process, refer to Chapter 19.)

• *Other care measures.* Teach the patient to watch for and report symptoms indicating that PIH is progressing. These symptoms include visual disturbances, headaches, dizziness, excitability, apprehension, anxiety, nausea, or vomiting.

TEACHING PATIENTS ABOUT OBSTETRIC AND GYNECOLOGIC TESTS

TEST AND PURPOSE	TEACHING POINTS
Amniocentesis • To determine fetal age and maturity, especially pulmonary maturity • To detect fetal abnormalities, particularly chromosomal and neural tube defects • To evaluate isoimmune disease (Rh incompatibility) • To diagnose fetal metabolic disorders • To identify the sex of the fetus	• Explain to the patient that this test evaluates fetal health and maturity and also identifies the sex of the fetus. • Describe the pretest preparation: the placenta and fetus will be located by ultrasonography. Just before the test, ask the patient to void to minimize the risk of puncturing the bladder and aspirating urine instead of amniotic fluid. • Describe what happens during the test: the patient will lie down on her back with her legs extended. The doctor will do an abdominal examination to reconfirm the position of the fetus and to assess its heartbeat. Next, he'll cleanse the abdominal skin with an antiseptic solution and inject a local anesthetic. Then he'll insert a special needle through the abdominal wall into the uterus and aspirate an amniotic fluid specimen. • Describe what happens after the test: the doctor will apply a sterile dressing over the puncture site. Mention that the fetal heartbeat and the patient's blood pressure, heart rate, and respirations will be monitored for about ½ hour. • Advise the patient to report any discomfort, fever, leakage of fluid, or change in fetal activity after the test.
Antepartal external fetal monitoring • To assess placental function during stress and nonstress situations • To measure fetal heart rate as an indicator of fetal health	• Explain to the patient that this test assesses fetal health and measures fetal ability to withstand the stress of contractions induced before actual labor begins. Tell her who will perform the test and where, and that it takes about 2 hours. Assure her that fetal monitoring is painless and noninvasive and that it won't harm the fetus or interfere with the normal progress of labor. Inform her that the test can also be performed without stimulated contractions, to assess fetal health. • If not contraindicated, instruct the patient to eat a meal just before the test to reduce bowel sounds and to increase fetal activity. Have the patient empty her bladder before the test. • Explain what happens during the test: the patient will be placed in a semi-Fowler or left lateral position with her abdomen exposed. An ultrasound transducer will be attached over the area with the most distinct fetal heart sounds. *For the nonstress test:* tell the patient that she'll hold a pressure transducer in her hand and be asked to push it each time she feels the fetus move. *For the stress test:* tell her that she'll receive a low-dose infusion of oxytocin until she experiences three or four uterine contractions within 10 minutes, each lasting longer than 30 seconds.

(continued)

TEACHING PATIENTS ABOUT
OBSTETRIC AND GYNECOLOGIC TESTS *(continued)*

TEST AND PURPOSE	TEACHING POINTS
Colposcopy • To visualize the cervix and vagina • To evaluate vaginal or cervical lesions • To confirm malignancy after a positive Pap test	• Explain to the patient that this test allows close study of the vagina and cervix, and thus provides more information than a routine pelvic examination. Tell her who will perform the test and where, that it's safe and painless, and that it takes 5 to 10 minutes. • Describe the procedure: the patient will be placed in the lithotomy position. Next, the doctor will insert a vaginal speculum and swab the cervix to remove any mucus. After viewing the cervix and vagina with the colposcope, he may biopsy areas that appear abnormal. • If biopsy is performed, tell the patient to abstain from intercourse and not to insert anything into the vagina until the biopsy site heals.
Hysterosalpingography • To confirm tubal abnormalities, such as adhesions and occlusion • To confirm uterine abnormalities, such as fistulas, adhesions, and the presence of foreign bodies	• Explain to the patient that this test confirms uterine and fallopian tube abnormalities. Tell her who will perform the test and where, and that it takes about 15 minutes. • Describe what happens during the test: the patient will be placed in the lithotomy position. Next, the doctor will insert a vaginal speculum and swab the cervix to remove any mucus. Then he'll insert a cannula into the uterus and slowly inject a radiopaque dye. If this triggers cramping, the doctor will temporarily stop the injection until the cramps subside. After the dye's injected, the uterus and fallopian tubes will be viewed fluoroscopically, and radiographs will be taken. Also mention that the test may increase the likelihood of pregnancy. As the dye flows through the tubes, it may break up adhesions, stimulate cilia that promote passage of the ovum, or alter cervical mucus to be more receptive to sperm. • Tell the patient to report signs of infection after the test, such as fever, pain, increased pulse rate, malaise, and muscle ache.
Pelvic ultrasonography • To detect foreign bodies and distinguish between cystic and solid masses (tumors) • To evaluate fetal viability, position, gestational age, and growth rate • To guide amniocentesis by determining placental location and fetal position • To detect multiple pregnancy	• Describe the test to the patient, and tell her why it's being performed. Tell her who will perform the test and where, and that it takes about ½ hour. Reassure the pregnant patient that the test won't harm the fetus. • Have the patient drink 6 to 8 glasses of fluid 1½ to 2 hours before the test. Instruct her *not* to void before the test. A full bladder serves as a landmark to define other pelvic organs. • Explain what happens during the test: the patient will be positioned on her back and her abdomen will be coated with mineral oil. Then the technician will guide a transducer over the abdomen to visualize the uterus, vagina, and adjoining organs. • Tell the patient that she will be allowed to empty her bladder immediately after the test.

SURGERY

Because surgery involving the female reproductive organs can challenge the patient's femininity, your preoperative teaching must be sensitive and thorough. For example, you'll need to carefully explain why the doctor must excise implants in endometriosis, while keeping in mind the patient's concerns about infertility. (See "Endometriosis," in this chapter, for more information.)

In this section, you'll discover your teaching responsibilities in A & P repair, laparoscopy, laparotomy, and vaginal hysterectomy.

A & P (anterior-posterior) repair

Explain to the patient that this surgery repairs weakened vaginal walls. Inform her that she'll receive a cleansing douche and perineal care the morning of surgery. Also prepare her for rectal enemas to cleanse fecal material from the bowel.

Tell the patient that she'll have an indwelling (Foley) catheter in place for 1 to 4 days after surgery. She'll need to lie flat or in a low Fowler position to prevent increased intraabdominal pressure from pulling on the sutures. Also tell her that she'll receive a clear liquid diet for about 5 days to allow the bowel to rest and heal. Instruct the patient to avoid Valsalva's maneuver and to use a laxative, if ordered, to avoid straining from constipation.

Laparoscopy

Tell the patient that this procedure allows the doctor to visually inspect the organs in the pelvis. Explain how he'll insert the laparascope through a small abdominal incision and then, if appropriate, perform minor surgery—such as removal of an endometrioma or small fibroids—by passing instruments through the scope.

If air is injected into the abdominal cavity during the procedure, tell the patient to lie in a prone position with a pillow under her abdomen. Warn the patient to expect some shoulder pain from air irritating the diaphragm. Also have her carefully observe the incision site for signs of infection, such as redness, warmth, or increased tenderness. Advise the patient to temporarily refrain from douching and intercourse, as her doctor orders.

Laparotomy

This procedure refers to any surgical incision into the abdominal cavity. Explain the purpose of the surgery, for example, removal of an ovarian cyst or ectopic pregnancy, tubal ligation, or hysterectomy.

Preoperatively, tell the patient that she'll receive a perineal shave and, if ordered, a cleansing vaginal douche. Also tell her that she'll have a Foley catheter in place for several days after surgery. Warn the patient to expect some serosanguineous vaginal discharge.

Advise the patient to avoid tub baths and douches after surgery until her vaginal incisions heal. Usually, she'll be able to resume her normal activities in about 6 weeks.

Vaginal hysterectomy

Explain to the patient that this surgery involves removal of the uterus and possibly the ovaries and fallopian tubes, through the vagina.

Inform the patient that she'll receive a cleansing vaginal douche before surgery. Instruct her to avoid tub baths and douches after surgery until her vaginal incisions heal. Have her call the doctor if she has heavy bleeding, abnormal cramps, hot flashes, or changes in her bowel habits. Usually, the patient will be able to resume her normal activities, including intercourse, in about 6 weeks. Mention that she'll no longer menstruate.

TEACHING PATIENTS ABOUT OBSTETRIC AND GYNECOLOGIC DRUGS

DRUG	ADVERSE REACTIONS	INTERACTIONS*
Estrogen-progestogen combinations (oral contraceptives)		
estrogen with progestogen (Brevicon, Demulen, Enovid, Loestrin, Modicon, Norinyl, Ortho-Novum, Ovcon, Ovral, Ovulen, Tri-Norinyl)	*Reportable:* abdominal pain, arm or leg weakness, breakthrough bleeding, breast lumps, shortness of breath, sudden chest pain, depression, dysuria, severe headache, hypertension, incoordination, jaundice, worsening myopia, rash, slurred speech, syncope, urinary frequency, curdlike vaginal discharge, visual disturbances *Other:* acne, anorexia, bloating, breast tenderness, dizziness, edema, headache, hirsutism, skin hyperpigmentation, lethargy, altered libido, nausea, photosensitivity, stomach cramps, vomiting	• Tell the patient that foods and beverages don't influence the safety or effectiveness of oral contraceptives. • Advise against taking mineral oil, which may decrease drug absorption.
Estrogens		
estradiol (Estrace) **estrogens, conjugated** (Premarin) **ethinyl estradiol** (Estinyl, Feminone) **quinestrol** (Estrovis)	*Reportable:* abdominal pain, acne, amenorrhea, arm or leg weakness, breakthrough bleeding, breast lumps, shortness of breath, sudden chest pain, depression, dysmenorrhea, dysuria, severe headache, jaundice, lethargy, altered menstrual flow, rash, slurred speech, urinary frequency, curdlike vaginal discharge, visual disturbances *Other:* anorexia, bloating, breast tenderness, dizziness, edema, headache, hair loss, leg cramps, nausea, photosensitivity, vomiting	• Tell the patient that foods and beverages don't influence the safety or effectiveness of estrogens. • Advise against taking mineral oil, which may decrease drug absorption.
Gonadotropins		
chorionic gonadotropin, human (Android HCG) **menotropins** (Pergonal)	*Reportable:* bloating, stomach or pelvic pain *Other:* (for chorionic gonadotropin, human) depression, edema, fatigue, gynecomastia, headache, irritability, pain at injection site, early puberty; (for menotropins) diarrhea, nausea, vomiting	• Tell the patient that foods, beverages, and over-the-counter drugs don't influence the safety or effectiveness of gonadotropins.

*Interactions include foods, alcohol, and over-the-counter drugs.

TEACHING POINTS

• Explain to the patient that this drug prevents conception.
• Advise her to take the drug at the same time each day to minimize side effects and enhance its effectiveness. Taking the drug at night may reduce headache and nausea. Or, recommend taking it with meals to reduce nausea.
• Discourage smoking when taking this drug to reduce the risk of MI, CVA, pulmonary emboli, and thrombophlebitis.
• Teach the patient how to perform breast self-examination.
• Instruct the patient to weigh herself at least twice a week and to report any sudden weight gain or edema to her doctor.
• If the patient suspects that she's pregnant, tell her to discontinue the drug immediately and notify her doctor. Use of this drug during pregnancy may cause birth defects and increase the risk of vaginal cancer in a daughter when she reaches childbearing age.
• Advise the patient to avoid prolonged exposure to sunlight and to use a sunscreen when outdoors.
• If the patient misses a dose, tell her to take the dose as soon as she remembers it. If she doesn't remember until the next day, she should take two tablets at once, then continue the regular schedule.

• Explain that this drug corrects estrogen deficiency and should help treat menopause (or osteoporosis). Instruct the patient to carefully read the package insert information and to ask her doctor or pharmacist to clear up any questions.
• Discourage smoking when taking this drug to reduce the risk of myocardial infarction (MI), cerebrovascular accident (CVA), pulmonary emboli, and thrombophlebitis.
• Teach the patient how to perform breast self-examination.
• Advise using a sunscreen when outdoors because estrogens can cause photosensitivity.
• If the patient suspects that she's pregnant, tell her to discontinue the drug and notify her doctor. Use of this drug during pregnancy may cause birth defects.
• To administer the drug vaginally, instruct the patient to insert the applicator into the tube of medication and squeeze the tube to fill the plunger. Then she should lubricate the applicator with water-soluble jelly, insert it into the vagina, and push the plunger to deposit the medication. Tell her to use a sanitary napkin to avoid staining her underpants.
• To relieve nausea, advise taking the drug with meals.

• Explain to the patient that this drug induces ovulation, improving the chances of conception. Warn about the possibility of multiple births.
• Advise the patient to engage in intercourse daily from the day before she takes the drug until ovulation occurs. Teach her the signs of ovulation, such as thick, mucoid vaginal discharge, localized pain on one side, and a 1- to 1½-degree rise in temperature.
• If the patient experiences severe lower abdominal pain at 8 to 12 weeks of gestation, tell her to notify her doctor immediately to rule out ectopic pregnancy.

(continued)

**TEACHING PATIENTS ABOUT
OBSTETRIC AND GYNECOLOGIC DRUGS** (continued)

DRUG	ADVERSE REACTIONS	INTERACTIONS*
Gonadotropin inhibitor		
danazol (Danocrine)	*Reportable:* acne, clitoral enlargement, decreased breast size, depression, dizziness, edema, headache, hematuria, hirsutism, hoarseness, jaundice, oily skin and hair, sleep disturbances, visual disturbances, weight gain *Other:* appetite changes; lethargy; mood changes; muscle cramps; nausea; nervousness; vaginal bleeding, burning, dryness, or itching	• Tell the patient that foods, beverages, and over-the-counter drugs don't influence the safety or effectiveness of danazol.
Nonsteroidal anti-inflammatory agents		
ibuprofen (Advil, Motrin, Nuprin) **meclofenamate sodium** (Meclomen) **naproxen** (Anaprox, Naprosyn) **suprofen** (Suprol)	*Reportable:* unusual bleeding, bloody or tarry stools, bloody urine, bruises, fever, skin rash, sore throat, decreased urine output, wheezing, yellowing of skin and eyes *Other:* diarrhea, dizziness, drowsiness, heartburn, indigestion, nausea, vomiting	• Tell the patient not to take this drug with aspirin, acetaminophen, or alcohol. Have her take the drug on an empty stomach—1 hour before meals or 3 hours after meals—for best absorption.
Progestins		
medroxyprogesterone acetate (Provera) **norethindrone** (Micronor) **norgestrel** (Ovrette)	*Reportable:* abdominal pain; amenorrhea; arm or leg weakness or pain; breakthrough bleeding; breast tenderness, enlargement, or secretion; shortness of breath; chest pain; depression; dizziness; dysmenorrhea; headache; jaundice; melasma; skin rash; slurred speech; visual disturbances *Other:* appetite changes, lethargy, nausea, ankle and feet swelling, vomiting, weight changes	• Tell the patient that foods, beverages, and over-the-counter drugs don't influence the safety or effectiveness of progestins.

*Interactions include foods, alcohol, and over-the-counter drugs.

TEACHING POINTS

• Explain to the patient that this drug helps treat endometriosis.

• If the patient misses a dose, tell her to take the dose as soon as she remembers it; however, she must not double-dose.

• Advise her not to store this drug in the bathroom, since moisture will cause drug breakdown.

• Tell the patient to use nonhormonal methods of birth control diligently throughout drug therapy even though she won't experience any menstrual periods. If she suspects that she's pregnant, tell her to discontinue the drug immediately and notify her doctor. Use of this drug during pregnancy causes female infants to develop male characteristics.

• If not contraindicated, advise the patient to eat a high-calorie, high-protein diet.

• Instruct the patient to wear cotton underpants and to wash after intercourse, to help decrease the risk of vaginitis.

• Reassure her that masculinizing side effects usually disappear when the drug is discontinued.

• To prevent nausea, advise the patient to take this drug after meals or with a snack.

• Explain to the patient that this drug should help relieve dysmenorrhea.

• If the patient misses a dose, tell her to take the dose as soon as she remembers it. However, if it's almost time for the next dose, tell her to skip the missed dose; she must not double-dose.

• If the patient experiences gastric upset, tell her to take the drug with meals or with an antacid.

• If this drug makes the patient dizzy or drowsy, advise her not to drive or operate machinery.

• Inform her that ibuprofen is available without a prescription.

• If the patient is hypersensitive to aspirin, warn her not to take this drug.

• Explain to the patient that this drug helps treat amenorrhea and dysfunctional uterine bleeding. Instruct her to read the package insert information and to ask her doctor or pharmacist to clear up any questions.

• If the patient suspects that she's pregnant, tell her to discontinue the drug immediately and call her doctor. Use of this drug during pregnancy may cause birth defects.

• If the patient misses a dose, tell her to take the dose as soon as she remembers it; however, she must not double-dose.

• Teach the patient how to perform breast self-examination.

• Discourage smoking when taking this drug to reduce the risk of MI.

13

Endocrine System

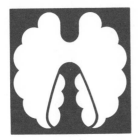

Endocrine System

Introduction

Teaching patients with endocrine disorders can be challenging but rewarding. Typically, these patients must learn to manage a complex and changing therapeutic regimen for the rest of their lives. Often they'll have to make major life-style changes before their disorder can be brought under control. Even then, they must be alert for acute crises that can develop rapidly, requiring emergency treatment.

Given enough time, even a mild endocrine imbalance can cause serious complications. And if complications become chronic, they can have a profoundly negative effect on the patient and may even shorten his life. Consider, for example, the persistent discomfort experienced by patients with uncontrolled Graves' disease or the devastating complications that can result from unchecked diabetes mellitus.

Most problems stemming from endocrine dysfunction can be avoided, or at least minimized, by strict patient compliance with the prescribed treatment regimen. This requires that the patient and his family understand the disorder and know how to manage it. Your ability to teach them what they need to know can make all the difference in how well the patient ultimately manages his disorder.

You'll need to schedule brief but frequent teaching sessions. Endocrine dysfunction can shorten the patient's attention span and also cause fatigue and anxiety. It may also limit the amount of information he'll be able to absorb in one session. Also be sure to include a family member in your teaching sessions; someone in the family should know what to do if the patient can't take care of himself.

Begin your teaching by clearly explaining the disorder. Then discuss the complications that can occur if the disorder isn't controlled. Emphasize that, unlike many chronic illnesses, endocrine disorders *can* be controlled. By complying with therapy, the patient can lead a near-normal life.

Review the key tests used to diagnose endocrine disorders. These tests may include measurement of serum and urine hormone levels, provocative testing (such as the oral glucose tolerance test), and X-rays of the affected endocrine gland.

Finally, you'll need to review guidelines that will help the patient and his family manage the disorder at home. These guidelines should cover diet therapy and medications for suppressing endocrine gland function or for replacing deficient hormones. Other important topics include recognition, treatment, and prevention of acute crises, and adjunctive measures, such as surgery or radiation therapy.

DISORDERS

Adrenocortical Insufficiency

Preventing life-threatening adrenal crisis is your overriding concern for patients with adrenocortical insufficiency. Toward this end, you'll need to teach about the disorder, dietary changes, activity precautions, and self-medication.

Covering these topics will probably be relatively easy compared to teaching about the precipitating factors, signs, and emergency treatment of adrenal crisis. After all, many patients don't appreciate the delicate balancing act performed by the endocrine system. They must understand that even moderate stress or minor infections can upset this balance and precipitate adrenal crisis. Teaching the patient to recognize potential precipitating factors and to respect the hazards they pose will help him prevent this extremely dangerous complication.

Describe the disorder
Explain to the patient that adrenocortical insufficiency is a chronic disorder in which the adrenal glands fail to produce enough cortisol and aldosterone. These hormones, secreted by the adrenal cortex, regulate fluid balance and glucose formation.

Explain the patient's type of adrenocortical insufficiency. In *primary adrenocortical insufficiency* (also called Addison's disease), vital tissue in the adrenal cortex is gradually destroyed. Possible causes include infection, trauma, cancer, hemorrhage, and chemotherapeutic drugs. Tell the patient with primary insufficiency that

90% of the adrenal gland is usually destroyed before symptoms appear.

If your patient has *secondary adrenocortical insufficiency,* explain that his condition results from reduced pituitary secretion of adrenocorticotropic hormone (ACTH). This hormone normally stimulates the adrenal cortex to produce cortisol and aldosterone. Secondary adrenocortical insufficiency can result from any condition that affects the hypothalamus and pituitary gland, both of which are responsible for regulating ACTH secretion. Long-term use of potent steroids is another possible cause.

Point out possible complications
Reinforce the importance of strict compliance with prescribed treatment by pointing out the effects of adrenal crisis: profound hypoglycemia and circulatory collapse. Without prompt emergency treatment, adrenal crisis will prove fatal. (See *What Happens in Adrenal Crisis,* pages 404 and 405.)

Teach about tests
Teach the patient about diagnostic tests, such as cortisol and ACTH studies, to confirm adrenocortical insufficiency and to identify its type. Explain that these tests require multiple blood samples and venipunctures. Some tests may also require a 24-hour urine sample.

Instruct the patient to follow a normal diet (with a daily sodium intake of 2 to 3 g) for 3 days before the plasma cortisol test. Advise him to avoid stressful situations and excessive or strenuous physical activity for at least 48 hours before the test. (Stress and excessive or strenuous physical activity can alter cortisol levels significantly.) If a stressful situation develops unexpectedly during the 48 hours before the test, tell the patient to notify his doctor so that the test can be postponed. Review any medications that might have to be withheld before the test.

Tell the patient that cortisol levels will first be measured in serum and urine samples. Explain that two blood samples will be drawn—one between 6 a.m. and 8 a.m., the other between 4 p.m. and 6 p.m. Also explain that the urine sample for a metabolite of cortisol is collected over 24 hours. Review the collection procedure with the patient, emphasizing the importance of keeping the sample refrigerated or on ice during the collection period. Make sure the patient understands that if he discards a urine sample by mistake, the test results will be invalid.

Inform the patient that a rapid ACTH test may be required after measurement of cortisol levels. Explain that this test, which takes about 1 hour, challenges the adrenal gland to secrete cortisol. It requires a blood sample drawn by venipuncture, followed by I.M. or I.V. injection of synthetic ACTH. More blood samples will be drawn 30 to 60 minutes later to see if the ACTH injection stimulated the adrenal gland to produce cortisol.

Explain that blood samples may be drawn to measure plasma ACTH levels. This test helps determine if adrenocortical insufficiency is primary or secondary. If the doctor orders a low-carbohydrate diet before the test, give the patient clear instructions to follow the diet for 48 hours before the test.

If the doctor orders the metyrapone test to determine if the pituitary gland can secrete ACTH, explain to the patient that this test is done over 3 days. On the first day, the patient will collect a 24-hour urine sample to be tested for urinary 17-hydroxycorticosteroids. On the second day, he'll take oral metyrapone, a synthetic compound that inhibits the enzyme responsible for synthesizing corticosteroids, every 4 hours (six doses altogether), to stimulate the pituitary to secrete ACTH. On the third day, he'll collect a second 24-hour urine sample for urinary 17-hydroxycorticosteroids.

Teach about treatments
● *Activity.* Explain to the patient the importance of planning physical activ-

CHECKLIST

> ## TEACHING TOPICS IN ADRENOCORTICAL INSUFFICIENCY
>
> ☐ An explanation of the type of disorder: primary or secondary
>
> ☐ Warning signs and prevention of adrenal crisis
>
> ☐ Serial diagnostic tests to evaluate hormone levels
>
> ☐ Dietary modifications, with special emphasis on sodium and glucose needs
>
> ☐ Activity restrictions and need for rest
>
> ☐ Hormone replacement therapy

ity. Because of his condition, he won't have glucose readily available for energy, so he'll tire easily. Advise him to avoid strenuous physical activity in hot or humid weather because profuse sweating depletes the body of fluid and sodium.

● *Diet.* Stress the importance of following the prescribed diet to meet glucose and sodium requirements. Make sure the patient understands his meal plan. To prevent hypoglycemia, caution him to avoid long fasts during periods of normal activity. If he's anorectic, advise him to eat six small meals a day to increase his caloric intake. His sodium intake should also be liberal. Tell him to avoid salt substitutes or salt-restricted products and to limit his consumption of foods rich in potassium.

● *Medication.* If adrenocortical hormone supplements are ordered, advise the patient to take them exactly as prescribed. Urge him never to change the dosage or stop the medication unless his doctor permits. If he's having a problem that appears to be related to the supplements, instruct him to notify his doctor. (See *Teaching Patients about Endocrine Drugs*, pages 432 to 435.)

● *Other care measures.* Review with the patient and his family the warning signs and prevention tips for adrenal

WHAT HAPPENS IN ADRENAL CRISIS

In adrenal crisis, a life-threatening complication of adrenocortical insufficiency, rapid decline in cortisol and aldosterone levels results from atrophy or destruction of the adrenal gland. These hormonal declines cause widespread effects throughout the body, as shown in

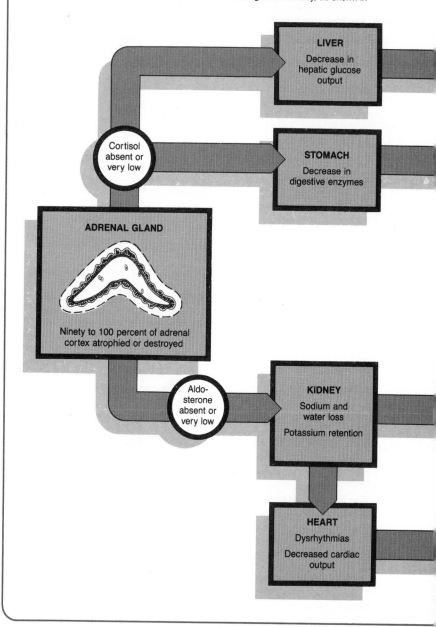

LIVER
Decrease in hepatic glucose output

Cortisol absent or very low

STOMACH
Decrease in digestive enzymes

ADRENAL GLAND
Ninety to 100 percent of adrenal cortex atrophied or destroyed

Aldosterone absent or very low

KIDNEY
Sodium and water loss
Potassium retention

HEART
Dysrhythmias
Decreased cardiac output

the illustration. Without emergency treatment, adrenal crisis may rapidly progress to coma and death.

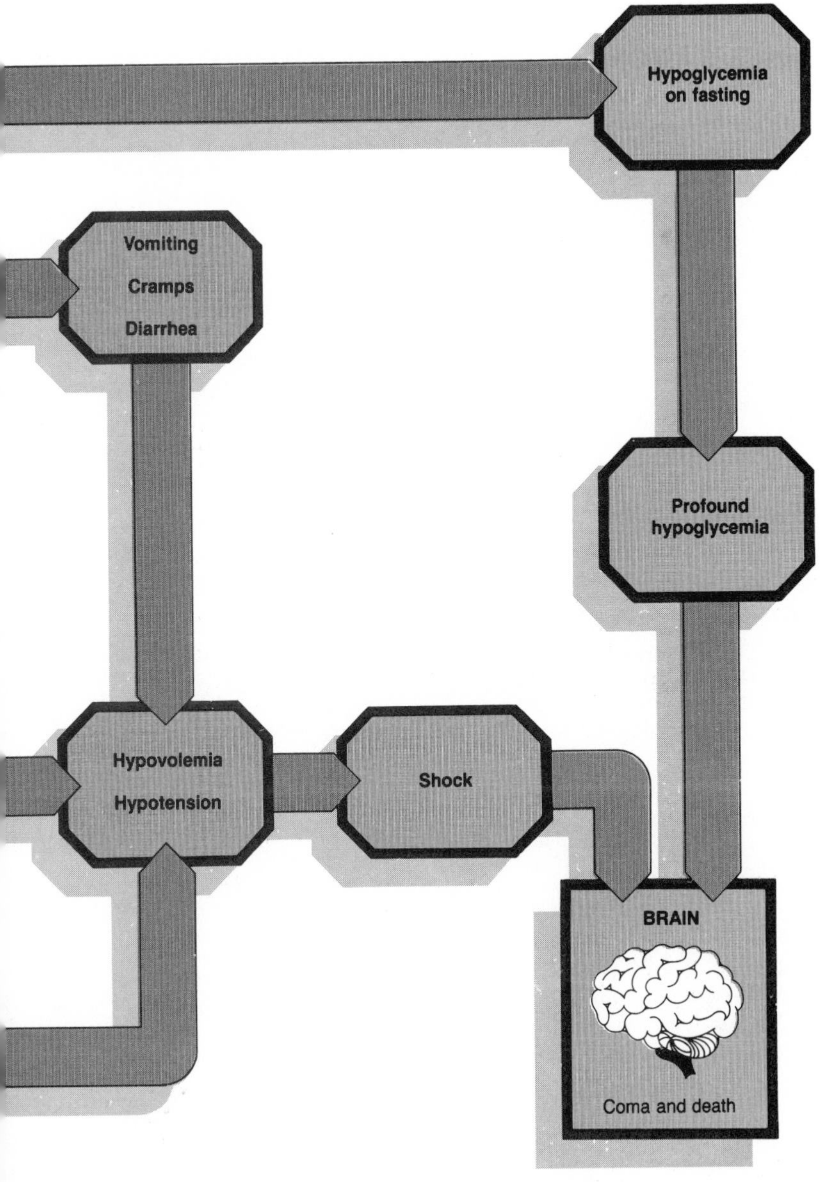

Hypoglycemia on fasting

Vomiting

Cramps

Diarrhea

Profound hypoglycemia

Hypovolemia
Hypotension

Shock

BRAIN

Coma and death

406

PREVENTING ADRENAL CRISIS

Dear Patient:

Even though you're following your treatment plan carefully, unexpected situations can create additional stress and worsen your condition. Because your adrenal glands can no longer meet such increased demands, you should anticipate potentially stressful situations and know what to do to prevent adrenal crisis.

Observe precautions

Always wear a Medic Alert identification bracelet or necklace that contains the following information: a clear statement of your disorder, the telephone number and name of a family member or friend to contact in an emergency, and your doctor's name and telephone number. Also, carry a clearly labeled emergency kit at all times, especially when you travel. The kit should contain a syringe, a needle, and 100 mg of hydrocortisone plus instructions for their use.

Be sure to avoid strenuous physical activity in hot, humid weather. If you begin to sweat heavily, increase your fluid and salt intake.

Follow your doctor's directions for increasing your daily prescribed dosage of glucocorticoids during times of stress, such as an emotional crisis, overexertion, infection, illness, or injury.

Recognize warning signs

Notify your doctor *immediately* (or go directly to the emergency department of the nearest hospital) if you develop any of these warning signs of adrenal crisis:
• weakness
• dizziness
• weak pulse
• fatigue
• cool, clammy skin
• nausea and vomiting or abdominal pain.

If you can't contact your doctor or get to a hospital at once, give yourself a subcutaneous injection of 100 mg of hydrocortisone. Then seek medical help.

Plan for a crisis

Instruct family members to give you a subcutaneous injection of 100 mg of hydrocortisone if they find you unconscious or physically unable to take your oral medication. They should then seek medical help immediately.

crisis (see *Preventing Adrenal Crisis*). If this complication does develop, they should know how to administer hydrocortisone. Finally, because adrenocortical insufficiency is a chronic disorder, recommend that the patient see his doctor regularly.

Diabetes Mellitus

To manage diabetes mellitus successfully, the patient must understand and comply with his prescribed treatment regimen. After all, preventing or at least minimizing complications requires that the patient understand the chronicity and complexity of his disorder. Above all, he must realize the importance of controlling his blood glucose levels.

When teaching the diabetic patient, you'll need to cover a broad range of topics: dietary changes, skin and foot care, self-monitoring of glucose levels, an exercise program, sick-day precautions, and possibly weight reduction and self-medication. And often when you teach you'll need to cover how—and when—to administer replacement doses of insulin.

Despite your best efforts, getting the patient to achieve diabetic control can be quite difficult. After all, diabetic control often requires major and permanent life-style changes. Although you can't ensure the patient's compliance with these changes and other treatment measures, you can improve its likelihood by helping him understand the relationship between good diabetes management and health and recognize the degree of diabetic control being achieved.

Describe the disorder
Explain to the patient that diabetes mellitus is a chronic disorder in which the pancreas fails to produce enough insulin to control blood glucose levels.

CHECKLIST

TEACHING TOPICS IN DIABETES MELLITUS

☐ An explanation of the pathology underlying Type I or Type II diabetes (depending on which type the patient has)

☐ The relationship between good diabetes management and health

☐ Preparation for the oral glucose tolerance test and any other scheduled diagnostic tests

☐ Dietary restrictions, such as exchange lists and the timing of meals and insulin injections

☐ Exercise program and precautions

☐ Medications and how to administer them properly

☐ Techniques for obtaining blood and urine samples

☐ Self-testing of glucose and ketone levels

☐ Sick-day precautions

☐ Foot and skin care

☐ Signs and symptoms of hyperglycemia and hypoglycemia

☐ Preventive measures for reducing long-term complications, such as visiting a podiatrist and ophthalmologist regularly

☐ Sources of additional information and support

In Type I, or insulin-dependent, diabetes, the pancreas fails to produce any insulin in response to elevated blood glucose levels. This type of diabetes occurs most commonly in children but may occur at any age.

Type II, or non-insulin-dependent, diabetes occurs in two forms: the pancreas produces some insulin but not enough to control glucose levels, or the pancreas produces a normal amount of insulin, but the peripheral cell membranes don't have enough insulin receptors to activate all of it. Type II accounts for 80% of all diabetes cases and most commonly occurs in obese patients over age 40. It's thought to be hereditary.

Point out possible complications

To help ensure compliance with treatment, point out to the patient that hypoglycemia and other severe complications can result from untreated or poorly managed diabetes mellitus. Two of these complications—diabetic ketoacidosis (DKA) and hyperglycemic hyperosmolar nonketotic coma (HHNC)—can be fatal without prompt treatment.

In DKA, the glucose-deprived cells use an alternate energy source that produces glycerol (a glucose substance) and ketones. The accumulation of ketones causes metabolic acidosis. In HHNC, blood glucose levels quickly exceed 800 mg/dl for some unknown reason, producing profound dehydration.

Emphasize that hypoglycemia, another acute complication, usually results from an error in management, such as excessive exercise or insulin or insufficient food intake. Untreated, it can cause brain damage and death.

Explain that chronic complications of diabetes are common and greatly affect the patient's quality of life. They include retinopathy, neuropathy, nephropathy, and cardiovascular disease. Although the cause of their development isn't clearly understood, the current suspect is inadequate blood glucose control.

Teach about tests

The diagnostic tests ordered for a suspected diabetic patient will depend on his signs and symptoms. Explain to him that his doctor will order tests to measure glucose levels in his blood, necessitating several blood samples.

If a fasting plasma glucose test is ordered, instruct the patient not to eat or drink anything except water for 12 hours before the test. If a postprandial plasma glucose test is ordered, explain that this test will measure his glucose levels after he's eaten a meal of about 100 g of carbohydrates. If his glucose levels exceed 120 mg/dl 2 hours after the test meal, the diagnosis of diabetes

mellitus is confirmed.

Inform the patient that his insulin levels may be measured, along with his blood glucose levels, to evaluate pancreatic function.

If necessary, teach the patient about the oral glucose tolerance test, which evaluates the body's response to ingestion of glucose. Explain that he'll be put on a diet that ensures a daily intake of 150 to 300 g of carbohydrates for 3 days before the test. Then, for 12 hours before the test, he'll need to fast. Instruct the patient to avoid caffeine, alcohol, strenuous exercise, and smoking during the fasting and testing periods, since these factors can cause misleading test results. Discuss any medications that must be withheld during the test period. Mention that the test itself may last up to 5 hours. Inform him that he'll be given a sweet solution to drink at the start of the test; urge him to drink the entire solution. In the diabetic patient, blood glucose levels will remain elevated for 2 to 3 hours after he drinks the solution.

Teach about treatments

• *Activity.* Regular exercise reduces blood glucose levels, thus lowering insulin requirements. However, the diabetic patient must carefully regulate the amount of exercise he gets according to his food and insulin consumption.

Obtain exercise guidelines from the doctor, then review them with the patient. Encourage him to follow the guidelines to the letter. He should avoid anaerobic exercises, such as weight lifting, because they don't use up glucose. Instead, he should engage in aerobic exercises, such as walking, jogging, cycling, or swimming.

Warn the patient to take safety precautions when exercising. For example, he should always carry a source of simple carbohydrates, as well as an identification tag that gives his name, condition, and medications, just in case he becomes hypoglycemic while exercising. Also, advise him to eat a snack before exercising, if appropriate.

If the patient is taking insulin, advise him not to inject it into a part of his body that he'll use during exercise. Instruct him to avoid exercising at the peak of insulin activity or before meals, and to refrain from drinking alcohol before or during exercise. Also instruct him never to exercise alone.

Caution the patient to stop exercising immediately if he experiences chest pain, severe dyspnea, palpitations, dizziness, weakness, or nausea. If any of these symptoms persist, he should see his doctor at once.

Emphasize to the patient that a balanced program of exercise and rest will help stabilize his blood glucose levels.

• **Diet.** Stress the importance of carefully following the prescribed diet to prevent rapid changes in blood glucose levels. Make sure the patient understands his specific meal plan, and urge him to stick to it. Advise him to eat about the same number of calories each day and to spread out his meals and snacks evenly throughout the day.

Keep in mind that controlling caloric intake is a key factor in regulating blood glucose levels. So, encourage the patient to cut down on the amount he eats. Remember, the less drastic the change in his eating habits, the better the chances he'll comply.

Consider where the patient usually eats his meals. A diabetic patient who eats most of his meals in restaurants will need special instructions. Emphasize that no matter how large the servings at a restaurant, he must restrict himself to eating only the amount specified in his meal plan.

Find out which foods the patient likes and write them on index cards. Color-code the cards by food groups, then explain how many foods per color group he may have for each meal.

If the patient is taking insulin, instruct him to time and limit his meals to match the amount of insulin he injects each day. This will help prevent abrupt shifts in blood glucose levels and possible complications. If exchange lists are included in the treatment regimen, help the patient incorporate them into his daily life by having him plan meals using these lists. Instruct him to avoid foods high in sugar, saturated fats, and cholesterol. His doctor will tell him whether or not he should abstain from drinking alcohol.

In Type II diabetes, diet alone may be enough to control blood glucose levels. Simply eating less will lower the amount of glucose produced and thus the amount of insulin needed to control blood glucose. If the patient is overweight, however, emphasize the importance of weight reduction. An obese patient will need to produce more insulin to control his glucose levels than a patient of normal body weight will. Discuss ways to help the overweight Type II diabetic patient cut down on his caloric intake.

Determine how much fluid the patient drinks daily—and what kinds of fluids he drinks. Then advise him of any changes he should consider. For example, a diabetic patient who drinks several cans of soda daily needs to be taught that he's consuming calories but getting little nutritional benefit in return. If he drinks alcohol regularly and doesn't seem willing to stop or at least cut down, explain that alcohol contains calories that must be counted as part of his daily intake. Also encourage him to seek counseling.

After evaluating the patient's usual elimination patterns, explain that some changes may occur because of treatment. For example, constipation may result if he stops eating certain foods. Teach him to relieve constipation by eating fruits and vegetables.

• **Medication.** If the patient is being discharged on insulin, teach him and a family member, if possible, the correct injection technique (see *Giving Yourself a Subcutaneous Insulin Injection,* pages 410 and 411). If he'll be taking two different kinds of insulin, show him how to mix them in a syringe (see *Mixing Insulins in a Syringe,* page

410

GIVING YOURSELF A SUBCUTANEOUS INSULIN INJECTION

Dear Patient:

To inject insulin subcutaneously, wash your hands thoroughly and remove your prescribed insulin from the refrigerator if it's stored there. Then follow these steps.

1

Warm and mix the insulin by rolling the vial between your palms.

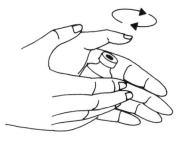

Caution: Never shake the vial. Check the expiration date; then read the label to make sure the medication is the correct strength and type. Use an alcohol swab to cleanse the rubber stopper on top of the vial.

2

Select an appropriate site. (Refer to the guide your nurse gave you, showing you how to rotate your injection sites correctly. To help you remember which site to use, write them on a calendar.)

Pull the skin taut; then clean it with an alcohol swab or a cotton ball soaked in alcohol, using a circular motion.

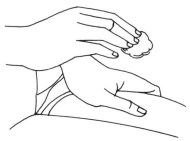

3

Before drawing up the insulin, inject an equal amount of air into the vial. That way you won't create a vacuum in the vial, and it'll be easier to withdraw your insulin.

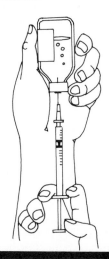

4

If air bubbles appear in the syringe after you fill it with insulin, tap the syringe lightly to remove them. Draw up more insulin, if necessary.

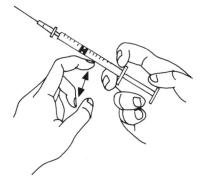

5

Using your thumb and forefinger, pinch the skin at the injection site. Then quickly plunge the needle into the fat fold at a 90-degree angle, up to its hub.

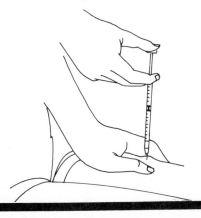

As you hold the syringe with one hand, pull back on the plunger slightly with your other hand to check for a backflow of blood. If blood appears in the syringe, discard everything and start again. If no blood appears, inject the insulin slowly.

6

Place the alcohol swab or cotton ball over the injection site; then press down on it lightly as you withdraw the needle.

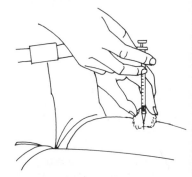

Snap the needle off the syringe, and dispose of both needle and syringe properly.

Important: If you travel, keep a bottle of insulin and a syringe with you at all times. The insulin doesn't need to be refrigerated as long as you keep it away from heat.

MIXING INSULINS IN A SYRINGE

Dear Patient:

Your doctor has prescribed regular and either intermediate or long-acting insulin to control your diabetes. To avoid giving yourself separate injections, you can mix these two types of insulin in a syringe and administer them together. Here's what to do.

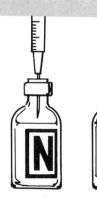

1

Wash your hands; then prepare the mixture in a clean area. Make sure you have alcohol swabs, both types of insulin, and the proper syringe for your prescribed insulin concentration. Then mix the contents of the vials by rolling each one gently between your palms.

2

Using an alcohol swab, clean the rubber stopper on the vial of intermediate or long-acting insulin. Then draw air into the syringe by pulling the plunger back to the prescribed number of insulin units. Insert the needle into the top of the vial, making sure the point doesn't touch the insulin (as shown at the top of the next column). Push in the plunger and withdraw the syringe.

3

Clean the rubber stopper on the regular insulin vial with an alcohol swab. Then pull back the plunger on the syringe to the prescribed number of insulin units, and inject air into the vial. With the needle still in the vial, turn the vial upside down and withdraw the prescribed dose of regular insulin.

4

Clean the top of the intermediate or long-acting insulin vial. Then insert the needle into it without pushing the plunger down. Invert the vial and withdraw the prescribed number of units for the *total* dose. (For example, if you have 10 units of regular insulin in the syringe and you need 20 units of intermediate or long-acting insulin, pull the plunger back to 30 units.)

OBTAINING BLOOD FOR GLUCOSE TESTING

Dear Patient:

To obtain a drop of blood so you can check your glucose level, use a lancet or a mechanical device (Autoclix). You'll also need alcohol wipes.

1

Choose a site on the end of any fingertip. Wash your hands thoroughly and dry. Or wipe the fingertip with alcohol, and let the alcohol evaporate.

2

Squeeze the fingertip with the thumb of the same hand. Place the fingertip (with your thumb still pressed against it) on a firm surface, such as a table.

3

If you're using a lancet, twist off the protective cap. Then grasp the lancet and quickly pierce the fingertip.

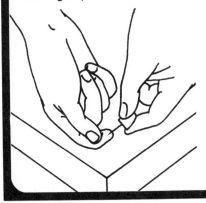

Remove your thumb from the fingertip to release pressure and permit blood flow.

If you're using the Autoclix, depress its plunger to insert a new lancet, and remove the lancet's cap. Then place the lancet at the puncture site and gently press the Autoclix to release the lancet into your fingertip.

4

Milk the finger gently until you get a hanging drop of blood that looks large enough to cover the reagent area of the test strip.

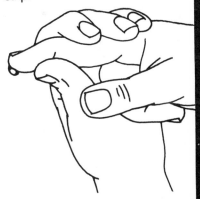

Be patient. If blood doesn't flow immediately from the puncture site, keep milking the finger before trying another site.

TESTING BLOOD FOR GLUCOSE

Dear Patient:

Two types of reagent strips are commonly used to test blood glucose levels visually: Chemstrip bG and Visidex II. (You can also use a glucose meter to measure levels electronically. If you do, be sure to follow the manufacturer's directions precisely.) The following instructions will help you use reagent strips to check your blood glucose levels. The procedure is identical for both types of strips. Here's what to do:

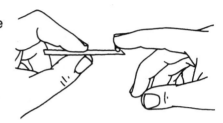

Let the blood completely cover the reagent area *without* rubbing or smearing it. If the blood smears, start over with a new strip.

1

Begin by assembling the necessary equipment: a lancet, a vial with reagent strips, cotton balls, a watch or clock with a second hand, and a pen.

3

As you put the drop of blood on the reagent area, look at your watch or a clock. Wait exactly 60 seconds. Make sure you keep the strip level.

2

Remove a reagent strip from its vial. Then replace the cap, making sure it's tight. Obtain a drop of blood from the end of any fingertip, following the directions the nurse gave you. Carefully lift the strip to the drop of blood. (The strip has a shiny, slippery undersurface; the blood will roll off if you don't place it on the strip correctly.)

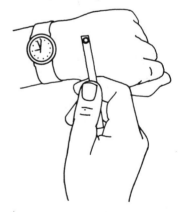

After 60 seconds, gently wipe all the blood off the strip with a clean, dry cotton ball. Wipe the strip three times, using a clean side of the cotton ball each time. Then wait another 60 seconds.

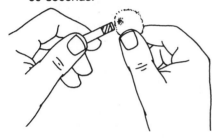

If the colors fall between two blocks, take the average of the two numbers. *Example:* If the colors fall between the two blocks labeled 120 and 180, your blood glucose level is approximately 150 mg/dl.

If the reading exceeds 240 mg/dl, wait another 60 seconds. Then compare the reagent area with the blocks in the 3-minute row.

Note: The reagent strip and vial shown at the bottom of the previous column *do not* appear in their actual colors.

4

Now determine your blood glucose level by holding the reagent strip next to the area of color blocks on the vial. Then match the colors that have appeared on the strip with the two color blocks (in the 2-minute row) on the vial. *Example:* If both colors match the block labeled 120, your blood glucose level is approximately 120 mg/dl.

5

Write the date, time, and your initials on the reagent strip and store it in an empty vial. Make sure the cap is on tight. The colors on the reagent area will last for up to a week.

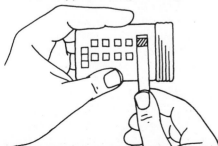

MANAGING DIABETES DURING ILLNESS

Dear Patient:

Minor illnesses—a cold, flu, infection, or upset stomach—can drastically alter your ability to control your blood glucose levels. As your body attempts to compensate for the stress of the illness, your blood glucose levels may rise. To prevent this, maintain your usual insulin schedule and pattern of meals and snacks, if possible, and follow these guidelines:

• Check your blood glucose levels every 4 hours.
• Test your urine for glucose and ketones every 4 hours.
• *Never* skip an insulin injection.
• Call the doctor if you can't eat or keep any food or liquids down, if you can't eat normally for more than 24 hours, or if you have a fever.
• If you live alone, arrange for someone to check on you several times during the day.

In addition, you can use this list of foods and liquids to guide you through the different stages of an illness. Just follow the instructions for your stage of illness. You don't have to start with stage 1 and progress through the remaining stages. You could, for example, start with stage 3, depending on your symptoms. Also, if your symptoms get worse and you can't tolerate recommended foods, you can drop back one stage until you feel better.

Stage 1
Your symptoms: severe nausea and vomiting, severe diarrhea, fever

Allowable foods and beverages: orange, grapefruit, or tomato juice; soup; broth; tea; coffee; cola

Special instructions: Sip a teaspoon of liquid every 10 to 15 minutes. If you can't tolerate this, call your doctor. Advance to stage 2 when nausea and diarrhea stop (or almost stop) and you're no longer vomiting.

Stage 2
Your symptoms: little or no appetite, occasional diarrhea, fatigue, fever

Allowable foods and beverages: cream soup, mashed potatoes, cooked cereal, plain yogurt, bananas, fruit-flavored gelatins, juice, broth, regular soft drinks

Special instructions: Take ½ to 1 cup of food or beverage every 1 to 2 hours. Because fever causes you to perspire and lose body fluids, you should also continue to sip an unsweetened beverage (tea or coffee without sugar, water, or diet soft drinks, for example) every 10 or 15 minutes. You're ready to advance to stage 3 when you've consumed the suggested amount of food and liquids several times, and your symptoms are improving.

Stage 3

Your symptoms: limited appetite, small meals tolerated, sluggishness, slight fever, able to sit up or walk

Allowable foods and beverages: Use your diabetic meal plan to guide you through this stage of your illness. (If you don't have one, talk to a diet counselor.) You can skip the protein and fat foods listed on your meal plan.

• Milk list: You can eat one of these foods instead of drinking 1 cup of milk—½ cup of eggnog or sweetened custard; or 1 cup of cream soup or plain yogurt.

• Bread and cereal list: You can eat one of the following foods instead of one bread or starch serving—¼ cup of sherbet; ½ cup of cooked cereal, mashed potatoes, ice cream, or fruit-flavored gelatin; ¾ cup of regular soft drink; 1 cup of noodle soup; or five salted crackers.

• Vegetable list: You can eat ½ serving from the bread and cereal serving list.

• Fruit list: You can eat any of these foods instead of one fruit serving—¼ cup of grape or prune juice; ⅓ cup of apple juice; ½ cup of unsweetened applesauce, regular soft drink, or orange or grapefruit juice; ½ of a banana or popsicle; or 2 teaspoons of honey.

Special instructions: Eat as many meals and snacks as your meal plan calls for. Advance to stage 4 when your appetite increases and you can eat these meals without any problems. If you still have a fever, drink several extra glasses of water, tea or coffee without sugar, or diet soft drink each day.

Stage 4

Your symptoms: general sick feeling, stomach upset by heavy or spicy foods

Allowable foods and beverages: Use food lists on your regular meal plan. Choose foods that don't give you problems. For protein, you might want to try cottage cheese, broiled fish, or baked chicken. Eat fruit, vegetables, starch, and protein in moderation.

Special instructions: Eat at regular meal and snack times. Use your regular diabetic meal plan if you have no problems with the easier-to-digest foods for a day.

TAKING CARE OF YOUR FEET

Dear Patient:

To avoid serious complications from your diabetes, follow these foot care instructions.

Routine care

Wash your feet daily with mild soap and warm water. (Don't use hot water, to prevent burns.) Dry your feet carefully, especially between the toes. If your skin is dry, apply lanolin ointment. If your feet tend to sweat, apply a mild foot powder, but make sure it doesn't cake.

Cut your toenails straight across and file them carefully to eliminate rough edges. Do this under good light after washing your feet. If your nails are too thick to cut, or if they tend to crack when you cut them, have a podiatrist cut them.

Inspect your feet daily— around the nails, between the toes, and the soles too. Look for corns, calluses, redness, swelling, bruises, or breaks in the skin.

Corns and calluses

To treat corns or calluses, soak your feet, rub them gently with a towel, and apply lanolin ointment. Repeat once or twice a day until corns or calluses improve. If they don't, see a podiatrist. *Caution*: Never use over-the-counter corn remedies and never cut corns or calluses with a razor or knife.

Special precautions

Keep these precautions in mind to prevent foot injuries.
- Make sure new shoes fit comfortably and support, protect, and cover your feet completely. Break them in gradually.
- Never go barefoot.
- Don't use hot-water bottles, heating pads, or ice on your legs or feet.
- If a foot injury causes a break in the skin, wash the affected area with soap and water immediately. Cover it with a dry sterile gauze bandage. Change the bandage daily and inspect for redness, swelling, and drainage.

Notifying your doctor

Call your doctor if any foot injury doesn't improve in 72 hours. Also call him if you notice any of these signs of impaired circulation when examining your feet:
- new sores or ulcers that take unusually long to heal
- unusual, persistent warmth or coolness
- numbness or muscle weakness
- swelling that doesn't go down after you raise your leg.

412). Give him a site rotation chart and stress the importance of rotating injection sites regularly.

If the patient is taking oral hypoglycemics, make sure he understands that they have been ordered as adjunctive therapy and aren't meant to replace dietary restrictions.

Instruct the patient to take his prescribed medication exactly as ordered. Emphasize that he should never change the dosage or stop taking his medication without first consulting his doctor.

• *Procedures.* Teach the patient how to collect a blood sample (see *Obtaining Blood for Glucose Testing,* page 413). Also teach him how to test urine or blood glucose levels (see *Testing Blood for Glucose,* pages 414 and 415). Also demonstrate how to test urine ketone levels during periods of illness. Teach him how to interpret the results and what to do if they're abnormal.

• *Other care measures.* You'll need to teach the patient about other daily care measures and ways to deal with special problems. For instance, you'll need to teach him how to manage diabetes during illness (see *Managing Diabetes During Illness,* pages 416 and 417). You'll also need to teach the patient about the signs of hypoglycemia—anxiety, hunger, diaphoresis, nausea, lethargy, personality changes, and diplopia. Inform the patient that excessive insulin, inadequate food, and overexertion can induce hypoglycemia.

Teach the patient about precautions to prevent infection and complications. For example, tell him to avoid extreme temperature changes to reduce the risk of infection, especially respiratory tract infection. Teach him to provide meticulous skin and foot care (see *Taking Care of Your Feet,* page 418). Advise him to keep his hands and feet warm during cold weather. If necessary, he should wear two or more pairs of socks. Warn him not to use a hot-water bottle; he may burn himself because of reduced sensation.

Keep in mind that some diabetic patients develop neuropathies. Most often, they affect the patient's legs. Assess your patient carefully for such sensory deficits, and explain the importance of caring for the affected area. Also, teach him the signs and symptoms of impaired circulation, such as dependent edema, pallor, paresthesias, and hair loss on the affected limb.

Abnormal blood glucose levels may impair vision. As a result, when teaching the diabetic patient who has a vision problem, make sure the booklets and other teaching aids you give him have large type. Explain that he should always read with a strong light behind him. Also, advise him to have regular eye examinations.

Instruct the patient to be especially careful to avoid accidents. Remember, even a relatively minor injury—such as a stubbed toe—can be serious for a diabetic patient; he could develop an infection from circulatory problems. Recommend the use of a night-light or flashlight for the patient who habitually goes to the bathroom in the middle of the night.

If the patient works, ask him about his job. Is he likely to cut or bruise himself at work? If he is, advise him to be extremely cautious. Teach him how to treat such injuries in case they do occur.

If the diabetic patient travels for business or vacation, explain that he should make plans for meals and medication beforehand. Tell him that airlines, for example, will provide a diabetic diet if he gives them a day's notice. An insulin-dependent patient who's traveling outside his home state should take along an insulin prescription and syringes. In some states, you can't buy insulin and syringes over the counter. And in some countries, only U-40 and U-80 insulin are available.

If the patient is traveling by plane, tell him to keep his insulin and syringes with him in case baggage areas aren't heated or pressurized or his baggage is lost. If he's crossing time zones, teach him to adjust his schedule accordingly.

If you're teaching a diabetic patient

who lives alone, spend a little extra time with him; he may find it more difficult to comply with therapy than the patient who has a spouse or other family member to encourage him. Ask the patient how he deals with stress. Many people overeat when they're frustrated or anxious. A diabetic patient who tries to cope with stress in this way won't be able to control his blood glucose levels.

Keep in mind that diabetic patients, particularly men, may experience sexual dysfunction, such as impotence. Since most patients probably won't bring up this subject on their own, you should mention it. Encourage the patient to discuss any sexual problems he may be having.

If a female diabetic patient is pregnant or plans to become pregnant, refer her to a specialist who cares for diabetic patients of childbearing age.

Suggest that the patient join the local chapter of the American Diabetes Association. Explain that members of this organization help each other cope with their condition.

Graves' Disease

Although chronic, Graves' disease can be a relatively benign condition, providing the patient complies with therapy. Fortunately, the patient will probably be motivated to comply if he understands his disease and the importance of keeping his metabolic rate under control. After all, Graves' disease can be managed successfully with several therapies that will allow him to lead a nearly normal life. Graves' disease itself is a hormonal imbalance that may be controlled with medications that reduce thyroid hormone levels. Its resulting symptoms—weight loss, fatigue, and irritability—can be minimized through diet and restricted activity until a euthyroid state is achieved. For some patients, radioac-

tive iodine therapy or subtotal thyroidectomy may be necessary to decrease thyroid hormone production.

Describe the disorder
Explain to the patient that Graves' disease is a chronic condition in which the thyroid gland produces an excessive amount of thyroid hormone. Overproduction of thyroid hormone accelerates all bodily functions and activities.

Explain that the exact cause of Graves' disease is unknown, but that it may be related to an immune defect that causes formation of abnormal antibodies. According to the most widely accepted theory, these antibodies are actually protein substances that stimulate the thyroid gland to produce thyroid hormone regardless of whether the body needs it. This results in excessive circulating levels of thyroid hormone.

Inform the patient that elevated thyroid hormone levels increase the rate at which his body uses energy. This can lead to a wide range of symptoms affecting all body systems. In the cardiovascular system, for example, an accelerated heart rate can produce flushing, palpitations, congestive heart failure, and other cardiac symptoms. In the nervous system, effects include emotional instability, difficulty concentrating, and insomnia.

Point out possible complications
To stress the importance of complying with therapy, point out to the patient that serious complications can develop from untreated or poorly managed hyperthyroidism. For example, thyroid storm, an acute complication, can be fatal without prompt treatment. In thyroid storm, the patient's metabolic rate accelerates rapidly, producing a state of extreme hypermetabolism. The functions of all body systems become severely taxed. Body temperature may rise as high as 106° F. (41° C.); both heart and respiratory rates rise dramatically. Total systemic collapse be-

comes imminent.

Explain to the patient that compliance with therapy can also forestall common chronic complications of hyperthyroidism, such as cardiac dysfunction, weight loss, and diarrhea.

Teach about tests

You'll need to teach the patient about the tests commonly used to evaluate thyroid function. Explain that these tests require a small blood sample drawn by venipuncture. Studies will be done on thyroid hormone itself or on its by-products found in the blood.

Serum thyroxine (T_4) levels are used to screen for Graves' disease. Elevated levels confirm hyperthyroidism. A serum long-acting thyroid stimulating test may then be ordered to determine if the abnormal antibody thought to be responsible for Graves' disease is present. If it is, the hyperthyroidism is attributed to Graves' disease.

Occasionally, a T_3 resin uptake test is ordered to further evaluate thyroid function. An elevated T_3 level strengthens a diagnosis of hyperthyroidism. A thyroid scan may also be ordered to aid diagnosis.

If the only clinical finding suggesting Graves' disease is an eye abnormality, such as exophthalmos, then a thyrotropin releasing hormone (TRH) infusion test may be done. Explain to the patient that this test will help determine if Graves' disease is causing his symptoms. The test involves injection of the TRH, followed by a series of blood samples drawn periodically over the next hour.

Inform the patient that a thyroid scan or thyroid ultrasonogram may be done after the TRH infusion test. These studies show the structure of the thyroid gland and may reveal abnormalities in its size or shape. (See *Teaching Patients about Endocrine Tests*, page 431.)

Teach about treatments

● *Activity.* Instruct the patient to restrict physical activity, since any form of exertion will only increase his met-

---

CHECKLIST

TEACHING TOPICS IN GRAVES' DISEASE

☑ ☐
☐ ☑
☑ ☐

☐ Pathophysiology of Graves' disease, including how excessive levels of thyroid hormone occur

☐ Complications, such as thyroid storm

☐ Blood tests and X-rays necessary to evaluate thyroid function

☐ Dietary measures to ensure sufficient caloric intake

☐ Activity restrictions to help counteract increased metabolism

☐ Relationship of stress to hormonal balance

☐ Medications and their administration

☐ Radioactive iodine therapy, if indicated

☐ Subtotal thyroidectomy, if indicated, and possible need for lifelong hormonal replacement therapy

☐ Eye care, if exophthalmos or visual changes occur

---

abolic rate and exacerbate his irritability. Encourage him to engage instead in activities that require minimal physical exertion—reading, for example—and to rest frequently. Reassure him that he'll be able to resume his customary activities when his metabolic rate returns to normal.

● *Diet.* Stress the importance of following the prescribed diet to prevent nutritional deficiencies, such as vitamin A and B deficiencies. Advise the patient to eat well-balanced meals each day, plus snacks, so that his caloric intake can keep up with the rapid expenditure of calories caused by hypermetabolism. (Once he's regained the weight he lost, he should cut his caloric intake back to normal.) Caution him to avoid caffeine, yellow and red food dyes, and artificial preservatives, since these substances will make him more irritable. If necessary, arrange for nutritional counseling.

● *Medication.* Teach the patient about

thyroid hormone antagonists, if prescribed. (See *Teaching Patients about Endocrine Drugs*, pages 432 to 435, for more information.) Also teach him about other prescribed drugs, such as propranolol to control cardiac effects and tranquilizers to control irritability and hyperactivity. Warn him to avoid taking aspirin and any aspirin-containing drugs, since they increase the metabolic rate.

● *Procedures.* Radioactive iodine therapy is an alternative treatment for Graves' disease if thyroid hormone antagonists are ineffective. If the patient's scheduled for this treatment, explain that its purpose is to decrease the thyroid's production of thyroid hormone by destroying thyroid tissue. Reassure him that the procedure is painless and won't harm other body tissue. But be sure he understands the risk of hypothyroidism, which can result from excessive destruction of thyroid tissue.

Tell the patient that the procedure entails drinking a tasteless, colorless, radioactive solution or swallowing a radioactive capsule. Review the precautions he'll need to take after the procedure. For example, tell him to avoid close contact with pregnant women, infants, and children for 1 week. During the first 48 hours after the procedure, he should flush the toilet immediately after urinating and use disposable plates and silverware, since his urine and saliva will be temporarily radioactive. Warn family members to avoid contact with the patient's bodily fluids, such as saliva, during this time. Reassure the patient and his family that the radioactive iodine poses no hazard once 48 hours have passed.

Inform the patient that symptoms of Graves' disease should subside in 3 to 4 weeks after therapy begins. If they don't, the patient may need a second round of therapy after several months.

● *Surgery.* If the patient is scheduled for a subtotal thyroidectomy, instruct him to increase his caloric intake to regain weight. (The operation may have to be delayed until he gains back any weight he lost. It may take up to 3 months of proper nourishment to prepare him for this surgery.) If a special preoperative diet (such as a high-protein diet) has been ordered, explain its purpose and urge strict compliance. Remind the patient to avoid caffeine and other stimulants, which will aggravate his condition.

During a subtotal thyroidectomy, more than 80% of the thyroid is removed, significantly reducing the gland's ability to produce thyroid hormone. Explain that the incision will be made in the patient's lower neck.

Explain the purpose of thyroid medication ordered preoperatively—to suppress secretion of thyroid hormone so that an excessive amount isn't released during surgery. Iodine preparations may also be ordered to decrease blood flow to the thyroid, thereby minimizing bleeding during surgery.

Before surgery, review preoperative and postoperative procedures. Be sure to explain preoperative preparation of the incision site.

Show the patient how to avoid putting stress on his incision postoperatively by placing his hands behind his head for support whenever he wants to turn. When rising to a sitting position, he should support his head with a pillow and put his hands together behind his head. If the patient has difficulty swallowing, he should report it immediately. Mention that cold drinks and ice will help relieve discomfort. Also mention that he'll be on a soft diet temporarily.

Tell the patient that his voice will be checked periodically for hoarseness after surgery. Advise him to talk as little as possible during the first few days postoperatively. If he has difficulty breathing, he should report it at once. Oxygen may have to be administered. He can expect to be out of bed on the first day after surgery.

Reassure him that he'll receive pain medication postoperatively. Inform him that sutures or surgical clips are usually removed on the second postoperative day, just before discharge.

To prepare the patient for discharge, teach him how to take care of his incision at home. Make sure he understands the importance of adequate rest and nutrition during recovery. Tell him to report signs of infection and hypothyroidism promptly to his doctor.

• **Other care measures.** Advise the patient and family to avoid stressful situations, which can exacerbate the patient's irritability. Advise keeping environmental stimulation to a minimum. For example, the patient should avoid watching television programs or movies that may cause him to become excited or upset. Reassure both the patient and his family that behavioral changes, such as irritability, anxiety, lack of concentration, and fatigue, are related to hyperthyroidism and will subside with treatment.

If ophthalmopathy is present, teach the patient the essentials of good eye care. Advise him to wear sunglasses and to avoid irritating his eyes. If eye drops are ordered, show him how to instill them. Instruct him to limit his fluid and salt intake to minimize fluid retention. Such retention will cause the eyeball to protrude even further.

Suggest that the patient sleep with his head elevated to aid drainage, thereby preventing fluid from accumulating behind the eyes. Instruct him to notify his doctor at once if visual changes, such as blurring, occur. Advise him to see an ophthalmologist regularly.

Hypoglycemia

Because hypoglycemia is a chronic disorder, its management can present an unceasing challenge to the patient. Most of all, the patient must learn to recognize the telltale symptoms of a hypoglycemic episode. And he must learn to provide prompt treatment to prevent possibly irreversible tissue damage.

CHECKLIST

TEACHING TOPICS IN HYPOGLYCEMIA

☐ An explanation of the patient's type of hypoglycemia: fasting or reactive

☐ Emergency treatment of a hypoglycemic episode

☐ Symptoms of hypoglycemia and hyperglycemia

☐ Preparation for diagnostic tests to help distinguish between fasting and reactive hypoglycemia, such as a fasting plasma glucose test

☐ Dietary modifications to prevent alterations in blood glucose levels

☐ Weight reduction, if necessary

☐ Medications and their administration

☐ Surgery, if necessary

☐ Prevention of hypoglycemic episodes

Although the patient may appreciate the urgency of promptly treating a hypoglycemic episode, he may have difficulty complying with the life-style changes involved in his treatment plan. That's because hypoglycemia can cause fatigue, an inability to concentrate, and considerable discomfort.

You'll need to support the patient in overcoming these barriers so that he can comply with necessary dietary changes, weight reduction (if necessary), drug regimens, and other characteristic treatment measures.

Describe the disorder

Explain to the patient that hypoglycemia occurs when glucose, the body's major energy source, isn't being produced fast enough or is being used too rapidly. Mention that a certain amount of glucose must always be present in the blood to meet the energy needs of vital tissues, such as brain cells. How low blood glucose levels must fall before triggering a hypoglycemic reaction varies greatly among individuals. Typically, a blood glucose level below

50 mg/dl causes symptoms.

Explain to the patient that the nature of his symptoms may reveal how rapidly glucose levels fall. For example, nervousness and an elevated heart rate and blood pressure can result from a rapid decline in glucose levels. Changes in mental status can result from a slow decline.

Explain the patient's type of hypoglycemia: fasting or reactive. In *fasting hypoglycemia*, blood glucose levels fall below normal about 5 hours after a meal, possibly causing changes in mental status and distressing pangs of hunger with prolonged fasting—during the night, for example. Untreated, fasting hypoglycemia may eventually cause seizures and loss of consciousness. These severe symptoms may resist even prompt treatment.

Fasting hypoglycemia most commonly results from alcohol or drugs, particularly insulin, oral hypoglycemics, and medications (such as salicylates) that exaggerate the effects of oral hypoglycemics. Some patients, though, have a rare form of fasting hypoglycemia caused by pancreatic tumors or liver disease.

Reactive hypoglycemia usually occurs within a few hours after a meal. Its characteristic symptoms are rarely severe, however, and resolve quickly with treatment. Three types of reactive hypoglycemia have been identified: alimentary hypoglycemia, hypoglycemia secondary to early Type II diabetes mellitus or impaired glucose tolerance, and idiopathic reactive hypoglycemia.

Alimentary hypoglycemia reflects digestive dysfunction, usually from extensive gastric surgery. In this type of reactive hypoglycemia, food passes through the stomach and enters the small intestine more rapidly than normal, causing glucose to be absorbed quickly. This produces hyperglycemia, which stimulates the release of an excessive amount of insulin. The insulin, in turn, causes blood glucose levels to drop abruptly. Alimentary hypoglycemia usually occurs within 1 to 3 hours after a patient eats a meal.

Reactive hypoglycemia secondary to early Type II diabetes mellitus or impaired glucose tolerance rarely occurs. It produces an abrupt drop in blood glucose levels 3 to 5 hours after a meal, but just why this happens remains a mystery. One theory: delayed and excessive insulin secretion, triggered by carbohydrate ingestion, causes the drop.

Idiopathic reactive hypoglycemia occurs more often than the other two types. Its hallmark is a rapid drop in blood glucose levels 2 to 5 hours after the patient eats a meal containing carbohydrates. The exact cause of idiopathic reactive hypoglycemia is unknown. Explain to the patient with this type of reactive hypoglycemia that his symptoms will subside with appropriate therapy within 20 minutes. Such symptoms include sweating, tremors, and dizziness. Reassure the patient that his condition doesn't predispose him to diabetes mellitus, as is commonly believed.

Point out possible complications

Emphasize the importance of preventing or promptly treating hypoglycemic episodes to avoid severe complications. Make sure your patient understands that the key danger with hypoglycemia is that once it occurs, he may suddenly lose his ability to think clearly. If this should happen while he's driving a car or operating machinery, it could cause a serious accident.

Explain that brain cells can't survive long without glucose. Prolonged or severe hypoglycemia will cause permanent brain damage and could be fatal.

Teach about tests

Explain to the patient that the diagnostic workup will depend on whether his symptoms are related to eating or fasting. Once the doctor determines this, serial blood glucose studies will be performed.

Inform the patient that blood tests

aim to confirm low blood glucose levels during a hypoglycemic episode. Review the symptoms of hypoglycemia with him, and tell him to notify you as soon as any of these symptoms occur, so that a blood sample can be drawn before treatment begins. If a fasting plasma glucose level is ordered, instruct the patient not to eat or drink anything except water for 12 hours before the test.

Inform the patient with suspected fasting hypoglycemia that the results of a fasting plasma glucose test may be inconclusive. If so, he'll need to be admitted to the hospital so that the fasting period may be extended another 24 to 72 hours. Explain that the liver can provide enough glucose to maintain adequate blood levels during a prolonged fast. But if his hypoglycemia results from an underlying pathology, such as an insulinoma, then test results will show it.

Tell the patient that insulin levels will be measured to evaluate pancreatic function. If an insulinoma is present, insulin levels will be elevated.

Teach the patient about other ordered diagnostic tests, such as an oral glucose tolerance test (OGTT), an I.V. glucose tolerance test, and a C-peptide assay. If the patient's scheduled for an OGTT, explain that this test helps diagnose reactive hypoglycemia. Explain that the doctor will place him on a diet that ensures a daily intake of 150 to 300 g of carbohydrates for 3 days before the test. Then, for 12 hours before the test, inform the patient that he'll need to fast. Also tell him to avoid caffeine, alcohol, strenuous exercise, and smoking during the fasting and testing periods, since these factors can cause misleading test results. Discuss any medications that must be withheld during the test period. Mention that the test itself will last 5 hours. Inform him that he'll be given a sweet solution to drink at the start of the test. Urge the patient to drink the entire solution, and instruct him to notify you immediately if symptoms of hypoglycemia occur. Make sure

he understands that the interval between ingestion of the glucose solution and the onset of symptoms can help determine what type of reactive hypoglycemia he has.

If the patient's scheduled for an I.V. glucose tolerance test, explain that this test helps detect fasting hypoglycemia caused by insulinomas and other tumors that secrete insulin or an insulin-like substance. Prepare the patient for the test in the same manner as for an OGTT. Point out, however, that instead of being given oral glucose to drink, he'll receive I.V. a substance known to stimulate insulin secretion (such as tolbutamide, glucagon, or leucine). Here again, the patient should be taught the importance of reporting hypoglycemic symptoms immediately. If such symptoms occurred, the test would be stopped, and he would be treated promptly.

If the patient's scheduled for a C-peptide assay, explain that this test helps diagnose fasting hypoglycemia. It also differentiates fasting hypoglycemia caused by an insulinoma from fasting hypoglycemia caused by insulin injections.

Teach about treatments

● *Diet.* Emphasize the importance of carefully following the prescribed diet to prevent a rapid drop in blood glucose levels. Discuss the patient's specific meal plan with him, and encourage him to stick to it. Advise him to eat small meals throughout the day. Mention that nighttime snacks may be necessary to keep his blood glucose at an even level. Also, instruct the patient to avoid alcohol and caffeine, since they may trigger severe hypoglycemic episodes.

Instruct the patient with reactive hypoglycemia to avoid simple carbohydrates and meals with a high carbohydrate content. Such meals load the body with glucose and may stimulate excessive production of insulin, triggering a hypoglycemic episode. Help the patient plan low-carbohydrate,

HYPOGLYCEMIA OR HYPERGLYCEMIA?

Use this list to help distinguish between hypoglycemia and hyperglycemia.

HYPOGLYCEMIA	HYPERGLYCEMIA
Causes	**Causes**
• Excessive insulin or exercise • Inadequate or delayed food intake	• Insufficient insulin • Failure to follow prescribed diet • Infection, fever, or emotional stress
Symptoms	**Symptoms**
• Diaphoresis • Faintness • Headache • Palpitations • Trembling • Impaired vision • Hunger • Difficulty awakening • Irritability • Personality changes	• Polydipsia and polyuria • Increased blood glucose and ketone levels • Weakness, abdominal pain, generalized aches • Deep, rapid breathing • Anorexia, nausea, and vomiting
Interventions	**Interventions**
• Give the patient food or liquid containing sugar (orange juice, cola, candy). • Don't give fluids if the patient is unconscious. • Call the doctor.	• Call the doctor immediately. • Give the patient *sugar-free* fluids (if he can swallow). • Test urine frequently for glucose and acetone.

high-protein meals. Go over the foods belonging to these food groups with him. Also, instruct him to add fiber to his diet. Explain that fiber delays the absorption of glucose from the GI tract.

If the patient is obese and has early-onset diabetes mellitus or impaired glucose tolerance, suggest ways that he can restrict his caloric intake and lose weight. If necessary, recommend that he join a support group.

The patient with fasting hypoglycemia, on the other hand, will need to increase his caloric intake. Explain to him that his body needs more glucose to counteract excessive insulin secretion. Meals and snacks should never be postponed or skipped. Otherwise, severe and possibly prolonged hypoglycemia may develop. Tell him to call his doctor for instructions if he doesn't feel well enough to eat.

• *Medication.* Teach the patient about prescribed drug therapy. For example, if an antianxiety drug such as diazepam is prescribed, warn the patient that it may cause drowsiness. Advise him to avoid potentially hazardous activities, such as driving a car or other activities that require alertness, until this adverse reaction subsides.

If medication has been prescribed to delay gastric emptying in reactive hypoglycemia, instruct the patient accordingly (see Chapter 8). Propranolol may also be ordered to alleviate symptoms of a hypoglycemic episode, such as hypertension, sweating, tachycardia, and palpitations.

If the patient has an inoperable insulinoma, explain that diazoxide helps treat fasting hypoglycemia by inhibiting insulin release. Together with a high-calorie diet, it will help maintain

MANAGING A HYPOGLYCEMIC EPISODE

Dear Caregiver:

A sudden hypoglycemic episode may affect the ability of the person in your care to recognize his symptoms and take appropriate action. It'll be up to you to manage the crisis for him. In such an emergency, you *must* raise his blood glucose levels immediately to prevent permanent brain damage and even death. So be sure you have sources of glucose available.

If the person is *unconscious* or has trouble swallowing, you'll have to give him a subcutaneous injection of glucagon, following the directions the nurse gave you. Then, you'll need to call the doctor immediately.

If the person is *conscious,* give him any of the following:

FOOD/FLUID	AMOUNT
Apple juice, orange juice, or ginger ale	4 oz
Regular cola or other soft drink	3 oz
Corn syrup, honey, or grape jelly	2 oz
Lifesavers	5
Jelly beans	6
Gumdrops	10

adequate blood glucose levels. (See *Teaching Patients about Endocrine Drugs,* pages 432 to 435.)

If chemotherapy has been ordered to treat inoperable tumors, explain the protocol to the patient and the possible adverse reactions to each drug.

Advise the patient not to take non-prescription medications, such as antihistamines, without his doctor's approval. Explain that many nonprescription medications contain ingredients that will mask symptoms of decreased blood glucose levels or induce hypoglycemia.

● **Surgery.** If your patient is scheduled for surgery to remove an extrapancreatic tumor or insulinoma causing fasting hypoglycemia, you'll need to prepare him for the operation. Review standard preoperative and postoperative procedures as you would with any patient scheduled for abdominal or thoracic surgery.

After surgery, provide appropriate discharge instructions. Most important, instruct the patient to notify his doctor if symptoms of hypoglycemia recur. He should also know the symptoms of hyperglycemia, such as increased urine output and thirst. (See *Hypoglycemia or Hyperglycemia?,* page 426). Hyperglycemia may occur postoperatively if some insulin-producing cells in the pancreas were destroyed during surgery.

● **Other care measures.** Teach the patient and his family the symptoms of hypoglycemia, such as tremors, palpitations, confusion, and sweating. Review treatment measures for hypoglycemic episodes and make sure they understand the importance of *immediate* care (see *Managing a Hypoglycemic Episode,* page 427). Also, teach them how to administer glucagon. Advise the patient and family to notify the doctor if hypoglycemic episodes don't respond to treatment or occur frequently.

Teach the patient how to prevent hypoglycemic episodes. Discuss his lifestyle and personal habits to help him identify precipitating factors, such as poor diet, stress, or mismanagement of diabetes mellitus. Explore ways in which the patient can change or avoid each precipitating factor you've identified. If necessary, teach him stress-reduction techniques and encourage him to join a support group. For the patient with reactive hypoglycemia, review the essentials of managing diabetes mellitus, if indicated. (See "Diabetes Mellitus," pages 407 to 420.) Finally, because hypoglycemia is a chronic disorder, encourage the patient to see his doctor regularly.

Hypothyroidism

Despite being relatively easy to manage and requiring few life-style changes, hypothyroidism can nevertheless have devastating effects if left untreated or managed improperly. Both acute and chronic complications may occur, affecting the quality of the patient's life and possibly even shortening his life span. That's why it's important for you to teach the patient about the chronic nature of his disorder. Most important, you'll need to stress the need for his compliance with lifelong thyroid hormone replacement therapy. Other areas you'll need to cover include dietary and activity precautions and possible adjunctive care measures.

Describe the disorder
Inform the patient that hypothyroidism is a chronic disorder in which the thyroid gland fails to secrete sufficient thyroid hormone. Explain the patient's type of hypothyroidism: primary or secondary.

Primary hypothyroidism results from gradual destruction of vital tissue within the thyroid gland. The most common cause of primary hypothyroidism *without* goiter is radioactive iodine therapy or surgery. Other causes include thyroid tumor, iodine imbalance, and excessive consumption of vegetables that interfere with thyroid function. The most common cause of primary hypothyroidism *with* goiter is Hashimoto's thyroiditis, in which lymphocytes mistake normal thyroid cells for foreign cells and destroy them.

Secondary hypothyroidism, which rarely occurs, results from the destruction of pituitary tissue responsible for producing thyroid-stimulating hormone (TSH). Without TSH stimulation, the thyroid gland is unable to produce thyroid hormone.

Explain to the patient how hypothyroidism affects the body. For example, explain that thyroid hormone deficiency causes a significant decrease in the body's ability to use energy. As a result, cells don't function effectively and use up what little energy is available to them. This causes the patient to tire easily.

Review the specific effects of thyroid deficiency on each body system, clarifying the patient's symptoms.

Point out possible complications

To underscore the importance of complying with therapy, point out to the patient the complications that might occur if hypothyroidism is poorly managed or left untreated. Myxedema, for example, is a major complication of hypothyroidism that develops gradually. In its early stages, it produces generalized symptoms, such as fatigue and lethargy. Later, changes involving the skin and hair may occur—for example, cool, dry skin; decreased sweat and oil production; thinning of scalp hair; and loss of body hair.

Impaired muscle function from myxedema predisposes the patient to complications, such as constipation and urinary tract infection. Decreased lung expansion raises the risk of respiratory infection. As myxedema worsens, profound hypotension, bradycardia, hypoventilation, and hypothermia may develop. The patient must understand that without prompt treatment this

---

---

complication can be fatal.

Other chronic complications of uncontrolled hypothyroidism are related to the accumulation of fatty substances in interstitial tissues and to decreased metabolism. Atherosclerosis leading to cardiovascular dysfunction is one such complication. Make sure the patient realizes the seriousness of these potential problems. Reassure him, however, that these complications can be prevented by carefully following prescribed treatment.

Teach about tests

To prepare the patient for diagnostic testing, explain to him that thyroid hormone deficiency is easily confirmed by measuring the thyroxine level in his blood. Additional blood studies will be necessary to see if the pituitary gland is producing enough thyrotropin to stimulate the thyroid. An elevated thyrotropin level confirms primary hypothyroidism.

A thyrotropin releasing hormone (TRH) infusion test may be ordered to measure the pituitary's reserve of thyrotropin if the patient's thyrotropin level is normal or borderline. Explain to the patient that this procedure requires the insertion of an I.V. catheter and the infusion of synthetic TRH through it. Tell the patient that several blood samples will be drawn over the course of an hour or so, and that the catheter will be removed after the last sample has been collected. If the pituitary responds to the TRH infusion by releasing an excessive amount of TSH, primary hypothyroidism is indicated; a blunted response indicates secondary hypothyroidism.

Teach about treatments

• *Activity.* Because patients with hypothyroidism have so little energy, they tend to be sedentary. As a result, you'll need to encourage your patient to increase his level of activity. But caution him to do so gradually because he risks impaired muscle function from myxedema. Discuss activities he enjoys and can fit into his life-style. (His doctor will have to provide guidelines for all such activities.)

Advise the patient to take precautions when exercising. Warn him to stop exercising and notify his doctor immediately if he feels chest pain or tightness, severe dyspnea, or palpitations.

• *Diet.* Stress the importance of following dietary restrictions. This will help the patient minimize weight gain, decrease cholesterol intake, and alleviate constipation. Remind him that thyroid hormone deficiency decreases his body's ability to use sugars and carbohydrates as sources of energy. It will also cause him to store fats.

Advise the patient to avoid foods high in saturated fats and cholesterol. Suggest that he talk with his doctor about whether or not he can drink alcohol. Explore ways to help him stick to a calorie-restricted diet. If appropriate, encourage him to join a support group.

Teach the patient how to increase the fiber content in his diet. If he has nonpitting edema, advise him to reduce fluid intake by one to two glasses daily, as prescribed.

• *Medication.* Inform the patient that thyroid hormone replacements are the primary treatment for hypothyroidism and will help him to achieve a normal metabolic rate and energy level. Explain that his therapy will be tailored to meet his individual needs, and that he'll need to take hormone replacements for the rest of his life. The dosage will depend on the severity of his hypothyroidism.

Explain to the patient that finding just the right dosage for him is a gradual process. But this will allow his body to adjust slowly to the changes resulting from the medications, thus preventing complications.

Instruct the patient never to take nonprescription medications without his doctor's approval. Explain that because hypothyroidism slows down his metabolism, the effects of any medications he takes will be prolonged. This creates the risk of drug toxicity. Advise him to inform all health care providers of his hypothyroidism so that any prescribed medications (especially narcotics, barbiturates, and digoxin) may be chosen carefully and the dosage reduced appropriately.

• *Other care measures.* Review the symptoms of hypothyroidism with the patient. Tell him to be especially alert for increased lethargy, sensitivity to cold, weight gain, facial puffiness, and changes in his skin or hair. Instruct him to report these symptoms immediately to his doctor.

At the same time, make sure he's familiar with the symptoms of hyperthyroidism, which would develop if his thyroid hormone dosage were too high. These symptoms include heat intolerance, increased sweating, nervous activity, difficulty concentrating, frequent defecation, skin changes, and feelings of apprehension.

Because hypothyroidism is a chronic disorder, encourage the patient to see his doctor regularly and to report any symptoms of infection, such as fever, malaise, diarrhea, or muscle pain. Remind the patient that hypothyroidism makes him vulnerable to infections.

TEACHING PATIENTS ABOUT ENDOCRINE TESTS*

TEST AND PURPOSE	TEACHING POINTS
Radioactive iodine uptake test • To assess thyroid function • To aid diagnosis of hyperthyroidism or hypothyroidism • In conjunction with other studies, to help distinguish between primary and secondary thyroid disorders	• Explain to the patient that this painless test evaluates thyroid function. Tell him who will perform the test and where. • Instruct him to fast after midnight before the test. • Explain what happens during the test: the patient will be given a radioactive iodine capsule or liquid. After 2, 6, and 24 hours, his thyroid will be scanned in the X-ray department to determine how much of the substance is present in the thyroid. Reassure him that the amount of radioactivity involved is extremely small and is harmless.
Thyroid scan (radionuclide thyroid imaging) • To evaluate the size, structure, and position of the thyroid gland • To evaluate thyroid function, in conjunction with thyroid uptake studies	• Explain to the patient that this test assesses the thyroid gland for abnormalities. Tell him who will perform the test and where. Reassure him that the test is painless. • Advise him to follow his doctor's guidelines for discontinuing medications before the test. Usually, he must avoid prescription and over-the-counter medications (particularly multivitamins and cough syrups) for at least 3 days. • Also instruct him to avoid iodized salt, iodinated salt substitutes, and seafood for 3 days before the test. • Explain what happens during the test: the patient will be given a radioisotope orally or intravenously. If he's given the drug orally, tell him that his thyroid gland will be X-rayed 24 hours later. If he's given the drug intravenously, it will be X-rayed within 20 to 30 minutes. Before the X-ray, instruct him to remove dentures and jewelry. Explain that he will be placed in a supine position with his neck extended. A special X-ray machine called a gamma camera will then be placed over his throat to visualize the thyroid gland.
Ultrasonography of the pancreas, or the parathyroid, thyroid, or adrenal glands • To evaluate the size and structure of the endocrine gland • To distinguish between a cyst and a solid tumor • To monitor response to therapy	• Explain to the patient that this test reveals the size and shape of the gland. Tell him who will perform the test and where, and that it takes about 30 minutes. Assure him that the test is painless. • For ultrasonography of the pancreas, instruct the patient to fast for 12 hours before the test: this reduces bowel gas, which hinders transmission of ultrasound. • Explain what happens during the test: the patient will be placed in a supine position. For ultrasonography of the thyroid or parathyroid glands, a pillow will be tucked under his shoulder blades to hyperextend his neck. Tell the patient that the skin over the gland will be coated with a water-soluble gel. Next, the technician will move the transducer over the area to study the gland.

---

*Refer to the entries in this chapter, pages 402 to 430, for information on serum and urine studies to detect endocrine dysfunction.

TEACHING PATIENTS ABOUT ENDOCRINE DRUGS

DRUG	ADVERSE REACTIONS	INTERACTIONS*
Antithyroid drugs		
methimazole (Tapazole) **propylthiouracil (PTU)**	*Reportable:* severe diarrhea, fever, jaundice, severe nausea or vomiting, mouth sores, pruritic rash, sore throat *Other:* mild diarrhea, dizziness, mild nausea or vomiting, skin discoloration or rash, loss of taste	• Tell the patient that foods and beverages don't influence the safety or effectiveness of methimazole or propylthiouracil. • Instruct him to avoid over-the-counter (OTC) drugs since many contain iodine, which can affect his thyroid condition. • Advise him to take methimazole or propylthiouracil at the same time every day for uniform absorption.
Corticosteroids		
prednisone (Orasone)	*Reportable:* abdominal pain, acne, back or rib pain, bloody or tarry stools, easy bruising, unusual fatigue, fever, hypertension, leg swelling, menstrual irregularity, extreme personality changes, purple striae, sore throat, vomiting, weakness, significant weight gain, wounds that won't heal *Other:* unusual appetite, diaphoresis, dizziness, euphoria or feeling of well-being, headache, indigestion, insomnia, mild mood swings, mild nausea, nervousness, restlessness, slight weight gain	• Advise against taking this drug with alcohol to avoid GI ulceration. • Instruct the patient not to take OTC drugs containing aspirin, unless the doctor specifically recommends them. Aspirin may increase the risk of GI ulceration. • Tell the patient to avoid OTC drugs and foods that contain sodium to reduce the risk of fluid retention.
Injectable hypoglycemics		
insulin	*Reportable:* difficulty breathing, frequent or severe hypoglycemia or hyperglycemia, itching, skin changes at injection site (such as redness, swelling, stinging, or itching) *Other:* mild hypoglycemia or hyperglycemia	• Tell the patient to avoid alcohol and aspirin (and other salicylates). Explain that salicylates and alcohol increase insulin's hypoglycemic effect. • Inform him that foods and other beverages and OTC drugs don't influence the safety or effectiveness of insulin.

*Includes foods, beverages, and over-the-counter (OTC) drugs.

TEACHING POINTS

• Explain to the patient that this drug will correct his hyperthyroidism. Tell him not to adjust the dosage or discontinue the drug abruptly without his doctor's approval.
• Teach him signs and symptoms of hypothyroidism (such as cold intolerance, edema, depression) and to report them if they occur. A dosage adjustment may be necessary.
• Advise the patient to store the drug in its original container.

• Explain to the patient that this drug helps correct his adrenal hormone deficiency. Instruct him not to adjust the dosage or discontinue the drug without his doctor's approval. Make sure he understands that abrupt withdrawal can be life-threatening.
• Warn the patient about cushingoid symptoms (such as edema, weight gain, facial or vision changes, humpback, and easy bruising). Tell him to notify the doctor if these signs or symptoms occur. A dosage adjustment may be necessary.
• Tell him to take the drug with milk or food to reduce gastric irritation.
• Advise the patient to always wear a Medic Alert bracelet or necklace stating his need for glucocorticoids during stress.

• Explain that insulin helps control blood glucose levels. Emphasize that it's not meant to replace proper diet.
• Tell the patient never to adjust the dosage or stop the drug without his doctor's approval: a rapid elevation in blood glucose levels could occur. Also explain the importance of injecting insulin on schedule to avoid extreme fluctuations in blood glucose levels.
• Teach him how to administer insulin subcutaneously. Also teach him how to mix insulins in a syringe. Tell him not to change the order in which he mixes insulins. Stress the importance of administering insulin promptly after mixing to avoid loss in potency.
• Advise him to administer insulin at room temperature. Refrigeration isn't necessary unless room temperature is very cold or warm.
• Tell him to rotate injection sites. Show him appropriate sites and help him plan rotation.
• Teach the patient to press, not rub, the injection site after withdrawing the needle. Advise him never to change the brand of insulin, syringe, or needle and to use the correct syringe for his type of insulin concentration.
• Review blood and urine testing, using the procedure of the patient's choice. Emphasize the importance of monitoring blood glucose.
• Advise the patient to always wear a Medic Alert bracelet or necklace stating that he takes insulin to control diabetes.

(continued)

**TEACHING PATIENTS ABOUT
ENDOCRINE DRUGS** *(continued)*

DRUG	ADVERSE REACTIONS	INTERACTIONS*
Oral hypoglycemics		
acetohexamide (Dymelor) **chlorpropamide** (Diabinese) **glipizide** (Glucotrol) **glyburide** (Micronase) **tolazamide** (Tolinase) **tolbutamide** (Orinase)	*Reportable:* hypoglycemia, jaundice *Other:* epigastric fullness, facial flushing, headache, heartburn, nausea, rash, vomiting	• Tell the patient to avoid alcohol and aspirin (and other salicylates). • Advise him to take this drug before meals, if possible, for full benefit.
Thyroid hormones		
levothyroxine (Synthroid) **liothyronine** (Cytomel) **thyroid USP**	*Reportable:* change in appetite, abnormal bleeding or bruising, chest pain, diarrhea, fever, severe headache, heat intolerance, insomnia, leg cramps, nervousness, palpitations, skin rash, sweating, tremors, weight loss *Other:* constipation, drowsiness, dry skin, headache, menstrual irregularities, nausea, transient alopecia	• Advise the patient to take this drug at the same time every day for uniform absorption. • Tell him that foods, beverages, and OTC drugs don't influence the safety or effectiveness of thyroid hormones.
Miscellaneous		
glucagon	*Reportable:* difficulty breathing, hypersensitivity (such as rash or skin eruptions) *Other:* nausea, vomiting	• Because glucagon is an emergency drug administered to treat hypoglycemic crisis, interactions with foods, beverages, and OTC drugs aren't applicable.
propranolol (Inderal)	*Reportable:* depression, dizziness, dyspnea, skin rash, very slow heart rate, wheezing *Other:* decreased libido, diarrhea, fatigue, headache, insomnia, nasal stuffiness, nausea, vivid dreams and nightmares, vomiting	• Tell the patient that OTC drugs don't influence the safety or effectiveness of propranolol. • Instruct him to take propranolol with foods to increase drug absorption.

*Includes foods, beverages, and over-the-counter (OTC) drugs.

TEACHING POINTS

• Explain to the patient that this drug helps control blood glucose levels. Emphasize that it's not meant to replace proper diet.
• Tell him to take the drug exactly as prescribed and not to adjust the dosage or stop taking it without his doctor's approval.
• If this drug causes gastrointestinal upset, tell the patient to take it with meals.

• Advise him to monitor blood glucose levels daily. Show him how to check blood or urine for glucose, using the procedure of his choice.
• Tell him to notify the doctor if he experiences increased stress or illness. A dosage adjustment may be necessary, or he may require insulin.

• Explain to the patient that this drug helps correct his thyroid hormone deficiency. Tell him to take the drug exactly as prescribed and not to adjust the dosage or discontinue the drug abruptly without his doctor's approval.
• Advise him not to switch drug brands once

his condition stabilizes and to avoid generic preparations.
• Warn the patient that partial hair loss may occur but will only be temporary.
• Tell the patient to store the drug in its original container.

• Explain to the patient that glucagon raises blood glucose levels when hypoglycemia can't be corrected with oral glucose.
• Review symptoms of hypoglycemia (weakness, headache, anxiety, and vision changes).
• Teach the patient and his family how to administer glucagon subcutaneously. Have them demonstrate the procedure, using sterile water.

• Stress the importance of obtaining medical help immediately if the patient doesn't respond to glucagon therapy.
• Inform the patient and his family that once reconstituted, glucagon may be stored in the refrigerator up to 3 months. Instruct them to check the expiration date regularly and to keep the correct type of syringes available.

• Explain to the patient that propranolol should lower his blood pressure, control rapid heart rate, and minimize hand tremors.
• If medication is to be taken daily, missed doses should be made up within 8 hours. If medication is to be taken more often than once daily, missed doses should be made up as soon as possible. However, instruct him not to double-dose. Also, warn him that severe cardiovascular complications may develop if he stops taking the drug suddenly

rather than tapers the dosage. Tell the patient to make sure he has enough medication on hand to get through weekends and vacations.
• Teach the patient to take his pulse rate before taking the drug and to notify the doctor if his pulse is below 60 beats/minute.
• If the patient experiences insomnia, suggest that he take the drug no later than 2 hours before bedtime.

14 Hematology

Hematology

Introduction

Except for anemia, most hematologic disorders rarely occur. Because of this, you may encounter difficulty finding reliable, up-to-date information for teaching the hematology patient. Similarly, the patient may face an equally difficult situation: he must learn enough about his disorder to judge whether he's getting appropriate care or not.

A new baseline
Keep in mind that some hematologic disorders, such as sickle cell anemia and hemophilia, are chronic and prone to acute exacerbations. That means you'll have to evaluate how much the patient knows about his condition each time he's hospitalized. Establishing a new teaching baseline is an important responsibility in these disorders.

Frequent teaching sessions
The complexity of hematologic disorders may make teaching pathophysiology and rationales for treatment somewhat more difficult than with other disorders. But by spacing out your teaching sessions, you can give the patient the information he needs without overloading him.

Frequent evaluation will be important to determine what points you need to reinforce and when you can introduce new information. Because the patient and family must absorb a lot of information, you may have to proceed at a slower pace than normal.

Compliance difficult
Teaching a patient with a hematologic disorder may be difficult, too, because his problem isn't visible and his symptoms are often intermittent. The child with hemophilia, for example, can easily forget to take certain precautions or may deliberately ignore them in order to avoid explaining his limitations to his playmates. For some patients, incorporating the necessary precautions into their life-style will be a lifelong struggle.

Special teaching needs
Most hematologic disorders require in-depth teaching about their course and ongoing treatment. The patient will have to learn about precautions, for example, and about taking medication at home. In fact, the hemophilia patient may have to learn to give himself clotting factor by I.V. infusion at home. Because home care measures like these are complicated, patient teaching becomes especially important. In many institutions, this kind of teaching is done by a hematology nurse. Naturally, you'll want to check your institution's protocol before you begin teaching the patient about home care.

DISORDERS

Hemophilia

This rare bleeding disorder affects about 1 in 4,000 males. Today, fortunately, early recognition and treatment of bleeding episodes can prevent most of the complications that were common before clotting factor concentrates and home I.V. infusion programs were developed. Your teaching should emphasize this point. You'll also need to teach the patient about the nature of his condition and explain measures he can take to manage bleeding episodes.

Describe the disorder
Explain that three stages normally occur during clotting. First, the injured blood vessels constrict to slow down the flow of blood. Then, platelets rush to the injury site to plug up leaking capillaries. Next, clotting factors (special plasma proteins) are activated to form a firm fibrin clot. This clot is constantly broken down and reformed until healing is complete.

In a person with hemophilia, an injured blood vessel will constrict and platelets will plug up the capillaries as usual, but because one of the blood's 10 clotting factors is missing or abnormal, the clotting process goes awry. In your teaching, you can compare the 10 clotting factors to a row of dominoes: if you remove one domino, the chain will be broken and the dominoes will stop falling when they reach the empty space. When the clotting process is interrupted like this, the result is a soft, mushy clot that doesn't do the job very well.

Make it clear to the patient with hemophilia that he doesn't bleed faster than anyone else. But because of the missing clotting factor, he may have prolonged or delayed oozing after certain injuries. Identify for him the deficient or absent clotting factor that's causing the abnormal bleeding. Mention that the most common deficiencies are factor VIII deficiency (hemophilia A, or classical hemophilia) and factor IX deficiency (hemophilia B, or Christmas disease).

Explain to the patient that hemophilia nearly always affects males because the defective gene is on the X chromosome. Women have two X chromosomes, so they have two chances to get an X chromosome with the normal gene. Men have an X and a Y chromosome, so they have only one chance to get the normal gene. (The Y chromosome has nothing to do with production of factors VIII and IX.) If a woman has an X chromosome with a hemophilia gene on it, she's considered a carrier. Clarify the inheritance pattern that results in hemophilia. (See *Questions Parents Ask about Inheritance Patterns in Hemophilia*, page 440.)

Explain that the normal range for all 10 clotting factors is 50% to 150% of a baseline figure, obtained by analyzing blood samples from 20 to 30 nonhemophiliacs. The average amount of factors VIII and IX in these blood samples is measured and that number is considered 100%.

Describe the severity of the patient's condition. Most people won't have abnormal bleeding unless their clotting factors fall below 30%. Between 6% and 30% is considered mild hemophilia. Patients whose clotting factors fall within this range usually experience abnormal bleeding only after surgery, tooth extractions, or major injuries. They may go for years without requiring treatment.

When clotting factor levels range from 1% to 5%, the hemophilia is considered moderate in severity. These patients may have abnormal bleeding after relatively mild trauma, such as hard bumps or sprains. The frequency of bleeding episodes ranges from once a month to once every several years.

Patients with severe hemophilia have clotting factors below 1% of the normal level. These patients may experience spontaneous bleeding, especially into joints, as well as prolonged bleeding from injuries.

Even in nonhemophiliacs, small blood vessels in the synovial membranes rupture from time to time. But normally the bleeding stops almost immediately. In someone with severe hemophilia, however, the vessel will continue oozing until the pressure in the joint becomes great enough to stop the bleeding, which usually takes several days. The only other way the bleeding will stop is if the hemophiliac receives an infusion of the missing clotting factor. Patients with severe hemophilia may have bleeding episodes as often as once a week.

Point out possible complications

Emphasize the importance of complying with treatment by pointing out that life expectancy for the patient with hemophilia is now normal. Still, damage from abnormal bleeding poses a serious threat. Any bleeding must be detected early and treated promptly. To prevent significant blood loss and chronic joint disease, the patient must recognize the signs and symptoms produced by bleeding in different parts of the body.

Teach about tests

The usual battery of tests for any patient with a suspected bleeding disorder includes a bleeding time, a platelet count, coagulation screening tests, and clotting factor assays. Once hemophilia is diagnosed, the usual tests required are specific clotting factor assays and an occasional inhibitor screen, all of which can be done on a venous blood sample. Other tests may be required to evaluate complications caused by bleeding. For example, a computed tomography (CT) scan would be done for

---

CHECKLIST

TEACHING TOPICS IN HEMOPHILIA

- [ ] Explanation of the normal clotting process and why it goes awry
- [ ] Severity of the patient's disorder, and type and frequency of bleeding episodes
- [ ] Inheritance patterns
- [ ] Recognition of bleeding episodes and how to get treatment day or night
- [ ] Need for early treatment to prevent complications, such as arthritis
- [ ] Avoidance of contact sports
- [ ] Explanation of clotting factor concentrates or other medications and how to administer them
- [ ] Importance of vaccination against hepatitis
- [ ] Risk of AIDS
- [ ] Avoiding aspirin and all medications that contain aspirin
- [ ] First-aid measures and preventive dental care
- [ ] Location of nearest hemophilia treatment center

---

suspected intracranial bleeding, arthroscopy or arthrography for certain joint problems, and endoscopy for GI bleeding.

Teach about treatments

● *Activity.* Discuss the benefits of regular, moderate exercise with the patient. Strong muscles protect joints and help decrease the incidence of hemarthrosis. Isometric exercises designed to strengthen surrounding muscles—for example, quadriceps exercises after knee joint bleeding—will help prevent muscle weakness and recurrent bleeding into a joint.

Some activities, however, should be avoided because of the risk of serious bleeding. All hemophiliacs, including those with only mild hemophilia, must avoid rough contact sports (such as

INQUIRY

QUESTIONS PARENTS ASK ABOUT INHERITANCE PATTERNS IN HEMOPHILIA

There has never been anyone with hemophilia in our family. How did our son get hemophilia?

In 25% of families with hemophilic children, there's no family history of the disorder. Apparently, there's a very high mutation rate in the genes responsible for the production of factors VIII and IX. The mutation may have taken place in your son, in you (the mother), or even further back in the family tree.

What are my chances of having another child with hemophilia?

If you're a carrier, each of your sons will have a 50-50 chance of being born with hemophilia, and each daughter a 50-50 chance of being a carrier. Your hemophilia treatment center can give you information on carrier testing and prenatal diagnosis.

Because my son has hemophilia, does that mean his children will also have it?

No, but it's possible that his grandchildren will have hemophilia. All of his sons will be normal and will not pass on the defective gene. But all of his daughters will be carriers, which means their sons may have hemophilia.

INHERITANCE PATTERNS IN HEMOPHILIA

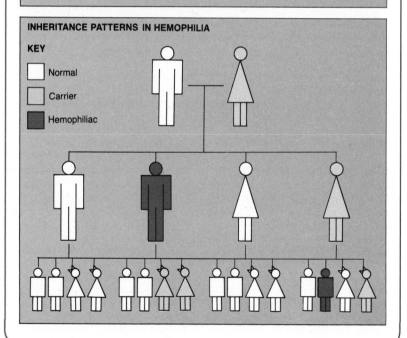

football and boxing) that carry a high risk of head injury. Patients with chronic joint disease should also avoid sports, such as soccer and basketball, that put stress on the joints. The National Hemophilia Foundation has published a pamphlet, *Sports in Hemophilia,* that discusses the benefits and injuries that may occur with each sport.

Encourage the hemophiliac and his family to take up swimming, hiking, and biking. If the patient is a child, review appropriate safety precautions with the parents.

• *Medication and procedures.* The primary treatment for hemophilia is I.V. infusion of the missing clotting factor. This treatment may be ordered to prevent bleeding from surgery or tooth extraction or to control bleeding from trauma. Teach the patient and his parents how to recognize when treatment is needed, and inform them of the approximate amount of clotting factor to use. Explain why prompt treatment is important and why the short half-life of clotting factors may require repeated infusions.

Patients with severe or moderate hemophilia A would receive an infusion of factor VIII, also called the antihemophilic factor (AHF). Factor VIII comes in two forms: a single-donor, frozen concentrate, called cryoprecipitate, that's usually administered by I.V. drip; and a commercially prepared, freeze-dried concentrate extracted from large pools of plasma contributed by paid donors. This form is reconstituted in a small amount of sterile water and is usually given I.V. push.

Patients with mild hemophilia A are often treated with desmopressin instead of clotting factor concentrates. This drug stimulates the release of stored factor VIII and temporarily doubles or triples the patient's factor VIII level. Desmopressin is administered I.V. every day or every other day for three or four doses.

To treat or prevent bleeding in patients with severe or moderate hemophilia B, freeze-dried prothrombin complex concentrate, which contains factor IX, is usually administered. This comes in a powder reconstituted with 20 to 30 ml of sterile water. It's given I.V. push.

Patients with mild hemophilia B may be treated with fresh-frozen plasma to reduce the risk of exposure to hepatitis and other viruses. It takes at least 30 minutes to infuse each unit; adult patients would characteristically receive four or five units per infusion.

You'll need to teach all patients with hemophilia how to care for their veins after performing a venipuncture. Impress on them the importance of preserving their veins for lifelong therapy. Instruct them not to apply pressure until the needle is removed; putting pressure on the needle as it's being withdrawn will cause damage to the vein. After the needle has been withdrawn, firm pressure should be applied at the site with one finger for 3 to 5 minutes. The arm should be kept straight, not bent.

Instruct patients to remind medical personnel to use stainless steel butterfly needles, whenever possible, and to remove them after each infusion. The reason for this: plastic inside-the-needle catheters may inflame and scar the vein, especially if they're left in place for several days. Even in the case of hospitalized patients receiving infusions every 12 hours, a needle should never be left in a vein. Instead, a new venipuncture should be performed for each infusion. The only exception would be cases where patients require continuous I.V. fluids or antibiotics or where venipuncture is especially difficult to perform, such as in a small child.

Teach patients with severe or moderate hemophilia—or their parents—how to mix and administer clotting factor concentrates at home. (See *Caring for the Hemophilic Child,* page 442.) This will prevent delays in treatment and, in the case of minor bleeding episodes, may save the patient a trip to

442

CARING FOR THE HEMOPHILIC CHILD

Dear Parents:

Your child has hemophilia, a lifelong bleeding disorder. But with proper care, he'll be able to lead a nearly normal life, attending school regularly and taking part in most play activities. However, he should avoid rough contact sports, such as football, and other activities that may cause head or joint injuries.

Dealing with injuries

If your child is injured, administer first aid as you would for anyone else. *Your child won't bleed any faster than normal.* He'll just bleed longer. He may have prolonged or delayed oozing that can cause pain and disability if it's not treated promptly. Injuries to the head, neck, or eye are especially serious. If your child says he has pain, starts limping, or stops using an arm or leg, assume that he's bleeding into a joint or muscle and arrange for prompt treatment.

Be alert for signs of intracranial bleeding—nausea, vomiting, headache, irritability, and drowsiness—especially if your child suffered a blow to his head in the last 4 or 5 days. If he vomits blood or material that looks like coffee grounds, or if he passes stools that are black and sticky (tarry), suspect bleeding into the stomach or intestines. Blood in the urine indicates kidney bleeding and should be treated by giving him fluids and administering clotting factor. Whenever your child has been injured or appears to be bleeding abnormally, call your doctor or hemophilia treatment center immediately.

Infusing clotting factors

When your child is 4 or 5 years old, you may want to learn how to give his clotting factor infusions at home. Home care allows your child to be treated as quickly as possible after signs and symptoms of abnormal bleeding are noticed.

Because your child will be receiving blood products, he'll be exposed to hepatitis. Be sure he receives the hepatitis B vaccine as well as his other immunizations.

Important precautions

Make sure your child wears a Medic Alert bracelet or necklace at all times. Never give him aspirin. It may increase the frequency or severity of his bleeding episodes. Look at all medication labels for these words—"aspirin," "acetylsalicylic acid," or "ASA."

his doctor's office or the hospital. Most parents are taught to mix and administer clotting factor concentrate by the time their hemophilic child enters school. To qualify for home care, the child must have reasonably accessible veins and must be able to hold still. Hemophilic children usually learn self-infusion between the ages of 8 and 12. (See *Learning Self-Infusion*, pages 444 and 445.)

Teach patients (or their parents) how to calculate the proper dosage of clotting factor concentrate needed for bleeding episodes. (See *Teaching Patients about Hematologic Drugs*, pages 458 to 463.) Also emphasize the importance of contacting their doctor or treatment center for major bleeding problems, such as gastrointestinal bleeding, head injuries, and prolonged joint bleeding. Home care is not meant to replace medical care.

Instruct patients how to keep accurate treatment records. These should include at least the following basic information: the problem that required treatment, the nature of the treatment itself, and its outcome. Advise patients to send this information to their treatment center at least once a month. For minor bleeding episodes, most patients are taught to infuse clotting factor concentrate and then to record the treatment. For major bleeding episodes, no documentation should be done until after the clotting factor concentrate has been infused and the doctor has been called for further instructions.

Teach patients about possible complications of the treatment itself. Hepatitis, for example, is transmitted through blood products. Make sure the patient understands the importance of receiving Heptavax-B, the hepatitis B vaccine. Patients should also know that there are two or more non-A, non-B hepatitis viruses for which no tests or vaccines exist.

To prevent the spread of hepatitis to family members and others, all needles and other home care equipment must be disposed of properly. Instruct patients to put needles in a hard plastic or cardboard container and return them to the hospital or clinic for disposal. Tell them to discard other disposable equipment in a plastic bag.

You'll also need to address other potential complications of treatment. For example, the patient will undoubtedly have heard about the risk of contracting acquired immune deficiency syndrome (AIDS) through blood products. To allay the patient's fears, inform him that all donated blood and plasma are now screened for antibodies to the HTLV-III virus, which is believed to cause AIDS. Also, all freeze-dried products are now routinely heat-treated to kill the HTLV-III virus. With these precautions, it's highly unlikely that a hemophiliac will contract AIDS through blood products.

Of course, hemophiliacs who received clotting factor concentrate before the development of heat treatment already may have been exposed to the virus. This is also true of some patients who received cryoprecipitate and plasma before blood donors were screened as carefully as they are today. These patients need your reassurance. Point out to them that very few people who have been exposed to the virus are actually susceptible to it, and that currently less than 1% of all hemophiliacs exposed to the virus have developed AIDS. Granted, it's difficult to reassure people about something as frightening and widely publicized as AIDS. If a patient of yours seems especially anxious about contracting AIDS, refer him to the nearest hemophilia center for follow-up information and counseling.

Ten to twenty percent of patients with severe hemophilia will develop inhibitors. This means that their body makes such an abnormal factor VIII or IX that it recognizes the normal factors as foreign proteins. In response, the body produces antibodies, called inhibitors, against normal factors VIII and IX. The antibodies destroy the clotting factor as fast as it's infused. Because of this risk, tell patients to call their doctor if

LEARNING SELF-INFUSION

Dear Patient:

These instructions will help you infuse clotting factors at home. Remember, if you're infusing clotting factors for a minor bleeding episode, record the episode and the infusion and bring this information with you on your next visit to the doctor. If you're infusing clotting factors for a major bleeding episode, call your doctor afterward to inform him of the episode.

1
Gather the equipment: clotting factor concentrate and sterile water, syringe, butterfly needle, tourniquet, alcohol swabs, gauze pads, and tape.

2
Wash your hands thoroughly with soap and water.

3
Remove the flip-top lids on the clotting factor concentrate bottle and the sterile water bottle. Swab the stoppers with alcohol.

4
If you're using *nonvacuum bottles*, inject air into the sterile water bottle and withdraw the water, as shown at the top of the next column.

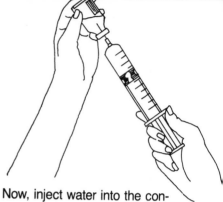

Now, inject water into the concentrate bottle, directing it against the side of the bottle to prevent foaming.

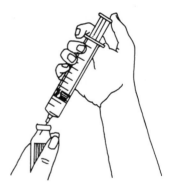

Withdraw air to relieve pressure, then withdraw the needle and cap it.

If you're using *vacuum bottles*, insert the double-ended needle into the water bottle. Then invert the needle and bottle and insert the other end of the needle into the concentrate bottle. Direct the stream of water against the side of the bottle to prevent foaming.

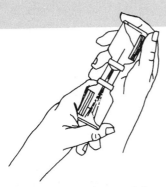

Take the water bottle off first to release the rest of the vacuum. Then remove the needle. Rotate the bottle gently until the powder is fully dissolved. Clean the stopper of the concentrate bottle with a second alcohol swab. Then inject air into the concentrate bottle and withdraw the reconstituted concentrate through the provided filter needle into the syringe.

5

Apply the tourniquet around your forearm about 3″ above the venipuncture site. Cleanse the site with alcohol and dry it with a gauze pad. Then, remove the cap on the end of the butterfly needle, and insert the needle through the skin at a 30- to 45-degree angle into the center of the vein.

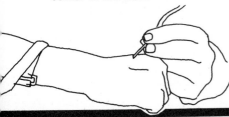

When you see blood return, level the needle off and advance it slightly so it won't slip from the vein.

6

Remove the tourniquet and tape the needle. Then remove the cap from the needle and attach the tubing to the syringe. Pull back gently on the plunger of the syringe to fill the tubing with blood. Infuse the concentrate slowly (3 to 5 ml/minute).

7

When the infusion is finished, place a gauze pad over the site and remove the needle. *Don't apply pressure to the site as you remove the needle. It can damage the vein.*

8

After removing the needle, apply firm pressure to the venipuncture site for 3 to 5 minutes.

9

To prevent the spread of infection, put used needles in a special box or plastic container, and return them to the hospital or clinic. Wrap other equipment in plastic, and discard.

COMMON PARENTAL REACTIONS TO HEMOPHILIA

Hemophilia can dramatically influence the way parents react to their affected child.

Overprotectiveness

When parents learn that their child has a bleeding problem, it's only natural for them to want to protect him from getting hurt. This may cause them to become overprotective, to the point where they interfere with the child's exploratory behavior and physical activities essential to his development. The child, depending on his personality, may respond to protectiveness with dependence, passivity, and fearfulness, *or* with rebellion, anger, and dangerous behavior.

Often just telling parents that, no matter how careful they are, they can't keep their child from having bleeding episodes will help them overcome their natural inclination to be overprotective.

Remind parents to ask themselves if they're treating their hemophilic child any differently than their other children. If they don't have other children, they can watch how friends and neighbors treat their children. Parents can also keep track of how often they say "watch out" or "be careful."

Permissiveness/indulgence

Parents may also adopt a permissive or indulgent attitude toward their hemophilic child. Perhaps they feel sorry for him because he has hemophilia or because they've restricted so many of his activities. If so, they may try to make it up to him by giving in to him on other matters or by showering him with toys, treats, and special privileges. They may let him get away

with not doing chores or not following the same rules as other children.

Unfortunately, these parents aren't helping their child. Their permissiveness may instill in the child a total disregard for rules that will almost certainly lead to trouble later in life. He may become prone to temper tantrums and manipulative behavior or grow up to become a lazy adult, passive and easily bored, who expects his parents or society to care for him.

Explaining to the parents how permissiveness or indulgence can do their child more harm than good may help them overcome these perfectly normal tendencies. The child needs attention and encouragement, of course, but giving in to unreasonable demands and excusing him from responsibilities won't help him function in school and in society.

Encouraging hypochondriasis

Another common parental reaction may lead to hypochondriasis in the child. Parents may become overly concerned about the risk of abnormal bleeding episodes. If the child gets too much attention whenever he has a bleeding episode or if he's encouraged to stay home from school, he may think of himself as ill or defective. He's also likely to start using his hemophilia to get out of school or other responsibilities. Stress to parents the need for regular school attendance.

Hemophilia is a lifelong disorder. Bleeding episodes should be treated matter-of-factly and not be allowed to interfere with daily activities.

Withdrawal and rejection

The most devastating parental reactions are withdrawal and rejection. If parents reject their child because he has hemophilia, the child will develop feelings of inferiority, a poor self-image, and a fear of failure.

Fortunately, complete withdrawal or rejection is rare among parents of hemophilic children. Parents are usually shocked and upset when their child's disorder is first diagnosed, but most eventually adjust. Meeting with professionals from a hemophilia treatment center and with other parents of hemophilic children may make the adjustment easier. Of course, a father who had hoped that his son would someday be a professional football player will have more trouble adjusting. Asking the parents about their hopes and plans for their son before diagnosis may help you better understand their ability to adjust.

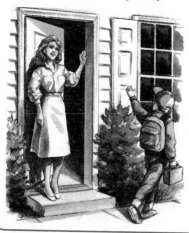

their infusions don't seem to be controlling bleeding episodes.

All patients, especially those on home care, should be taught how to recognize and treat adverse reactions to blood products. The most common reaction to freeze-dried concentrate is flushing, headache, or tingling. This isn't a serious reaction; slowing the infusion rate will usually cause the symptoms to abate.

Hives—the most common reaction experienced by patients receiving cryoprecipitate or plasma—results from an allergy to a plasma protein. It's usually treated with diphenhydramine or another antihistamine. Patients who develop hives frequently should receive an antihistamine about 45 minutes before their infusions.

The same plasma proteins that cause hives may occasionally cause anaphylaxis. Patients on home care not only need to recognize the signs and symptoms of such a reaction, but also should learn how to administer epinephrine. Occasionally, patients will develop fever and chills because of an allergy to white blood cell antigens. These reactions most often occur with plasma infusions. Reassure the patient that these reactions usually aren't serious and that discomfort may be relieved with acetaminophen.

Teach all hemophiliacs to avoid taking aspirin and any medications containing aspirin. Aspirin decreases platelet function significantly, which would only exacerbate hemophilia. It can increase not only the frequency but also the severity of bleeding episodes and must be strictly avoided.

• *Other care measures.* Although clotting factor infusions are the major treatment for bleeding episodes, general first-aid measures should also be taught to the parents of hemophilic children. These measures would be the same for the hemophiliac as for anyone else. Remember to reassure parents that their child won't bleed any faster than normal.

Mention that application of pressure is usually the only treatment needed for surface cuts and nosebleeds. Deeper cuts may stop temporarily with pressure, but if they're deep enough to require suturing, clotting factor infusions will be necessary to prevent rebleeding. Ice packs and elastic bandages may help alleviate pain from hemarthrosis. These measures are no substitute, however, for clotting factor infusions.

Emphasize the importance of obtaining a Medic Alert necklace or bracelet. It will help ensure that clotting factor infusions are administered as soon as possible after major accidents.

Preventive dental care is important for everyone, of course, but especially so for the patient with hemophilia. Make sure he understands that dental caries can be filled and teeth extracted, but emphasize that clotting factor infusions are required before these procedures. Poor dental hygiene also introduces the risk of bleeding from inflamed gums.

Because hemophilia is a rare disorder, but one that can be managed at home, the patient obviously has much to learn. You can't possibly cover everything in just a few sessions while the patient is in the hospital. That's why you should refer the patient to the nearest comprehensive hemophilia center for evaluation and follow-up teaching. Inform family members that carrier testing and prenatal diagnosis are available at these centers; they too should receive genetic counseling and appropriate testing. If you don't know of a center in your area, contact the National Hemophilia Foundation.

Finally, remember that emotional problems can be more disabling than physical ones. So, for example, you may need to tactfully remind parents that overprotectiveness, permissiveness, and even withdrawal are common parental responses to hemophilia that may cause serious social or emotional problems. (See *Common Parental Reactions to Hemophilia.*) If appropriate, offer to refer the family for counseling.

Iron Deficiency Anemia

Patient teaching for iron deficiency anemia—the most prevalent nutritional disorder in the United States—should focus on promoting compliance with therapy. Because this disorder is fairly common, patients often don't take it seriously enough. Convincing them that iron deficiency can lead to severe problems will help ensure strict compliance with treatment regimens, including supplements to dietary iron and continued medical follow-up.

Describe the disorder
Explain to the patient that when the body's demand for iron isn't met, its iron reserves can be rapidly depleted. Fewer circulating red blood cells (RBCs) cause both hemoglobin concentration and the blood's oxygen-carrying capacity to decrease. Consequently, the patient develops signs and symptoms of anemia. Make sure the patient is aware that the body's demand for iron will increase after blood loss and at certain life stages.

CHECKLIST

TEACHING TOPICS IN IRON DEFICIENCY ANEMIA

☐ Explanation of iron deficiency anemia (including roles played by iron and red blood cells, hemoglobin, and tissue oxygenation)

☐ Explanation of the cause of the patient's anemia

☐ Frequent blood tests to determine serum iron level

☐ Foods high in iron

☐ Daily iron supplements

☐ Importance of follow-up visits

Naturally, you'll need to tailor your teaching about iron deficiency anemia to the patient's age. If the patient is an infant, teach the parents that their child's iron stores will be depleted by age 4 to 6 months. After that, the infant will need formula that's supplemented with iron. Explain that babies who drink a lot of cow's milk are at high risk for iron deficiency anemia.

If the patient is a teenager, explain that he's at risk for iron deficiency because of increased nutritional demands during adolescence. With many patients in this age group, poor nutrition only compounds the problem.

Women may develop an iron deficiency because of blood loss during menstruation. Inform these patients that even though menstruation may not appear to cause significant blood loss, it can still cause iron deficiency anemia in someone whose iron stores are low to begin with. If the patient is pregnant, explain that much of her body's supply of iron is being diverted to the fetus for erythropoiesis.

All patients should be informed that anemia is the final stage of iron deficiency. Anemia occurs only after the body's iron stores and its supply of transport iron have been depleted.

Point out possible complications
Explain that failure to comply with therapy will result in a chronic lack of oxygen, possibly producing such signs and symptoms as chronic fatigue, chronic dyspnea, inability to concentrate, irritability, and susceptibility to infection. Also, if tissues don't receive enough oxygen, the body will compensate by increasing heart rate and cardiac output. However, some patients are well compensated and exhibit no signs or symptoms.

Teach about tests
Explain that laboratory tests requiring small amounts of venous blood will be done to confirm a diagnosis of iron deficiency anemia. The severity of the de-

ficiency can also be determined by these tests. A complete blood count will be necessary to evaluate hemoglobin levels and detect morphologic changes in RBCs. Tests to determine the iron concentration of the blood also will be done.

Periodically during treatment, blood counts, including reticulocyte counts and RBC indices, must be obtained to assess the patient's degree of recovery. No special preparation is required for these tests.

Teach about treatments

• *Diet.* Although diet alone can't treat iron deficiency anemia, it does play an important role in therapy. Even with a patient who has developed this disorder because of blood loss or increased nutritional demands—during pregnancy or adolescent growth, for example—insufficient dietary iron may be a contributing factor.

Encourage the patient to include iron-rich foods—such as beef, poultry, leafy green vegetables, whole grain breads and cereals, grapes, and berries—in his daily diet. Since ascorbic acid helps the body absorb iron, instruct him to eat plenty of fruit and to drink fruit juices. If big meals make the patient feel tired, suggest that he eat small, frequent meals instead.

• *Medication.* Explain that iron replacement therapy will be started to correct the anemia. Oral iron is prescribed most often; it's the safest, most effective, and least expensive treatment. Parenteral iron supplements may have to be given if the patient fails to take oral medication as prescribed or experiences adverse reactions, such as nausea or constipation. (See *Teaching Patients about Hematologic Drugs*, pages 458 to 463.)

• *Procedures.* Explain to the patient with severe iron deficiency anemia that he may need transfusions of packed RBCs. Mention that this treatment will increase the amount of circulating hemoglobin in his blood and improve tissue oxygenation. Packed RBCs are given by I.V. infusion, which may take up to 2 hours.

• *Other care measures.* Encourage the patient to keep follow-up appointments with his doctor and to continue the prescribed therapy even after his condition improves. Once hemoglobin levels return to normal, therapy should continue for at least 2 more months to replenish the body's depleted iron stores. The patient should be warned that iron deficiency may recur.

Tell the patient to pace his activities and to allow for frequent rest periods. If he develops shortness of breath, weakness, light-headedness, or palpitations, suggest changing position or moving about slowly to minimize dizziness.

Stress the importance of immunizations for the child with iron deficiency anemia and prompt treatment of infection.

Sickle Cell Anemia

This chronic, inherited, hemoglobin disorder affects 1 in 400 black Americans. Shrouded by myth and misinformation, it requires especially sensitive teaching to reduce the patient's fear and anxiety. Since the disorder has no cure, your teaching will focus on palliative treatment, the prevention of crises and complications, and hereditary transmission.

Because the patient with sickle cell anemia may have periodic crises, he may become easily discouraged and depressed. This will often complicate patient teaching. So, before you can begin teaching, you may have to spend time simply listening to the patient express his feelings about his condition.

Because sickle cell anemia is a chronic disorder, you'll want to determine how much the patient already knows before you start teaching. If the patient has been hospitalized before for an acute exacerbation, point out to him

CHECKLIST

TEACHING TOPICS IN SICKLE CELL ANEMIA

- [ ] Explanation of sickle cell anemia, including its inheritance pattern and possible complications
- [ ] Symptoms of sickle cell anemia requiring immediate medical attention
- [ ] Precipitating factors for VOC
- [ ] Explanation of blood tests
- [ ] The importance of good nutrition, especially adequate intake of foods containing folic acid
- [ ] The importance of immunizations and of taking prescribed medication
- [ ] Home treatment of VOC
- [ ] The need for careful monitoring of the patient's condition
- [ ] Sources of help and information

that there's always more to learn about his condition. The more information he absorbs, the better prepared he'll be to seek early intervention and reduce complications in any future crisis.

Describe the disorder

Explain that sickle cell disease results from a hemoglobin abnormality. The abnormal hemoglobin S forms fibers within the hemoglobin when oxygen is removed from red blood cells (RBCs). This causes RBCs to become rigid, rough, and elongated. Eventually, they assume the crescent or sickle shape that gives the disorder its name.

These changes can destroy RBCs and impede blood flow through small vessels. That's where the sickled cells tend to clump together and interfere with circulation, depriving body organs and tissues of oxygen. Subsequent anoxia leads to the destruction of even more RBCs and further obstruction of small vessels. Chronic anemia results because RBCs survive in the circulation for only 15 to 20 days, compared to the normal 120 days.

To put to rest any misconceptions your patient and his family may have, teach them how sickle cell disease is inherited. (See *Questions Parents Ask about Sickle Cell Anemia.*) Explain that sickle cell trait refers to the presence of one hemoglobin S gene and one normal hemoglobin gene (hemoglobin A). Having this trait makes a person a carrier of the disorder. However, *both* parents must have the trait for a child to inherit the disorder.

Point out possible complications

Stress the importance of adhering to treatment by pointing out that patients with sickle cell anemia are susceptible to serious infection, especially meningitis, sepsis, and pneumonia. One cause of this is the spleen's inability to function properly, limiting the body's defenses against infection. Serious infection can set in suddenly and quickly get worse. Although young children are at greater risk, serious infection can occur at any age.

Also point out that vaso-occlusive crisis (VOC), the most common complication of sickle cell anemia, can result from infection as well as from dehydration, excessive fatigue, and anxiety. (See *What Happens in Vaso-Occlusive Crisis,* page 452.)

Teach about tests

Hemoglobin electrophoresis can confirm diagnosis of sickle cell anemia. All family members should be tested for sickle cell anemia or the sickle cell trait.

The only other tests the patient may need are routine blood counts, blood chemistry studies, and urinalysis to detect early signs of organ damage. Complications of sickle cell anemia, however, may require other blood tests and possibly X-rays.

Teach about treatments

• *Activity.* There's no reason for the patient with sickle cell anemia to shy away from physical activities promoting health and fitness, such as regular

QUESTIONS PARENTS ASK ABOUT SICKLE CELL ANEMIA

Must both parents have sickle cell trait for a baby to have sickle cell anemia?

Yes. Sickle cell anemia is a homozygous disorder. That means that one sickle gene is required from each parent for a baby to have sickle cell anemia.

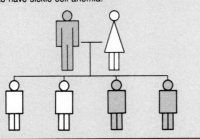

KEY

Normal hemoglobin

Sickle cell trait

Sickle cell anemia

If our baby has sickle cell anemia, does that mean that any other children we have may also be born with it?

Yes. If both parents have sickle cell trait, the chances *with each pregnancy* are one in four that the baby will have sickle cell anemia. Having one baby with sickle cell anemia does not increase the risk. The chances remain one in four with each pregnancy.

One of us has sickle cell anemia. Will our children also have it?

That depends on the hemoglobin genes of the other partner. If he or she has normal hemoglobin, without sickle cell trait or anemia, your children will all have sickle cell trait. If he or she has sickle cell trait, there's a 50% chance with each pregnancy that your child will have sickle cell anemia, and a 50% chance that your child will have sickle cell trait. If he or she has sickle cell anemia, all children will have sickle cell anemia.

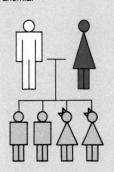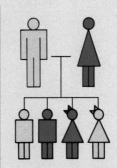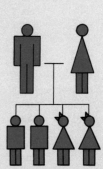

WHAT HAPPENS IN VASO-OCCLUSIVE CRISIS

In sickle cell anemia, vaso-occlusive crisis occurs when red blood cells release oxygen to the tissues. In response, abnormal hemoglobin S associates to form fibers that cause the red cells to assume a sickle shape. The sickled cells clump together and reduce or block blood flow to the area fed by the vessel. If this persists, microscopic obstructions eventually produce widespread ischemia. Increased oxygen demand, meanwhile, causes further sickling and compounds the problem. This, in turn, produces severe pain from tissue infarction and possible organ damage. Factors that increase tissue oxygen demand and thus may precipitate a crisis include infection, exposure to cold or high altitude, overexertion, and dehydration.

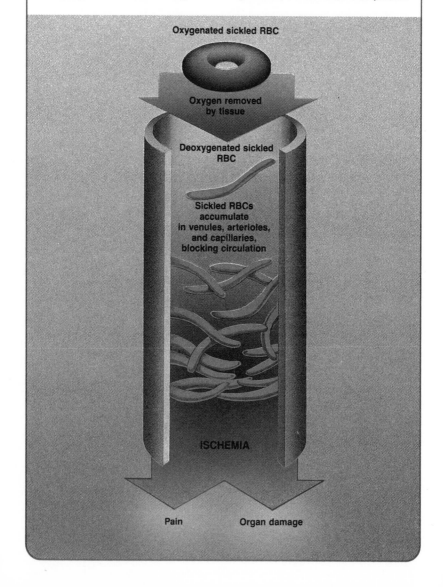

Oxygenated sickled RBC

Oxygen removed by tissue

Deoxygenated sickled RBC

Sickled RBCs accumulate in venules, arterioles, and capillaries, blocking circulation

ISCHEMIA

Pain   Organ damage

gym classes. But warn him to take frequent rest periods and, in general, not to overdo it since fatigue can contribute to the onset of VOC. One further caution: the patient with splenomegaly should be told to avoid contact sports to reduce the risk of splenic rupture.

• *Diet.* Good nutrition is an essential part of treatment for sickle cell anemia. Since folic acid deficiency will exacerbate anemia and may lead to bone marrow depression, teach the patient or his parents about dietary sources of folic acid, such as leafy vegetables, asparagus spears, broccoli, mushrooms, red beans, beef liver, peanut butter, oatmeal, and wheat germ. Also teach about the importance of maintaining adequate hydration. This will minimize the sickling of RBCs and also help prevent dehydration from the patient's inability to concentrate urine. Emphasize that fluid intake should be increased during hot weather.

• *Medication.* Teach parents the importance of preventing infection in the child with sickle cell anemia. Immunization against childhood diseases is a must, as is strict adherence to a prescribed medication regimen once an infection has developed. Polyvalent pneumococcal vaccine may be given at age 6 months and should be repeated at age 2 years. Boosters are needed every 4 years. Sometimes a low dose of prophylactic oral penicillin twice daily will reduce the risk of pneumococcal infections until age 6, after which it may no longer be necessary. *Hemophilus influenzae B* vaccine should be given at age 18 months.

Although parents must understand the importance of complying with these measures, they should also realize that prophylaxis isn't foolproof. They still have to watch for early signs and symptoms of infection. Of course, appropriate antibiotic therapy will be prescribed for infections. In many cases, the patient (especially a child) will have to be hospitalized for antibiotic therapy.

A daily folic acid supplement also may be prescribed because of the increased demands on bone marrow to replace sickled RBCs.

If a patient with sickle cell anemia receives regular transfusions, he may require deferoxamine, a chelating agent. This medication can help remove dangerous iron deposits caused by repeated transfusions. The patient can take deferoxamine at home, but first he or his parents will need detailed instructions on how to mix and administer it (subcutaneously or intravenously) at home. Before giving these instructions, consult your institution's procedures manual or talk to a hematology nurse.

The patient with sickle cell anemia may have to take analgesics to curb the pain of VOC. Recommend acetaminophen. Or, if the doctor prescribes a narcotic analgesic, tell the patient to follow his instructions and to report persistent pain.

• *Other care measures.* Teach the patient or his parents the following symptoms of VOC so he or they can recognize it early: abdominal, chest, muscle, or bone pain; dark urine; and a low-grade fever. Make sure that the parents know how to take their child's temperature correctly. Tell parents that the first VOC an infant experiences is often the so-called "hand-foot crisis," in which the infant's hands or feet, or both, swell and become painful. Explain that they can treat VOC at home by increasing fluid intake; applying warm, moist heat to the painful area; promoting rest; and giving oral analgesics as prescribed. Tell them to call the doctor if symptoms persist or worsen. If the patient must be hospitalized for VOC, explain that I.V. fluids and parenteral analgesics will most likely be ordered. Oxygen may be administered to some patients.

Teach the patient or his parents techniques to help prevent VOC. These include relaxation exercises, biofeedback, and self-hypnosis. Explain that repeated episodes of VOC can lead to permanent organ damage.

Also teach the patient or his parents other symptoms that must be reported immediately. For example, teach parents of young children that acute splenic sequestration—the trapping of blood in the spleen—is a rare but serious complication and a medical emergency. It most often occurs in children between 8 months and 2 years old. Its symptoms include increased pallor, lethargy, and abdominal pain.

Other warning symptoms in sickle cell anemia include fever over 101° F. (38.3° C.), stiff neck, difficulty speaking or walking, numbness, weakness, or priapism.

Explain to parents that urinary frequency, caused by the child's inability to concentrate urine, may occur. Bedwetting often starts around age 6. Also advise them to have their child's eyes examined yearly by an ophthalmologist to detect early signs of retinal damage.

Because delayed growth and late puberty are common, reassure adolescents that they'll grow and mature. Tell them they should catch up with their friends by age 17 or 18. Also tell them the importance of meticulous leg and foot care, because leg ulcers may occur during the late teens.

Since sickle cell anemia affects all body systems and many aspects of a patient's life-style, it requires multidisciplinary care involving hematologists, social workers, nurses, and psychologists. Encourage the patient and his family to take full advantage of available resources, such as a comprehensive sickle cell treatment center.

Thrombocytopenia

In this congenital or acquired disorder, you'll need to emphasize the importance of taking precautions against accidental bleeding—without unduly frightening the patient. You'll also need to explain just what platelets are and

how they function before you can move on to a fuller discussion of thrombocytopenia. Understanding this disorder will help the patient and his family to cope with its limitations, to take realistic but not excessive precautions, and to be responsive to treatment recommendations.

Describe the disorder

Explain that thrombocytopenia may result from decreased or defective production of platelets in the bone marrow or from increased destruction of platelets in the bloodstream. The cause may be unknown, or it may be one of numerous associated conditions, such as infection, use of quinidine or certain other drugs, aplastic anemia, systemic lupus erythematosus or other primary immune disorder, or vitamin B_{12} or other deficiency. Tell the patient the cause of his thrombocytopenia, if it's known. Then explain that platelets (or thrombocytes) are the smallest blood cells and that they're essential for normal blood clotting.

Describe the normal clotting process for the patient. After an injury, the blood vessels constrict in an attempt to stop the bleeding. Platelets rush to the injured area, stick to the edges of the torn vessels, then clump together to form a plug that temporarily stops the bleeding until a clot can form. Explain that a clot builds within the platelet plug; without the platelet plug, a clot cannot form. Mention that even in the absence of injury, platelets help maintain vascular integrity by filling small gaps in blood vessel walls. This prevents blood from leaking out of vessels.

In thrombocytopenia, decreased platelet function not only impairs blood clotting after a vascular injury, but also allows red blood cells to escape from the circulatory system through small gaps in undamaged vessels. This produces the petechiae, ecchymoses, and mucous membrane bleeding commonly seen with this disorder.

Inform the patient that a normal platelet count is between 150,000 and

400,000 platelets per microliter of blood. Usually, though, abnormal bleeding won't occur, even with surgery, unless the platelet count drops below 100,000 per microliter.

Review the severity of the patient's disorder and describe the symptoms of abnormal bleeding. If his platelet count is between 30,000 and 50,000, for example, tell him to expect bruising with minor trauma.

If the patient's platelet count is between 10,000 and 30,000, tell him to expect spontaneous bruising and petechiae, most prominently on his arms and legs. A woman with a platelet count in this range may have menorrhagia.

If the patient's platelet count is below 10,000, tell him that he may experience spontaneous bruising or—after minor trauma—mucosal bleeding, generalized purpura, epistaxis, hematuria, and GI or intracranial bleeding. Tell this patient the symptoms of intracranial bleeding—persistent headache, mood change, nausea, vomiting, and drowsiness. Instruct him to report any of these symptoms immediately, even if he hasn't suffered a head injury. Because capillary or mucosal bleeding may lead to GI bleeding, as well as epistaxis, menorrhagia, or gingival or urinary tract bleeding, explain the significance of black, tarry stools or "coffee-ground" emesis. Prompt reporting of these signs can help prevent serious blood loss from a tiny ulcer or another lesion in the patient's stomach or intestine.

Point out possible complications
Stress the importance of complying with treatment recommendations and activity restrictions by pointing out the dangers of abnormal bleeding.

Teach about tests
The patient with thrombocytopenia may need to have his platelet count measured frequently. While this relatively simple test requires only a small sample of venous blood, a larger sample

---

CHECKLIST

TEACHING TOPICS IN THROMBO- CYTOPENIA

- ☐ Explanation of platelets' role in clotting
- ☐ Explanation of the possible causes of the patient's thrombocytopenia
- ☐ Severity of thrombocytopenia
- ☐ Signs and symptoms of serious bleeding
- ☐ Platelet counts and other diagnostic tests
- ☐ Activity restrictions
- ☐ Administration of corticosteroids
- ☐ Platelet infusions and possible reactions
- ☐ Explanation of splenectomy, if performed

---

would be required for platelet antibody studies. If your patient needs these additional tests, explain that antibody studies help determine why his platelet count is low and may help direct treatment.

Occasionally, a patient will also need platelet survival studies. These tests help differentiate between ineffective platelet production and platelet destruction.

Patients with severe thrombocytopenia usually need to undergo a bone marrow aspiration to determine the number, size, and cytoplasmic maturation of the megakaryocytes. This information may shed light on the cause of the thrombocytopenia and rule out a malignant process.

Teach about treatments
● *Activity.* The lower the patient's platelet count, the more cautious he'll have to be in his activities. Teach him that even minor bumps or scrapes may result in bleeding. Emphasize the importance of avoiding contact sports and other activities that involve a high risk of head injury. If the patient has severe thrombocytopenia, tell him to avoid

sports or other strenuous physical activities in which he might twist a joint, strain a muscle, or sustain hard blows or kicks.

● *Medication and procedures.* Corticosteroids are most often used to treat thrombocytopenia, especially if the disorder results from immune destruction of platelets. (See *Teaching Patients about Hematologic Drugs*, pages 458 to 463.)

Thrombocytopenic patients who have episodes of abnormal bleeding often receive I.V. infusions of platelets. Explain to the patient that these infusions usually stop abnormal bleeding caused by a low platelet count. However, in patients with immune destruction of platelets, platelet infusions are minimally effective and are used only for life-threatening bleeding.

If the patient receives repeated platelet infusions, he may develop antibodies to the white blood cells contained in the platelets. These antibodies can cause fever and chills. If this happens, reassure the patient that although these reactions are uncomfortable, they're not serious. Acetaminophen may help decrease or prevent these symptoms. The patient can also develop antibodies to plasma proteins, which may result in hives. Administering an antihistamine before a platelet infusion will characteristically prevent this type of reaction.

Inform the patient that after a platelet infusion, blood may need to be drawn for a platelet count, especially if he has received repeated infusions. Explain that the platelet count will show whether the infusion is working or whether the infused platelets are being destroyed.

● *Surgery.* Splenectomy may be necessary to correct thrombocytopenia caused by platelet destruction that doesn't respond to corticosteroids or that requires long-term corticosteroid therapy to maintain a safe platelet count. Since the spleen acts as the primary site of platelet removal and antibody production, a splenectomy

usually significantly reduces platelet destruction.

The patient scheduled for this surgery should be told where the spleen is located and what type of incision to expect. Warn him that fever and abdominal distention may develop postoperatively. Explain that antipyretics may be ordered for fever; abdominal distention may require insertion of a rectal tube, application of an abdominal binder, or administration of an antiflatulent.

● *Other care measures.* Encourage good dental hygiene to prevent the need for tooth extractions or restorations. Tell the patient to use a soft toothbrush. Also demonstrate proper flossing technique; the patient should avoid using a sawing motion that cuts the gums. (If his platelet count drops below 30,000, he may have to stop flossing.) Warn the patient to avoid using toothpicks.

If the patient experiences frequent nosebleeds, instruct him to use a humidifier at night. Also instruct him to keep the insides of his nostrils moist by applying Neosporin Ointment twice a day.

Inform the patient that surgery, I.M. injections, dental procedures, certain diagnostic tests, and trauma can cause serious bleeding. For this reason, he needs to tell all doctors and his dentist of his condition before any procedures are performed.

Advise the patient to carry an identification card to alert others that he has thrombocytopenia. A Medic Alert identification bracelet or necklace is also a good idea.

Finally, teach the patient to monitor his condition by examining his skin for ecchymoses and petechiae. Ideally, he should make sure that someone else checks areas that he has difficulty seeing. Tell him to report any bleeding from the mucous membranes or GI tract, as well as any new petechiae or ecchymoses. If the patient's female, tell her to report increased menstrual flow, if appropriate.

TEACHING PATIENTS ABOUT HEMATOLOGIC TESTS*

TEST AND PURPOSE	TEACHING POINTS
Bleeding time • To assess hemostasis • To detect congenital and acquired platelet function disorders	• Explain that the test measures the time it takes to form a clot and stop bleeding. The test usually takes 10 to 20 minutes. • Explain what will happen during the test: the test site (the forearm) is cleansed with antiseptic. A blood pressure cuff is applied to the upper arm and two tiny cuts are made on the forearm. Filter paper is then used to blot drops of blood until a platelet plug forms and oozing stops.
Bone marrow aspiration and biopsy • To assess the number, size, and cytoplasmic maturation of megakaryocytes, red cell precursors, and white cell precursors • To determine if thrombocytopenia, leukopenia, or anemia results from decreased or abnormal production and to determine possible cause • To assess iron stores • To identify an infiltrative process	• Explain that the test evaluates blood cells made in bone marrow and takes 5 to 10 minutes. • Explain what will happen during the test: the skin over the iliac crest (bony protrusion just above buttock) will be cleansed with antiseptic solution and anesthetized. A hollow needle with stylet is introduced into the bone marrow cavity. The stylet is removed, a syringe attached, and a small volume (0.5 ml) of blood and marrow aspirated. For biopsy, a small skin incision (3 to 4 mm) is made so a larger hollow needle can be introduced and a tiny core of bone marrow removed through the needle. Warn the patient that he may experience brief discomfort when marrow is aspirated. Explain that pressure will be applied for 10 to 15 minutes afterward. Tell the patient he can expect slight soreness over the puncture site but should report bleeding or severe pain.

Prenatal studies
• To detect genetic disorders, such as hemophilia or sickle cell disease, when there's a known family history
	• Explain that in some families it is now possible to determine whether a fetus has a specific genetic disorder.
	• Explain that blood samples are often required from multiple family members.
	• Prenatal studies may include chorionic villi sampling, amniocentesis, or fetoscopy. In *chorionic villi sampling,* the patient lies in lithotomy position while the doctor uses bimanual palpation to locate the uterus and an ultrasound scanner to locate the placenta. The patient may feel a crampy sensation as the doctor passes a catheter through the vagina into the uterus and applies suction to the catheter to remove a sample of embryonic tissue. Afterward, tell the patient to report any discomfort, fever, or fluid leakage.
	   In *amniocentesis,* the patient lies in lithotomy position while the doctor assesses fetal position and heartbeat. He then inserts a needle through the abdominal wall into the uterus, removes amniotic fluid, and applies a sterile dressing. Afterward, fetal heartbeat and maternal vital signs are monitored for ½ hour. The patient should report any discomfort, fever, fluid leakage, or change in fetal activity.
	   In *fetoscopy,* the doctor injects a small needle through the abdominal wall into the uterus and into a fetal blood vessel to obtain a blood sample. Afterward, monitoring is the same as for amniocentesis.

*Most hematologic tests require a serum, plasma, or whole blood sample but do not involve teaching beyond explaining the test's purpose and the collection technique.

TEACHING PATIENTS ABOUT HEMATOLOGIC DRUGS

DRUG	ADVERSE REACTIONS	INTERACTIONS*
Androgens		
fluoxymesterone (Halotestin) **methyltestosterone** (Android) **nandrolone decanoate** (Deca-Durabolin) **oxymetholone** (Anadrol-50) **stanozolol** (Winstrol) **testosterone**	*Reportable:* black stools, breast swelling (in men), confusion, dependent edema, dizziness, masculinizing effects (in women), nausea, precocious puberty in children, premature epiphyseal closure, priapism, red skin or other change in skin color, skin rash, urinary urgency (in men), vomiting *Other:* abdominal pain, anorexia, changed sexual desire, diarrhea, insomnia, pain and redness (from I.M. injection), sore mouth (from buccal administration)	• Tell the patient to avoid drugs and foods containing sodium. • Advise him that alcohol and other foods and over-the-counter products don't influence the safety or effectiveness of androgens.
Corticosteroids		
betamethasone (Celestone) **cortisone** (Cortone) **dexamethasone** (Decadron) **hydrocortisone** (Cortef) **prednisolone** **prednisone** (Deltasone) **triamcinolone** (Aristocort)	*Reportable during therapy:* abdominal pain or burning, acne, back pain, bleeding, delayed healing, edema, frequent urination, irregular heartbeat, menstrual disturbances, moon face, muscle weakness or cramps, skin rash, tarry stools, vision disturbances, vomiting *Reportable after therapy:* abdominal pain, back pain, dizziness, fainting, low-grade fever, muscle or joint pain, nausea, prolonged anorexia, shortness of breath, unusual weakness or weight loss, vomiting *Other:* increased appetite, indigestion, mood changes, nausea, restlessness, weight gain	• Tell the patient to avoid alcohol and sodium-containing foods or drugs. • Also tell him to avoid ephedrine, aspirin, and nonsteroidal anti-inflammatory drugs, such as ibuprofen.

*Interactions include food, alcohol, and over-the-counter products.

TEACHING POINTS

• Explain that androgens (male hormones) are prescribed to stimulate bone marrow production of blood cells. Explain the specific purpose for the patient.
• Mention that these drugs aren't usually prescribed for long periods for females because of masculinizing effects.
• Encourage fluids in patients with elevated serum calcium levels.
• Tell the patient to take a missed dose as soon as possible, unless it's almost time for the next dose. Tell him *not* to double-dose.

• Remind diabetic patients to closely monitor urine or blood glucose levels and to report changes. Androgens may elevate blood glucose levels.
• If the patient's taking buccal tablets, instruct him not to swallow the tablet but to let it dissolve. Remind him to avoid eating, drinking, or smoking immediately after taking the drug.
• Tell the patient to take oral preparations before or with meals to reduce GI upset.

• Explain the purpose of taking corticosteroids—for example, immunosuppression in thrombocytopenia.
• Make sure the patient knows whether therapy will be brief or long-term and what possible adverse reactions to expect.
• Tell women to let the doctor know if they are pregnant, plan to become pregnant, or are breast-feeding.
• Tell the patient *never* to stop taking medication without consulting the doctor, who may want to decrease the dose gradually. Abrupt withdrawal may cause serious adverse reactions.
• Warn patients receiving high doses of possible cushingoid effects. Reassure them that these effects will subside after therapy ends.
• Recommend that patients wear an identification bracelet describing treatment.
• Tell patients to keep medications out of the reach of children and to flush unused medication down the toilet.
• Advise patients to watch caloric intake to prevent weight gain. Encourage them to take

the drug with meals to prevent GI upset.
• Stress the importance of informing doctors of steroid therapy before undergoing immunizations, skin tests, surgery, or treatment for serious injuries or infections.
• Instruct patients how to handle a missed dose. *For an every-other-day schedule,* take the missed dose if you remember it early in the day; then continue as scheduled. If you remember late in the day, take it the next morning and skip the following day, returning to the every-other-day schedule.
For an every-day schedule, take the missed dose as soon as you remember and continue the schedule. If you don't remember until the next day, *do not double up.* Skip the missed dose and continue with the schedule.
For a several-times-a-day schedule, take the missed dose as soon as you remember. If it's close to the next one, you *may* double the dose.
• Tell the patient that after the drug is stopped, it may take a while for its effects to subside.

(continued)

**TEACHING PATIENTS ABOUT
HEMATOLOGIC DRUGS** (continued)

DRUG	ADVERSE REACTIONS	INTERACTIONS*
Hemostatics		
aminocaproic acid (Amicar)	*Reportable:* anuria, chest pain, diarrhea, dysuria, leg pain, nausea, severe muscle pain or weakness, thrombosis, unusually slow or irregular heart rate *Other:* dizziness, headache, nasal congestion, red eyes, rhinitis, skin rash	• Tell the patient that foods, alcohol, and over-the-counter products don't influence the safety or effectiveness of aminocaproic acid.
antihemophilic factor (AHF) (Factorate, Hemofil, Koate-HT)	*Reportable:* chills, difficulty breathing, fever, flushing, hives	• Tell the patient that foods, alcohol, and over-the-counter products don't influence the safety or effectiveness of AHF.
prothrombin complex concentrates (factors II, VII, IX, and X) (Konyne, Proplex)	*Reportable:* chest pain, chills, cough, fever, flushing, hives, respiratory distress, thrombosis *Other:* headache	• Tell the patient that foods, alcohol, and over-the-counter products don't influence the safety or effectiveness of this drug.
Iron-chelating agents		
deferoxamine mesylate (Desferal)	*Reportable:* erythema, hypotension, urticaria *Other:* abdominal discomfort, diarrhea, leg cramps	• Tell the patient that foods, alcohol, and over-the-counter products don't influence the safety or effectiveness of this drug.

*Interactions include foods, alcohol, and over-the-counter products.

TEACHING POINTS

• Inform the patient that this drug treats excessive bleeding.
• Warn against taking the drug within 6 to 12 hours of infusing prothrombin complex concentrates. Instruct the patient to check first with the treatment center.
• Emphasize the importance of taking medication for the prescribed length of time, even after bleeding has stopped.

• Recommend a soft diet to prevent clot disruption.
• Encourage parents to check the dosage with the treatment center as their child grows.

• Explain that AHF treats bleeding when factor VIII is deficient or absent.
• Teach the patient sterile I.V. infusion technique.
• Teach dosage calculations: multiply the patient's weight in kilograms by the percent desired. Then multiply this figure by 0.4 to find the number of AHF units needed. The doctor will specify the percent desired (higher for a major bleeding episode, so the dose will be larger).
• Emphasize the importance of keeping and

submitting treatment records.
• Also emphasize the importance of blood precautions, including proper disposal of I.V. equipment, to prevent transmission of blood-borne disease.
• Advise the patient to call the treatment center if problems arise.
• Tell the patient to use only concentrates labeled "heat treated."
• Instruct him to keep concentrates in the refrigerator.

• Explain that prothrombin complex treats bleeding when clotting factors II, VII, IX, and X are absent or deficient.
• Teach the patient sterile I.V. infusion technique. Emphasize the importance of slow infusion (no more than 3 ml/minute) to reduce the risk of thrombosis.
• Tell the patient to stop the infusion immediately if chest pain or difficulty breathing occurs.
• Teach the patient how to calculate dosage: multiply his weight in kilograms by the percent desired. Then multiply this figure by 0.6 to get the needed dosage. The doctor will

specify the percent desired (higher for a major bleeding episode so the dose will be larger).
• Emphasize the importance of keeping and submitting treatment records.
• Also emphasize the importance of blood precautions, including proper disposal of I.V. equipment, to prevent transmission of blood-borne disease.
• Remind the patient to call the treatment center if problems arise.
• Tell the patient to use only concentrates labeled "heat treated."
• Instruct him to refrigerate concentrates.

• Inform the patient that this drug helps remove dangerous iron deposits from his body. Explain the specific causes of this to the patient.
• Remind him not to take iron supplements.
• Tell him not to cook in a cast-iron skillet since some iron would be absorbed into food.
• Because protocols for home infusion programs differ, consult a hematology nurse before teaching the patient about home infusion.

• Remind the patient to call the doctor if problems develop with his home infusion program.
• Recommend periodic eye examinations for patients on long-term treatment and those at risk for cataracts.
• Explain the need for periodic urine and blood tests to assess his response to treatment.

(continued)

**TEACHING PATIENTS ABOUT
HEMATOLOGIC DRUGS** *(continued)*

DRUG	ADVERSE REACTIONS	INTERACTIONS*
Iron supplements		
ferrous gluconate (Fergon) **ferrous sulfate** (Feosol)	*Reportable:* bluish lips, nails or palms; drowsiness; pale, clammy skin; red or tarry stools with bloody streaks; severe diarrhea with vomiting and cramping; unusual weakness; weak or fast heartbeat *Other:* constipation, dark urine or stools, diarrhea, nausea, vomiting	• Warn the patient not to drink alcohol with iron supplements. • Tell the patient not to take antacids or ingest dairy products, tea, whole grain breads, eggs, or coffee within 1 hour of taking iron. • Instruct him to take iron with vitamin C, if possible, to improve absorption.
Vitamins		
cyanocobalamin (vitamin B_{12})	*Reportable:* anaphylaxis, difficulty breathing *Other:* diarrhea, itching	• Advise the patient not to drink excessive amounts of alcohol; absorption of cyanocobalamin may decrease. • Tell him not to take large doses of vitamin C (more than 1 g) within 1 hour of taking cyanocobalamin. • Tell him that foods and other over-the-counter drugs don't influence the safety or effectiveness of cyanocobalamin.
folic acid (vitamin B_9)	*Reportable:* fever, skin rash *Other:* yellow urine	• Tell the patient that foods, alcohol, and over-the-counter products don't influence the safety or effectiveness of folic acid.

*Interactions include foods, alcohol, and over-the-counter products.

TEACHING POINTS

• Explain the purpose of replacement therapy.
• Warn parents to keep iron supplements out of the reach of children. *Note:* Even small doses of adult iron can be fatal to children.
• Review proper administration.
• Tell the patient to come to the emergency department immediately if *any* reportable signs occur.
• Identify dietary sources of iron.
• Emphasize the importance of taking the prescribed course of iron, even if the patient's condition improves. Explain that replacing iron stores takes at least 2 months after hemoglobin levels return to normal.
• Point out that, although iron is best absorbed on an empty stomach, gastric irritation may require taking it with meals.
• Stress the importance of medical follow-up.
• Explain that long-term, excessive iron supplementation, especially without medical follow-up, may cause toxicity.
• Warn the patient that stools will probably be black but that this is expected.

• Explain that this vitamin helps treat pernicious anemia. Stress the need for lifelong therapy.
• Tell the patient that the doctor may wish to evaluate treatment with blood tests and checkups.

• Explain that folic acid is given for sickle cell anemia because of increased demands on the patient's bone marrow.
• Advise the patient that if he misses one or more doses, he should take the next dose at the regularly scheduled time.
• Tell the patient not to store folic acid in the bathroom medicine cabinet. Heat or moisture may ruin it.
• Tell him to expect bright yellow urine.

15

Immune System

Immune System

Introduction

The chronicity that marks many immune disorders adds a special challenge to your teaching efforts. After all, your patient may feel that he's gradually losing control of his life. He may feel the strain of family or social pressures. He may also fear losing his job or facing economic hardship. Or, worse yet, he may fear an unfavorable or untimely prognosis.

Obviously, emotional concerns like these can pose barriers to learning about an illness and its treatment. Overcoming them is a must if your teaching's to be effective. To do this, you'll need to follow these guidelines.

Proceed at the patient's pace

Pay careful attention to the signals a patient sends you. Do his words or gestures suggest that he's denying the existence of his illness? Does he seem to get angry at anyone who brings up the subject? Or does your patient seem concerned about what can be done about his illness or about where his life will now head?

Once you're clear about your patient's baseline responses to his illness, you'll be able to judge the pace at which he can learn.

Focus on key concerns

Typically, the patient isn't overly concerned with the pathophysiology of his illness. He's more concerned with the way in which his symptoms, prognosis, and complications will affect his daily life. However, the patient's active involvement in learning about basic pathophysiology and the resulting symptoms will help him understand how he'll need to adapt his life-style and why he'll need to adhere closely to his treatment regimen.

Underscore the importance of treatment

In immune disorders, compliance with treatment can sometimes spell the difference between a minor disruption in life-style and major complications. In rheumatoid arthritis, for example, the patient who adheres to his prescribed drug therapy, balances rest and activity, and protects his joints may avoid contractures and deformity. In systemic lupus erythematosus, the patient who rests adequately, takes prescribed corticosteroids, and follows other treatment measures may live a near-normal life and avoid life-threatening complications.

However, in disorders like acquired immune deficiency syndrome (AIDS), compliance with treatment doesn't have the same benefit for the patient. Nevertheless, his compliance does help him maintain the quality of his life for as long as possible.

DISORDERS

Acquired Immune Deficiency Syndrome

If you're like many nurses, you might feel overwhelmed when initially teaching a patient with acquired immune deficiency syndrome (AIDS). After all, this fatal syndrome currently has no cure. And its newsworthiness has put every grudging inch of medical progress in the public spotlight. However, these very reasons underscore the need for in-depth teaching of the person behind the headlines, the *individual* patient who faces an unfavorable and untimely prognosis. To help him maintain an optimum quality of life for as long as possible, you'll need to convince him of the value of preventive measures and supportive treatments. For exam-

---

CHECKLIST

TEACHING TOPICS IN A.I.D.S.

☐ Explanation of normal immune response and how the AIDS virus affects it

☐ The current status of AIDS research

☐ Tests to support diagnosis and confirm complications

☐ Treatment for any complications

☐ Activity and dietary modifications

☐ Symptoms of opportunistic infections and cancers

☐ Prevention of AIDS transmission, including safe sexual practices

☐ Measures to prevent infection

☐ Availability of support groups and other services

---

ple, the patient must take precautions to avoid infection and must comply with treatment for existing infection. Your teaching can help him understand this by pointing out that his damaged immune system leaves him vulnerable to opportunistic infections, which may be fatal.

Teaching the AIDS patient won't be easy. His initial feelings of anxiety and shock may later be accompanied by feelings of isolation and abandonment, resulting from contact with people who fear contagion or disapprove of homosexuals or I.V. drug users—the two groups most commonly afflicted by AIDS. Because the patient's emotions can interfere with his learning ability, you'll need to pace your teaching to match his receptivity to learning. And you may need to repeat much of the information you plan to teach him.

Because AIDS is a relatively new disorder, you may feel somewhat unprepared to answer some of the patient's questions about his illness. Therefore, you'll want to keep up to date on AIDS research so that you can teach more effectively. You should also explore your own feelings—possibly fears—about caring for AIDS patients to help you better establish the trusting and caring relationship necessary for successful teaching.

Describe the disorder

Explain that AIDS results from a virus—human T-cell lymphotropic virus, type III (HTLV-III)—that impairs immune function. This virus selectively attacks and disables specialized white blood cells called T_4 helper lymphocytes, gradually depleting their number and impairing their response to infection (see *How the AIDS Virus Affects Immunity*).

Explain to the patient that various opportunistic infections and cancers can occur with AIDS—most commonly *Pneumocystis carinii* pneumonia and Kaposi's sarcoma—because of his impaired immune function. Inform him that many opportunistic diseases can

HOW THE A.I.D.S. VIRUS AFFECTS IMMUNITY

Normal immune function
1. When viruses enter a healthy body, they're detected and identified as antigens by macrophages. Macrophages process the antigens and present them to T cells and B cells.
2. The antigen-activated T cells proliferate and form several kinds of T cells. Helper T cells stimulate B cells, whereas suppressor T cells control the extent of T cell help for B cells. Lymphokine-producing T cells are involved in delayed hypersensitivity and other immune reactions. Cytotoxic, or killer, T cells directly destroy antigenic agents. Memory T cells are stored to recognize and attack the same antigen on subsequent invasions.
3. The B cells proliferate, forming memory cells and plasma cells that produce antigen-specific antibodies, which then attack and kill the invading virus.

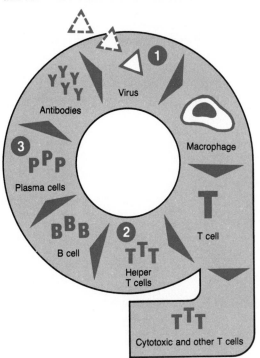

Altered immune function
1. The HTLV-III virus infects helper T cells and impairs their ability to recognize antigens, which allows the HTLV-III virus to proliferate within the T cells.
2. Cell-mediated immunity is weakened, making the patient vulnerable to bacterial, viral, and fungal infections and certain malignancies, all of which can be fatal. Meanwhile, the damaged T cells produce more HTLV-III virus, which invades other T cells, compounding the problem.

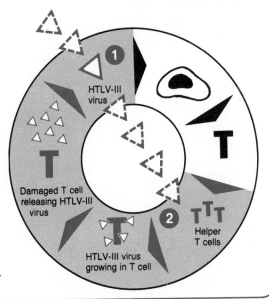

be treated but that his immune system still won't function normally. Even though he may be cured of one of these diseases, he remains susceptible to others that can be fatal.

Point out that no cure for AIDS currently exists but that recent discoveries hold promise for the future. Also mention that major research hospitals conduct experimental drug trials for which they require volunteers.

Point out possible complications

Emphasize the importance of following the recommended treatment plan to limit the number of infections the patient incurs. Make sure he clearly understands that preventing assaults on his damaged immune system can help him preserve the quality of his life for as long as possible.

Teach about tests

Tell the patient that positive results from the HTLV-III antibody blood test (ELISA) indicate exposure to the virus but don't confirm diagnosis of AIDS. If ELISA results are positive, a follow-up blood test called the Western blot analysis is done. Positive results confirm exposure to HTLV-III. Together with a laboratory-confirmed diagnosis of opportunistic infection or certain malignancies, they support the diagnosis of AIDS.

If necessary, teach the patient about tissue biopsies to confirm diagnosis of opportunistic infections. He may require such procedures as bronchoscopy, colonoscopy, or bone marrow aspiration.

Teach about treatments

• *Activity.* Tell the patient to alternate periods of rest and activity and to lie down whenever he gets tired. Stress the importance of adequate sleep and rest to reduce his risk of infection. Recommend a regular program of moderate exercise to help the patient maintain optimal health. As his condition deteriorates, his exercise pro-

gram will have to be modified.

• *Diet.* Explain to the patient that loss of appetite and weight accompany AIDS. Stress that maintaining adequate nutrition helps prevent infection. Encourage eating small, frequent, high-calorie, high-protein meals, and emphasize the importance of drinking at least 1,500 ml of fluid each day (about six glasses of water). Advise the patient to spend minimal energy preparing food. Suggest that he cook large quantities and freeze portions for later use or that he ask others to help with food preparation.

Tell the patient to rest before meals to conserve energy and increase his appetite. Encourage him to eat with friends or family to make eating more enjoyable and prevent feelings of isolation. If he continues to lose weight, show him how to keep a calorie count, and teach him about commercial dietary supplements.

If the patient has mouth sores or an oral infection, he may need a soft diet. If he has diarrhea, recommend a low-fat, lactose-reduced, low-fiber diet. Teach the patient how to select and prepare appropriate foods to fit these diets.

• *Medication.* Explain to the patient that even though no drug has succeeded in restoring immune function in AIDS, doctors have had success in using drugs (as well as radiation and surgery) to treat associated conditions. For example, *P. carinii* pneumonia, a parasitic infection, is usually treated with co-trimoxazole or pentamidine. Kaposi's sarcoma, which appears on the surface of the skin or in the mouth, can be treated with radiation, chemotherapy, or certain experimental drugs.

• *Other care measures.* Make sure you emphasize the importance of prevention or early detection and treatment of infections. (See *Preventing Infection—and Recognizing Its Symptoms.*)

Stress the urgency of preventing the spread of AIDS. Explain to the patient why he mustn't donate blood, sperm, organs, or tissues. Make sure he un-

PREVENTING INFECTION—AND RECOGNIZING ITS SYMPTOMS

Dear Patient:

Because AIDS impairs your body's ability to fight infection, prevention of infection is extremely important. However, if you do come down with an infection, always remember that early recognition and treatment are equally important. They can prevent worsening of your condition and improve the quality of your life.

Preventing infection

To help you prevent infection, follow these guidelines:
• Avoid crowds and people with known infections, such as herpes, influenza, candidiasis, chickenpox, and giardiasis.
• Get an adequate amount of sleep, and rest often during the day.
• If you've lost your appetite, you'll still need to eat regularly to maintain good nutrition. Try small, frequent meals.
• Practice good hygiene, especially oral care. Don't use commercial mouthwashes because their high alcohol and sugar content may irritate your mouth and provide a medium for bacterial growth.
• Don't use any nonprescribed intravenous drugs. However, if you do use them, *don't* share needles.
• Avoid travel to foreign countries.

Recognizing symptoms of infection

If you notice any of the following symptoms of infection, be sure to contact your doctor as soon as possible:
• persistent fever or sweating at night (but not necessarily every night) that's unexplained by a cold or flu
• swollen lymph nodes in your neck, armpits, or groin that last more than 2 months and aren't explained by any other illnesses
• profound and persistent fatigue that's not relieved by rest and not explained by increased physical activity, longer work schedules, drug use, or a psychological disorder
• weight loss of more than 10 lb in less than 2 months that's unrelated to diet or exercise and possibly accompanied by loss of appetite
• persistent, unexplained diarrhea
• a white coating or spots on your tongue or throat, possibly accompanied by soreness, a burning sensation, or difficulty swallowing
• blurred vision and/or persistent and severe headaches
• rash or skin discoloration that persists or spreads
• unexplained bleeding or bruises.

derstands that he can transmit the AIDS virus to other men or women through sexual intercourse. Tell him that if a female partner acquires AIDS and then becomes pregnant, her child is also at risk of developing AIDS. Teach the patient about safe sexual practices, which exclude anal, oral, or vaginal penetration. Mention that consistent use of condoms may reduce the risk of transmission but that this hasn't been proven. Warn the patient not to share toothbrushes, razors, or other implements that may be contaminated with his blood.

Because the patient requires considerable emotional support, make him aware of AIDS organizations and the kinds of help they offer: information on and referrals to appropriate services, such as medical and psychological care centers; support groups for AIDS patients and those close to them; and counseling on third-party payment of health care costs and on government financial aid. Volunteer peer counselors also can provide ongoing emotional support.

Rheumatoid Arthritis

Successful management of rheumatoid arthritis (RA) depends largely on the patient's willingness to comply with his treatment plan, thereby preventing complications. It also depends on his willingness to experiment with self-care measures and assistive devices to enhance the comfort and quality of his life.

To promote the patient's compliance, you can point out to him that RA can be controlled with medication, diet, and a balanced program of exercise and rest. However, because magical cures for arthritis are commonly advertised, you'll need to emphasize that treatment should be directed only by a qualified team of health professionals. You'll also need to emphasize that

symptoms can vary widely among patients, although most report periods of exacerbation and remission.

Describe the disorder

Tell the patient that rheumatoid arthritis is a chronic, systemic inflammatory disorder that can progress slowly or rapidly. Its early symptoms usually include pain, tenderness, swelling, or stiffness in the synovial joints (in the shoulder, elbow, wrist, hand, hip, knee, and foot).

Inform the patient that RA's course varies from person to person but usually involves periods of exacerbation and remission. Mention that its cause isn't known but that researchers suspect it involves an autoimmune response to the patient's own immunoglobulin G (IgG). Apparently, RA develops when synovial lymphocytes (B cells) act as if the patient's IgG were an antigen. They produce antibodies, which stimulate formation of immune complexes within the joint. These complexes initiate and sustain an inflammatory response, resulting in damage to the joint lining and cartilage (see *Results of Immune Complex Formation*, pages 472 and 473). Subsequently, pannus formation—fibrotic changes and hypertrophy of the synovial membranes—develops in these joints. Inflammatory damage may also occur in tendons, ligaments, and eventually bone. This results in joint deformities, subluxations, contractures, pain, and loss of function.

Point out possible complications

Describe the complications that can result from poorly managed RA. Joint pain, for instance, can become excruciating, and joint damage and severe deformities can become irreversible, if the patient fails to follow his drug regimen. In addition, muscle strength and joint mobility can be reduced if he doesn't follow his prescribed exercise program. Weakness in hip flexor and quadriceps muscles can also lead to gait problems, demanding extra energy and placing further stress on the patient's other joints.

Teach about tests

Inform the patient that the rheumatoid factor (RF) test for anti-IgG antibody is positive in about 95% of patients with RA but that no single laboratory test provides conclusive diagnosis. Explain that a complete blood count may be performed to detect anemia, a frequent finding in RA, and an erythrocyte sedimentation rate may be determined to detect inflammation. Explain that these three tests require small blood samples.

Synovial fluid analysis also helps diagnose RA. Explain to the patient that this test helps determine the cause of joint inflammation and swelling. Tell him who will perform the test and where, and describe the procedure for aspiration, which is usually performed on the knee joint. If appropriate, explain that aspiration not only provides fluid for laboratory analysis but also may decrease pain and prevent joint destruction. Warn the patient that even though he'll be given a local anesthetic, he may feel transient discomfort as the needle penetrates the joint. Tell him to report any increased pain or fever (indications of joint infection) after the test.

Inform the patient that X-rays of the affected joints may be performed to assess joint damage. They may be repeated at varying intervals to monitor bone erosion and joint deformity.

Teach about treatments

• *Activity.* Emphasize the need to balance rest and activity. Recommend that the patient sleep 8 to 10 hours a night and lie down for ½ hour twice during the day. Tell him to maintain correct body position during rest, with his joints extended rather than flexed. Advise using a firm mattress supported by a bed board and placing a small, flat pillow under his head. Caution against placing a pillow under his

---

CHECKLIST

TEACHING TOPICS IN RHEUMATOID ARTHRITIS

☐ Explanation of the chronicity and variable symptoms of rheumatoid arthritis

☐ Importance of strict compliance with treatment to prevent complications, such as worsening pain and deformity

☐ Preparation for blood tests and, if ordered, synovial fluid analysis

☐ Administration of salicylates or other medication, such as nonsteroidal anti-inflammatory drugs

☐ A balanced program of rest and activity

☐ An exercise program to reduce stiffness and promote mobility

☐ Importance of joint protection, including the need for good body mechanics and use of assistive devices

☐ Dietary considerations, including devices to ease meal preparation

☐ Application of heat or cold to reduce stiffness, swelling, or pain

☐ Sexual activity

☐ Sources of information and support

---

knees. If splints are prescribed, remind him that they're to be worn in bed and whenever possible during the day.

Stress the importance of using good body mechanics at all times to avoid pain and joint stress. Warn him to avoid bending, stooping, or remaining in one position for a prolonged period. Instruct him to work with his fingers extended as much as possible to avoid exaggerating flexion deformities. To avoid joint stress, tell him to sit in a straight-backed chair with a seat high enough for his feet to remain flat on the floor. Suggest that he consider buying a raised seat for his toilet.

Advise the patient to pace himself and to set realistic goals for activities. Point out symptoms that signal when he should curtail activity: increased pain or fatigue and progressive loss of dexterity in involved joints. Explain that his prescribed exercise program helps preserve joint mobility and strengthen muscle groups that aren't used in normal activities. It will include gentle range-of-motion exercises, usually done daily.

Inform the patient that applying heat will relieve stiffness before exercise or other activity. Warn him to avoid strenuous exercise during acute inflammatory episodes.

• *Diet.* Stress the importance of a bal-

RESULTS OF IMMUNE COMPLEX FORMATION

The formation of immune complexes triggers several different processes in the bloodstream. These include phagocytosis, the release of vasoactive substances, and the activation of coagulation. Excess circulating immune complexes are deposited in the tissues, initiating an

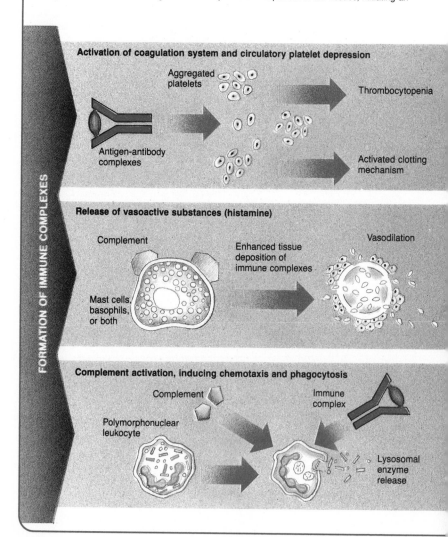

FORMATION OF IMMUNE COMPLEXES

Activation of coagulation system and circulatory platelet depression

Aggregated platelets

Antigen-antibody complexes

Thrombocytopenia

Activated clotting mechanism

Release of vasoactive substances (histamine)

Complement

Mast cells, basophils, or both

Enhanced tissue deposition of immune complexes

Vasodilation

Complement activation, inducing chemotaxis and phagocytosis

Complement

Polymorphonuclear leukocyte

Immune complex

Lysosomal enzyme release

anced diet and ensure that the patient knows how to select foods from the four basic food groups to meet his daily requirements. Explain that foods high in vitamins, proteins, and iron promote tissue building and repair. Advise the patient to eat frequent, small meals if his appetite is poor.

If the patient's overweight, tell him that he's placing extra stress on his joints. Encourage him to lose weight.

• **Medication.** Explain to the patient

inflammatory response. This response produces glomerulitis in the renal basement membrane, vasculitis in the blood vessels, and arthritis in joint synovia (as shown here).

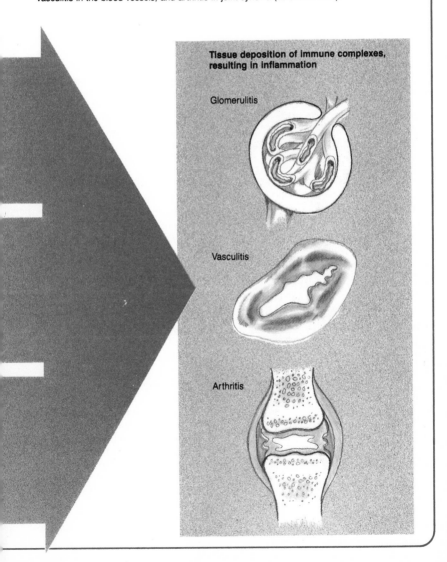

Tissue deposition of immune complexes, resulting in inflammation

Glomerulitis

Vasculitis

Arthritis

that drug therapy aims to control inflammation and pain and arrest progression of the disease. Point out that he may need to take several drugs to achieve the desired results. Salicylates, the mainstay of therapy, reduce inflammation and relieve pain. Gold salts,

penicillamine, nonsteroidal anti-inflammatory drugs, antimalarials, immunosuppressants, and corticosteroids may also be helpful. (See *Teaching Patients about Immune Drugs,* pages 478 to 483.)

To help the patient remember his medication schedule, you may need to devise a medication calendar for him. Instruct him to notify the doctor if his symptoms worsen during drug therapy. If his hands are weak or deformed or if their movement causes pain, tell him to ask his pharmacist not to use childproof caps on medication bottles.

• ***Other care measures.*** If arthritis affects the patient's feet, tell him that pain may be relieved by having special pads or metatarsal bars inserted in his shoes. If he has a severe foot deformity, he may need custom-made shoes.

Suggest that the patient sit while preparing meals to save wear and tear on affected weight-bearing joints. Mention that counter-top appliances, such as slow cookers and toaster ovens, can eliminate bending to use an oven. Advise using lightweight plastic dishes for meals, aluminum pots and pans for cooking, and a wheeled dolly or plant stand for moving heavy items across counters. Point out that using double-handled pots and pans will allow the patient to use both hands for lifting. He can also drive a few rustproof nails into a cutting board to hold food so that he can use both hands for cutting. He can attach a raised lip along one edge of the board to secure bread for buttering. To open jars, he can use a rubber gripper or vise-grip opener; for cans, an electric can opener.

Discuss application of local heat and cold to relieve pain and inflammation, and suggest that the patient try different methods to find out what works best for him. Point out that he needn't buy costly devices to apply heat or cold because home methods are usually effective. For moist heat, he can stand in a warm shower, soak in a tub, or apply wet towels to stiff or painful joints. For dry heat, he can wrap a heating pad in a towel before placing it against his skin. If he has diminished sensation, tell him never to set the heating pad on high and to check often for burns.

Because heat can increase joint pain and synovial fluid volume and trigger muscle spasms, the patient may benefit more from cold application. Suggest using moist towels or ice bags.

Besides teaching the patient about assistive devices and physical treatments, you'll need to address his sexual concerns. For example, tell him that he can still enjoy a satisfying sexual relationship even though his arthritis may change the way he looks and moves. He should let his partner know what feels good and what causes discomfort. Advise him to plan sexual activity for when he feels best. Also advise him to pace his activities beforehand to avoid fatigue, to perform range-of-motion exercises to relax joints, to take a warm bath or shower to relax, and to take analgesics to relieve joint pain.

Inform the female patient of childbearing age to let her doctor know if she plans to become pregnant. He may adjust her medication dosage.

Warn the patient that many advertised devices and treatments claim to cure arthritis or relieve its pain. However, these can be expensive, ineffective, and even harmful if they interfere with prescribed therapy. Encourage him to notify you, his doctor, or the local chapter of the Arthritis Foundation *before* he tries any alternative treatment. Note that the Arthritis Foundation also provides support services.

Systemic Lupus Erythematosus

Teaching the patient with systemic lupus erythematosus (SLE) is likely to be an ongoing process. In the early stages, you'll need to prepare the patient for the sometimes lengthy diagnostic

---

CHECKLIST

TEACHING TOPICS IN S.L.E.

☐ Explanation of the disorder, including its unpredictable exacerbations and remissions

☐ Prevention of complications

☐ Need for repeated diagnostic tests

☐ Corticosteroids or other prescribed drugs

☐ Avoiding fatigue and balancing rest and activity

☐ Apheresis to treat life-threatening complications and acute flare-ups, if necessary

☐ Measures to prevent infection and skin breakdown

☐ Avoiding sun and cold exposure

☐ Stress-reduction techniques

---

workup. Once the diagnosis is made, you'll focus on the disorder's long-term management, especially the importance of adhering to the prescribed drug regimen, monitoring and reporting warning symptoms, and practicing self-care measures. If the patient's especially prone to flare-ups, you'll need to address any aggravating factors, such as excessive activity or stress, and help correct them.

Compliance with treatment can reduce the risk of complications and improve the quality of life for the patient with SLE. Despite these possible benefits, teaching him may not always be easy. That's because the disorder's chronicity and unpredictability can act as a barrier to learning. Typically, you'll have to help the patient adjust to the prospect of lifelong treatment and periodic flare-ups before he'll be receptive to your teaching.

Describe the disorder

Tell the patient that SLE is a chronic disorder that causes structural changes in the connective tissue, the fibers that support many other body tissues. Its unpredictable course includes exacerbations interspersed with long periods of complete or near-complete remission. The disorder may produce only mild effects. However, it may also be life-threatening because of its effects on the heart, blood vessels, kidneys, lungs, and central nervous system.

Explain that the cause of SLE isn't known but that researchers believe antibodies develop against the body's own tissues—mostly deoxyribonucleic acid (DNA), but sometimes ribonucleic acid (RNA), clotting factors, and blood cells. This autoimmune response generates immune complexes, which damage connective tissue and cause inflammation. (See *Results of Immune Complex Formation,* pages 472 and 473.) Explain that because these immune complexes may be present in any part of the body, he may have different symptoms at different times—and with varying severity.

Point out possible complications

Emphasize to the patient that failure to follow the prescribed treatment plan can cause a flare-up, but that even total compliance doesn't rule one out. Gaining this understanding can help the patient avoid unwarranted self-recrimination.

Explain that emotional stress and inadequate rest may make the patient more prone to a flare-up. Point out that exposure to sunlight—including reflected sunlight—may lead to a flare-up, severe urticaria, and bullous lesions. Even brief exposure (20 minutes or less) may produce a rash. Stress the importance of minimizing exposure to infection, since the patient has increased susceptibility.

Teach about tests

Inform the patient that definitive diagnosis of SLE may take months of observation, many laboratory tests, and sometimes a trial of drugs. Explain that he needs to provide a precise history of his symptoms to aid diagnosis.

Tell the patient that blood tests will be performed to evaluate his immune system and to detect certain antibodies. One such test, the antinuclear antibody test, yields positive results in about 95% of SLE patients. Also, a positive lupus erythematosus factor test strongly suggests SLE, especially if clinical symptoms are present. However, the anti-DNA antibody test remains the most specific test for SLE because it rarely gives positive results in other disorders. Tell the patient that these blood tests may be repeated periodically to monitor the effectiveness of therapy.

Explain to the patient that a complete blood count, an erythrocyte sedimentation rate, a urinalysis, a chest X-ray, an electrocardiogram, and renal function tests may be performed to evaluate SLE's effects. If a renal biopsy is scheduled to determine the extent of renal involvement, tell the patient to fast for 6 hours before the test. Explain that the biopsy involves inserting a needle through the skin on his flank and obtaining a small tissue sample from his kidney. Inform the patient that he'll be sedated for the test. He'll lie on his stomach with a sandbag under his abdomen and be asked to hold his breath while the needle is inserted. Explain that he'll remain in bed up to 24 hours after the test.

Teach about treatments

● *Activity.* Tell the patient with joint stiffness and inflammation that a program of moderate exercise and specific range-of-motion exercises promotes optimal health and maintains joint mobility. Recommend the use of moist or dry heat before exercising to decrease discomfort. Warn him to avoid exercising to the point of fatigue to avoid flare-ups. Advise him to restrict his activity if he's experiencing a flare-up and to resume activity slowly after one.

Because fatigue commonly occurs in SLE, recommend that the patient sleep 10 to 12 hours each night and rest periodically during the day. Make sure he understands the need to curtail his activities before he tires.

• *Diet.* Explain that no specific diet will improve or cure SLE but that foods high in protein, vitamins, and iron help maintain optimum nutrition and prevent anemia. If the patient has lost weight, advise him to increase his caloric intake with between-meal snacks or commercially available high-protein, high-calorie supplements.

• *Medication.* Drug therapy aims to control symptoms of SLE. Corticosteroids, for example, form the backbone of treatment to slow SLE's progressive symptoms. Salicylates or nonsteroidal anti-inflammatory drugs may be used to treat fever and arthritic symptoms. Antimalarial drugs may be used to combat skin manifestations and joint involvement. And immunosuppressants may be prescribed when other drugs fail to control the disorder. (See *Teaching Patients about Immune Drugs*, pages 478 to 483.)

Tell the patient that as his condition improves, drug dosages will be lowered gradually. Remind him that any deviations from his prescribed regimen can exacerbate his disorder.

• *Procedures.* If the patient has life-threatening complications or an acute flare-up that's unresponsive to corticosteroids, a procedure called therapeutic apheresis may be performed. To prepare the patient for this procedure, explain that a needle will be inserted in each arm and that his blood will be pumped through a machine to remove the circulating immune complexes that are exacerbating his disorder. Tell him that his pulse and blood pressure will be monitored and that he should report any tingling sensations around his mouth or in his hands or feet.

• *Other care measures.* Caution the patient to avoid exposure to sunlight—even sunlight that's reflected from sand or snow. Advise him to use a sunblock or to wear protective clothing. Wide-brimmed hats, sunglasses, and hypoallergenic cosmetics also lower the risk of reactions to sun exposure.

Make sure the patient understands the need to prevent infection. Advise him to avoid crowds and people with known infections and to consult his doctor about influenza and pneumococcal vaccines. Caution against excessive bathing because it can dry or break down the skin, leaving it vulnerable to infection. However, each day he should cleanse and pat dry areas where two skin surfaces touch, such as the underarm or genital areas. Tell him to regularly inspect these areas for signs of infection or skin breakdown.

Stress the importance of meticulous mouth care to prevent or treat oral lesions. Advise the patient to use a soft toothbrush and to avoid commercial mouthwashes because of their high sugar content and the irritating and drying effect of the alcohol base. Tell him to call his doctor if he notices white plaques in his mouth; they could indicate a fungal infection. Suggest soft, bland foods if he has open sores. Emphasize the importance of regular dental care to prevent infection.

Inform the patient that emotional extremes and stress can worsen symptoms. Advise him to maintain a calm, stable environment if possible. Teach him relaxation exercises and other stress-reduction techniques.

If the patient has Raynaud's phenomenon (a common occurrence in SLE), tell him to protect his hands and feet against cold weather to prevent vasospasm. Instruct him to avoid cold water and to wear gloves when handling cold items, such as frozen foods.

Explain to the female patient that she may experience menstrual irregularities during flare-ups but will resume her normal cycle during remissions. Advise her to discuss contraceptive methods or pregnancy plans with her doctor. Patients often feel better during pregnancy, but flare-ups can occur postpartum.

Finally, tell the patient to call the doctor if fever, cough, or skin rash occurs or if chest, abdominal, muscle, or joint pain worsens.

TEACHING PATIENTS ABOUT IMMUNE DRUGS

DRUG	ADVERSE REACTIONS	INTERACTIONS*

Aspirin and salicylates

aspirin
(Bayer Aspirin, Ecotrin)

aspirin and caffeine
(Anacin)

buffered aspirin
(Ascriptin, Bufferin)

choline magnesium trisalicylate
(Trilisate)

magnesium salicylate
(Doan's Pills)

salsalate
(Disalcid)

sodium salicylate

Reportable: abdominal pain, asterixis of hands, unusually deep breathing, chest tightness, confusion, diaphoresis, diarrhea (severe), drowsiness (severe), hallucinations, hearing loss, hematochezia, hematuria, nausea (severe), polydipsia, seizures, tachypnea, tinnitus, visual disturbances, vomiting, wheezing
Other: heartburn, indigestion

• Tell the patient to avoid taking acetaminophen, antacids, other aspirin or salicylate products, or cellulose-containing laxatives unless his doctor approves.
• Advise the patient to avoid alcohol while taking this drug.
• Tell the patient that foods and nonalcoholic beverages don't influence the drug's safety or effectiveness.

Corticosteroids

prednisone
(Deltasone, Orasone)

Reportable: abdominal pain, acne, back or rib pain, easy bruising, fever, hypertension, melena, menstrual irregularity, psychoses, sore throat, unusual tiredness, vomiting, weight gain (marked)
Other: diaphoresis, increased facial and body hair, mood swings (mild), nausea (mild), polyphagia, weight gain (slight)

• Tell the patient to avoid products containing aspirin, unless his doctor specifically recommends them, because they increase the risk of GI ulceration.
• Tell him to avoid alcohol because it increases the risk of GI ulceration.
• Advise the patient to avoid foods or over-the-counter drugs containing sodium because they may increase the risk of fluid retention.

*Interactions include food, alcohol, and over-the-counter drugs.

TEACHING POINTS

• Explain to the patient that this drug should help relieve pain or reduce inflammation.

• If the patient is taking this drug for arthritis, inform him that he may not experience relief for several weeks. Mention that his doctor may order biweekly serum tests until the drug reaches optimal levels in his blood.

• Warn him not to substitute acetaminophen preparations, which lack an anti-inflammatory effect.

• Tell the patient to take the drug at the same time every day. If he misses a dose, tell him to take it as soon as he remembers. But if it's almost time for the next dose, tell him to skip the missed dose.

• If the drug causes gastric upset or heartburn, instruct the patient to take it with food or a full glass of water.

• Describe the general symptoms of GI bleeding, and tell the patient to report them if they occur. Also tell him to be especially alert for tinnitus, usually the first symptom that the salicylate dose may be too high.

• Warn the patient not to break up or chew long-acting aspirin or enteric-coated tablets, because this will cause excess stomach irritation and will destroy the long-acting effect.

• Caution the patient to store the drug tightly capped and in a moisture-free area to prevent chemical breakdown. Tell him not to use aspirin or buffered aspirin that has a strong vinegary odor, because this means the drug has broken down.

• Stress the need to check the contents of all over-the-counter products he buys. Many products contain aspirin or salicylates and can cause toxicity by increasing serum salicylate levels. Tell the patient to ask the pharmacist or the doctor if he's unsure about a product's ingredients.

• If the patient's on a sodium-restricted diet, inform him that buffered aspirin, effervescent tablets, and sodium salicylate may contain large amounts of sodium.

• Explain to the patient that this drug should help control severe symptoms of his connective tissue disorder.

• Explain the expected effects of corticosteroid therapy.

• Tell the patient to take his medication at the same time each day. Warn him never to stop taking the drug abruptly.

• Describe the general symptoms of GI bleeding, and tell the patient to report them if they occur.

• Inform him that the drug may mask some signs of infection; discuss preventive measures.

(continued)

**TEACHING PATIENTS
ABOUT IMMUNE DRUGS** *(continued)*

DRUG	ADVERSE REACTIONS	INTERACTIONS*
Gold salts		
auranofin (Ridaura) **aurothioglucose** (Solganal) **gold sodium thiomalate** (Myochrysine)	*Reportable:* abdominal cramps, alopecia, anorexia, bleeding tendencies, bloody or cloudy urine, diarrhea, dizziness, dyspnea, fainting, itching, jaundice, mouth sores, nausea, rash, metallic taste, weakness	• Tell the patient to avoid over-the-counter nonsteroidal anti-inflammatory drugs, such as ibuprofen, because they may increase the risk of kidney damage. • Tell the patient that foods and beverages don't influence the safety or effectiveness of gold salts.
Immunosuppressants		
azathioprine (Imuran)	*Reportable:* bleeding tendencies, chills, fever, heartburn, jaundice, sore throat *Other:* anorexia, nausea, rash, vomiting	• Tell the patient that foods, beverages, and over-the-counter drugs don't influence the safety or effectiveness of azathioprine.
cyclophosphamide (Cytoxan)	*Reportable:* bleeding tendencies, chills, dyspnea, dysuria, fever, heartburn, hematuria, jaundice, sore throat *Other:* alopecia, anorexia, nausea, skin and fingernail darkening, vomiting	• Tell the patient that foods, beverages, and over-the-counter drugs don't influence the safety or effectiveness of cyclophosphamide.
methotrexate (Folex, Mexate)	*Reportable:* bleeding tendencies, chills, diarrhea, dyspnea, fever, heartburn, hematochezia, jaundice, mouth sores, sore throat *Other:* anorexia, nausea, vomiting	• Tell the patient to avoid alcohol, salicylates, and vitamin preparations containing folic acid.

*Interactions include food, alcohol, and over-the-counter drugs.

TEACHING POINTS

• Explain to the patient that gold salts should help control his joint inflammation. Inform him that he may not see improvement in his condition for several months. Mention that concurrent treatment with anti-inflammatory agents may be necessary, especially for the first few months.

• Explain that the doctor will order frequent blood tests to monitor for drug toxicity.
• Stress the importance of good oral hygiene to maintain comfort.
• Tell the patient to avoid exposure to sunlight.

• Explain to the patient that this drug should help control severe symptoms of rheumatoid arthritis (RA) and prevent joint damage.
• Inform him that he may be more susceptible to infection while he's taking the drug; discuss preventive measures.
• Discuss the general symptoms of infection and bleeding, and tell the patient to report them if they occur.
• Advise female patients to use birth control measures during and for 4 months after therapy.
• Tell the patient to take the drug with meals to reduce nausea and vomiting.

• Explain to the patient that this drug should help control severe symptoms of RA and prevent joint damage.
• Tell him to drink at least 2½ quarts of fluid a day and to urinate as often as possible.
• Inform him that he may be more susceptible to infection while he's taking the drug; discuss preventive measures.
• Discuss the general symptoms of infection and bleeding, and tell the patient to report them if they occur.
• Advise female patients to use birth control measures during and for 4 months after therapy.
• Tell the patient to take the drug with meals to reduce nausea and vomiting.

• Explain to the patient that this drug should help control severe symptoms of RA and prevent joint damage.
• Because the drug suppresses the immune response, inform the patient that he may develop infections while he's taking it.
• Discuss the general symptoms of infection and bleeding, and tell the patient to report them if they occur.
• Advise female patients to use birth control measures during and for 4 months after therapy.
• Stress the importance of good oral hygiene to maintain comfort.
• Tell the patient to take the drug with meals to reduce nausea and vomiting.

(continued)

TEACHING PATIENTS
ABOUT IMMUNE DRUGS (continued)

DRUG	ADVERSE REACTIONS	INTERACTIONS*
Nonsteroidal anti-inflammatory agents		
fenoprofen (Nalfon) **ibuprofen** (Advil, Motrin, Nuprin) **indomethacin** (Indocin, Indocin SR) **ketoprofen** (Orudis) **meclofenamate** (Meclomen) **naproxen** (Anaprox, Naprosyn) **piroxicam** (Feldene) **sulindac** (Clinoril) **tolmetin** (Tolectin)	*Reportable:* edema, fever, hematochezia, hematuria, jaundice, melena, oliguria, rash, sore throat, wheezing *Other:* diarrhea, dizziness, drowsiness, heartburn, indigestion, nausea, vomiting	• Tell the patient not to take this drug with aspirin, acetaminophen, or alcohol. • Tell him to take the drug on an empty stomach—1 hour before meals or 3 hours after meals—for best absorption.
Miscellaneous drugs for arthritis		
hydroxychloroquine (Plaquenil)	*Reportable:* anxiety, dizziness, visual disturbances, weakness *Other:* abdominal cramps, anorexia, diarrhea, headache, nausea, vomiting	• Tell the patient to avoid alcohol, because it increases the risk of hepatotoxicity. • Tell the patient that foods, non-alcoholic beverages, and over-the-counter drugs don't influence the safety or effectiveness of hydroxychloroquine.
penicillamine (Cuprimine, Depen)	*Reportable:* anorexia, bleeding tendencies, chills, fever, infections, mouth sores, nausea, rash, stomach upset, taste disturbance or loss, weakness	• Tell the patient not to take iron or iron preparations because they may impair the drug's effectiveness. • Tell him to take the drug on an empty stomach—1 hour before or 3 hours after a meal.

*Interactions include food, alcohol, and over-the-counter drugs.

TEACHING POINTS

• Explain to the patient that this drug should help relieve his arthritis, joint inflammation, or pain associated with sprains, strains, bursitis, tendinitis, or gout. Inform him that he may not notice improvement in his condition until he has taken the drug for a month.
• If the drug causes gastric distress, tell him to take it with meals or an antacid, if his doctor approves.
• If the patient misses a dose, tell him to take it as soon as he remembers. However, if it's almost time for the next dose, tell him to skip the missed dose; he shouldn't double-dose.
• If the drug makes him drowsy or dizzy, advise him not to drive or operate machinery.

• Explain to the patient that this drug may arrest his progressive RA or may relieve skin and joint symptoms associated with SLE. Inform him that he may not see the full benefit of therapy for 6 months.
• Stress the need for regular eye examinations during therapy.

• Explain to the patient that this drug should help control joint inflammation. Inform him that he may not see the benefits of therapy for several months.

16

Eyes and Vision

Eyes and Vision

Introduction

Because an eye disorder may threaten vision—perhaps our most valued sense—it's likely to cause the patient considerable anxiety. This makes meeting your teaching responsibilities a challenge from the start. What's more, as eye disorders are increasingly treated on an outpatient basis, you'll have limited time to teach. So to ensure effective teaching, you'll have to make the most of every moment to provide information and to reinforce what you've taught.

A framework for teaching
In this chapter we'll discuss patient teaching for cataracts, glaucoma, and retinal tear or detachment—eye disorders that affect millions every year. To help the patient understand these and other eye disorders, you may need to briefly discuss pathophysiology—for example, why intraocular pressure rises or how a cataract matures. With this background, the patient can begin to appreciate the role of treatment.

Tests and treatments
When a patient's admitted for diagnostic tests, you'll need to stress that he'll usually experience only minimal discomfort. Inform him that he may be given drops to dilate the pupil or anesthetize the eye before testing.

Teaching for surgery or laser treatments usually begins in the doctor's office and is wrapped up there on the first postoperative visit. When the patient's admitted, you'll have to reinforce this teaching.

Successful home care
Much of your teaching for eye disorders will focus on home care. For example, you'll need to stress the importance of using prescribed medication. Many patients feel squeamish about putting drops or ointment into their eyes. Also, patients may have impaired vision, which makes using medications even more difficult.

The patient may also have to wear an eye patch or eye shield at home. After teaching him how to apply it, you'll need to stress the importance of wearing it for as long as prescribed.

After outlining home care for the patient, be sure to explain any adverse effects to help avoid noncompliance. For example, when therapy requires patching one eye, tell the patient that he'll lose binocular vision and thus depth perception. Advise him to be extra careful when performing daily activities—especially using stairs.

To evaluate the success of home care, you'll need to encourage regular checkups with the doctor. Otherwise, the patient may be tempted to stop treatment if his symptoms clear.

DISORDERS

Cataracts

Preparation for upcoming surgery ranks as your chief teaching goal for the patient with cataracts. Typically, you'll be dealing with an elderly patient who may have grown accustomed to impaired vision and may have second thoughts about undergoing surgery. This patient may also know something about cataract surgery from acquaintances or the news media. Besides reassuring the patient, you'll need to teach him about the surgery and help correct any misconceptions. Don't be surprised if the patient initially appears unreceptive to your teaching. He may feel he already knows everything he needs to know.

You'll need to teach the patient how to administer eye drops and how to apply an eye patch or eye shield, if prescribed. What's more, you'll need to emphasize the importance of adhering to postoperative restrictions so he can protect his newly improved vision.

Your teaching efforts, though, are pitted against a potential problem: limited time. Since most patients are admitted the morning of surgery and discharged within a few hours after surgery, you'll have to efficiently plan and carry out your teaching.

Describe the disorder
Tell the patient that a cataract is a common cause of vision loss. Explain that it's a gradually developing opacity of the lens or lens capsule of the eye, usually associated with aging. It's not a growth on the lens or film over the eye, as he may suspect.

Point out possible complications
If the cataract isn't surgically removed, the patient will experience progressive vision loss. An untreated cataract can also cause the lens to swell, resulting in glaucoma. Rarely, an untreated cataract can cause an infection of the iris.

Teach about tests
Typically, the patient will have had direct ophthalmoscopy with dilation, visual acuity testing, and a slit-lamp examination to confirm the diagnosis of a cataract. Tell him that these tests may be repeated before surgery to evaluate the cataract's maturation and after surgery to evaluate the outcome. (See *Teaching Patients about Eye Tests,* pages 499 and 500.)

Teach about treatments
Explain to the patient that surgery is the only way to successfully treat a cataract. Tell him that the surgeon will remove the lens that has the cataract and will probably implant an intraocular lens to replace it. Or the surgeon will recommend a contact lens or glasses after surgery instead.

If the surgeon implants an intraocular lens, tell the patient he'll probably

---

CHECKLIST

TEACHING TOPICS IN CATARACTS

☐ An explanation of the disease

☐ Risk of progressive vision loss without surgery

☐ Surgical lens removal

☐ Preparation for intraocular lens implant or fitting for corrective contact lens or glasses

☐ Postoperative instructions, including activity restrictions, medication, and schedule for follow-up tests and examinations

☐ Eye drops and their administration

☐ Eye patch application, if necessary

☐ Eye shield application, if necessary

HOW TO PATCH YOUR EYE

Dear Patient:

Your doctor wants you to wear an eye patch. Here's how you can apply one:

1

First, wash your hands thoroughly.

2

Now, close the eye you intend to patch. Fold two or three sterile gauze pads in half and place them on top of each other over your eye.

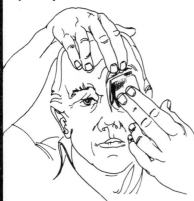

3

Grasp the sterile eye patch in the center, and place it over the gauze pads.

Then, apply tincture of benzoin compound on your cheekbone and forehead above the affected eye.

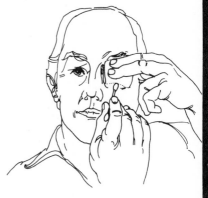

4

Secure the patch with two parallel strips of nonallergenic tape. Tape from the midforehead to your cheekbone.

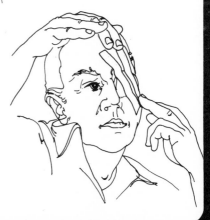

488

POSTOPERATIVE CATARACT INSTRUCTIONS

Dear Patient:

To prevent complications after your cataract surgery, your doctor wants you to follow these instructions:

Doctor's appointment

Your next doctor's appointment is on _____ at _____ o'clock.

Medication
Your doctor has prescribed the following eye drops for you:

Medicine #1: _____.
Use ____ drops ____ times a day in your _____ eye.

Medicine #2: _____.
Use ____ drops ____ times a day in your _____ eye.

What you shouldn't do:
• Bend over.
• Lift anything heavy.
• Read excessively, since this requires back and forth eye movements that can disturb your stitches.
• Drive for long periods.
• Shampoo your hair until the doctor approves, since soap may irritate your eye.

What you should do:
• Kneel to pick things up instead of bending over.

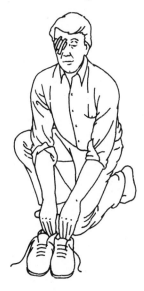

• Lift your feet to put on your shoes.
• Wear your eye patch or shield, as the doctor instructs.
• Sleep on the same side as the unaffected eye.

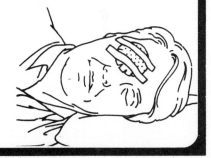

have clear distance vision at once. However, he'll need reading glasses or a contact lens for near vision. If the surgeon uses the other approach, tell the patient he'll be fitted for a contact lens or glasses about 4 to 8 weeks after surgery. Until then, tell him that his vision will be blurred (unless he receives temporary cataract glasses).

Inform the patient that you'll be giving him eye drops preoperatively to reduce the risk of infection and to dilate the pupil. Advise him to call you if he needs to get out of bed after receiving the eye drops; he'll have trouble seeing with a dilated pupil. If the patient will receive a local anesthetic, describe what he'll see and hear during surgery.

Tell the patient he'll be allowed out of bed immediately after surgery and then be discharged when he recovers from the anesthetic—usually within a few hours. If the doctor prescribes a patch for 24 hours after surgery, teach the patient how to apply it (see *How to Patch Your Eye*, page 487). Most doctors also instruct the patient to wear a plastic or metal eye shield at night for 3 to 6 weeks to prevent bumping or rubbing the eye during sleep. Teach the patient how to apply a shield on his eye. Warn him to move about cautiously; covering one eye causes loss of depth perception.

Discuss other postoperative instructions, including eye drop administration and activity restrictions. (See *How to Administer Eye Drops*, pages 494 and 495.) Usually, the doctor will order antibiotic and steroid eye drops but will advise only minor activity restrictions.

Glaucoma

Whether the patient has acute angle-closure or chronic open-angle glaucoma, he'll need your teaching to help him understand how this disorder raises intraocular pressure, risking permanent vision loss. However, your teaching approach will reflect the type

---

CHECKLIST

TEACHING TOPICS IN GLAUCOMA

☐ An explanation of the disorder: acute angle-closure or chronic open-angle glaucoma

☐ Intraocular pressure: what it is and why it needs to be lowered

☐ Preparation for gonioscopy, slit-lamp examination, or other nonroutine eye tests

☐ Importance of using prescribed eye drops in chronic open-angle glaucoma to prevent vision loss

☐ Administration of eye drops

☐ Argon laser trabeculoplasty and post-treatment instructions

☐ Surgical iridectomy for acute angle-closure glaucoma; trabeculectomy for chronic open-angle glaucoma

---

of glaucoma. For example, if the patient has acute angle-closure glaucoma, an ophthalmologic emergency, you'll need to calmly and succinctly explain treatment measures. You'll stress the importance of immediate drug therapy to lower intraocular pressure, followed by surgery (usually within 48 hours) to preserve vision. If the patient has chronic open-angle glaucoma, you'll have more time to provide and reinforce teaching. That's because chronic open-angle glaucoma (the more common type) is usually diagnosed during intraocular pressure measurement in a routine eye examination. However, if the patient was asymptomatic at diagnosis, you may be challenged to convince him that daily care is crucial in controlling intraocular pressure. He'll need to learn how to give himself eye drops and follow a medication schedule. Equally important, he'll have to adhere to regular medical checkups to monitor his intraocular pressure.

In both types of glaucoma, the patient may fear blindness—and not without cause. Treatment typically can't restore vision that's already lost,

COMPARING TYPES OF GLAUCOMA

To differentiate acute angle-closure and chronic open-angle glaucoma, you must first understand how aqueous humor normally circulates. Aqueous humor—a transparent fluid produced by the ciliary body epithelium—flows continuously from the posterior chamber, through the pupil, to the anterior chamber. It then flows peripherally and filters through the trabecular meshwork to the canal of Schlemm, and from there enters venous circulation.

In acute angle-closure glaucoma, the iris adheres more tightly to the lens. This increases pressure in the posterior chamber, causing the peripheral iris to balloon forward into the anterior chamber. Decreasing the size of the anterior chamber, in turn, narrows the angle between the surface of the iris and the trabecular meshwork. If this angle closes, drainage of aqueous humor abruptly stops, causing intraocular pressure to increase sharply.

In chronic open-angle glaucoma, aqueous outflow is obstructed somewhere in the trabecular meshwork, canal of Schlemm, or aqueous veins. (The angle of the iris remains normal.) This obstruction causes an insidious rise in intraocular pressure. Chronic open-angle glaucoma causes 90% of all glaucoma cases and is commonly familial.

NORMAL FLOW OF AQUEOUS HUMOR

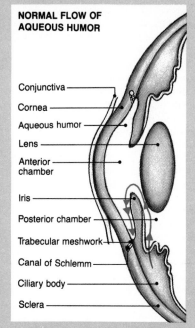

Conjunctiva

Cornea

Aqueous humor

Lens

Anterior chamber

Iris

Posterior chamber

Trabecular meshwork

Canal of Schlemm

Ciliary body

Sclera

ACUTE ANGLE-CLOSURE GLAUCOMA

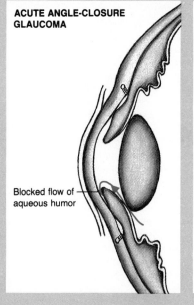

Blocked flow of aqueous humor

CHRONIC OPEN-ANGLE GLAUCOMA

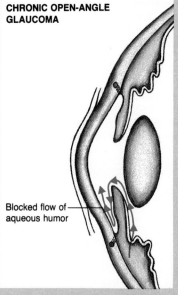

Blocked flow of aqueous humor

but it can prevent any further loss of sight. Your effective teaching can help ensure that the patient diligently follows his treatment plan.

Describe the disorder

Explain that glaucoma is characterized by an increase in intraocular pressure, which compresses the capillaries that nourish the optic nerve. This increased pressure can eventually damage the optic nerve (see *Questions Patients Ask about Glaucoma*).

If the patient has *acute angle-closure glaucoma*, tell him that such symptoms as eye pain, light sensitivity, blurred vision, seeing halos, and nausea and vomiting occur when intraocular pressure rises suddenly. This usually happens in one eye at a time when the iris obstructs the flow of aqueous humor. Mention that aging typically contributes to this obstruction by causing thickening of the lens and pushing the iris forward.

If the patient has *chronic open-angle glaucoma*, explain how intraocular pressure insidiously rises when the flow of aqueous humor is obstructed somewhere else within the drainage system. That's why he's had only mild symptoms—such as occasionally seeing halos or blurred peripheral vision—or perhaps no symptoms at all. Make sure the patient understands that the absence of symptoms doesn't rule out pathology.

Point out possible complications

If the patient has chronic open-angle glaucoma, point out that if he doesn't use his eye drops as prescribed and visit the doctor regularly for intraocular pressure checks, he'll experience progressive vision loss. The patient with acute angle-closure glaucoma may also risk vision loss if he doesn't undergo regular eye examinations after surgery.

Teach about tests

Typically, the patient had visual acuity and tonometry testing, and direct

---

INQUIRY

QUESTIONS PATIENTS ASK ABOUT GLAUCOMA

What is intraocular pressure?

Intraocular pressure is the force exerted by the fluids within your eyeball known as aqueous humor and vitreous humor. Aqueous humor—the clear fluid in the front of your eye—is continually being produced and reabsorbed. Vitreous humor—the jellylike substance in the back of your eye—stays constant in volume.

What causes increased intraocular pressure?

Intraocular pressure increases when aqueous humor doesn't drain normally or when excessive aqueous humor is being produced. A sudden increase usually results when aqueous outflow is obstructed by narrowing of the opening between the iris and the lens. A slow increase usually results when aqueous outflow is obstructed somewhere else within the eye's drainage system or when excess aqueous humor is being produced.

How will this affect my vision?

If intraocular pressure isn't decreased and permanently brought under control, you stand to lose your vision. Persistently high intraocular pressure impairs the blood supply to the optic nerve, eventually causing blindness.

---

ophthalmoscopy to confirm the diagnosis. Tell him that these tests may be repeated to monitor the progress of therapy. Also prepare him for visual field examination, gonioscopy, and slit-lamp examination to verify the type of glaucoma, the extent of impaired vision, and the progress of therapy. (See *Teaching Patients about Eye Tests*, pages 499 and 500.)

Teach about treatments

• *Medication.* If the patient has acute angle-closure glaucoma, explain that eye drops, such as pilocarpine, will reduce intraocular pressure by constricting the pupil. This pulls the iris away from the lens, allowing the aqueous humor to drain. If the doctor orders systemic medications, possibly carbonic anhydrase inhibitors (such as acetazolamide) or hyperosmotic agents (such as mannitol), explain their effects, too. Tell the patient that these systemic medications aim to rapidly reduce intraocular pressure before surgery; he won't need to continue taking them after surgery. (See *Teaching Patients about Eye Drugs*, pages 502 to 505.)

If the patient has chronic open-angle glaucoma, teach him how to instill eye drops (see *How to Administer Eye Drops*, pages 494 and 495). Also teach a family member or another caregiver in case the patient can't do this for himself. Emphasize the importance of using the eye drops daily—whether the patient has symptoms or not—to control intraocular pressure. Tell him to keep an extra bottle of medication on hand at all times. Warn the patient that he may have trouble seeing in the dark, in early morning, or at dusk with his constricted pupil. Advise him to add lights in his home, if necessary, and to avoid driving or walking after dark. Suggest that the patient confine reading and other close activities to daylight hours. Also recommend that he wear a Medic Alert bracelet or necklace that states he has glaucoma.

When the doctor prescribes oral carbonic anhydrase inhibitors for severe chronic open-angle glaucoma, compliance may be especially difficult for the patient. Tell him not to stop therapy even if he experiences drug-induced nausea or paresthesias.

• *Procedures.* Argon laser trabeculoplasty can replace surgery for some patients with chronic open-angle glaucoma. By relieving aqueous humor buildup, this noninvasive procedure

may also reduce or eliminate the need for lifelong glaucoma medication. However, you'll need to inform the patient that more than one treatment may be necessary. Tell him that each treatment takes less than 30 minutes, and describe what he should expect. First, the doctor will place a topical anesthetic in the eye and apply a special lens. The patient will then sit facing the doctor with his chin supported on a rest. He'll be asked to focus his gaze on a certain area during the treatment. Tell the patient that he'll be able to return home a few hours after each treatment. Before he goes home, though, make sure he knows how to instill his own eye drops. (Usually, the doctor will order steroid eye drops.) Tell him he can resume all activities within 48 hours, but mention that he may have transient blurred vision and a slightly red eye during this period. Remind the patient to return for a checkup 24 hours after treatment and at scheduled intervals thereafter.

Argon laser peripheral iridotomy may benefit the patient with acute angle-closure glaucoma by creating an opening between the anterior and posterior chambers for aqueous outflow. Your teaching for this treatment resembles that for argon laser trabeculoplasty (see also *Lasers in Ophthalmology*).

• *Surgery.* Explain to the patient with acute angle-closure glaucoma that surgical iridectomy creates an opening in the iris, allowing aqueous humor to flow freely from the posterior to the anterior chamber. Note that he may eventually need this surgery on both eyes. (The doctor may start miotic eye drops to help prevent onset in the normal eye.)

Tell the patient that he'll probably be allowed out of bed immediately after surgery. Describe the dressing that he may have over his eye postoperatively. The doctor may also advise him to wear a patch until his first checkup, usually 24 hours after discharge. Advise him to move about cautiously since patch-

LASERS IN OPHTHALMOLOGY

Ideally suited to the precision work required in ophthalmology, lasers are being used ever more frequently to treat various eye disorders. How do these former science fiction wonders work? Quite simply, by using mirrors. Lasers first generate focused, or monochromatic, light waves and then increase their power by bouncing them off a series of mirrors. The result: a finely focused, high-energy beam. Depending on the type of laser (gas or solid-state), this beam shines at a specific wavelength and color. An argon laser, for example, produces a blue-green beam with a short wavelength that's highly absorbed by the colors red and orange, making it ideal for surgery on the highly vascular retina.

In argon laser trabeculoplasty, the beam is directed at the trabecular meshwork; in argon laser iridotomy, at the iris. As the beam comes in contact with tissue, light energy is absorbed and converted to heat, creating a burn (photocoagulation). The laser beam can create small, nonpenetrating scars or burn completely through tissue, depending on the eye disorder being treated.

In chronic open-angle glaucoma, creating multiple scars around the trabecular meshwork relieves aqueous humor buildup, reducing intraocular pressure. In acute angle-closure glaucoma, laser energy is used to burn through the peripheral iris, creating an opening between the anterior and posterior chambers for aqueous outflow.

Laser treatment can also prevent retinal detachment by repairing peripheral retinal thinning, holes, or tears. And surrounding an existing localized detachment with laser burn scars can limit its size and prevent further damage.

Before laser treatment, a special lens is placed over the fundus of the eye to prevent the patient from closing his eye. The lens also absorbs some of the thermal energy generated by the laser. Laser treatment avoids surgical complications (such as hemorrhage and infection), is relatively painless, and can be done on an outpatient basis. It's especially useful for treating older adults who are poor surgical candidates or who are reluctant to undergo major eye surgery.

ing one eye will cause loss of depth perception. If he doesn't have a dressing or patch, mention that he'll have blurred vision until the postoperative eye drops wear off. Instruct him to visit the doctor to have his intraocular pressure measured, usually the day after surgery, a week later, and at intervals after that. Tell him not to lie on his affected side until the doctor allows this.

Most patients with chronic open-angle glaucoma don't require surgery, except when drug therapy fails to control intraocular pressure or compliance is inadequate. Then, you'll have to prepare the patient for trabeculectomy—a surgical filtering procedure that creates an opening for aqueous outflow. In trabeculectomy, the surgeon dissects a flap of sclera, removes a portion of the trabecular meshwork, then performs a peripheral iridectomy to create a filtering bleb, or opening for aqueous outflow, under the conjunctiva.

After explaining this procedure, tell the patient that he'll probably be allowed out of bed immediately after surgery. Describe the dressing that he may have over his eye. The doctor may also advise him to wear a patch until his first checkup, usually 24 hours after discharge. If the patient doesn't have a dressing or patch, warn him that he'll experience blurred vision until the postoperative eye drops wear off. When he's in bed, instruct him not to lie on his affected side. Mention that some doctors also recommend an eye shield at night for 3 to 4 weeks postoperatively. As ordered, tell the patient if he'll need eye drops after surgery. If the patient has glaucoma in both eyes, advise him to keep the drops for each eye separate.

• *Other care measures.* If the patient has chronic open-angle glaucoma, you may need to explain care measures besides medication. For example, you may need to advise him to avoid excessive fluid intake, heavy lifting, and undue straining.

494

HOW TO ADMINISTER EYE DROPS

Dear Patient:

Your doctor has prescribed these eye drops for you:

Medicine #1: _____.
Use _____ drops _____ times
a day in your _____ eye.

Medicine #2: _____.
Use _____ drops _____ times
a day in your _____ eye.

Here's how to give yourself eye drops:

1
Wash your hands thoroughly.

2
Hold the medication bottle up to the light and examine it. If the medication's discolored or contains sediment, don't use it. Take it back to the pharmacy, and have them examine it. If the medication looks OK, warm it to room temperature by holding the bottle between your hands for 2 minutes.

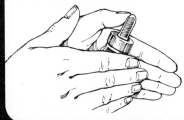

3
Moisten a rayon ball or tissue with water, and clean any secretions from around your eyes. Use a fresh rayon ball or tissue for each eye.

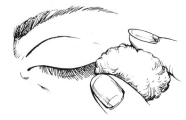

4
Now, stand or sit before a mirror, or lie on your back, whichever's most comfortable for you. Squeeze the bulb of the eyedropper to fill the dropper with medication.

5
Tilt your head slightly back and toward the eye you're treating. Pull down your lower eyelid.

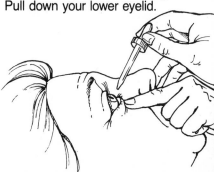

6

Position the dropper over the conjunctival sac you've exposed between your lower lid and the white of your eye. Steady your hand by resting two fingers against your cheek or nose.

7

Look up at the ceiling. Then squeeze the prescribed number of drops into the sac.

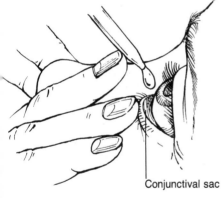

Conjunctival sac

Also take care not to touch the dropper to your eye, eyelashes, or finger. Wipe away excess medication with a clean tissue.

8

Release the lower lid. Try to keep your eye open and not blink for at least 30 seconds. Apply gentle pressure to the corner of your eye at the bridge of your nose for 1 minute to prevent the medication from being absorbed through your tear duct.

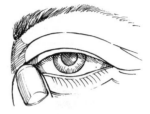

9

Repeat the procedure in the other eye, if the doctor orders.

10

Recap the bottle and store it away from light and heat.

If you're using more than one kind of drop, wait for 5 minutes before you use the next one.

Important: Call your doctor immediately if you notice any of these side effects: _____

_____.

And remember, never put medication in your eyes unless the label reads "For Ophthalmic Use" or "For Use in the Eyes."

Retinal Tear and Detachment

Because a retinal tear (with or without detachment) demands immediate treatment, your patient teaching must be brief and reassuring. And, at times, uncommonly convincing. Why? If the patient has experienced only minor symptoms, such as visual floaters or light flashes, he'll probably be stunned by the need for urgent treatment and the risk of partial or total vision loss. After treatment, your teaching addresses restrictions to ensure healing without complications.

Describe the disorder
Explain that a *retinal tear* is a split in the retina—the part of the eye that perceives light. Then, when vitreous humor leaks between the retina's sensory and pigment layers, the retina becomes *detached* from its blood supply.

Point out possible complications
Explain to the patient that without surgery a retinal tear can progress to a retinal detachment and, in turn, to severe loss of vision.

Teach about tests
Prepare the patient for indirect ophthalmoscopy with scleral depression and slit-lamp examination to measure the tear or detachment. (See *Teaching Patients about Eye Tests*, pages 499 and 500.)

Teach about treatments
• *Procedures.* Depending on the retinal tear or detachment's size and location, the doctor may perform cryotherapy (cold therapy), photocoagulation (laser therapy), or diathermy (heat therapy). For each, explain to the patient that the procedure triggers a sterile inflammatory reaction, causing the edges of the retinal tear to fuse together. He'll probably be able to go home a few hours after the procedure. Suggest acetaminophen for any discomfort. Then, make sure he knows how to give himself eye drops (see *How to Administer Eye Drops*, pages 494 and 495) or eye ointment.

Instruct the patient to avoid vigorous physical activity, bending over, straining, and lifting heavy objects, as they increase intraocular pressure. Remind him to return for a checkup.
• *Surgery.* For the patient with retinal detachment, you'll also have to explain scleral buckling. (See *Retinal Detachment: Its Causes and Cure.*) Preoperatively, the doctor will probably order bed rest and patching of both eyes to minimize eye movement. He may also recommend special positioning of the patient's head to prevent the detachment from extending to the macula. Explain these measures to the patient.

Postoperatively, inform the patient that he'll be on bed rest with bathroom privileges for several days, then gradually progress to ambulation. Instruct him not to lie on the affected side. If the patient has an eye patch prescribed, warn him to move about carefully because of loss of depth perception. Tell him you'll apply cold compresses to de-

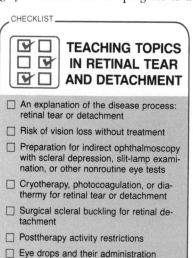

CHECKLIST

TEACHING TOPICS IN RETINAL TEAR AND DETACHMENT

- [ ] An explanation of the disease process: retinal tear or detachment
- [ ] Risk of vision loss without treatment
- [ ] Preparation for indirect ophthalmoscopy with scleral depression, slit-lamp examination, or other nonroutine eye tests
- [ ] Cryotherapy, photocoagulation, or diathermy for retinal tear or detachment
- [ ] Surgical scleral buckling for retinal detachment
- [ ] Posttherapy activity restrictions
- [ ] Eye drops and their administration

crease swelling and discomfort.

Because the patient will have to instill his own eye drops after discharge, teach him the proper technique. Instruct him to avoid vigorous physical activity, bending over, straining, and lifting heavy objects for 6 weeks, or as ordered. Also suggest that he avoid crowds to minimize undue jostling and

avoid reading and writing, which demand rapid eye movement. Advise him to wear dark glasses to reduce light sensitivity. Instruct the patient to promptly report any severe or increasing pain; this may indicate increased intraocular pressure or uveitis. Remind him to return for checkups, as ordered.

RETINAL DETACHMENT: ITS CAUSES AND CURE

When a hole or tear in the retina allows vitreous humor to seep between the retina's sensory and pigment layers, the retina becomes separated—or detached—from its choroidal blood supply. Without adequate circulation, the retina can't function properly, resulting in vision loss. In the older adult, vitreous degeneration or vitreous body collapse can cause a retinal hole or tear, which can lead to retinal detachment. Contributing factors include myopia, cataract surgery, and trauma.

Retinal detachment may also result from seepage of fluid into the subretinal space (due to inflammation, tumors, or systemic diseases, such as accelerated hypertension or circulatory disorders) or from traction that's placed on the retina by vitreous bands or membranes (due to proliferative diabetic retinopathy, posterior uveitis, or a traumatic intraocular foreign body).

Retinal detachment rarely occurs in

children but may result from retinopathy of prematurity, tumors (retinoblastoma), or trauma.

A two-step cure
To treat retinal detachment, the surgeon must first repair the retinal hole or tear and then restore the retina's blood supply. Using cryotherapy (cold therapy), photocoagulation (laser therapy), or diathermy (heat therapy), he creates a sterile inflammatory reaction that seals the retinal hole or tear and causes retinal readherence. The surgeon then performs scleral buckling: he places a silicone plate (or sponge) called an *explant* over the site of readherence and holds it in place with a circling band. The pressure exerted on the explant indents or "buckles" the eyeball and gently pushes the choroid and retina closer together. This reunites the retina with its choroidal blood supply.

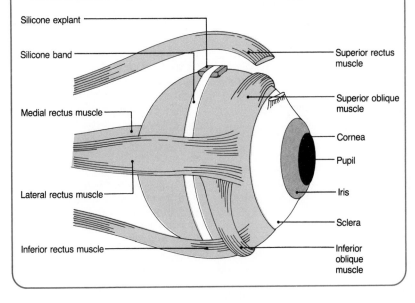

HOW TO USE EYE OINTMENT

Dear Patient:

Your doctor has prescribed this eye ointment for you:

Name of medicine: _____.
Use this ointment ____times a day in your ____eye.

Here's how to use it yourself:

1
Wash your hands thoroughly. Then hold the ointment in your hand for several minutes to warm it before use.

2
Moisten a rayon ball or tissue with water and clean any secretions from around your eyes. Use a fresh rayon ball or tissue for each eye.

3
Now, stand or sit before a mirror or lie on your back, whichever's most comfortable.

4
Gently pull down your lower eyelid. Tilt your head back slightly and look at the ceiling.

5
Squeeze a small amount of ointment (about ¼″ to ½″) inside

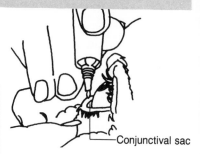

Conjunctival sac

the conjunctival sac between your lower lid and the white of your eyeball. Steady your hand by resting two fingers against your cheek or nose.

6

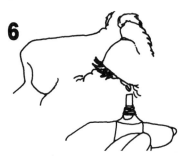

Close your eye gently to pinch off the ointment. Then withdraw the tube and roll your eyeball in all directions with your eyes closed. Repeat the procedure in the other eye, if ordered.

7
Recap the medication. If you're using more than one ointment, wait about 10 minutes before you use the next one. Don't worry if you have blurred vision temporarily after you use the ointment; this is normal.

TEACHING PATIENTS ABOUT EYE TESTS

TEST AND PURPOSE	TEACHING POINTS
Fluorescein angiography • To document retinal circulation as an aid in evaluating intraocular abnormalities, such as retinopathy, tumors, and inflammatory disorders	• Explain that this test evaluates the eyes' small blood vessels and that it takes about 30 minutes to perform. • Tell the patient that dilating drops will be instilled before the test. • Explain that during the test the patient will sit facing a camera, with his chin placed in a support and with his forehead resting against the bar. The camera will take photographs of the eye before and after the patient receives an I.V. injection of sodium fluorescein. Warn him that he may have brief nausea and a feeling of warmth as the dye's injected. Instruct him to open his eyes wide, stare straight ahead, and blink normally. Also remind him to keep his teeth together and to breathe normally during the test. • Tell the patient that his near vision will be blurred for up to 12 hours and that his skin and urine may appear yellow for 24 to 48 hours after the test.
Gonioscopy • To evaluate the angle of the eye's anterior chamber	• Explain that this test takes 5 to 10 minutes and involves placing a special lens in the eye—the goniolens—and then performing a slit-lamp examination. • Tell the patient that his cornea will be anesthetized and a thin layer of 2% methylcellulose solution will be applied to separate the lens from the cornea. • Explain that the patient will sit on one side of the slit lamp, with his chin placed in a support and with his forehead resting against the bar. The doctor will sit on the other side of the lamp and look into the patient's eye. Instruct the patient to remain still during the test.
Ocular ultrasonography • To aid evaluation of a fundus clouded by an opaque medium, such as a cataract • To aid diagnosis of retinal detachment and vitreous disorders • To locate intraocular foreign bodies • To diagnose and differentiate between intraocular and orbital lesions, and to monitor their progression	• Explain that this safe, painless test evaluates the eye's structures and takes about 5 minutes to perform. • Describe the preparation for the test: for an A-scan, the patient's eye will be numbed with anesthetic drops and a clear-plastic eye cup will be placed directly on the eyeball. Water-soluble jelly will then be applied to the eye cup. For a B-scan, he will have water-soluble jelly applied to his eyelid. • Explain that during the test a small transducer will be placed on the eye cup or the eyelid. This will direct high-frequency sound waves at structures in the patient's eye. After striking these structures, the waves reflect back as echoes. An A-scan will convert these echoes into waveforms; a B-scan, into a pattern of dots. • Tell the patient that he may be asked to move his eyes or change his gaze during the test.
Ophthalmoscopy (direct and indirect) • To detect and evaluate disorders of the fundus, including the optic disk, retinal blood vessels, macula, and retina	• Explain that this painless test examines the internal eye and takes less than 5 minutes to perform. • Tell the patient that dilating drops will be instilled before the test. • If the patient is scheduled for *direct ophthalmoscopy*, explain that he'll be seated in a chair and asked to focus on a distant object. Then the doctor will shine a light in the patient's eye with a small, hand-held instrument and examine the internal eye.

(continued)

TEST AND PURPOSE	TEACHING POINTS
Ophthalmoscopy (direct and indirect) *(continued)*	• If the patient is scheduled for *indirect ophthalmoscopy*, explain that he'll be asked to look up and focus on the ceiling. The doctor will hold an indirect ophthalmoscope about an arm's length away from the patient's eye and use a head-lamp to provide ample light.
Slit-lamp examination • To detect and evaluate abnormalities of anterior segment tissues and structures	• Explain that this painless test evaluates the front of the eye and that it takes 5 to 10 minutes. • If appropriate, tell the patient that dilating drops will be instilled before the test. • Describe what will happen during the test: the patient will sit on one side of the slit lamp, with his chin placed in a support and with his forehead resting against the bar. The doctor will sit on the other side and look into the patient's eyes. Instruct the patient to remain still during the test.
Tonometry • To measure intraocular pressure • To aid diagnosis and follow-up evaluation of glaucoma	• Explain that this painless test measures intraocular pressure and takes only a few minutes to perform. • Tell the patient that his eyes will be anesthetized before the test so that he won't feel the tonometer's pressure. • Instruct him not to cough or squeeze his eyelids together during testing to prevent an increase in intraocular pressure. • If the patient is scheduled for *applanation tonometry*, explain that he'll sit at the slit lamp, with his chin placed in a support and with his forehead resting against the bar. Instruct him to look straight ahead and to breathe normally during the test. • If the patient is scheduled for *indentation tonometry*, tell him to lie supine and look upward at a spot on the ceiling. Instruct him to breathe normally during the test. • After the test, tell the patient not to rub his eyes for at least 20 minutes to prevent corneal abrasions. Mention that any slight itching in the eye should subside within 24 hours.
Visual acuity • To test distance and near visual acuity • To identify refractive errors in vision	• Explain that this test evaluates the patient's vision and takes only a few minutes. • Describe what will happen during the test: the patient will sit 20′ (6 m) from the Snellen chart and be asked to read the smallest line possible on the chart to test distance visual acuity. Then he'll be asked to read a Jaeger card (a card with print in graded sizes) at approximately 14″ (35.6 cm) to test near visual acuity. Tell him that one eye at a time will be tested, then both eyes together, and that he'll be tested both with and without corrective lenses.
Visual field examination • To detect or monitor visual field loss	• Explain that this test detects or evaluates areas of visual loss. • Explain that the patient will be asked to focus on the center of his visual field. In *kinetic (Goldmann) perimetry*, he'll be asked to identify an object brought from the periphery toward the center. In *static (Humphrey) perimetry*, he'll be asked to identify test points flashed at random over the visual field. Tell the patient that one eye at a time will be tested.

SURGERY

Today, eye surgery is often performed as an outpatient procedure—a dramatic change from just a few years ago. No longer must a patient remain on bed rest for an extended period postoperatively and have both eyes patched. Instead, he's usually in and out of the hospital the same day and expected to provide eye care for himself at home. To accommodate the patient's changing needs, your teaching will reinforce what the patient has learned about surgery from his doctor, correct any misconceptions, and review home care measures. For example, if the patient must wear an eye patch or shield postoperatively, you'll need to show him how to apply it.

What you teach each patient will depend, of course, on his special needs. In this section, you'll find out about teaching considerations for enucleation and eye muscle surgery. In the entries earlier in this chapter, you'll find similar information for lens removal, iridectomy, trabeculectomy, and scleral buckling.

Enucleation

Besides providing emotional support, you'll need to clearly explain this surgery to the patient. Tell him that the doctor will remove his eyeball and implant a synthetic ball to fill out the socket. This ball will provide a permanent stump to support an artificial eye, or prosthesis. The doctor will then insert a temporary prosthesis. (Later, when postoperative swelling resolves, the doctor will insert a permanent prosthesis.) Assure the patient that he won't experience much pain after surgery. In fact, he'll probably be allowed out of bed on the first day and be discharged within several days. Describe the pressure dressing that he'll wear over the operated eye for 24 to 48 hours. Tell him that subsequently he'll need to wear a patch to keep the socket clean until he returns for a checkup—usually 1 to 2 weeks after surgery. Teach him how to apply a patch (see *How to Patch Your Eye*, page 487). Instruct him to immediately report bleeding or signs of infection, such as headache, fever, or unusual discharge.

When the patient is fitted with a permanent prosthesis, make sure he recognizes that having vision in only one eye will cause loss of depth perception. Advise him to use caution when performing daily activities until he adjusts to this. And stress the importance of regular eye examinations to protect vision in the remaining eye.

Eye muscle surgery

Typically, this surgery aims to correct eye muscle incoordination in strabismus—a common eye disorder in preschoolers. Your teaching, of course, must reflect the child's age as well as his parents' concerns. Usually, the child will be admitted the morning of surgery and discharged after recovery from anesthesia. After surgery, you'll need to teach the child or his parents how to use eye ointment or drops. Since the child usually won't be wearing a patch postoperatively, describe the serosanguineous drainage that may run down his cheek; this is perfectly normal. Mention that the child's eyes may be red for up to 2 weeks. Suggest that he wear dark glasses if he experiences burning or tearing.

Within several days after surgery, the child can usually return to his normal routine. However, explain that some children continue to have diplopia as their eyes adjust to their new placement. Inform the child and his parents that corrective glasses and eye exercises may be necessary postoperatively. Instruct them to promptly report unusual drainage, eye pain, headache, or fever. Remind them to return for their scheduled postoperative visit.

TEACHING PATIENTS ABOUT EYE DRUGS

DRUG	ADVERSE REACTIONS	INTERACTIONS*
Adrenergics		
dipivefrin hydrochloride (Propine) **epinephrine bitartrate** (Epitrate) **epinephrine hydrochloride** (Epifrin) **epinephryl borate** (Epinal)	*Reportable:* palpitations, tachycardia *Other:* blurred vision, brow ache, headache, ocular stinging or burning, pallor, sweating	None
Beta-adrenergic blocking agents		
betaxolol hydrochloride (Betoptic) **timolol maleate** (Timoptic)	*Reportable:* bradycardia, breathing difficulty, headache, skin rash *Other:* blurred vision, hypotension, ocular pain, ocular stinging or burning	None
Carbonic anhydrase inhibitors		
acetazolamide (Diamox) **dichlorphenamide** (Daranide) **methazolamide** (Neptazane)	*Reportable:* bloody urine, confusion, lower back pain, malaise, urinary difficulty *Other:* anorexia, diarrhea, drowsiness, gastric upset, metallic taste, tingling of extremities, urinary frequency	Tell the patient that foods, beverages, and over-the-counter drugs don't influence the safety or effectiveness of carbonic anhydrase inhibitors.
Cholinergics		
Direct-acting agents **carbachol** (Isopto Carbachol) **pilocarpine** (Isopto Carpine, Pilocar)	*Reportable:* abdominal cramps, breathing difficulty, diarrhea, increased salivation and tearing, nausea, vomiting *Other:* blurred vision, brow ache, conjunctival injection and irritation, dull headache, eye ache	None

*Includes foods, beverages, and over-the-counter drugs.

TEACHING POINTS

• Explain to the patient that the prescribed drug should control his chronic glaucoma.
• Tell him to discard the solution if it changes color. Also tell him to keep it refrigerated, protected from light, and tightly closed when not in use.

• Explain that blurred vision may occur for a few minutes after application. Advise the patient not to drive until his vision clears.
• Tell the patient that stinging and burning should diminish with continued therapy. If they don't, have him call the doctor.

• Explain to the patient that the prescribed drug should control his chronic glaucoma.

• Warn diabetics that betaxolol and timolol may mask signs of hypoglycemia.

• Explain to the patient with chronic glaucoma that the prescribed drug should control his condition. Explain to the patient with acute glaucoma that it will reduce intraocular pressure before surgery.
• Tell the patient that this drug initially causes urinary frequency but that this symptom should subside with continued therapy.
• Instruct him to consume fluids and foods high in potassium, such as orange juice and bananas.

• If the patient's taking a single dose, advise him to take it in the morning after breakfast. If he's taking more than one dose a day, tell him not to take the last dose after 6 p.m.
• Advise him to take the drug with meals if he has gastric upset.
• Tell him to drink plenty of fluids during therapy to prevent formation of calculi.

• Explain to the patient that this cholinergic should control his glaucoma.

• Tell him that blurred vision usually disappears after 10 to 14 days of therapy.

(continued)

**TEACHING PATIENTS ABOUT
EYE DRUGS** *(continued)*

DRUG	ADVERSE REACTIONS	INTERACTIONS*
Cholinergics *(continued)*		
Indirect-acting agents **demecarium** (Humorsol) **echothiophate iodide** (Phospholine Iodide) **isoflurophate** (Floropryl) **physostigmine** (Eserine Sulfate)	*Reportable:* abdominal cramps, diarrhea, increased salivation and tearing, increased urination, nausea, vomiting *Other:* blurred vision, brow ache, eye irritation, headache, twitching of eyelids	None
Cycloplegics		
atropine sulfate **cyclopentolate** **hydrochloride** (Cyclogyl) **homatropine** **hydrobromide** (Homatropine) **scopolamine** **hydrobromide** (Isopto Hyoscine) **tropicamide** (Mydriacyl)	*Reportable:* confusion, delirium, eye pain, flushing, hyperactivity, tachycardia *Other:* blurred vision, photophobia, transient ocular stinging or burning	None
Hyperosmotic agents		
glycerin (Glyrol, Osmoglyn)	*Reportable:* confusion, irregular heartbeat *Other:* dizziness, headache, increased thirst, mouth dryness, nausea, vomiting	None
Mydriatics		
hydroxyamphetamine (Paredrine) **phenylephrine** **hydrochloride** (Neo-Synephrine)	*Reportable:* headache, hypertension, trembling *Other:* blurred vision, brow ache, photophobia, transient ocular stinging or burning	None

*Includes foods, beverages, and over-the-counter drugs.

TEACHING POINTS

• Explain to the patient that this cholinergic should control his chronic glaucoma.
• Tell him to avoid exposure to organophosphate insecticides and pesticides during therapy to avoid intensifying adverse reactions.

• Explain to the patient that the prescribed drug should help the doctor examine his eyes by paralyzing the muscles that regulate accommodation.
• Warn the patient that his vision will be temporarily blurred until the drug wears off.
• Recommend sunglasses to relieve photophobia. However, tell the patient to call his doctor if this symptom persists for more than 24 hours.

• As appropriate, explain that this drug should control chronic glaucoma or, in acute glaucoma, should reduce intraocular pressure before surgery.
• Tell the patient to lie down briefly after taking the drug to help relieve headache.
• To make this drug more palatable, tell the patient to mix it with a small amount of unsweetened lemon, orange, or lime juice. Then he should pour the mixture over cracked ice and sip it through a straw.

• Explain to the patient that the prescribed drug will dilate the pupil.
• Warn the patient that his vision will be temporarily blurred until this drug wears off.
• Advise him to wear sunglasses to relieve temporary photophobia.

17

Infection

Infection

Introduction

In many disorders, your teaching can help the patient understand his illness and the need for treatment. And it can improve the likelihood of a timely recovery. In infectious disorders, though, your teaching can mean this and more. That's because many infectious disorders are easily transmitted. So, by explaining modes of transmission to the patient and teaching him measures to prevent contagion, you can benefit the community as a whole. And you can arm the patient with information that may help him prevent subsequent infection.

What the patient needs to know

Typically, your patient will want to learn about his own infection before learning how he can prevent its recurrence or its spread to others. You'll begin by teaching him about the body's natural defenses against infection, the type and severity of his infection, and the possible complications. You'll also need to teach him about the role of diagnostic tests, especially those that require him to collect a sample of sputum, stool, or urine.

Perhaps most important, you'll emphasize the need for him to complete the prescribed course of antimicrobial drug therapy, even if his symptoms subside. After all, once the patient begins to feel better, he may think that it's unimportant for him to continue taking his medication. By pointing out potential complications, you'll show him that it is indeed important to complete the prescribed antimicrobial drug regimen.

In certain infectious disorders, you may need to explain important self-care measures, such as application of dressings, meticulous I.V. line care, or correct use of mouthwashes and gargles. You'll also need to teach the patient and his family essential precautionary measures, especially correct hand-washing technique and proper disposal of contaminated secretions and dressings.

What is infection?

Explain that infection is the replication of microorganisms in the patient's own tissues. Inform him that the body's natural defenses—normal flora residing in nonsterile areas, such as the skin, the eyes, and the respiratory, GI, and GU tracts—provide a barrier that repels small numbers of invading microorganisms. (See *Natural Barriers to Infection*, page 509.) However, if inadequate nutrition, poor hygiene, or existing illness weakens the body's physical and chemical defenses, microorganisms increase in number. They then enter the body and cause infection.

THE DISORDER

Types and Transmission of Infection

Depending on the patient's infection, explain the type of microorganism that's causing it. (See *Reviewing Types of Infection,* pages 510 and 511, for further information.)

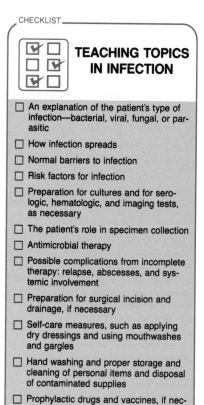

CHECKLIST

TEACHING TOPICS IN INFECTION

☐ An explanation of the patient's type of infection—bacterial, viral, fungal, or parasitic

☐ How infection spreads

☐ Normal barriers to infection

☐ Risk factors for infection

☐ Preparation for cultures and for serologic, hematologic, and imaging tests, as necessary

☐ The patient's role in specimen collection

☐ Antimicrobial therapy

☐ Possible complications from incomplete therapy: relapse, abscesses, and systemic involvement

☐ Preparation for surgical incision and drainage, if necessary

☐ Self-care measures, such as applying dry dressings and using mouthwashes and gargles

☐ Hand washing and proper storage and cleaning of personal items and disposal of contaminated supplies

☐ Prophylactic drugs and vaccines, if necessary

Modes of transmission

Depending on the patient's infection, explain the mode of transmission: contact, common vehicle, airborne, or vector-borne.

● *Transmission by contact.* Infection may be transmitted through three types of contact: direct, indirect, and droplet spread. *Direct contact* occurs when the infected person and susceptible host have physical contact, allowing transfer of the microorganism. For example, direct contact occurs when a patient with a herpes simplex lesion on his lip kisses another person. Besides herpesvirus infections, direct contact also commonly spreads staphylococcal, streptococcal, and rhinoviral infections.

Indirect contact involves transmission of a microorganism by a contaminated inanimate object. For example, suppose that a person with hepatitis B nicks his face while shaving, leaving infected blood on the blade. If another person uses this razor and also nicks himself, he may acquire the hepatitis B virus.

The third method of contact—*droplet spread* of microorganisms—occurs through the air, but only over short distances, when an infected patient talks, coughs, or sneezes. The microorganisms don't remain suspended in the air, and they generally infect only those people within 3′ (about 1 m) of the source. Measles is a droplet-spread infection.

● *Transmission by common vehicle.* This type of transmission occurs when a single, inanimate substance serves as a vehicle for transmission to several people. Most often, this common substance is food or water, as occurs in hepatitis A or salmonellosis. However, contaminated blood and I.V. fluids have also been implicated in these same diseases.

● *Airborne transmission.* Occurring when the infecting organism remains suspended in the air for long periods and travels more than 3′, this type of transmission involves droplet

NATURAL BARRIERS TO INFECTION

The human body has a number of inter-related physical and chemical defenses against invading pathogens.

Nonimmunologic defenses
The skin forms an effective mechanical barrier against microorganisms. In addition, specific body functions, including epithelial cell turnover, defecation, urination, saliva-tion, sneezing, the respiratory tract's mucociliary elevator, and lacrimation, also help eliminate microorganisms.

The normal pH of the skin and the GI and GU systems can destroy or inhibit the growth of microorganisms. Lysozymes, antimicrobial enzymes found in tears, saliva, and nasal secretions, eliminate bacteria. And normal body flora stimulate antibody formation to help prevent colonization by microorganisms.

Immunologic defenses
When pathogenic microorganisms penetrate the body's nonimmunologic barriers, two types of immune response—antibody-mediated (humoral) immunity and cell-mediated immunity—combine to reinforce the defense by white blood cells. Both types of immunity involve lymphocytes that share a common origin in stem cells of the bone marrow.

In *humoral immunity,* antigen-stimulated B cells differentiate into plasma cells, producing immunoglobulins (antibodies) that disable bacteria and viruses before they can enter host cells. These antibodies circulate in the blood, providing specific protection in several ways. For example, they neutralize bacterial toxins, such as those that cause diphtheria, cholera, tetanus, gas gangrene, and botulism. Antibodies also induce or enhance phago-cytosis, bacteriolysis, and agglutination through activation of the complement system. Complement (the primary humoral mediator of inflammation) recruits addi-tional phagocytes and lyses bacteria. This is especially important in defending against capsular organisms, such as *Strep-tococcus pneumoniae,* that resist phagocy-tosis. In bacteriolysis, particularly significant in meningococcal and gonococcal infec-tions, complement and antibody work together to destroy bacteria. In agglutina-tion, specific antibodies (agglutinins) interact with insoluble particles—such as gram-negative bacteria—causing them to localize or clump together and thus mak-ing them more vulnerable to phagocytosis. In addition, antibodies prevent microorgan-isms from attaching to mucous mem-branes.

Cell-mediated immunity, involving T cells, is another important means of defense, especially against viruses, mycobacteria, fungi, and intracellular parasites. T cells move directly to attack invaders, particularly within cell walls. Subgroups of T cells trigger the response to infection by spurring B cells to manufacture antibodies, by directly killing antigens, and by producing lymphokines. (These are proteins that induce the inflammatory response by at-tracting lymphocytes, macrophages, and other blood cells to the battleground and that mediate the delayed hypersensitiv-ity reaction.) Another T cell subgroup regulates both T and B types of immune response.

Macrophages also affect both types of immune response by presenting antigens in the proper orientation to B cells for recognition and to T cells for destruction. Macrophages themselves are activated by lymphokines to destroy antigens.

Each time a microorganism, such as a bacterium, invades the body, both T and B cells preserve a "memory" of this encounter, providing long-term immunity to many diseases.

---

nuclei or resuspended dust. Common airborne infections include chicken pox and tuberculosis.

• *Vector-borne transmission.* Re-ferring to transmission by insects, this type may be either *mechanical* or *in-ternal.* Mechanical transmission oc-curs in such infections as shigellosis, in which microorganisms are trans-ferred from a fly's body surface to the patient through a break in the patient's skin. Internal transfer occurs in such infections as malaria, in which an in-fected mosquito transmits *Plasmo-dium* sporozoites to the patient through a bite.

Portal of entry

Inform the patient that microorgan-isms must enter the body to cause in-fection. Explain that they may enter through the skin, such as when the hep-

REVIEWING TYPES OF INFECTION

Microorganisms, such as bacteria, viruses, fungi, and parasites, are responsible for most human diseases.

Bacterial infections

Always present in the environment, bacteria grow independently without the aid of other cells. *Staphylococcus aureus,* one common bacterium, normally inhabits the skin surface but can cause boils (furuncles) and infection of hair follicles (folliculitis). It's also responsible for wound infections, abscesses, osteomyelitis, bacterial pneumonia (often preceded by an influenza-like illness), food poisoning, and bacteremia. And it's thought to be linked with toxic shock syndrome. The most serious staphylococcal illnesses are nosocomial infections associated with skin breakdown resulting from surgery or invasive devices, such as I.V. catheters.

One way of classifying bacteria is by their shape. Certain spherical bacteria called cocci (or diplococci, if they exist in pairs) cause meningococcal meningitis (*Neisseria meningitidis*), gonorrhea *(Neisseria gonorrhoeae),* and pneumococcal pneumonia *(Streptococcus pneumoniae).*

Bacterial cocci that grow in chains, called streptococci, commonly affect the skin and subcutaneous tissue, causing erysipelas, impetigo, and cellulitis, usually occurring in areas of injury, surgery, or ulceration. And streptococcal pharyngitis (strep throat), resulting from group A streptococci, may lead to scarlet fever, otitis media, acute sinusitis, rheumatic fever, and acute glomerulonephritis.

Rod-shaped bacteria (bacilli) are classified as gram-positive rods and gram-negative rods. In the gram-positive group, *Clostridium* commonly inhabits the soil and the GI tracts of animals and humans. *Clostridium* causes several types of human disease, including botulism, gas gangrene, pseudomembranous colitis, and tetanus. *Corynebacterium,* another group of gram-positive bacilli, exists most commonly as the normal flora of the skin, mucous membranes, and respiratory tract. However, it may also cause diphtheria and, less frequently, pulmonary infection or septicemia.

A second group of bacilli—gram-negative rods—are called enteric bacteria, which, for the most part, act as the normal GI flora. However, the most common of these cause nosocomial infections. They include *Escherichia coli, Pseudomonas aeruginosa, Klebsiella pneumoniae, Enterobacter* species, and *Proteus* species. However, *Escherichia coli* is also the most common cause of urinary tract infections unrelated to hospitalization. (*Escherichia coli* causes traveler's diarrhea, too.)

Other gram-negative bacteria include *Salmonella,* responsible for food poisoning and typhoid fever; *Shigella,* which causes dysentery; and *Vibrio cholerae,* responsible for cholera. *Hemophilus influenzae,* another gram-negative bacilli, is a major cause of meningitis in children. This microorganism may also cause epiglottitis, bronchitis, pneumonia, otitis media,

STAPHYLOCOCCUS AUREUS

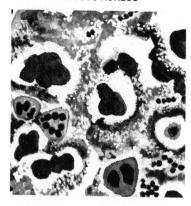

HERPES SIMPLEX VIRUS

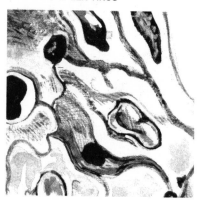

cellulitis, and sinusitis.

Mycobacteria, another category of bacteria, cause tuberculosis (*Mycobacterium tuberculosis*) and leprosy (*M. leprae*). Infection with other, atypical mycobacteria species, such as *M. avium* complex and *M. kansasii*, occurs more often today. For example, *M. avium* complex causes opportunistic infection in patients with acquired immune deficiency syndrome (AIDS).

Viral infections

Unable to multiply outside of living tissues, viruses cause infections that vary from minor to life-threatening. Viral respiratory infections account for over half of all acute illnesses, and they're the major cause of morbidity in developing countries. Viruses, in fact, cause more than 90% of upper respiratory tract infections. Major viruses causing respiratory disease include the influenza virus, parainfluenza virus, respiratory syncytial virus, and rhinoviruses. Viruses in this group also cause systemic diseases, such as mumps and measles.

Viruses of the enteroviral family—such as poliovirus, coxsackievirus, echovirus, and reovirus—are spread by infected feces. The resulting infections may range from asymptomatic to mild fever with rash to pronounced neurologic symptoms associated with meningitis and encephalitis.

Five herpesviruses are important pathogens to man: herpes simplex viruses, types 1 and 2 (cold sores and genital lesions); Epstein-Barr virus (infectious mononucleosis); cytomegalovirus (influenza-like syndrome and potential congenital abnormalities); and varicella-zoster virus (chicken pox and shingles). These viruses may remain latent and may cause recurrent disease.

Several viruses can cause hepatitis. Hepatitis A, primarily a food- or water-borne illness, is usually mild and self-limiting, with no carrier state. Hepatitis B—blood-borne or sexually transmitted—is much more serious. About 10% to 20% of infected patients become carriers.

Fungal infections

Fungi are primitive organisms that feed on living plants, animals, and decaying organic material. They cause infections that range from a mild, superficial nail infection caused by a dermatophyte to the overwhelming, often fatal disseminated disease caused by candidiasis in the severely immunosuppressed patient. Other diseases caused by fungi include cryptococcosis, histoplasmosis, coccidioidomycosis, and aspergillosis.

Parasitic infections

Parasitic diseases, caused by protozoa (malaria, trypanosomiasis, and leishmaniasis) or helminths (schistosomiasis), are major causes of illness throughout the world.

Protozoa also cause diseases occurring with increasing frequency in the United States (toxoplasmosis, pneumocystis infection, giardiasis, and trichomoniasis).

CANDIDA ALBICANS

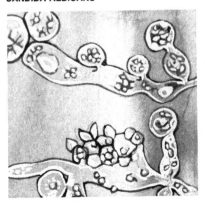

TRICHOMONAS VAGINALIS

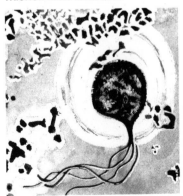

atitis B virus is introduced by a hypodermic needle. Also, *Candida* may be transmitted through the skin by I.V. catheters, and *Staphylococcus aureus* may infect skin damaged by a burn or wound.

Microorganisms may also enter through the mucous membranes when deposited on the conjunctiva (rhinovirus), inhaled and absorbed through the respiratory tract (*Mycobacterium tuberculosis*), or ingested through the GI tract (*Salmonella*). And they may enter the GU tract by retrograde flow through a urinary catheter (*Escherichia coli*). Certain microorganisms, such as cytomegalovirus, may enter in a transplanted kidney.

Explain to the patient that infection doesn't always occur at the entry site. For example, measles can be transmitted through the respiratory tract or through the conjunctivae by touching an affected patient and then rubbing the eye. However, its most notable sign is a rash.

Complications

Reinforce the need for strict adherence to prescribed antimicrobial therapy by pointing out the possible complications of noncompliance: relapse, abscess formation, and systemic involvement. Explain to the patient that, in some infections, inadequate drug therapy may delay accurate identification of the causative microorganism, postponing proper treatment.

Relapse
Explain that relapse commonly results when the patient halts antimicrobial therapy because he's asymptomatic or feeling better. Unfortunately, premature cessation of therapy lowers antibiotic blood levels, allowing microorganisms to multiply and promoting emergence of antibiotic-resistant bacterial strains.

Abscess
Tell the patient that a local infection, such as cellulitis, may progress to an abscess if he interrupts or stops antimicrobial therapy. Although a cutaneous abscess may not be life-threatening, it often causes pain and disfiguring scars.

Emphasize that abscesses in other parts of the body are usually more serious. For example, if the patient has bacterial pneumonia, tell him that inadequate therapy may lead to development of a lung abscess, which may rupture into the pleural space and cause an accumulation of pus. If the patient has pyelonephritis, inform him that inadequate therapy may predispose him to a perinephritic abscess or, in extreme cases, pyonephrosis—which may require nephrectomy. Once developed, an abscess almost always requires drainage—usually involving surgical intervention. Teach the patient that adequate antimicrobial therapy doesn't always prevent abscess formation but that it will at least limit the size of an abscess.

Systemic complications
Stress that erratic dosing or premature cessation of treatment may lead to systemic complications. If the patient's at a high risk for sepsis, explain how he and his family may recognize its early warning signs. (See *Early Signs of Septic Shock.*)

Also inform the patient that even minor local infections, if treated inadequately or not at all, may spread through the bloodstream or the lymphatic system to produce serious complications. For example, an untreated bladder infection may ascend the ureters and affect the kidneys, producing pyelonephritis. Cellulitis may involve the local veins, producing life-threatening suppurative thrombophlebitis.

Finally, teach the patient that local abscesses may spread infection to distant sites. For example, a patient with a lung abscess is at a high risk for developing a brain abscess.

EARLY SIGNS OF SEPTIC SHOCK

Without prompt, vigorous treatment, septic shock—an ominous complication of infection—may rapidly progress to death. Septic shock most often results from a bacterial infection. But other infections caused by viruses, rickettsiae, chlamydiae, or protozoa may also cause it.

Even small local infections, if untreated or treated inadequately, may spread locally or via the bloodstream. And once pathogens invade the bloodstream, infection may develop in virtually any body site, such as the bones (osteomyelitis), the joints (arthritis), the heart valves (endocarditis), the retina (endophthalmitis), or the brain

(brain abscess). Such infections, often referred to as the late complications of sepsis, may follow an episode of bacteremia in just days or weeks.

Tell the patient or his family to contact the doctor right away if the patient has any of these early warning signs of life-threatening sepsis:
- decreased urination
- sudden fever (over 101° F. [38.3° C.])
- chills
- nausea
- vomiting
- diarrhea.

DIAGNOSTIC TESTS

If appropriate, explain to the patient that he'll undergo tests to detect the causative microorganism. (See *Teaching Patients about Tests and Treatments for Common Infectious Disorders*, pages 514 to 521.) Stress that more than one test may be necessary. Such tests may include cultures, serologic and hematologic studies, and imaging tests.

Cultures

Explain to the patient that cultures can reliably identify causative bacteria, fungi, and, at times, viruses. Emphasize that their accuracy hinges on collecting a specimen without contamination. Explain that contamination may occur during collection, during transfer of the specimen to the container, or during transport to the laboratory. As appropriate, teach the patient how to avoid contamination at each step of the collection process.

Review the collection procedure for sputum, feces, or urine, and answer any questions. (See *How to Collect a Sputum Specimen for Culture*, page 523.) For collection of all specimens except stool, explain that the container should be sterile. For sputum and urine collection, provide the patient with a plastic container with a leakproof lid. For urine collection, tell the patient to follow the directions in the collection kit.

Instruct the patient to bring all specimens to the laboratory as soon as possible, preferably within 1 hour of collection. Delay may result in deterioration of the organisms, overgrowth of contaminants, or decreased or increased bacteria—all of which affect the accuracy of test results.

If the patient's having a throat culture, inform him that you'll be obtaining the specimen and that you'll use a swab to collect drainage from the affected area of the throat. Warn him that he may gag slightly during swabbing.

As necessary, explain the purpose and procedure for cultures of blood,

TEACHING PATIENTS ABOUT TESTS AND TREATMENTS FOR COMMON INFECTIOUS DISORDERS

DISORDER	DIAGNOSTIC TESTS
Gastrointestinal system	
Esophageal candidiasis	• Inform the patient that a barium swallow detects abnormalities in his esophagus. Explain the procedure and tell him to fast after midnight before the test. • If the patient's scheduled for endoscopy, explain the procedure and tell him to fast for 12 hours before testing.
Gastroenteritis	• Inform the patient that a physical examination, including a rectal examination, can rule out other causes of diarrhea, such as inflammatory bowel disease. • Explain that a stool culture identifies pathogenic organisms in the GI tract. Tell the patient that blood or leukocytes in the stool may indicate *bacterial gastroenteritis*. Teach him how to collect stool samples. If appropriate, explain that stool samples will be collected at 2- to 3-day intervals to check for parasites. Mention that a saline laxative may be required to evacuate the part of the bowel where protozoa concentrate. Also mention that he'll have a blood test to detect antibodies formed in response to certain parasites. • If scheduled, prepare the patient for a sigmoidoscopy. Teach him about positioning for the test.
Oral candidiasis	• Inform the patient that an examination of scrapings from the white plaques in his mouth may reveal the causative organism.
Viral hepatitis	• Explain that diagnosis usually includes a physical examination. Anorexia, jaundice, dark urine, clay-colored stools, and tenderness under his rib cage suggest viral hepatitis. • Inform the patient that liver function tests, such as serum alkaline phosphatase and bilirubin, help determine the extent of liver damage and monitor the infection. Serologic tests, such as hepatitis B surface antigen and hepatitis B antibodies, may help pinpoint the viral cause. Explain that these tests require a blood sample. Tell him who will perform the venipuncture and when. • If liver biopsy is necessary, explain the procedure. Advise bed rest after the test to minimize the risk of bleeding.
Musculoskeletal system	
Osteomyelitis	• Tell the patient that he'll undergo X-rays to detect soft-tissue swelling and bone involvement (periosteal elevation and lysis or sclerosis of bone). • If appropriate, prepare him for a bone scan, which may confirm osteomyelitis earlier than X-rays. • Explain that a complete blood count can reveal the presence of infection and that a blood culture can identify the causative organism. If an abscess has formed, tell the patient that a culture of the drainage may help isolate the organism and guide antibiotic therapy.

TREATMENTS

• Inform the patient that esophageal candidiasis is treated with nystatin. Or, if severe, it's treated with I.V. amphotericin B.

• If the patient has *viral gastroenteritis,* reassure him that this illness is usually self-limiting and requires no special treatment.
   If he has *bacterial gastroenteritis* and requires antibiotics, emphasize the need to complete the prescribed course of therapy.
   If he has *parasitic gastroenteritis,* also emphasize the importance of completing the prescribed course of therapy. Because some parasitic disorders are communicable, tell the patient that family members and any sexual partner may require concurrent treatment.
• Inform the patient that good hydration may improve his feeling of well-being. Tell him to avoid milk and milk products for a week or more following acute infection. Also advise him to replace lost fluids and electrolytes with clear fluids, such as broth and ginger ale.
• To relieve anal irritation, recommend warm sitz baths or witch hazel compresses.
• Teach the patient proper hand-washing techniques.
• Emphasize the importance of notifying the doctor if the patient has increasing abdominal pain or bright red blood in his stool, since intestinal hemorrhage and perforation are possible complications of bacterial gastroenteritis.

• To treat oral candidiasis, instruct the patient to hold nystatin liquid in his mouth, to swish it around, and then to swallow it. Explain that nystatin vaginal tablets are sometimes used for oral therapy. Reassure him that they're safe for oral use. He should hold them in his mouth until they're completely dissolved.

• Inform the patient that no specific drug treatment exists for viral hepatitis.
• Tell the patient with *type A hepatitis* that the infection spreads via the fecal-oral route and that he should observe proper hand-washing techniques to prevent contagion. Tell the patient with *type B hepatitis* that the infection's a blood-borne as well as a sexually transmitted disease. Tell him to avoid activities that could mingle his blood with others, such as sharing razors or toothbrushes, and to inform any sexual partner of his illness.
• Teach the patient about passive and active immunoprophylaxis with immune serum globulin, hepatitis B immune globulin, and hepatitis B vaccine.
• Explain that a high-calorie diet will help increase his resistance to infection. If his appetite is best in the morning, suggest a big breakfast. Emphasize the importance of vitamin supplements.
• Tell the patient he needn't restrict activity unless symptoms worsen when he's active.

• Inform the patient that antibiotic therapy is specific to the causative organism.
• Tell him to immobilize the affected limb to decrease pain and to protect the bone from further injury.
• If appropriate, prepare him for surgery to remove the infected bony area; also instruct him about dressing changes and the proper use of crutches or splints. He should report any sign of malposition of the limb, joint stiffness, pain, or fever.
• Teach him that some organisms causing osteomyelitis, such as *Staphylococcus aureus,* may be transmitted. If drainage occurs, tell him to discard soiled dressings in a closed plastic bag and to wash his hands.

(continued)

TEACHING PATIENTS ABOUT TESTS AND TREATMENTS
FOR COMMON INFECTIOUS DISORDERS *(continued)*

DISORDER	DIAGNOSTIC TESTS
Nervous system	
Herpes zoster (shingles)	• Inform the patient that this disorder is caused by the same virus (varicella zoster) that causes chicken pox. • Explain that diagnosis usually relies on examination of fluid-filled lesions occurring along the path of a nerve. If necessary, the doctor may use a small needle to withdraw fluid from a lesion to examine it for the presence of varicella zoster. Reassure the patient that this procedure takes less than 5 minutes and usually causes only minimal discomfort.
Meningitis	• Inform the patient that he'll have several tests to determine the cause of his symptoms. Tell him to expect a physical examination, including a neurologic assessment and an eye examination. Explain that cultures of blood, urine, sputum, throat or nasal secretions, or cerebrospinal fluid (CSF) may identify the causative organism. Tell him that a complement fixation test may also help diagnose viral meningitis. • If he's scheduled for a blood culture, inform him who will perform the venipuncture and when. • Tell him that he'll have a lumbar puncture to obtain CSF for a white blood cell count and differential and for protein and glucose levels. Explain that a Gram stain and culture can further identify the causative organism and assure appropriate treatment. Instruct him to lie flat in bed for 4 to 24 hours after the test to prevent a headache. • Explain that he may have other tests to locate the primary sites of infection, such as X-rays of the chest, skull, and sinuses and computed tomography scan to rule out cerebral hematoma.
Reproductive system	
Sexually transmitted diseases (chancroid, Chlamydia, gonorrhea, herpes simplex, syphilis, and trichomoniasis)	• Tell the patient that diagnosis of sexually transmitted infections depends on a physical examination and laboratory tests. In syphilis and herpes simplex, the presence of lesions can be diagnostic. • In some sexually transmitted infections, diagnosis requires a microscopic examination of a smear (trichomoniasis) or culture from the infection site (gonorrhea, chancroid). Teach patients that a specimen will be obtained from the cervix (in females), urethral exudate (in males), anal canal, or oropharynx. • Explain that urinalysis may help diagnose trichomoniasis.

TREATMENTS

• Inform the patient that drug therapy isn't usually necessary if he has no underlying immune deficiency.
• Tell the patient to avoid scratching. To relieve itching, instruct him to apply cool, wet compresses to the lesions; to take tepid baths; and to apply calamine lotion and other antipruritics, as ordered. If lesions rupture, tell the patient to apply cold compresses, as ordered, and to wear loose-fitting clothing over the affected area.
• Reassure the patient that herpetic pain will eventually subside and that the disorder usually doesn't recur. Tell him the doctor may order analgesics to reduce neuralgia but probably won't prescribe narcotic analgesics because of the danger of addic-

tion. Teach the patient about other medications that may be ordered, such as corticosteroids, tranquilizers, sedatives, or antidepressants.
• Advise the patient to notify the doctor if lesions appear on other body areas, if pain persists after the lesions heal, or if facial paralysis, dizziness, hearing loss, or visual disturbances develop.
• Advise against skin contact with anyone who hasn't had chicken pox. Explain that shingles is a recurrence of an already-present virus, but that it can't be transmitted as shingles. However, someone who comes into contact with the patient's lesions and is susceptible to chicken pox may develop that disease.

• Tell the patient with *bacterial meningitis* that drug therapy will vary, depending on the causative organism. In *pneumococcal* or *meningococcal meningitis*, the patient will receive I.V. penicillin. In meningitis caused by *Hemophilus influenzae*, he'll receive ampicillin and chloramphenicol. (The chloramphenicol will be discontinued if the organism is found to be sensitive to ampicillin.) Explain that drug therapy (usually I.V.) continues for at least 10 days. If drug therapy is administered intrathecally, tell the patient that he'll have a lumbar puncture to inject the drug into the CSF. Inform him that oral antibiotics usually follow I.V. antibiotics. Explain the importance of completing this therapy to eradicate the organism.
• If the patient has *viral meningitis*, tell him that it's not always possible to identify the causative virus. Inform him that treatment is usually nonspecific. One exception

is herpes simplex meningoencephalitis, which is usually treated with I.V. acyclovir. If appropriate, teach the patient about antiviral therapy.
• Teach the patient with viral or bacterial meningitis about other drug treatments, such as analgesics for muscle aches and headache and antipyretics for fever. Advise him to remain on bed rest and then to slowly increase his activities until he regains his full strength.
• Tell him to notify the doctor if he has symptoms of recurrence: headache, nausea, vomiting, mental status changes, or difficulty with balance.
• If nasal or sputum cultures are positive, teach the patient about respiratory isolation, proper hand-washing techniques, and disposal of respiratory secretions. Tell the parents of a child with *H. influenzae* to consult their doctor about immunizing their other children.

• Tell the patient that antimicrobial therapy treats most sexually transmitted infections: penicillin for syphilis and gonorrhea; tetracycline for chlamydial infection; metronidazole for trichomoniasis; and erythromycin for chancroid. As with all infections, treatment is specific to the causative organism. Emphasize the importance of completing the prescribed course of therapy. Herpes simplex may be treated with topical or oral acyclovir, although

the efficacy of such treatment for recurrent infection is uncertain.
• Impress upon the patient the importance of medical follow-up because relapse is common. Also, to prevent spreading the disease and reinfection, emphasize the importance of examination and simultaneous treatment for sexual partners.
• Tell female patients with herpes simplex to have a Pap smear twice a year to check for cervical cancer.   *(continued)*

TEACHING PATIENTS ABOUT TESTS AND TREATMENTS FOR COMMON INFECTIOUS DISORDERS *(continued)*

DISORDER	DIAGNOSTIC TESTS

Reproductive system *(continued)*

Toxic shock syndrome	• Explain to the patient that the disorder, most often affecting females, results from a toxin produced by *Staphylococcus aureus*. Tell her that diagnosis depends on several findings, including a fever exceeding 104° F. (40° C.); systolic pressure of less than 90 mm Hg; a desquamate rash; and at least three of the following: vomiting or diarrhea, myalgias or fivefold increase in creatine phosphokinase, hyperemia of mucous membranes, renal insufficiency, hepatitis, thrombocytopenia, or central nervous system disturbances. • Inform the patient that examination of vaginal secretions can detect the causative organism and a blood culture can detect *S. aureus* in the bloodstream.

Cardiovascular system

Bacterial endocarditis **Myocarditis**	• In *bacterial endocarditis*, inform the patient that a blood culture can detect the causative organism. Other blood tests (such as rheumatoid factor, erythrocyte sedimentation rate, serum immune complex assays, and complement) may support the diagnosis. • Tell the patient he'll have frequent blood tests for viral antibodies and cardiac enzyme levels to detect the causative organism and to determine the extent of cardiac damage. • Explain to the patient that a chest X-ray may be ordered to determine the size of his heart and that an EKG may be performed to determine the extent of cardiac damage. • Teach the patient about echocardiography, which can demonstrate the size and location of cardiac vegetations in bacterial endocarditis or heart muscle function in *myocarditis*. (See Chapter 6 for additional teaching points.) • If the patient requires cardiac catheterization, explain that this procedure evaluates heart valve function and can rule out angina as a cause of chest pain.

Renal and urologic system

Cystitis **Pyelonephritis**	• Tell the patient that a urine culture can detect the organism causing his symptoms and determine appropriate therapy. Explain that a urine culture may be repeated 1 week after completion of drug therapy to evaluate its effectiveness. • Inform him that a urinalysis can reveal red or white blood cells in the urine, indicating infection. Teach the patient about proper collection of samples. • If the patient is scheduled for excretory urography to evaluate the structure of the urinary system, tell him that a contrast medium injected into a vein will concentrate in the urine. Then he'll have X-rays taken of the kidneys, ureters, and bladder. Instruct him to restrict liquids for 8 hours before the test.

TREATMENTS

• Explain that drug therapy is specific to the causative organism. Stress the importance of completing the course of drug therapy to prevent recurrence.
• Teach the patient about the importance of volume replacement to maintain blood pressure. Stress the importance of liberal fluid intake—at least six to eight glasses of water daily.
• Educate the patient about risk factors, particularly cautioning against the use of hyperabsorbent tampons. Advise her to choose tampons made entirely of cotton.

• In *bacterial endocarditis,* tell the patient that antibiotic therapy is the cornerstone of treatment. Explain that its duration depends on the heart valve involved, the microorganism causing the infection, microbial sensitivities, the size of vegetations, and the duration of his illness. Explain that therapy usually lasts at least 4 weeks.
• In *myocarditis,* inform the patient that *strict* bed rest is essential until his EKG shows improvement.

• Instruct the patient to notify the doctor if he develops a fever while taking antibiotics. Explain that fever may indicate a drug reaction or microbial resistance to therapy.
• Tell the patient to take aspirin for fever and discomfort, as ordered. Also encourage adequate fluids, unless restricted by an associated condition.
• Tell the patient to resume activities slowly and to avoid strenuous sports during his recovery.

• Tell the patient with *cystitis* that a 7-day course of antibiotic therapy can eradicate the infection. (More than 90% of these infections are caused by *Escherichia coli* and are sensitive to many antibiotics, such as ampicillin or a sulfonamide.)
• If single-dose therapy has been ordered, tell the patient that this therapy's as effective as more prolonged therapy.
• Tell the patient with *pyelonephritis* that a 10- to 14-day course of co-trimoxazole, a cephalosporin, or ampicillin usually provides adequate therapy.
• Advise the patient to drink extra fluids—at least eight glasses a day—to prevent side effects of the antibiotic, to help combat infection, and to promote good hydration.

• Instruct the female patient to prevent bacterial contamination of the urinary tract by wiping the perineum from front to back after each bowel movement. Also instruct her to void after sexual intercourse to prevent infection. In some repeated urinary tract infections in women, a single-dose antibiotic may be prescribed after intercourse to prevent reinfection.
• Teach the patient to use warm sitz baths to relieve perineal discomfort.
• Tell the patient to report symptoms that recur or don't improve after a few days of therapy. Such symptoms include painful urination, urinary urgency and frequency, and malaise.

(continued)

**TEACHING PATIENTS ABOUT TESTS AND TREATMENTS
FOR COMMON INFECTIOUS DISORDERS** (continued)

DISORDER	DIAGNOSTIC TESTS
Respiratory system	
Common cold **Laryngitis** **Pharyngitis**	• Explain that viruses commonly cause upper respiratory infections, although bacteria may also cause them—for example, *streptococcal pharyngitis (strep throat)*. • In suspected streptococcal pharyngitis, tell the patient that a throat culture can identify the causative microorganism. Tell him that a swab used to collect drainage from his throat may make him gag. Reassure him that the procedure takes less than 30 seconds and causes only minor discomfort.
Pneumonia **(bacterial, fungal, and viral)**	• Tell the patient that a chest X-ray helps diagnose pneumonia and, in about 6 weeks, evaluates treatment. • Explain that a sputum culture is the most useful test to determine the cause of pneumonia. To obtain expectorated sputum, instruct the patient in deep coughing. If necessary, explain that suctioning may be required, or he may be asked to inhale nebulized saline solution to obtain sputum. • Tell the patient that a blood culture may also identify the causative organism. Tell him that other blood tests may detect antibodies to aid diagnosis of some forms of pneumonia, such as mycoplasmal or legionella. • Inform him that secretions may be obtained by bronchoscopy to find the cause of pneumonia. This procedure involves the insertion of a lighted instrument into the trachea and bronchi via the nose or mouth. He'll receive medication to help him relax and to relieve discomfort. Advise him to fast for 6 hours before the test. Afterwards, when his gag reflex returns, he can have food and water.
Skin	
Bacterial infection	• Tell the patient that culture of the skin lesions (aspiration of pus or the leading edge of advancing skin lesion) helps confirm bacterial skin infection. Tell the patient that the diagnosis can sometimes be made by examining a Gram-stained specimen from the skin lesion. • Explain that blood tests can rule out systemic involvement.
Fungal infection	• Explain to the patient that diagnosis of a fungal skin infection includes microscopic examination, Gram stains, and cultures. Explain that fungi often live in nails or the outer epidermis and cannot be cultured or stained with usual techniques.

TREATMENTS

• Inform the patient that upper respiratory viral infections usually require no specific antiviral therapy. One exception is *influenzal pharyngitis,* occurring during an influenza-A epidemic. It's treated with amantadine, given early in the illness.
• In *streptococcal pharyngitis,* instruct the patient to complete the full (usually 10-day) course of treatment with penicillin.
• Inform the patient that treatment is symptomatic for most upper respiratory infections and typically includes analgesics and throat lozenges to relieve pain and nasal sprays to unblock nasal passages and promote drainage. Instruct the patient using nose drops to bend his head down after instilling the drops.

• Advise the patient to use warm saline gargles to relieve sore throat. For a cough, suggest over-the-counter cough drops or dextromethorphan preparations or pre-scribed medication containing codeine.
• Instruct the patient with laryngitis to rest his voice until hoarseness subsides.
• Advise rest, acetaminophen for aches and pains, and extra fluids (tea, juice).
• Inform the patient that most upper respi-ratory infections are transmitted by direct contact. To block their transmission, reinforce the importance of proper hand washing and avoiding finger-to-nose or finger-to-eye contact. Instruct the patient to promptly discard used tissues into a wastebag.

• Tell the patient that most pneumonias can be treated at home. Explain that drug therapy depends on symptoms, X-ray find-ings, and sputum analysis. If these findings fail to detect the cause, erythromy-cin may be prescribed. It's effective against pneumococci and *Mycoplasma pneumoniae,* which cause Legionnaire's disease and *Hemophilus influenzae* pneumonia.
• Teach the patient with a chronic fungal pneumonia, such as histoplasmosis or coccidioidomycosis, about treatment with oral ketoconazole.

• Tell the patient to drink plenty of fluids (at least six to eight glasses daily) and to take analgesics for chest pain and cough suppressants for a nonproductive cough.
• Tell him that fatigue and weakness may persist. Encourage him to return slowly to his normal activity level.
• Encourage deep breathing to maintain full lung expansion and adequate ventilation.
• Tell the patient to contact the doctor if such symptoms as cough, fever, or short-ness of breath do not improve or if they recur.

• Inform the patient that he'll receive oral antibiotics, usually penicillin, since bacterial infections are often caused by staphylo-cocci.
• Instruct him to wash the infected area with soap and water. Also advise him to use good hand-washing techniques after

contact with the infectious drainage, and to use a separate towel and washcloth from other family members.
• Show the patient how to cover draining lesions with a dressing. Teach him proper dressing-change techniques, emphasizing proper disposal of old dressings.

• Explain that most fungal skin infections are chronic and may require months of treatment with oral drugs, such as griseo-fulvin and ketoconazole. Encourage him to continue his treatment as prescribed.
• Advise him to contact the doctor regu-larly, since the prescribed oral drugs

are potentially toxic.
• Teach about local treatments ordered (such as selenium sulfide suspension). In-struct the patient to bathe and dry himself thoroughly before applying the suspension and to wash it off in the morning, as ordered.

cerebrospinal fluid, urine (by suprapubic aspiration), gastric or duodenal aspirates, or tracheobronchial secretions. Reassure the patient that, if necessary, he'll receive medication to help him relax and to relieve discomfort.

Hematologic and Serologic Tests

Hematologic tests help detect current infection, whereas serologic tests may supply evidence of past or current infection by revealing an antigen or antibody in serum or other body fluids.

Hematologic tests

If the patient's scheduled for a white blood cell (WBC) count and differential, explain that an elevated WBC count usually signals infection, such as tonsillitis or abscess. The WBC count will return to normal as infection subsides. Tell him a low WBC differential may indicate a viral infection, such as influenza or mononucleosis.

Serologic tests

Tell the patient that serologic tests may diagnose viral infections, such as rubella, hepatitis, and mononucleosis; bacterial infections caused by syphilis and streptococci; and some fungal infections. Make sure he understands that serum samples will be taken during both acute and convalescent stages of the disorder to monitor infection.

Explain to the patient that the diagnostic workup may include a test for C-reactive protein (CRP), a protein produced by the liver and excreted into the bloodstream during acute inflammation. Inform him that CRP is a nonspecific method of evaluating the severity and course of inflammatory disorders and of monitoring treatment.

Tell the patient about other nonspecific serologic tests that may help diagnose febrile disorders. For example,

a febrile agglutination test helps diagnose disorders caused by *Salmonella, Rickettsia, Francisella tularensis,* or *Brucella* microorganisms.

Imaging Tests

Prepare the patient for any additional tests scheduled to help diagnose his infection, including X-rays, computed tomography (CT) scans, and echocardiography. Inform him that X-ray examinations of his chest, sinuses, GI tract, kidneys, and joints or a gallium scan can help locate the source of his infection. If the patient's scheduled for a CT scan, inform him that this noninvasive test can detect cerebral and epidural abscesses and sinus and nasopharyngeal infections. If he's scheduled for echocardiography, explain that this test can demonstrate cardiac abnormalities that predispose infection, such as valvular growth.

TREATMENTS

Medication

Stress strict adherence to the patient's prescribed antimicrobial therapy. Remind him to take his medication on schedule and to take every dose, even if he feels better. (See *Teaching Patients about Antimicrobial Drugs,* pages 528 to 539.) Inform him that he may also be given analgesics for pain and antipyretics for fever.

I.V. antibiotics

If the patient's receiving I.V. antibiotics at home, teach him or a caregiver how to administer the prescribed drug

HOW TO COLLECT A SPUTUM SPECIMEN FOR CULTURE

Dear Patient:

The best time to collect a sputum specimen is early morning because secretions have accumulated overnight. Unless the doctor has told you to restrict fluids, be sure to drink plenty of fluids the night before specimen collection to increase your sputum production. Once you're ready to collect the specimen, simply follow these directions.

1

Keep the specimen container close by. Before collecting the specimen, rinse your mouth with water, if necessary, but don't brush your teeth or use mouthwash. Also, wash your hands thoroughly.

2

Open the container and prepare to cough the specimen into it. Take several deep abdominal breaths until you feel the mucus "moving." (Using a nebulizer containing only saline solution or using chest physiotherapy may ease the movement of mucus.) When you're ready to cough, take a comfortably deep abdominal breath (feeling your abdomen push out), bend forward, and make a soft, staged, shortened cough into the container.

3

Press the lid closed. Be careful not to touch or contaminate the inside of the container with your hands. Also be careful not to contaminate the outside of the container with sputum.

4

Holding the container upright, remove the bottom lid. Carefully pull out the specimen tube, the label, and the specimen tube cap, taking care not to spill the collected sputum or to contaminate the cap.

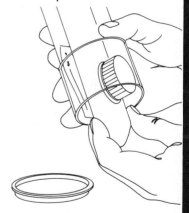

5

Screw the cap onto the specimen tube, and thoroughly wash your hands. Label the tube, and take it to the doctor or laboratory as soon as possible.

through a peripheral I.V. line. Teach him about site care, the preparation and injection of a dilute heparin solution, and how to check catheter patency. Similarly, demonstrate how to prepare the antibiotic, set up the tubing, and infuse the solution. Also demonstrate how to maintain catheter patency after infusion.

Also teach the patient the signs of phlebitis—a common complication from injury or irritation at the insertion site. Signs include redness, swelling, pain, and a burning sensation at or around the site. Explain how to remove the catheter, and advise him to apply a warm washcloth or an ice pack to reduce tenderness and to take antipyretics to relieve any discomfort. For swelling, tell him to elevate his limb.

Inform the patient that he can obtain supplies from a medical equipment dealer or a home care agency that has an I.V. therapy program. If appropriate, have the patient's family obtain an infusion pump or controller before discharge so that you can teach them how to use the device.

Prophylaxis

Explain that prophylactic drugs may be given before exposure to infection (such as antibiotics before surgery), during the time of exposure (such as chloroquine before and during travel to an area where malaria is endemic), or after exposure (such as penicillin after exposure to gonorrhea). Instruct the patient to take prescribed drugs precisely as ordered.

If appropriate, ask about other family members who may require immunization against contagious diseases, such as hepatitis A or B, rubella, and *Hemophilus influenzae*. Stress the importance of immunizations, and advise keeping a record of them. Mention reportable reactions, such as high fever, severe local swelling, or manifestations of the disease. Suggest measures to decrease symptoms, such as acetaminophen for fever or an ice pack for injection site pain.

Surgery

If the patient's scheduled for incision and drainage (I & D) to treat an abscess, explain that the surgeon makes an incision in the infected area to drain the accumulated pus. Mention that adequate drainage of pus may eliminate the infection, thereby also eliminating inflammation and pain. Reassure him that analgesics can relieve his pain until symptoms subside.

If the patient has a deep-seated infection that can't be eliminated by I & D, explain that more radical surgery may be necessary. Infective thrombophlebitis, for example, may require ligation of the vein or excision of an infected segment to prevent infected emboli from seeding other organs. A splenic or renal abscess may require splenectomy or nephrectomy.

As appropriate, explain the surgical procedure and tell the patient what to expect afterward. For example, if he's having continuous wound irrigation after surgery, explain that a catheter placed in the incision allows infusion of an antibiotic solution to help the wound heal properly. Tell him he'll have a bulky, wet dressing over the area.

Emphasize the need to prevent contamination. Remind the patient to avoid touching an open wound except with sterile gloves or a sterile dressing. However, if the wound is sewn shut, tell him that he may change dressings without gloves. If the patient has an infected wound, instruct him to change the dressing when it becomes wet. (See *How to Apply Dry Dressings*, pages 526 and 527.) To prevent the spread of infection, advise him to place used dressings in a plastic bag, to tie the bag, and to discard it in another bag.

Instruct the patient to notify the doctor immediately if he experiences symptoms of continued, progressive, or recurrent infection, such as heat, redness, pain, swelling, tenderness, fever, or increased drainage.

Other Care Measures

Explain additional care measures, including diet and ways to prevent contagion or recurrence of infection.

Diet

Explain that adequate nutrition helps to combat infection and prevent recurrence. During active infection, recommend a high-protein, high-calorie diet, including meat and fish, cheese, vegetables, and nuts, to provide energy for the patient's increased needs. Stress that adequate nutrition is essential even if he doesn't feel like eating. Tell him to weigh himself regularly to monitor any weight loss. If he has fever or severe vomiting or diarrhea, instruct him to replace lost fluids. If appropriate, recommend extra fluids—eight glasses of water each day. Advise limited activity and extra rest.

Preventing contagion

If the patient's infection is contagious, teach him about ways to prevent its spread. Point out the organism's mode of transmission, and offer concrete methods for blocking such transmission. For example, impress upon the patient—and his family—that hand washing is the most effective method to prevent contagion. Teach them to carefully wash their hands with soap and water and to rinse them thoroughly before and after any contact with the infected area. Emphasize that nasal and oral secretions may harbor a respiratory virus and that fluid from a cold sore may harbor herpes simplex virus. Discourage the patient from sharing toothbrushes and razors—possible sources of contamination. Inform him that some organisms, such as hepatitis B virus, can be transmitted by sharing such personal items. Teach proper storage and cleaning of contaminated washcloths, towels, pillowcases, and brushes. Also tell him to discard any used dressings or tissues in a closed bag. Suggest he use disposable items—razors, paper cups, paper towels.

Depending on the patient's infection, provide appropriate additional instructions.

• If the patient has an oral or throat infection, teach him how to use a mouthwash and gargle to reduce symptoms of inflammation and to expose the affected area to the anti-infective solution.

• If he has a sexually transmitted disease, such as syphilis, stress the importance of avoiding sexual contact. Tell him to notify all sexual partners so they may also be treated.

• If the patient has measles (a droplet-spread disease), urge him to stay more than 3' away from susceptible people.

• To prevent food poisoning, advise the patient to store food at the proper temperature to avoid multiplication of microorganisms. Explain the importance of drinking only pasteurized milk.

• Tell the patient with an airborne infection, such as chicken pox, to cover his mouth when coughing and to wear a mask in the presence of susceptible people.

THE BEST DEFENSE

In infectious disorders, thorough patient teaching provides the best defense against complications and contagion. After all, the patient who understands his type of infection, its mode of transmission, and his role in its diagnosis and treatment will be best prepared to manage his condition. And he'll be in a position to prevent the spread of his infection to others.

HOW TO APPLY DRY DRESSINGS

Dear Patient:

As directed by the doctor, you'll need to change your dressing _____ times a day. Here's how.

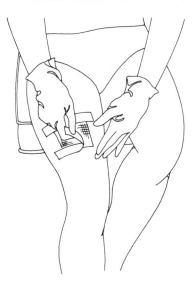

1

First, gather several 4" × 4" gauze pads, cleansing solution (such as povidone-iodine), and sterile lukewarm water (boiled for 5 minutes) to wet the gauze pads. Also collect a sterile bowl (washed, rinsed, and immersed in boiling water for 5 minutes), baby oil, surgical tape, scissors, a plastic bag, and rubber gloves.

2

Wash your hands, and put on rubber gloves. Then, to remove the tape, hold your skin taut and pull the old tape strips toward the wound (as shown at the top of the next column). Remove *all* the old tape. If the tape sticks, soften it with baby oil.

3

Now, slowly remove the old dressing. Does it stick to the wound? If so, stop and moisten the dressing with sterile luke-warm water. When the dressing's loose, remove it. Then discard it in the plastic bag.

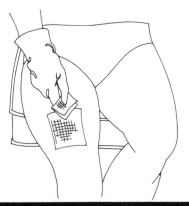

4

Before you clean the wound, examine it carefully for any changes since the last dressing change, especially an increase in swelling, redness, drainage or pus, or odor. If you think the wound looks worse, contact your doctor.

5

Take one of the gauze pads and saturate it with sterile water and cleansing solution. Then fold the pad into quarters. Holding the pad as shown, gently wipe from the top of the wound to the bottom in one motion. Then discard this pad in the plastic bag.

6

Saturate another gauze pad, fold it into quarters, and wipe the wound again, this time on one side first and then on the other. Do this several times to clean the entire wound area that the dressing will cover. Then use another clean gauze pad to pat the wound dry. Remove the rubber gloves and discard them in the plastic bag.

7

Next, apply a clean gauze pad over the area. Depending on the amount of drainage, use several layers of pads. As the nurse has demonstrated, secure the pads with tape or with

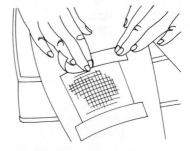

Montgomery straps (lengths of adhesive tape used in place of taping directly to the skin to make dressing changes easier). Be sure you've collected all soiled material in the plastic bag. Tie the bag, and dispose of it properly.

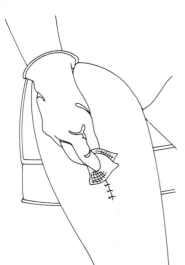

TEACHING PATIENTS ABOUT ANTIMICROBIAL DRUGS

DRUG	ADVERSE REACTIONS	INTERACTIONS*
Antifungals (oral)		
flucytosine (Ancobon, Ancotil)	*Reportable:* fever; rash; sore throat; unusual bleeding, bruising, fatigue, or weakness *Other:* diarrhea, headache, nausea, vomiting	• Tell the patient that foods, beverages, and over-the-counter (OTC) products don't influence the safety or effectiveness of this drug.
ketoconazole (Nizoral)	*Reportable:* dark or amber urine, gynecomastia, pale stools, yellowing of eyes or skin *Other:* diarrhea, dizziness, drowsiness, itching, nausea, rash, vomiting	• Tell the patient not to drink alcohol while taking this drug to prevent hepatotoxicity. • Inform him that foods, nonalcoholic beverages, and OTC products don't influence the safety or effectiveness of this drug.
Antifungals (topical and other local)		
clotrimazole (Gyne-Lotrimin, Lotrimin, Mycelex) **miconazole** (Monistat 7 Vaginal Cream) **nystatin** (Mycostatin, Nilstat) **tolnaftate** (Tinactin)	*Reportable:* hives; itching; skin blistering, burning, peeling, redness, rash, or swelling; vaginal burning (with vaginal use) *Other:* abdominal cramps, diarrhea, nausea, vomiting	• Inform the patient that foods, beverages, and OTC products don't influence the safety or effectiveness of these drugs.
Antiparasitics		
Anthelmintic agents **mebendazole** (Vermox) **praziquantel** (Biltricide)	*Reportable:* none *Other:* abdominal pain, diarrhea, dizziness, drowsiness, fever, headache, itching, nausea, rash, vomiting	• Unless contraindicated, tell the patient to avoid a low-fat diet. • Inform him that other foods, beverages, and OTC products don't influence the safety or effectiveness of these drugs.

*Includes foods, beverages, and over-the-counter (OTC) drugs.

TEACHING POINTS

• Instruct the patient to complete the prescribed course of therapy. Inform him that therapy may take weeks or months.

• Tell the patient to take capsules over a 15-minute period to reduce nausea and vomiting.

• Instruct the patient to complete the prescribed course of therapy. Inform him that therapy may take weeks or months.
• If the patient has achlorhydria, he'll need special directions for taking ketoconazole: instruct him to dissolve each tablet in 4 ml aqueous solution of 0.2N hydrochloric acid and, to avoid contact with his teeth, to sip the

mixture through a straw. Tell him to follow the dose with a glass of water.
• Reassure the patient that nausea, common early in therapy, will subside. To minimize nausea, tell him that, with the doctor's permission, he may divide the daily dosage into two doses and take them with meals or snacks.

• Instruct the patient to complete the prescribed course of therapy. Remind him to take every dose.
• Tell the patient to store the drug away from direct heat or light.
• If the patient is taking clotrimazole lozenges, advise him to allow each one to dissolve slowly and completely in his mouth. This may take 15 to 30 minutes. Instruct him *not* to chew or swallow the lozenges whole.
• Instruct parents not to give lozenges to children under age 4.
• If the patient's taking the liquid form of clotrimazole, advise him to swish the dose in his mouth for as long as possible and then to swallow.

• If the patient's using a topical cream, show how to apply it on the affected area and surrounding skin and to rub it in gently. Warn the patient *not* to cover the area with an occlusive wrapping or dressing. Advise the patient to keep the drug away from the eyes.
• If the patient's using the vaginal form, advise her to wear cotton panties (or panties or pantyhose with cotton crotches) that are freshly laundered. If she experiences vaginal discharge while using this drug, advise her to wear a sanitary napkin to protect her clothing.
• Advise the patient to continue therapy during menstruation and to wash the vaginal applicator thoroughly after each use.

• Instruct the patient to complete the prescribed course of therapy. Remind him to take every dose.
• If the patient's taking mebendazole, tell him that tablets may be chewed, swallowed whole, or mixed with food.
• If he's taking praziquantel, advise him to swallow tablets whole and not to chew them. The drug's bitter taste may cause gagging or vomiting.
• If the patient's being treated for pinworms

or roundworms, instruct him to wash the perianal area and to change undergarments daily. Also instruct him to wash his hands and clean his fingernails thoroughly before meals and after bowel movements.
• Teach him that pinworms may be easily transmitted to others, especially in a family. Therefore, all family members should be treated simultaneously.
• Advise the patient to drive or operate machinery cautiously.

(continued)

**TEACHING PATIENTS ABOUT
ANTIMICROBIAL DRUGS** *(continued)*

DRUG	ADVERSE REACTIONS	INTERACTIONS*
Antiparasitics *(continued)*		
Antimalarial agents **chloroquine** (Aralen) **primaquine** **pyrimethamine** (Fansidar) **quinine** (Quinamm)	*Reportable:* dark urine, dizziness, dyspnea, hearing loss, hives, itching, severe headache, rash, tinnitus, unusual fatigue or weakness, vision changes (especially blurring) *Other:* abdominal cramps, anorexia, diarrhea, mild headache, nausea, vomiting	• Tell the patient taking chloroquine to avoid alcohol (increased risk of hepatotoxicity). • Inform the patient that foods, nonalcoholic beverages, and OTC products don't influence the safety or effectiveness of these drugs.
metronidazole (Flagyl)	*Reportable:* dryness or discharge not present before therapy; hives; numbness, tingling, pain, or weakness in the hands or feet; seizures; rash; vaginal irritation *Other:* abdominal pain, anorexia, constipation, dark or reddish brown urine, diarrhea, dizziness, dry mouth, headache, nausea, unpleasant metallic taste, vomiting	• Tell the patient to avoid alcohol and alcohol-containing OTC products (such as cough and cold remedies) for 48 hours after taking this drug. • Inform the patient that foods, nonalcoholic beverages, and alcohol-free OTC products don't influence the safety or effectiveness of this drug.
Antituberculars		
ethambutol (Myambutol)	*Reportable:* blurred vision; chills; color blindness; decreased vision; eye pain; joint pain, swelling, and warmth *Other:* dizziness, GI upset, itching, rash	• Tell the patient that foods, beverages, and OTC products don't influence the safety or effectiveness of this drug.
isoniazid (INH) (Laniazid, Nydrazid)	*Reportable:* anorexia; clumsiness or unsteadiness; dark urine; nausea; numbness, tingling, burning, or pain in the hands and feet; unusual fatigue or weakness; vomiting; yellowing of eyes or skin *Other:* dizziness, GI upset, gynecomastia	• Instruct the patient to avoid taking aluminum- or magnesium-containing antacids within 1 hour of taking isoniazid. These antacids may decrease drug absorption. • Tell him not to drink alcohol to prevent hepatotoxicity. • Tell the patient to take the drug on an empty stomach, if possible. Inform him that certain foods, such as Swiss cheese or tuna fish, may rarely cause a reaction (such as sweating, chills, increased heartbeat).

*Includes foods, beverages, and over-the-counter (OTC) drugs.

TEACHING POINTS

• Instruct the patient to complete the prescribed course of therapy. Remind him to take every dose.
• To decrease GI upset, advise the patient to take the prescribed drug with or after meals, with milk or antacids.
• Advise the patient taking chloroquine to drive or operate machinery cautiously.

• Instruct the patient to complete the prescribed course of therapy. Remind him to take every dose.
• To minimize GI upset, tell the patient to take this drug with meals.
• Tell the female patient of childbearing age to practice birth control during therapy; some studies have shown that metronidazole causes cancer in mice and rats.
• Tell the patient with trichomoniasis that sexual partners should be treated simultaneously to avoid reinfection.

• Instruct the patient to complete the prescribed course of therapy. Remind him to take every dose.
• Tell the patient to visit his doctor regularly while he's taking this drug.
• Reassure him that any visual disturbances will disappear several weeks to months after cessation of therapy.

• Instruct the patient to complete the prescribed course of therapy. Remind him to take every dose.
• Stress the need to completely eradicate tuberculosis. Tell the patient that therapy may last for 1 year or longer.
• If GI upset occurs, tell the patient to take this drug with food or with antacids that do not contain aluminum or magnesium.
• Inform the diabetic patient that isoniazid may cause spurious results on some urine glucose tests. Tell him to check with his doctor before changing his diet or medication dosage.

(continued)

**TEACHING PATIENTS ABOUT
ANTIMICROBIAL DRUGS** *(continued)*

DRUG	ADVERSE REACTIONS	INTERACTIONS*
Antituberculars *(continued)*		
rifampin (Rifadin, Rimactane)	*Reportable:* anorexia, chills, difficulty breathing, dizziness, fever, headache, muscle and bone pain, nausea, unusual fatigue or weakness, vomiting, yellowing of eyes or skin *Other:* diarrhea; reddish orange to reddish brown urine, saliva, sputum, stools, sweat, and tears	• For best results, instruct the patient to take this drug with a full glass of water on an empty stomach—1 hour before or 2 hours after meals. • Tell him not to drink alcohol to prevent possible hepatotoxicity. • Also tell him that OTC products don't influence the safety or effectiveness of this drug.
Antivirals		
acyclovir (Zovirax)	**With oral form** *Reportable:* bloody urine, confusion, hives, rash, trembling *Other:* diaphoresis, headache, light-headedness **With topical form** *Reportable:* none *Other:* itching; mild pain, burning, or stinging; rash	• Tell the patient that foods, beverages, and OTC drugs don't influence the safety or effectiveness of this drug.
amantadine (Symmetrel)	*Reportable:* confusion, difficulty urinating, fainting, hallucinations, mood or other mental changes *Other:* anorexia, anxiety, difficulty concentrating, dizziness, insomnia, irritability, light-headedness, nausea, nightmares, oral or nasal dryness, skin blotches	• Tell the patient not to drink alcohol, which can worsen CNS symptoms. • Inform the patient that foods, nonalcoholic beverages, and OTC products don't influence the safety or effectiveness of this drug.
Cephalosporins		
cefaclor (Ceclor) **cephalexin** (Keflex)	*Reportable:* abdominal pain and distention; diarrhea (severe, watery, perhaps bloody); fever; hives; itching; nausea; rash; unusual fatigue, thirst, weakness, or weight loss; vomiting; wheezing *Other:* mild diarrhea, mild GI upset, sore mouth or tongue	• Tell the patient that foods, beverages, and OTC drugs don't influence the safety or effectiveness of these cephalosporins.

*Includes foods, beverages, and over-the-counter (OTC) drugs.

TEACHING POINTS

• Instruct the patient to complete the prescribed course of therapy, and remind him to take every dose. Therapy may last months or even years.
• If the patient experiences GI upset, tell him to take rifampin with food.
• Warn the patient that this drug may cause permanent discoloration of soft contact lenses. He should avoid wearing soft contact lenses while taking the drug. Hard lenses aren't discolored.
• Because rifampin may make oral contraceptives less effective, tell the patient to use an alternate method of birth control.

• Inform the patient that this drug effectively controls herpes simplex infection but doesn't cure it. Explain that it won't prevent the spread of infection. Tell him not to engage in sexual activity if he or his partner has symptoms of herpes.
• Instruct the patient to complete the prescribed course of therapy. Remind him to take every dose.
• Urge the patient to recognize early symptoms of infection (such as tingling, itching, or pain) so he can take acyclovir before infection fully develops.
• Advise the patient to use a finger cot or rubber glove when applying creams to avoid spreading infection to other body sites or to other people.
• Tell the female patient with genital herpes to visit her doctor regularly. Explain that women with genital herpes are at an increased risk for cervical cancer, so regular Pap smears are important for early detection.
• Teach the patient to keep herpetic areas clean and dry. Advise wearing loose-fitting clothing to avoid irritating the sores.
• If the patient doesn't notice improvement after using the drug for 1 week, advise him to contact the doctor.

• Instruct the patient to complete the prescribed course of therapy. Remind him to take every dose.
• Advise the patient to drive or operate machinery cautiously.
• Warn the patient that sudden sitting up or standing may cause dizziness. Advise him to change positions slowly.
• If the patient has a dry mouth, nose, or throat, advise him to chew sugarless gum or dissolve ice chips in his mouth.
• Reassure the patient with skin blotches that these usually disappear from 2 to 12 weeks after stopping the drug.
• If the patient has insomnia, tell him to take the dose several hours before bedtime.

• Instruct the patient to complete the prescribed course of therapy. Remind him to take every dose.
• Tell him to take the drug with food or milk to decrease GI upset.
• Tell him to store the reconstituted suspension form in the refrigerator and to shake well before using. Inform him that the suspension form is stable for 14 days if refrigerated.
• Advise the diabetic patient that this drug may cause false-positive results on some urine glucose tests. Advise him to check with the doctor before changing his diet or medication dosage.
• If the patient develops diarrhea from taking this drug, tell him to contact the doctor before taking an antidiarrheal.

(continued)

**TEACHING PATIENTS ABOUT
ANTIMICROBIAL DRUGS** *(continued)*

DRUG	ADVERSE REACTIONS	INTERACTIONS*
Ophthalmic anti-infectives		
chloramphenicol (Chloromycetin, Chloroptic) **natamycin** (Natacyn) **neomycin, polymyxin-B, and bacitracin** (Neosporin) **neomycin, polymyxin-B, and hydrocortisone** (Cortisporin) **sulfacetamide** (Sodium Sulamyd)	*Reportable:* fever; itching, rash, redness (not present before therapy); sore throat; unusual bleeding or bruising (with chloramphenicol); unusual fatigue or weakness *Other:* blurred vision, burning, or stinging after application	• None significant
Penicillins		
Aminopenicillins **amoxicillin** (Amoxil) **ampicillin** (Omnipen, Polycillin) **cyclacillin** (Cyclapen-W)	*Reportable:* abdominal cramps, severe diarrhea, signs of hypersensitivity (hives, itching, rash, wheezing), unusual thirst or weight loss *Other:* mild diarrhea, nausea, sore mouth or tongue, vomiting	• If the patient's using ampicillin or cyclacillin, tell him to take the drug on an empty stomach—1 hour before a meal or 2 hours after it. If he's using amoxicillin, tell him to take the drug without regard to mealtimes. • Inform the patient that beverages and OTC drugs don't influence the safety or effectiveness of aminopenicillins.
Natural penicillins **penicillin G potassium** (Pentids) **penicillin V potassium** (Pen-Vee K, V-Cillin K)	*Reportable:* signs of hypersensitivity (hives, itching, rash, wheezing) *Other:* darkened or discolored tongue, mild diarrhea, nausea, vomiting	• Tell the patient to take this drug on an empty stomach—1 hour before meals or 2 hours after. Also tell him to avoid acidic juices and other beverages while taking penicillin G. • Mention that OTC products don't influence the safety or effectiveness of the prescribed drug.
Penicillinase-resistant agents **cloxacillin** (Tegopen) **dicloxacillin** (Dynapen)	*Reportable:* signs of hypersensitivity (hives, itching, rash, wheezing) *Other:* mild diarrhea, nausea, vomiting	• Tell the patient to take this drug on an empty stomach—1 hour before or 2 hours after meals. • Mention that beverages and OTC products don't influence the safety or effectiveness of the prescribed drug.

*Includes foods, beverages, and over-the-counter (OTC) drugs.

TEACHING POINTS

- Instruct the patient to complete the prescribed course of therapy. Remind him to take every dose.
- Demonstrate the proper method for instilling eye drops or ointment. Tell the patient to cleanse the eye area of exudate before applying medication.
- Also warn him not to share eye medications with family members. If a family member develops similar symptoms, instruct him to contact the doctor.
- If the patient's using sulfacetamide, tell him to wait at least 5 minutes before administering other eye drops.
- If the sulfacetamide solution is discolored (dark brown), tell him not to use it.

- Instruct the patient to complete the prescribed course of therapy. Remind him to take every dose.
- If amoxicillin causes GI upset, advise the patient to take it with meals.
- Tell the female patient taking ampicillin to avoid using oral contraceptives. Suggest another method of birth control.
- If the patient is taking the suspension form of this drug, remind him to check the drug label for storage directions.

- Instruct the patient to complete the prescribed course of therapy, even if he feels better. Remind him to take every dose.

- Instruct the patient to complete the prescribed course of therapy, even if he feels better. Remind him to take every dose.

(continued)

**TEACHING PATIENTS ABOUT
ANTIMICROBIAL DRUGS** (continued)

DRUG	ADVERSE REACTIONS	INTERACTIONS*
Sulfonamides		
co-trimoxazole (trimethoprim-sulfamethoxazole) (Bactrim, Septra) **sulfamethoxazole** (Gantanol) **sulfisoxazole** (Gantrisin)	*Reportable:* aching joints or muscles; fever; itching; pallor; skin blistering, peeling, rash, or redness; sore throat; unusual bleeding, bruising, fatigue, or weakness; yellowing of eyes or skin *Other:* anorexia, diarrhea, dizziness, headache, nausea, photosensitivity, vomiting	• Instruct the patient to take this drug on an empty stomach—1 hour before or 2 hours after meals. • Mention that beverages and OTC products don't influence the safety or effectiveness of the prescribed drug.
Tetracyclines		
demeclocycline (Declomycin) **doxycycline** (Doxy-Caps, Vibramycin) **minocycline** (Minocin) **tetracycline** (Achromycin, Tetracyn)	*Reportable:* diarrhea; increased pigmentation of skin or mucous membranes; unusual thirst, fatigue, or weakness; urinary frequency or increased volume *Other:* abdominal cramps or burning, discolored tongue, dizziness, genital or rectal itching, light-headedness, nausea, photosensitivity, sore mouth or tongue, vomiting	• Tell the patient to take tetracycline on an empty stomach—1 hour before or 2 hours after meals. • Tell him not to take tetracycline with milk. • Advise against taking aminosalicylate calcium, antacids, calcium supplements, or magnesium-containing preparations (such as Epsom salts or sodium bicarbonate) within 2 hours of taking tetracycline. • Advise against taking iron preparations (including iron-containing vitamins) within 3 hours of taking tetracycline.
Urinary tract agents		
nalidixic acid (NegGram)	*Reportable:* blurred vision, change in color vision, decreased vision, double vision, halo vision *Other:* diarrhea, drowsiness, itching, nausea, photosensitivity, vomiting	• Advise the patient to take this drug on an empty stomach—1 hour before or 2 hours after meals. • Tell him that beverages and OTC products don't influence the safety or effectiveness of this drug.
nitrofurantoin (Macrodantin)	*Reportable:* breathing difficulty, chest pain, chills, cough, dizziness, drowsiness, facial or oral burning or paresthesias, headache, pallor, unusual fatigue or weakness *Other:* anorexia, diarrhea, discolored teeth (liquid form), itching, nausea, rash, vomiting	• Tell the patient that foods, beverages, and OTC products don't influence the safety or effectiveness of this drug.

*Includes foods, beverages, and over-the-counter (OTC) drugs.

TEACHING POINTS

• Instruct the patient to complete the prescribed course of therapy. Remind him to take every dose.
• Tell the patient to drink a full glass of water with each dose and extra water throughout the day to prevent formation of urine crystals.
• Warn the patient to avoid direct sunlight and ultraviolet light to prevent photosensitivity.
• Tell him to notify his doctor before undergoing surgery requiring general anesthesia.
• Tell him that "DS" on a co-trimoxazole drug label means "double strength."

• Instruct the patient to complete the prescribed course of therapy. Remind him to take every dose.
• Tell the pregnant patient or the parent of the patient under age 8 that this drug may permanently discolor teeth, cause enamel defects, and retard bone growth.
• Teach the patient good oral hygiene. Check his tongue for signs of candidal infection. If superinfection occurs, instruct him to stop the drug and notify the doctor.
• Warn the patient to avoid direct sunlight and ultraviolet light. Instruct him to use a sunscreen if exposure is unavoidable, and tell him that photosensitivity may continue after he stops the drug.
• Instruct the patient to take the drug at least 1 hour before bedtime to prevent esophageal irritation.
• Instruct the patient to store reconstituted solutions in the refrigerator. Tell him they're stable for 48 hours.
• Advise him not to use medication that has changed color, taste, or appearance.

• Instruct the patient to complete the prescribed course of therapy. Remind him to take every dose.
• Reassure the patient that visual disturbances usually disappear with reduced doses.
• Instruct the patient to avoid unnecessary exposure to sunlight. Tell him that photosensitivity may continue up to 3 months after stopping the drug.
• Tell the diabetic patient that this drug may cause false-positive results on urine glucose tests. Advise him to contact his doctor before changing his diet or medication dosage.

• Instruct the patient to complete the prescribed course of therapy.
• Tell the patient to take the drug with food or milk to minimize GI upset.
• Warn him not to store pills in any metal container other than stainless steel or aluminum, since a precipitate may form.
• Inform the diabetic patient that this drug may cause spurious results on some urine glucose tests. Tell him to check with his doctor before changing his diet or medication dosage.
• Advise the patient taking the liquid form to rinse his mouth with water after swallowing to avoid staining his teeth. Reassure him that staining is temporary.

(continued)

TEACHING PATIENTS ABOUT
ANTIMICROBIAL DRUGS *(continued)*

DRUG	ADVERSE REACTIONS	INTERACTIONS*
Urinary tract agents *(continued)*		
methenamine hippurate (Hiprex, Urex) **methenamine mandelate** (Mandelamine)	*Reportable:* bloody urine, lower back pain, painful or burning urination *Other:* GI upset, nausea, rash	• Tell the patient not to take calcium carbonate and magnesium-containing antacids. They reduce methenamine's effectiveness by making urine alkaline. • Mention that foods and beverages don't influence the safety or effectiveness of these drugs.
Miscellaneous		
chloramphenicol (Chloromycetin)	*Reportable:* blurred vision; eye pain; fever; numbness, tingling, burning pain, or weakness in hands or feet; pallor; sore throat; unusual bleeding, bruising, or fatigue *Also reportable in children:* abdominal distention, drowsiness, gray skin, subnormal temperature, uneven breathing *Other:* diarrhea, nausea	• Instruct the patient to take this drug on an empty stomach—1 hour before or 2 hours after meals. • Inform the patient that beverages and OTC drugs don't influence the safety or effectiveness of this drug.
clindamycin (Cleocin)	*Reportable:* abdominal cramps or pain; nausea; severe diarrhea (possibly bloody); severe abdominal distention; unusual fatigue, thirst, weakness, or weight loss; vomiting *Other:* itching, mild diarrhea, rash	• Instruct the patient not to take antidiarrheals containing kaolin and pectin while taking this drug. They may decrease absorption of clindamycin. • Mention that foods and beverages don't influence the safety or effectiveness of this drug.
erythromycin (E-Mycin, Erythrocin, Ilosone, Pediamycin)	*Reportable:* dark or amber urine, fever, pale stools, severe abdominal pain, unusual fatigue or weakness, yellowing of eyes or skin (more common with Ilosone) *Other:* abdominal cramps, diarrhea, nausea, sore mouth or tongue, vomiting	• Instruct the patient to take this drug 1 hour before or 2 hours after meals. If prescribed, he can take enteric-coated, estolate, or ethylsuccinate forms without regard to meals. • Mention that beverages and OTC products don't influence this drug's safety or effectiveness.
trimethoprim (Trimpex)	*Reportable:* bluish fingernails, lips, or skin; difficulty breathing; fever; pallor; sore throat; unusual bleeding or bruising *Other:* abdominal cramps, anorexia, diarrhea, headache, itching, rash	• For best results, instruct the patient to take this drug 1 hour before or 2 hours after meals. • Mention that beverages and OTC products don't influence the safety or effectiveness of this drug.

*Includes foods, beverages, and over-the-counter (OTC) drugs.

TEACHING POINTS

• Instruct the patient to complete the prescribed course of therapy.
• Caution elderly patients against aspirating the medication, because it contains vegetable oil and may cause severe lipid pneumonia.

• Tell the patient to limit his intake of alkaline foods, such as vegetables, milk, and peanuts. To acidify his urine, tell him to drink cranberry, plum, and prune juices.

• Instruct the patient to complete the prescribed course of therapy. Remind him to take every dose.
• Inform the patient that he'll have regular blood tests during therapy.

• Tell the diabetic patient that this drug may cause spurious results on some urine glucose tests. Advise him to check with the doctor before changing his diet or medication dosage.

• Instruct the patient to complete the prescribed course of therapy. Remind him to take every dose.
• Tell him not to refrigerate the reconstituted solution, as it will thicken. Mention that the

drug is stable at room temperature for 2 weeks.
• If the patient's using the capsule form, advise him to take it with a full glass of water.

• Instruct the patient to complete the prescribed course of therapy. Remind him to take every dose.
• Advise the patient to take the drug with a

full glass of water.
• Tell him not to swallow chewable tablets whole.

• Instruct the patient to complete the prescribed course of therapy. Remind him to take every dose.
• If trimethoprim causes GI upset, tell the patient to take it with food.
• Tell the patient to notify his doctor if symptoms don't improve within a few days. Also

advise him to visit the doctor regularly while taking this drug.
• Tell the patient that if the drug causes anemia, the doctor may prescribe folic acid. If so, instruct him to take folic acid, as ordered, with trimethoprim and not to miss any doses.

18

Cancer

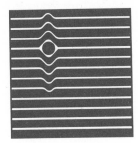

Cancer

Introduction

Despite the efforts of nurses and other health care professionals to educate the public about cancer, fear of this dreaded disorder still discourages many people from seeking early (and possibly lifesaving) treatment. Those who do seek treatment may have their worst fears confirmed when a definitive diagnosis is made. Your teaching can do much to reduce such fear and to encourage active participation in treatment and ongoing care. You'll need to provide patients and their families with the facts about cancer and, above all, to stress that this disorder can be managed successfully.

Because of the wide-ranging effects of cancer and its primary treatments—surgery, chemotherapy, and radiation therapy—you'll find that certain teaching topics recur in many neoplastic disorders. For example, certain types of cancer and most cancer treatments can dramatically alter the patient's life-style and thus challenge his identity. Many neoplastic disorders also require an exhaustive battery of tests to obtain a diagnosis, select and monitor treatment, arrive at a prognosis, and check for recurrence. What's more, many cancer patients are actively involved in their ongoing care and have physical care needs that continue after they leave the hospital.

To help the patient effectively deal with cancer, your teaching must address his psychological and emotional needs as well as his need for physical care. You'll have to help him master strategies for coping with his disorder, its treatment, and its effect on his life-style.

Helping your patient through a diagnostic workup poses a different kind of teaching challenge. The typically exhaustive battery of tests may bewilder your patient or make him feel powerless. Your teaching must help him gain a sense of control by combining calm reassurance and emotional support with thorough preparation for the tests he needs.

You can encourage your patient to participate in his ongoing care by explaining the recommended treatment and by teaching him how to manage common side effects, such as pain or gastrointestinal complaints. You can also help him make informed decisions about treatment by discussing available treatment options.

To ensure that the patient's physical care needs are met after he leaves the hospital, you'll need to focus much of your teaching on home care. Besides teaching the patient and his family how to perform home care procedures, you'll need to emphasize the importance of maintaining good nutrition and avoiding infection.

THE DISORDER

The diagnosis of cancer, whether for the first time or for a recurrence, can threaten anyone's sense of well-being. Patients who've just learned they have cancer often feel shocked, isolated, and confused by the diagnosis. They may have misconceptions as well as realistic fears about the disorder, its treatment, and its prognosis.

When cancer recurs, the effect can be equally shattering. These patients may suffer feelings of guilt and personal failure compounded by a sense of despair or rage. Often, their first reaction is "How can this be happening to me again?" Some patients may have put their experiences with cancer completely behind them, and its recurrence hits them almost as hard as the first diagnosis. Other patients may not be surprised when cancer recurs, but they still may endure some emotional ups and downs as they adjust to the diagnosis.

As a nurse, you'll teach patients who are experiencing cancer for the first time as well as patients whose cancer has recurred. And when you do, you'll encounter different—although related—teaching challenges. First-time cancer patients must learn how to face this dreaded disorder; patients with recurrent cancer must learn how to summon the strength to face it again. You can meet both learning needs by teaching patients the facts about cancer and by helping them realize that this disorder can be managed.

Teaching the Patient with Newly Diagnosed Cancer

Help your patient adjust to the diagnosis by giving him only the information he needs, requests, or is ready to learn. Answer his questions specifically, but don't bombard him with unimportant details. Also pay attention to the way you present information: a patient who has endured weeks of tension before learning the diagnosis may interpret vague descriptions of the disorder or broad reassurances as an attempt to avoid discussing death. Provide clear, accurate information in a factual but sensitive way, and give the patient time to absorb what you tell him. Remember, some patients respond to stress by hearing only what they want to hear. A patient who repeats the same questions or remembers only part of what you tell him may need more time to absorb the information. He may also need to hear certain information repeated.

CHECKLIST

TEACHING TOPICS IN CANCER

☐ An explanation of the disease process: primary or metastatic

☐ Preparation for biopsy and other scheduled tests

☐ An explanation of the recommended treatment, including its purpose, procedure, and possible side effects

☐ How to manage side effects and prevent complications of treatment

☐ Discussion of experimental treatments

☐ How to cope with life-style changes

☐ Pain control

☐ Home care measures to prevent protein-calorie malnutrition and infection

☐ Signs and symptoms of recurrence

☐ Availability of support groups, such as the American Cancer Society

Determine the patient's perception of cancer

Find out what your patient knows about cancer, its diagnosis, and its treatment. By determining his perception of cancer, you can set learning goals that fill gaps in the patient's knowledge and correct misconceptions. Also ask your patient about his experience with other people who have (or had) the disorder—a factor that may affect his attitude about his diagnosis. For example, a patient with colorectal cancer whose neighbor died of the same disorder may believe that this type of cancer is invariably fatal.

Also determine the patient's response to what the doctor has told him about his disorder and its treatment. You can expect cancer patients to share certain responses. For example, they usually fear rejection and isolation, death, the unknown, treatment, pain, or becoming a financial burden to their families. If your patient expresses any of these fears, don't dismiss them. Note the intensity of his response, and rely on your experience to judge whether a response is normal or unusual. If you have any doubts, consult a more experienced colleague or a professional counselor.

Correct misconceptions about cancer

A patient's misconceptions about cancer and its treatment are often far more disturbing than the facts. You can do a great deal to correct his misconceptions by debunking common myths about cancer. For example:

• *"Cancer is always fatal."* In fact, cancer survival rates have consistently improved since the turn of the century, when few patients survived. Today, three out of eight patients diagnosed as having cancer can expect to be alive 5 years later.

• *"Cancer is always excruciatingly painful."* Many patients can recall one or more friends or family members who suffered painful deaths from cancer. If your patient has a type of cancer that

doesn't normally produce pain, such as basal cell carcinoma, reassure him that he needn't fear pain. On the other hand, if he has a cancer that's characterized by pain, such as metastatic bone cancer, tell him what to expect. Explain that many effective treatments are available to help manage pain, although they may not eradicate it.

• *"Cancer is contagious."* Tell your patient that even though cancer is widespread—and this incidence is sometimes mistakenly termed as epidemic—no evidence exists that cancer is an infectious disorder.

• *"Cancer always mutilates the body."* The key word here is *always*. There's no question that cancer dramatically alters a patient's body image. Even if your patient has a type of cancer that doesn't change his physical appearance, he may still feel that his condition sets him apart from others. Of course, if his cancer destroys external body tissues or requires disfiguring surgery for treatment, your patient's body image will be altered more acutely.

Describe the disorder

Tell the patient that cancer refers to a group of disorders in which certain cells grow and multiply uncontrollably. Describe what type of cancer the patient has. If he has a *tumor*, explain that as cancer cells continue to multiply, the tumor will increase in size. A *localized* tumor remains confined to a specific area. A *metastatic* tumor invades neighboring tissues or spreads to other sites—most commonly, the lungs, liver, bones, and brain.

If your patient has *leukemia*, explain that this cancer originates in the bone marrow, where blood cells are made. As the cancer cells grow, they crowd out and inhibit the growth of platelets, white blood cells, and red blood cells. Eventually, the cancer cells spill into the bloodstream, where they travel throughout the body.

If your patient has *lymphoma*, explain that this cancer arises in the lym-

TEACHING THE PEDIATRIC CANCER PATIENT

Teaching a child with cancer requires expertise and sensitivity. Like an adult with cancer, a child may face pain, separation, altered body image, and death. However, you must adjust your teaching to the child's stage of development when you determine how much to tell him about his disorder. For example, a preschooler with cancer should know that he's sick and needs medicine to feel better. A school-age child should know that cancer is treatable, that he requires a lot of medicine, and that

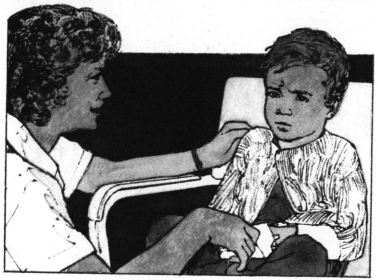

phatic system, a network of glands, vessels, and organs that provides a major defense against infection. The lymphatic vessels carry the cancer cells throughout the body.

Discuss possible causes

Tell the patient that cancer has no clear-cut cause, although a number of factors or agents have been linked to its development. For example:

• *Genetic predisposition.* If appropriate, inform the patient that certain cancers are familial. For example, a woman's risk of developing breast cancer increases if her mother, sister, or another close relative has or had the same disorder. This predisposition may result from common genes, environmental factors, or both.

• *Chemical carcinogens.* Cancer-causing agents may exist in the workplace, such as in nickel refineries; in certain drugs, such as diethylstilbestrol; and in the air, such as from asbestos dust. Exposure to a wide range of carcinogens is the most common external cause of cancer.

• *Radiation.* Ionizing radiation of all kinds—including X-rays and nuclear radiation—may cause cancer. Fair-skinned people are at an increased risk for skin cancer caused by ultraviolet radiation.

• *Tobacco and alcohol.* Cigarette smoking accounts for about 30% of all cancers. Typically, it's linked to cancers of the lungs, mouth, pharynx, larynx, esophagus, pancreas, and bladder. Pipe smoking is associated with lip cancer, and smokeless tobacco is linked to gum cancer. Smokers who also drink

it may take some time before he feels well again.

In general, don't try to shield a child from the seriousness of his disorder. Even young children seem to be aware of the seriousness of their disorder, although they may not be able to discuss it in adult terms. Strive for gentle, honest communication. Hiding the truth from a child might result in the loss of his trust and confidence. Try to create an atmosphere that encourages the child to ask questions and discuss worrisome issues.

Expect a child with cancer to regress at first and react to his disorder the way a much younger child would. However, eventually he should move on to a more appropriate developmental stage. If he doesn't, refer him for counseling.

Special problems of adolescence
A seriously ill adolescent has special adjustment problems because the main developmental task of adolescence—achieving independence—conflicts with the forced dependence associated with illness. Also, although he's old enough to understand his diagnosis and prognosis, he may not have yet developed adult coping mechanisms. He may become rebellious, angry, and uncooperative.

To counteract these problems, try to give

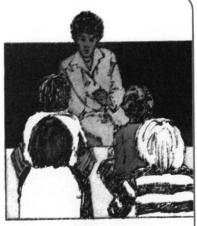

an adolescent patient as much control over his treatment as possible, even if you must deviate slightly from strict hospital protocol. When you can, give him a choice of body sites for blood tests, injections, or I.V.s, and plan treatment so you can accommodate his schedule. Your flexibility will foster his cooperation. Also, be sure to inform him and his parents of treatment options. When possible, schedule group teaching sessions with a peer support group, because an adolescent is extremely peer-oriented. Such a group provides social contact and support.

alcohol heavily run an increased risk of head, neck, and esophageal cancer.
• **Diet.** Excessive dietary consumption of protein and fats has been linked to colorectal cancer. Liver cancer may result from food additives, such as nitrates (commonly used in smoked and processed meat) and alfatoxin (a fungus that grows on stored grains, nuts, and other foods).

Discuss the prognosis

Most cancer patients continue to maintain hope for a cure as long as they're alive. With this in mind, try to help your patient form realistic expectations of treatment without supporting or providing false hope. When you teach your patient about the likelihood of a cure, stress that although cure rate statistics help determine which treatments are generally most effective, his individual response to treatment matters most. Inform him of other options if his initial treatment fails.

For many patients, a diagnosis of cancer means facing their mortality. Be sensitive to your patient's need to talk about death; he may not be able to share his feelings with his family. If you sense that he's having difficulty discussing this subject, try remarking that most patients think about death even when they're doing well. If he doesn't respond, arrange for him to speak to other cancer patients, or refer him for individual or group counseling.

A patient whose cancer progresses to an advanced or terminal stage may become increasingly discouraged and depressed—often sleeping for long periods, refusing food and visitors, and

QUESTIONS PATIENTS ASK ABOUT CANCER

Am I going to die?

Many people equate cancer with dying. However, cancer can often be controlled or cured with surgery, chemotherapy, radiation therapy, other new treatments, or a combination of these. Although cure rate statistics help determine which treatments are generally the most effective, your individual response to treatment is what matters the most.

Will I develop side effects from cancer treatment?

Every patient responds to cancer treatment differently. Some patients report few side effects, while others have a more difficult time. Fortunately, most side effects last only a short while and disappear after treatment ends. The health care team can suggest ways to help you cope with side effects to avoid disrupting your life-style as much as possible.

How can the doctor tell if the treatment is working?

By scheduling you for regular checkups. During these checkups, the doctor may take X-rays to see whether the cancer is shrinking in response to chemotherapy or radiation therapy. Or he may run certain tests to be sure that treatment is causing as little damage as possible to normal cells.

Your own reports of how you feel may be the best sign of the treatment's success. Tell the doctor if you notice any decrease in pain, bleeding, or other discomforts associated with your cancer.

After you complete treatment, the doctor will still want to see you regularly—but less often—to check for cancer recurrence. Be sure to come in for follow-up appointments, as scheduled.

expressing sadness and hopelessness. Support the patient as he comes to grips with the prospect of his death. Encourage him to reflect on his past accomplishments to help him find purpose in his life and view death from a more peaceful perspective. Give the patient and his family privacy to share their feelings and resolve any lingering conflicts. Remember, sometimes a patient is more prepared than his family to face the coming of death. Discuss hospice care with the patient and his family.

A patient whose cancer has been surgically removed or is in remission may also experience emotional turmoil. He may feel a combination of relief and anxiety about resuming his occupation or life-style. He may also feel anxious during periodic checkups. Encourage him to express his feelings and concerns. Also teach him to recognize signs and symptoms that may indicate recurrence, such as a weight change, bleeding, or continuing pain.

Teaching the Patient with Recurrent Cancer

A patient whose cancer has recurred may experience some of the same emotions he felt when his cancer was first diagnosed. But there's a difference: he's faced cancer already, endured treatment-related discomfort, seen his life-style disrupted, and probably come to grips with his mortality. Such a patient may believe "I've coped with this before; I can do it again." But if his memories of past treatment discourage or frighten him, he may wonder "Will the treatment really work this time?" or "How can I go through that again?" His apprehension about treatment can be aggravated by an exhaustive series of tests to outline the cancer's metastasis. He's likely to feel alone and anxious as he awaits the results. You'll need to tailor your teaching to meet his special needs for information and support.

Discuss how—and why—cancer recurs

Explain to the patient that even though treatment aimed to destroy his original cancer, cells in numbers too small for detection may sometimes survive. These cancer cells are detected later, after they've multiplied. If the patient had a tumor, explain how cells can break away and travel through the lymph system or bloodstream to start new cancer growths. The cancer that recurs is the same type as the original cancer—no matter where it appears. For example, if breast cancer recurs in the lung, it's not lung cancer, but breast cancer that has spread to the lung.

Determine the patient's expectations

Patients with recurrent cancer often have expectations about how they'll handle their disorder, based on their past experiences. Ask your patient about his first bout with cancer. How did he cope with the disorder before? What, if anything, would he like to do differently this time?

Frequently, recurrent cancer is treated similarly to the initial cancer—although perhaps more intensively. As a result, the patient will probably be familiar with the treatment-related effects he's likely to experience. However, if the doctor recommends a different type of treatment, make sure your patient knows what to expect. If the patient feels that the treatment's likely risks outweigh its benefits, support his decision to opt against it. In this way, you can provide comfort during a potentially lonesome and fearful time.

Encourage hope

Starting cancer treatment again will probably tax your patient's spirits as well as his body. That's why your teaching must also emphasize the importance of maintaining hope. At times, the patient may feel overcome by fear,

anxiety, depression, or even rage as he learns to cope with this setback. Encourage him to express such feelings. Stress that a positive attitude may help him control some of his emotional and physical reactions to treatment.

DIAGNOSTIC TESTS

Typically, a cancer patient must undergo an array of tests to confirm cancer, to select and monitor treatment, to predict prognosis, and to check for recurrence. At times, he may feel frightened or even powerless as he endures these tests and awaits their results.

Your teaching can provide information and much-needed support to help the patient through the diagnostic workup. By telling him which tests he'll undergo and when, you can help him maintain a sense of control. By clearly explaining the tests, you can prepare him for what to expect. By teaching him how to recognize and manage their side effects, you can help him assume an active role in post-test care. And by answering his questions about test results, you can help him make informed decisions about the future.

Test Selection and Sequence

Although test selection depends on the patient's history and physical examination, the diagnostic workup usually begins with routine blood and X-ray tests. Cytologic and histologic tests may follow to confirm or rule out malignancy. Further special tests, such as nuclear medicine scans and endoscopies, help determine the extent of ma-

REVIEWING COMMON TISSUE BIOPSIES

TYPE OF BIOPSY	PROCEDURE AND TARGET TISSUE
Aspiration 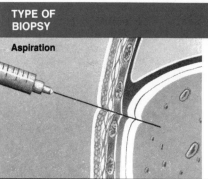	Aspiration of tissue specimen from bone marrow, liver, or breast, using a flexible or fine aspiration needle, needle guide, and aspiration syringe
Excision 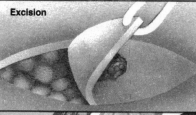	Surgical removal of entire lesion from any tissue, using a scalpel
Needle 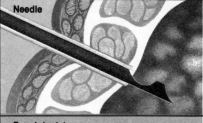	Removal of a core of tissue from bone, bone marrow, breast, lung, pleura, lymph node, liver, kidney, prostate, synovial membrane, or thyroid, using a cutting needle
Punch incision 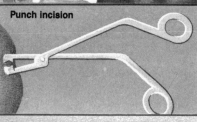	Removal of tissue specimen from core of lesion in skin or cervix, using a punch
Shave 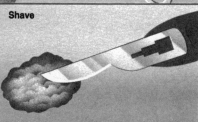	Tissue shaved from raised surface lesion on the skin, using a scalpel

ADVANTAGES AND DISADVANTAGES

• *Advantages:* avoids need for surgery; aspiration of fluid from a breast cyst combines diagnosis and treatment; is less painful than needle biopsy; can be done on an outpatient basis
• *Disadvantages:* disturbs cell architecture; permits study of individual cells but not of intercellular structure; may not furnish a representative specimen; may cause seeding of malignant cells (less likely with fine needle aspiration than with needle biopsy)

• *Advantage:* combines diagnosis and treatment of lesion
• *Disadvantage:* may require major surgery under general anesthesia

• *Advantages:* avoids need for surgery; usually furnishes a representative specimen; preserves cell architecture
• *Disadvantages:* may require excision or other treatment if specimen is malignant; may be traumatic to surrounding tissues; may not furnish a representative specimen; may cause seeding of malignant cells

• *Advantages:* avoids need for surgery; furnishes a representative specimen
• *Disadvantages:* may cause seeding of malignant cells; may require excision or other treatment if lesion is malignant

• *Advantages:* generally safe; combines diagnosis and treatment of benign lesion; yields good cosmetic results
• *Disadvantages:* may require excision or other treatment if lesion is malignant; may cause seeding of malignant cells

lignancy, predict prognosis, select and monitor treatment, and check for recurrence.

The sequence of tests in the diagnostic workup depends on the sensitivity and specificity of available tests. *Sensitivity* indicates how reliably the test gives a positive finding for a disease. *Specificity* indicates how often the test is negative when the disease is absent. A bone scan, for example, reliably gives a positive finding when bone cancer is present (high sensitivity). However, it also gives a positive finding in nonmalignant bone disorders (low specificity).

When teaching the patient about the following tests, explain that many tests are repeated at intervals to check his response to treatment. Emphasize that repeating a test doesn't necessarily indicate a setback in treatment.

Blood tests

Blood chemistry studies and a complete blood count are routinely ordered when cancer is suspected. Certain specialized blood tests, such as radioimmunoassays for tumor markers, provide important information about the extent of malignancy and the effectiveness of treatment.

When blood tests are ordered, tell the patient who will perform the venipuncture and when, and inform him of any pre-test restrictions. For example, he may have to fast for 6 hours before blood is drawn for blood chemistry studies.

Radiographic and imaging tests

Explain that radiographic and imaging tests allow visualization of internal structures and, at times, guide biopsy procedures. Although these tests can help detect and localize cancer, they can't confirm it. However, they can identify an underlying disorder that may require different treatment. For example, a myelogram can determine a brain or spinal cord infection as well as the presence of cancer cells.

Although most radiographic and imaging tests are painless, the equipment they require can be especially frightening to the patient. Be sure to describe what the patient will hear, feel, or see during the test. For example, describe the rapid-fire clacking sound of an X-ray machine, the characteristic burning sensation that follows infusion of contrast material, and the formidable appearance of a computed tomography (CT) scanner. Also inform the patient who will perform the test and when, and advise him of any pre-test restrictions.

Cytologic tests
Explain that these screening tests help detect suspected primary or metastatic disease and assess the effectiveness of treatment. However, they can't show the location and size of a malignancy and may require histologic tests for confirmation. Before the patient undergoes a cytologic test, make sure he understands the test's purpose and procedure. Also make sure he understands any pre-test restrictions.

Histologic tests
Typically, a histologic test is essential for definitive diagnosis before treatment begins. Describe the biopsy procedure to the patient, and explain that this test permits microscopic examination of a tissue specimen. (See *Reviewing Common Tissue Biopsies,* pages 548 and 549.) If the patient is scheduled for local anesthesia, tell him that he needn't restrict food, fluids, or medication. Inform him that he may feel weak or tired after the procedure but that he can resume his usual activities within a day or two. If he's scheduled for general anesthesia, advise him to fast from midnight the night before the test. Tell him who will perform the test and where; that it will take 15 to 30 minutes; and that pre-test blood studies, urinalysis, and X-rays may be required.

If you're preparing a patient for *open biopsy* (performed in the operating room), explain that the doctor will obtain a tissue specimen and send it immediately to the laboratory for rapid analysis. If the test results indicate malignancy, he may then perform curative surgery. This eliminates the need for two separate surgical procedures.

If you're preparing a patient for *bone marrow biopsy*, explain that this procedure can diagnose leukemia, determine whether cancer has spread to the bone marrow, and check his response to treatment. Describe the procedure to him: in aspiration biopsy, a fluid specimen in which bone spicules are suspended is removed from the bone marrow. In needle biopsy, a core of marrow cells is removed. Tell the patient that the procedure usually takes only 5 to 10 minutes and that test results are generally available in a few days. Inform him that more than one bone marrow specimen may be required and that a blood sample will also be collected for laboratory testing. Tell the patient which bone—sternum, anterior or posterior iliac crest, vertebral spinous process, rib, or tibia—has been selected as the biopsy site. Inform him that he'll receive a local anesthetic but will feel pressure when the biopsy needle's inserted and a brief, pulling pain as the marrow is removed. If appropriate, tell the patient that he'll receive a sedative before the procedure.

Lumbar puncture
If you're preparing a patient for lumbar puncture, explain that this test can detect cancer cells or infection in cerebrospinal fluid. Describe the procedure, and inform him that he'll receive a local anesthetic. After the test, advise the patient to lie flat and to increase his intake of fluids, to prevent post-test headache.

Endoscopic tests
Because endoscopic tests are often uncomfortable and embarrassing, the patient may feel especially anxious before and during the procedure. You can help reduce his stress by describing the pro-

TEACHING A CHILD
ABOUT BONE MARROW BIOPSY

To prepare a child for bone marrow biopsy, give her a biopsy kit: a syringe without a needle, cotton balls, and adhesive bandages. Then demonstrate the procedure by using a doll or stuffed animal. In this way, you can gain the child's confidence and answer any questions she may have. Be sure to describe any discomfort that she may feel during the procedure.

After the doctor positions the child on the table, have the parents stand at the child's head, while you stand at her side. When the doctor is ready to begin, hold the child's arms firmly, and continue talking to her quietly and reassuringly. Tell her that it's important to remain as still as possible during the procedure, so the needle doesn't go in the wrong place. Also tell the child that she will feel some pain when the doctor aspirates the bone marrow, that it's OK to cry or yell if she wants to, and that the pain will go away quickly.

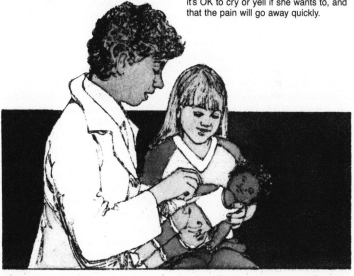

cedure fully and clearly. Inform the patient which endoscopic test he'll undergo—for example, bronchoscopy, mediastinoscopy, or colonoscopy. Next, explain the purpose of the test—for example, to obtain a biopsy specimen, to visualize internal structures, or to perform minor surgery. Tell him where the test will be done, how long it will last, and what he can expect to experience. Since patient preparation for endoscopic tests varies greatly, tailor your teaching to follow the doctor's orders. As ordered, instruct the patient to follow necessary dietary restrictions. If special bowel preparation is ordered, tell him how to proceed.

TREATMENTS

Whether the patient's scheduled for surgery, chemotherapy, or radiation therapy, he's likely to be apprehensive. After all, he may associate treatment with uncomfortable and, at times, disfiguring side effects. Although you can't expect to eliminate the patient's fear, you can help him adjust to treatment's effects with appropriate teaching. For example, you could explain to the patient who'll be receiving chemotherapy that not all people experience uncontrollable nausea and vomiting from it. In fact, some don't experience any. Also explain that drugs, relaxation exercises, and diet can minimize or prevent nausea and vomiting. Before radiation therapy, reassure the patient that he'll be protected from potentially harmful effects. When possible, put your patient in touch with patients who've had (or are undergoing) similar treatment.

Tell the patient that the goal of cancer treatment is to destroy malignant cells while minimizing damage to normal ones. To achieve this, a single treatment or a combination of treatments may be used. Explain that surgery and radiation therapy combat malignant cells locally or regionally, while chemotherapy combats them systemically. Make sure the patient understands that treatment selection depends on a variety of factors, including his type of cancer, its size and location, and his general health. In teaching about cancer treatments, you must be able to:
• explain the recommended treatment, including its purpose, procedure, and potential side effects
• prepare the patient and his family to recognize and manage side effects
• allow adequate time to answer their questions and provide support.

Surgery

Not surprisingly, many cancer patients fear surgery more than any other treatment. The three surgical procedures discussed here—mastectomy, laryngectomy, and colectomy (with creation of an ostomy)—can have a dramatic impact on a patient's self-image and functioning. (For information about amputation, a fourth surgical procedure for cancer, see "Surgery" in Chapter 10.) Before undergoing mastectomy, laryngectomy, or colectomy, the patient may wonder "How will I look after surgery?" and "How will surgery affect my life-style?" Your thorough, sensitive teaching can help the patient overcome his fear of disfigurement and prepare him to cope effectively with any life-style changes.

A review of types and techniques
Explain and compare the three major types of cancer surgery: curative, preventive, and palliative. *Curative surgery* is performed to remove the entire tumor, along with a margin of surrounding tissue and some nearby lymph nodes. *Preventive surgery* is performed to remove noncancerous growths that would probably become cancerous if left in place. *Palliative surgery* is performed to relieve symptoms, such as pain; it doesn't cure cancer. As appropriate, describe the specific surgical technique to the patient.
• *Local excision.* Explain that local excision involves removing only the malignancy. Usually, this is adequate for most skin cancers, which rarely spread to the lymph nodes.
• *Electrosurgery.* Explain that this technique uses a high-frequency electrical current—transmitted through a blade, needle, or disk electrode—to cut or coagulate tissue. It's performed for certain skin, mouth, and rectal cancers.
• *Cryosurgery.* Tell the patient that cryosurgery involves freezing and destroying a tumor with liquid nitrogen applied with a special probe. It's used most often to treat cancers of the brain, mouth, and prostate.

Mastectomy
A woman with breast cancer may fear its primary treatment, mastectomy, almost as much as the disorder itself—perhaps because mastectomy threatens her self-image more than any other surgery. To relieve your patient's fears, you'll have to do considerable teaching before and after surgery.

Before surgery, reinforce the doctor's

explanation of the procedure and clear up any misconceptions. If biopsy and curative surgery are to be performed during the same procedure, prepare the patient for the possible outcome. Make sure she understands which type of mastectomy will be performed. In a *lumpectomy*, the breast lump and a margin of normal tissue around it are removed. Usually, the surgeon also removes some of the axillary lymph nodes to screen for malignancy. In a *simple mastectomy*, the breast alone is removed. Some of the axillary lymph nodes may also be removed if cancer has spread beyond the breast. In a *modified radical mastectomy*, the breast, the axillary lymph nodes, and the lining over the chest muscles (but not the muscles themselves) are removed. In a *radical mastectomy*, the breast, the chest muscles under the breast, and all the axillary lymph nodes are removed, leaving a hollow chest area.

Explain that the surgery will be performed under general anesthesia. Tell the patient that shortly before surgery, the surgical area will be shaved, and she may be given a sedative. Show her where the incision will be made, and describe the dressing and the surgical drain she'll have in place for several days postoperatively. Warn the patient that she may feel some discomfort in her breast area after surgery. Some women experience paresthesias or pain in the chest or the shoulder, upper arm, or axillary areas. Others feel phantom breast pain—a temporary tingling or pins-and-needles sensation in the area of the removed breast tissue. Reassure the patient that she'll receive adequate pain medication.

Emphasize that proper home care can speed recovery and prevent complications. Stress the importance of performing prescribed exercises (see *Strengthening Exercises after Mastectomy*, pages 554 and 555). Also teach the patient how to minimize lymphedema by elevating the affected arm frequently, by avoiding restrictive clothing, and by massaging the affected arm to increase circulation. Since lymphedema makes the affected arm more susceptible to infection, emphasize measures to avoid infection or injury (see *Preventing Complications after Radical Mastectomy*, page 556).

After surgery, discuss the procedure with the patient and encourage her to share her feelings. If appropriate, put her in touch with another breast cancer patient from the American Cancer Society or Reach for Recovery. In this way, you can help her come to grips with the procedure and emotionally prepare her to see the incision when the dressing's changed.

Help the patient improve her body image by explaining how she can dress to conceal her mastectomy. After the breast area heals (2 to 6 months after surgery), she may want to use a breast prosthesis or explore the possibility of breast reconstruction. If your patient voices concerns about resuming sexual activity after mastectomy, help her develop strategies for coping. Encourage her to talk about the changes in her body with her partner. Tell her that she may resume sexual activity as soon as she feels she's ready.

Remember to consider the emotional needs of the patient's partner. He may be dealing with a variety of emotional responses, such as guilt, fear, and a sense of loss. If possible, include him in your teaching sessions to help him understand what the patient's experiencing. If necessary, refer the patient and her partner to a psychiatrist, clinical specialist, social worker, or social agency.

Laryngectomy

Typically, a patient facing laryngectomy must prepare to cope with two dramatic changes: since part or all of the larynx will be removed, he'll be temporarily unable to speak postoperatively. And since the upper part of the trachea will be removed, he'll be breathing through a permanent tracheostomy. As a result, a laryngectomy

STRENGTHENING EXERCISES AFTER MASTECTOMY

Dear Patient:

After your mastectomy, you'll need to exercise the affected arm and shoulder to prevent muscle shortening, to maintain muscle tone, and to improve blood and lymph circulation. Just follow these instructions:

Pendulum swing

To get ready for this exercise, place your unaffected arm on the back of a chair. Let your affected arm hang loosely.

1

Swing your arm from left to right. Be sure the movement comes from your shoulder joint and not your elbow.

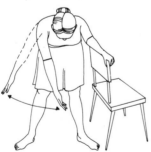

2

Swing your arm in small circles. Again, be sure the movement is coming from your shoulder

joint. As your arm relaxes, the size of the circle will probably increase. Then, circle in the opposite direction.

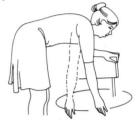

3

Swing your arm forward and backward from your shoulder, within your range of comfort.

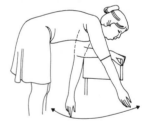

Wall climbing

Stand facing a wall, with your toes as close to the wall as possible and your feet apart.

1

Bending your elbows slightly, place your palms against the wall at shoulder level.

2

Then, flexing your fingers, work
your hands up the wall until
your arms are fully extended.
Work your hands back down to
the starting point.

Pulley

To begin this exercise, toss a
rope over a shower curtain rod
or a chin-up bar.

1

Hold an end of the rope in each
hand.

2

Using a seesaw motion and
with your arms outstretched,
slide the rope up and down
over the rod.

Rope turning

Attach a rope to the doorknob.
Then stand facing the door.

1

Take the free end of the rope in
the hand of the affected arm.
Place your other hand on your
hip.

2

With your arm extended and
held away from your body, turn
the rope, making as wide a
swing as possible. Start slowly,
and increase your speed as
your arm gets stronger.

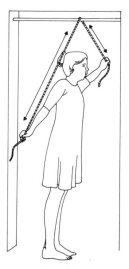

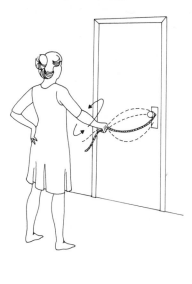

PREVENTING COMPLICATIONS AFTER RADICAL MASTECTOMY

Dear Patient:

Removal of lymph nodes and lymph vessels in a radical mastectomy may cause your arm to swell and increase your risk of infection. To prevent complications after your mastectomy, keep in mind this list of do's and don'ts when using or caring for the affected arm:

Do:
• Contact the doctor if your affected arm becomes red, warm, or unusually hard or swollen.
• Protect the hand and arm on your affected side.
• Order and wear a Medic Alert tag that's engraved: *Caution—lymphedema arm. No tests, no injections.*
• Use a thimble when sewing.
• Wear a loose rubber glove while washing dishes.
• Stay out of strong sunlight.
• Apply lanolin hand cream several times a day.
• Use an electric shaver to remove underarm hair.
• Apply insect repellent to avoid bites or stings.

Don't:
• Hold a cigarette.
• Cut cuticles or hangnails.
• Use strong detergents or abrasive compounds.
• Reach into a hot oven.
• Dig in the garden or work near thorny bushes.
• Allow anyone to draw blood, give an injection, or apply a blood pressure cuff on your affected arm.
• Wear tight-fitting jewelry or a wristwatch.
• Carry heavy bags or a heavy purse.
• Wear clothing with elastic at the wrists, elbows, or upper arms.

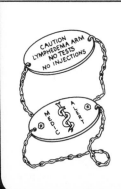

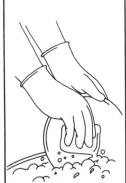

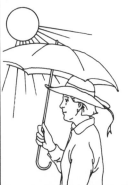

patient may be especially concerned about how he'll sound and look after surgery. His concerns may be compounded if he also requires a radical neck dissection—a procedure that may disfigure his face and neck. You'll need to teach the patient and his family about the changes in life-style and function that laryngectomy may produce.

Make sure the patient and his family understand the extent of the planned surgery. Reinforce the doctor's explanation and clear up any misconceptions. In a *partial laryngectomy*, the surgeon usually removes only the diseased vocal cord or portion of the larynx. When the suture line heals, the band of scar tissue is a vibrating surface capable of producing husky but acceptable speech. In a *total laryngectomy*, the surgeon removes the larynx, vocal cords, and thyroid cartilage. If the cancer has spread to surrounding tissues and glands, the surgeon will perform a *radical neck dissection* to remove the tumor and the involved lymph nodes. Tell the patient that the surgery will be performed under general anesthesia.

Next, carefully explain postoperative measures, including suctioning, nasogastric feeding, and tracheostomy tube care. Encourage the patient to express his concerns before surgery temporarily cuts off oral communication. Help him choose an alternate method of communication that he finds comfortable, such as pencil and paper, sign language, or a communication board. He may want to discuss his concerns about surgery with a patient with a laryngectomy.

Warn the patient that he may experience considerable postoperative pain. Encourage him to request pain medication early—before pain becomes unbearable.

After a partial laryngectomy, explain that the patient must not use his voice until his doctor permits (usually 2 to 3 days postoperatively). Then, caution him to whisper until healing is complete.

After a total laryngectomy, reinforce the speech therapist's teaching. Reassure the patient that speech rehabilitation (laryngeal speech, esophageal speech, artificial larynx, or various mechanical aids) can help him speak again.

After a radical neck dissection, stress the importance of performing postoperative exercises (see *Strengthening Exercises after Radical Neck Dissection*, page 562). If the patient will be using a prosthesis to conceal the effects of surgery, teach him how to apply and remove it, and to check the surgical area for signs of infection, such as redness or tenderness. Tell him to notify the doctor if he develops wheezing, stridor, fever, or a milky drainage from the stoma (especially after meals).

Teach the patient and his family how to care for the tracheostomy tube and stoma at home (see *Caring for Your Trach Tube and Stoma*, pages 558 to 561). Warn the patient to notify the doctor if he experiences constant shortness of breath—a possible sign of tracheostomy stenosis.

If the patient must continue nasogastric tube feeding at home, teach him and his family the procedure (see *How to Give an Intermittent Feeding* in Chapter 9). Also stress the importance of maintaining good oral hygiene.

As you discuss needed life-style changes like those above, be sure to emphasize that having a tracheostomy allows the patient to lead a full, healthy life. Advise him to contact the International Association of Laryngectomees (IAL), a division of the American Cancer Society. This volunteer organization has local chapters in most states and in many foreign countries. Among other services, IAL clubs provide the following:
• psychological counseling for new laryngectomees and their families
• fellowship with other laryngectomees who've overcome their handicap
• help in locating speech therapists
• help in locating needed equipment, such as stoma shields and bibs.

558

558 CARE

CARING FOR YOUR TRACH TUBE AND STOMA

Dear Patient:

As part of your laryngectomy, the doctor created a permanent tracheostomy—a small opening, or stoma, in your throat. Inserting a tube into the tracheostomy makes it easier for you to breathe, because it keeps your windpipe open. A tracheostomy (trach) tube has three parts: an inner cannula, an outer cannula, and an obturator.

How to clean the inner cannula

To prevent infection, remove and clean the inner cannula regularly, as your doctor orders.

1

First, gather this equipment: two small basins, a small brush, mild liquid dish detergent, water or saline solution, a gauze pad, scissors, and clean trach ties (twill tape). Or, open a prepackaged kit that contains the equipment you need. Now, wash your hands. Then, position a mirror so you can see your face and throat clearly.

2

Now, unlock the inner cannula and remove it by pulling steadily outward and downward. Pre-

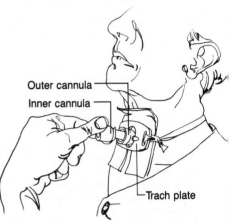

Outer cannula

Inner cannula

Trach plate

pare to clean the soiled cannula immediately for reinsertion. (Or put this soiled cannula aside and slip a clean, spare inner cannula inside the outer cannula.)

If you start to cough while removing the cannula, cover your stoma with a tissue and relax until the coughing stops.

3

Next, clean the soiled cannula. Here's a good method: soak the cannula in mild liquid dish detergent for 10 minutes, then clean it with a small brush.

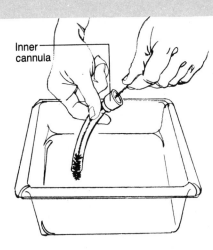

Inner cannula

You can obtain a special trach tube brush at a medical supply company or pharmacy. However, the small brushes used to clean percolators are just as effective and can be obtained easily and cheaply at hardware stores.

4

Now, shake off the cleaning solution, and put the cannula in a separate basin of water or saline solution. Gently swirl the cannula back and forth for about 10 seconds to rinse it. Then, remove the cannula from the basin, and shake off the excess water or saline solution. Reinsert the clean cannula immediately—don't dry it; the moisture that remains will help lubricate the cannula and make reinsertion easier.

5

After you lock the clean inner cannula in place, replace the soiled trach ties that secure the trach plate. Use scissors to carefully clip and remove one trach tie at a time. Knot the end of each clean trach tie to prevent fraying, then cut a ½″ slit in each tie. Thread the end that isn't knotted through the opening on the trach plate. Then, feed the end through the slit, as shown below, and gently pull the tie taut. Do the same for the other tie.

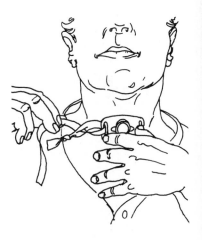

(continued)

CARING FOR YOUR TRACH TUBE AND STOMA
(continued)

6

Secure the ties at the side of your neck with a square knot. Leave enough room so you can breathe comfortably.

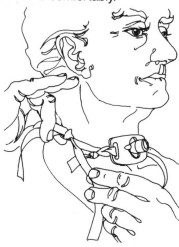

7

Finally, cut a slit in a nonshredding gauze pad, then a hole in the center just big enough to go around the trach tube. Carefully insert the gauze pad un-

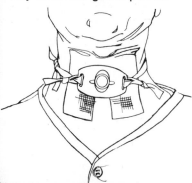

der the trach plate to help absorb any moisture.

How to reinsert your trach tube

Suppose you accidentally cough out your trach tube. *Don't panic.* Follow these simple steps to reinsert it.

1

First, remove the inner cannula from the dislodged trach tube. If you're using a cuffed tube, be sure you deflate the cuff first.

2

Next, take the obturator and insert it into the outer cannula. Make sure the cuff is deflated. Then reinsert the trach tube, with the obturator, into your stoma.

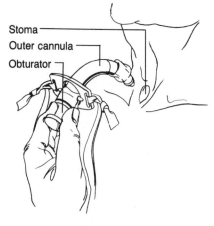

Stoma
Outer cannula
Obturator

3

Hold the trach plate in place while you remove the obturator.

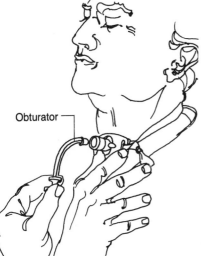

Obturator

Then, insert the inner cannula into the trach tube. Next, turn the inner cannula clockwise until it locks in place. Chances are you'll cough or gag while you're doing this, so be sure to hold onto the trach plate securely.

4

Now, insert the tip of a syringe into the tube's pillow port. Inflate the cuff, as your doctor orders. The inflated cuff will help prevent the tube from accidentally being dislodged again.

5

After inflating the cuff, secure the trach ties and tuck a gauze pad under the trach plate.

How to protect your stoma

Keep in mind this list of do's and don'ts to protect your stoma.

Do:
- Wash the skin around your stoma with a moist cloth several times a day.
- Apply petroleum jelly around the stoma to keep the skin moist.
- Wear a foam filter over your stoma in winter to warm the air you breathe. Wear a crocheted bib to shield your stoma and to cover the filter.
- Wear a stoma shield to protect your stoma when showering. Or simply direct the stream of water to hit below the level of the stoma.
- Bend at the waist to cough, and remember to cover your stoma with a tissue.

Don't:
- Clean your stoma with cotton swabs.
- Swim. Avoid getting water in your stoma.
- Use mineral oil to lubricate the outer cannula or to moisturize the skin around your stoma.

STRENGTHENING EXERCISES AFTER RADICAL NECK DISSECTION

Dear Patient:

After radical neck dissection, you'll need to exercise your affected side to restore muscle function in your arm, shoulder, and neck. Do these exercises twice a day in a relaxed posture. If you feel too much strain on your affected side, place that arm on a table or the back of a chair for support while doing the exercises.

1

Turn your head as far to the right as possible, and then as far to the left as possible.

2

Tilt your head to the left and then to the right; to the front and then to the back.

3

Place the hand of your unaffected arm on a bar stool or on the back of a chair. Let your affected (free) arm hang loosely. Then swing your arm forward and backward from your shoulder.

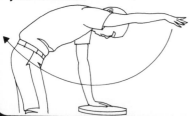

Now swing your arm in a circle. Be sure the movement is coming from your shoulder joint and not from your elbow.

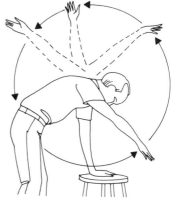

4

While sitting in a chair, rotate your shoulders forward and then backward.

5

While still sitting in a chair, grasp each elbow with the opposite hand. Then lift your shoulder toward your ear. Repeat with the opposite shoulder.

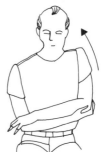

Colectomy

A patient facing colectomy (with creation of an ostomy) must prepare for dramatic changes in his body function and life-style. Such a patient needs your emotional support as well as practical instruction on how to care for himself after surgery. Your teaching will vary, though, according to the extent of surgery. If the entire colon is removed, you'll need to teach your patient how to care for an ileostomy (see the "Surgery" section in Chapter 8). If only a portion of the colon is removed, you'll need to teach your patient how to care for a colostomy.

Begin by explaining that a colostomy is a surgically created opening between the colon and the surface of the abdomen, through which he'll excrete body wastes. Show the patient drawings of the colon before and after surgery, and stress how much of the colon remains intact. Mention that the farther down the colon his colostomy is located, the more closely his stools will resemble those he had before surgery. Inform him that the stoma will be red, moist, and swollen postoperatively but that swelling will subside. Explain that the stoma has no muscles, so he won't be able to open and close it at will. However, he can learn to control his bowel movements by irrigating the colostomy. In the meantime, he'll need to wear a colostomy bag to collect any wastes that drain from the stoma.

After surgery, encourage the patient to look at his stoma and to participate in colostomy care and irrigation as soon as possible. Teach him how to remove, empty, and reapply his colostomy bag. Stress the importance of proper skin care, and show him how to keep the skin around the stoma clean, dry, and free from irritation. Demonstrate how to irrigate his colostomy correctly, and supplement this with return demonstration and written instruction (see *How to Irrigate Your Colostomy*, pages 564 to 567). Instruct the patient to notify the doctor if he has repeated trouble inserting the irrigation tube or if he develops persistent diarrhea or constipation, bloody or abnormal drainage, unusually colored or foul-smelling stools, or skin irritation around the stoma.

Encourage the patient to discuss how he feels about his colostomy. He may want to talk with a representative from a local ostomy association or the American Cancer Society.

Besides teaching the patient about colostomy care, you'll need to help him learn how to adapt his life-style. Be prepared to answer questions on a wide range of issues.

● *Activity.* Generally, the patient won't need to restrict his activities. However, advise him to avoid putting extra strain on his abdominal muscles and to check with his doctor before engaging in sports.

● *Clothing.* Tell the patient he can wear his regular clothes, as long as they don't lie directly over his stoma. Reassure him that colostomy bags aren't noticeable, because they're made to lie flat against the body.

● *Diet.* Teach the patient to avoid foods that may cause foul-smelling gas—for example, onions, eggs, cabbage, beer, and certain cheeses. If the patient must follow a special diet, reinforce the dietitian's teaching and answer any questions.

● *Odor control.* Reassure the patient that if he cares for his colostomy properly, he probably won't have an odor problem. For extra security, he may want to use a colostomy bag deodorant. Stress that he should notify the doctor if his stool smells extremely foul; this may signal infection, although it may also be related to diet. Inform him that eating oranges, parsley, or yogurt, or drinking buttermilk, orange juice, or cranberry juice may help control odor. Tell the patient that he may take bismuth subcarbonate, bismuth subgallate, chlorophyll, or activated charcoal to reduce odor, unless the doctor orders otherwise.

● *Sexuality.* Unless surgery has been extensive, inform the patient that a co-

HOW TO IRRIGATE YOUR COLOSTOMY

Dear Patient:

Your doctor may give you specific instructions for irrigating your colostomy. If he doesn't, you can use this step-by-step procedure as a guide.

1
First, sit on the toilet or on a chair next to the toilet. Remove the colostomy pouch.

2
Now, fasten one end of the belt to the gasket on the drainage bag. Hold the gasket with one hand while you wrap the belt around your waist with your other hand. Then, attach the other end of the belt to the gasket.

3
Carefully center the gasket around the stoma, and adjust the belt to fit.
    Dangle the bottom end of the drainage bag into the toilet.

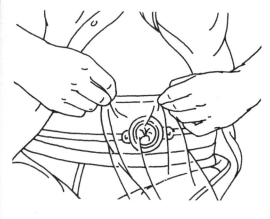

4
If you're using a stoma cone, gently twist together the end of the cone's tube and the end of the tube leading to the irrigator bag, until you hear a snap.

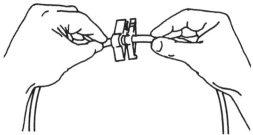

5

Fill the irrigator bag with about 1 quart of lukewarm water or irrigating solution, as your doctor orders. Hang the filled bag on a towel rack or a hook placed next to the toilet. During irrigation, the bag should be at your shoulder level.

6

Hold the end of the irrigator tube over the toilet. Open the control clamp and allow a small amount of water or irrigating solution to flow through the tubing. This will force any trapped air out of the tubing. Then close the control clamp.

(continued)

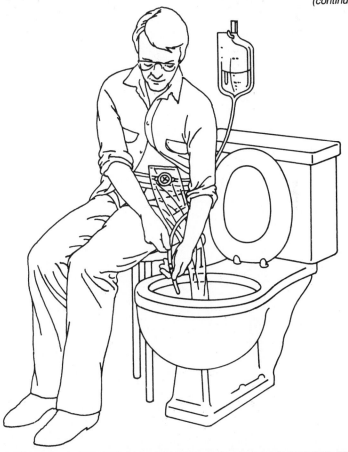

HOW TO IRRIGATE YOUR COLOSTOMY
(continued)

7

Next, squeeze a small amount of water-soluble lubricant onto a gauze pad and roll the first 3″ of the tube in it.

Now, slowly slide the tube through the open top of the drainage bag and into your stoma, as shown below. If you meet resistance, don't force the tube. Try to relax, and pull the tube out slightly. Unclamp the flow control and allow a small amount of water or irrigating solution to flow into the colon. Wait about 5 minutes and then try again to insert the tube. If you have repeated trouble inserting the tube, notify your doctor.

If the doctor wants you to irrigate your colostomy with a stoma cone instead of a tube, first lubricate the tip of the cone. Then insert the lubricated tip through the open end of the drainage bag and into your stoma, as shown at the top of the next page. To prevent back flow, always hold the cone in place against the stoma during irrigation.

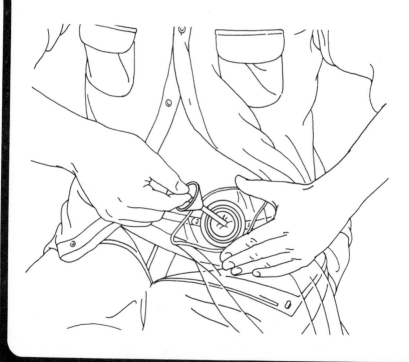

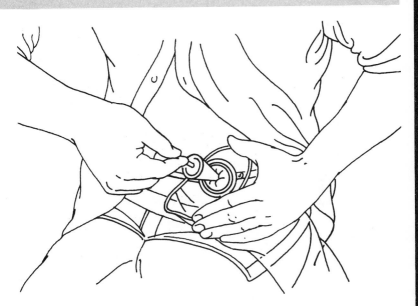

8

Open the flow clamp of the irrigator bag, and let the water or irrigating solution run slowly into your colon. This should take about 10 to 15 minutes. If you get stomach cramps, reduce the flow or stop the procedure until the cramps go away. After all the fluid has entered your colon, slowly remove the tube or cone from your stoma.

9

After the initial surge of water or irrigating solution returns, you can fold the drainage sleeve back, clamp it shut, and do whatever you want to until all the fluid and stool have returned. It will take about 30 minutes for the colon to empty completely.

10

After the colon empties, return to the toilet. Unhook the belt and remove the drainage bag. Then clean the area around your stoma with warm water, dry the area thoroughly, and apply a clean colostomy bag. Finally, wash, rinse, and store the irrigation equipment for reuse.

lostomy won't interfere with sexual function. However, a woman who's had surgery in the perineal area may experience some discomfort until the wound heals. A man who has a colostomy because of bladder or rectal cancer may have temporary or permanent impotence. Refer a patient who has problems adjusting sexually to a professional counselor, the local ostomy association, or the local chapter of the American Cancer Society.

• *Travel.* Reassure the patient that he'll be able to travel whenever and wherever he pleases. Suggest that he take along extra supplies, and remind him to use only drinking water when irrigating his colostomy. Tell him to check with his doctor before his departure and to obtain medication for diarrhea or constipation, if prescribed.

Chemotherapy

This treatment involves the administration of drugs that interfere with the replication of cancer cells. These drugs are given by mouth or by injection into the veins, muscles, or spinal fluid. Typically, they're given in specific cycles and sequences, so that the body can recover during the drug-free period. Tell the patient the type and sequence of drugs that he'll receive and whether they'll be administered in the hospital or at home. If he'll be receiving chemotherapy through an implanted infusion port (such as Infus-A-Port or Port-A-Cath), explain that no dressing or special care will be needed after the incision heals. Inform the patient of any harmful drug interactions (see *Special Alert: Chemotherapeutic Drug Interactions*).

Explain that side effects may occur during chemotherapy because the drugs can affect *any* rapidly growing cells in the body—normal cells as well as cancer cells. The normal cells most likely to be affected are in the bone marrow, digestive tract, reproductive organs, and hair follicles. Teach the patient how to manage common side effects of chemotherapy (see *How to Control Side Effects of Chemotherapy and Radiation Therapy*, pages 570 and 571).

Make sure the patient realizes that every person reacts differently to chemotherapy. Some people have few or no side effects; others have a more difficult time. Reassure him that if a drug causes severe side effects, the doctor can adjust the dosage. Explain that most side effects resolve before or shortly after treatment ends. However, the fatigue that some patients experience during chemotherapy may linger.

Radiation Therapy

Bombarding cancer cells with high-level radiation destroys their ability to grow and multiply. Although radiation also affects normal cells, these cells can usually recover quickly. Explain to the patient that radiation therapy may be used before surgery to shrink a tumor or after surgery (perhaps combined with chemotherapy) to stop the growth of any remaining cancer cells and to prevent recurrence.

Make sure the patient understands when and where he'll receive radiation therapy and who will administer it. Reinforce the doctor's explanation of the procedure, and answer any questions. Explain the type of radiation therapy—external or internal—that the patient will receive.

External radiation therapy

In this therapy, a machine directs high-level radiation at the cancer cells as well as at some of the normal surrounding tissue. Describe the machine that will be used—for example, the cobalt 60 or a linear accelerator.

Explain that a simulation test will be performed before radiation therapy to determine the exact location and size of the cancer. Tell the patient that he'll be asked to lie still on a table while an X-ray machine locates the area to be treated. Then his skin will be marked with water-soluble ink to define the treatment area. Emphasize to the patient that he mustn't scrub off the ink because it's important to treat the same area each time.

Tell the patient that each treatment session lasts about ½ hour; however, he'll receive radiation for only 1 to 5 minutes of that time. Reassure him that special lead shields will be placed between the machine and certain body areas to protect normal tissue and organs. Instruct him to remain still so that the radiation is delivered only to the target area. Reassure the patient that radiation therapy is painless and won't make him radioactive. Stress that he'll be under close observation during therapy and need only call out if he wants anything.

Teach the patient how to care for the skin in the treatment area. Instruct him not to apply soap, deodorant, lotion, perfume, topical medication, or extreme heat or cold to the area, and to avoid rubbing the skin. If he must shave the area, tell him to use an electric shaver instead of a razor. Advise him to protect the area from the sun with soft, lightweight clothing and a sunscreen, if his doctor permits. Suggest that he limit activities that might irritate the area, and warn him that the area may be sore or sensitive for some time after therapy.

If the patient has hair in the treatment area, inform him that he may lose some or all of it during radiation therapy. Reassure him that his hair will probably grow back after therapy is completed. In the meantime, he may want to wear a toupee or wig or to cover his head with a hat or scarf.

Internal radiation therapy

In this therapy, a small amount of radioactive material is implanted in a body cavity or directly into the tumor

---

SPECIAL ALERT: CHEMOTHERAPEUTIC DRUG INTERACTIONS

As a rule, foods, beverages, and over-the-counter drugs don't influence the safety or effectiveness of chemotherapeutic drugs. But you should teach your patient about a few important exceptions. Warn him about potentially serious interactions if he's taking any of these chemotherapeutic drugs.

Plicamycin (Mithracin). Tell the patient to inform the doctor if he's taking acetaminophen, antacids, or aspirin or salicylate products.

Procarbazine (Matulane). Advise against taking this drug with alcohol, caffeine-containing beverages, and tyramine-containing foods (such as cheese and beer). Tell the patient to inform the doctor if he's taking over-the-counter cough suppressants that contain dextromethorphan.

Methotrexate. Instruct the patient not to take this drug with alcohol or aspirin. Also advise him to avoid vitamin and mineral supplements that contain folic acid (vitamin B_9).

Mitotane (Lysodren). Tell the patient to check with his doctor before taking this drug with any over-the-counter central nervous system depressants, such as antihistamines or sleeping pills. Also advise against taking mitotane with alcohol.

---

itself. This permits access to the tumor while sparing most of the normal tissue surrounding it. Explain the type of implant that the doctor will use and where it will be placed. Inform the patient how long he'll be hospitalized and whether he'll be required to stay in a private room. Explain that hospital staff and visitors will need to limit the amount of time they spend in the patient's room to avoid excessive exposure to radiation. If the implant is temporary, tell the patient when it will be removed. If the implant is permanent, explain that it will lose a small amount of radioactivity each day, and that only

HOW TO CONTROL SIDE EFFECTS OF CHEMOTHERAPY AND RADIATION THERAPY

Dear Patient:

Follow these tips to help control some common side effects of chemotherapy and radiation therapy.

Mouth ulcers
• Until your mouth ulcers heal, avoid foods that are difficult to chew, such as apples; highly acidic beverages that irritate the mouth, such as citrus juices; extremely hot, cold, or spicy foods; alcohol; and tobacco.
• Eat soft, bland foods, such as soft-boiled or poached eggs or oatmeal. Also eat soothing foods, such as ice pops.
• Maintain good oral hygiene. Use a soft toothbrush. Rinse with a mouthwash of equal parts of Kaopectate and Benadryl Elixir. If you wear dentures, remove them when possible.

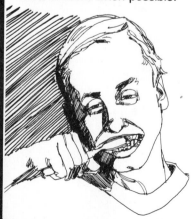

Nausea and vomiting
• Take antiemetic drugs regularly, as your doctor orders.
• Eliminate any unpleasant odors from your dining area. Also, brush your teeth before eating to refresh your mouth.
• Drink small amounts of cool, clear, unsweetened fluids, such as apple juice. Gradually progress to eating crackers or dry toast. Avoid eating sweets or fatty fried foods.
• Eat small, frequent meals, and avoid lying down for 2 hours after eating.
• Notify your doctor if vomiting is severe or lasts longer than 24 hours, or if you have decreased urine output, weakness, or a dry mouth.

Diarrhea
• Ask your doctor about anti-diarrhea medications.
• Eat low-fiber foods, such as bananas and cheese. Avoid high-fiber foods, such as raw vegetables and whole grain bread.
• After bowel movements, clean your perianal area and apply petroleum jelly.
• Notify your doctor if you have persistent diarrhea, decreased urine output, weakness, or a dry mouth.

Constipation
• Take a stool softener, such as Colace, or a laxative, as your doctor orders. Check with your doctor before using enemas.
• Drink plenty of fluids, unless your doctor orders otherwise.
• Eat high-fiber foods, such as raw vegetables and bran. Avoid gas-producing foods, such as cabbage, beans, and sweets.
• Set aside a specific time each day to have a bowel movement.

Heartburn
• Take oral medications with a glass of milk or a snack.
• Avoid spicy foods, alcohol, and smoking. Eat small, frequent meals.
• Use antacids, as your doctor orders.

Muscle aches or pain, weakness, numbness, or tingling
• Use acetaminophen or acetaminophen with codeine, as your doctor orders.
• Apply heat to the affected area.
• Plan frequent rest periods.
• Avoid any activity that aggravates your symptoms.
• Notify your doctor if symptoms persist or if pain localizes in a specific area.

Hair loss
• Have your hair styled in a short cut to make thinning hair less noticeable.
• Wash your hair gently with a mild shampoo, and avoid frequent brushing and combing.
• Cover your head with a hat or scarf, or wear a wig or toupee.

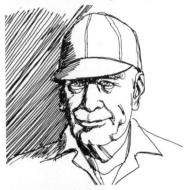

Sun sensitivity
• Use a sunblock (SPF 15) when you're out in the sun.
• Cover your scalp with a light hat or scarf.

Increased susceptibility to infection
• Avoid crowds and people with colds or infections.
• Use an electric shaver instead of a razor.
• Use a soft toothbrush to clean your teeth without injuring your gums.
• Notify your doctor if fever, chills, or excessive bruising or bleeding occurs.

a low level of radiation will remain when the patient leaves the hospital.

Managing side effects

Whether the patient's receiving external or internal radiation therapy, you'll need to teach him how to manage side effects. (See *How to Control Side Effects of Chemotherapy and Radiation Therapy*, pages 570 and 571.) Tell him to notify the doctor if side effects are persistent or especially troublesome, or if he develops fever, cough, or unusual pain. Since radiation therapy may increase susceptibility to infection, warn the patient to avoid persons with colds or other infections while he's receiving therapy.

In collaboration with the dietitian, teach the patient to maintain a balanced diet while he's receiving radiation therapy. Stress that good nutrition is a must, and provide tips to stimulate the patient's appetite if his desire for food lags during therapy. Also advise him to get plenty of rest; his body will need extra energy over the course of therapy.

New Treatments

When your patient and his family learn about new cancer treatments— through the news media, doctors, or friends—they may turn to you for clarification. As a result, you should be prepared to reinforce the doctor's explanation or to answer questions about how the new treatment works and whether it's appropriate for the patient. Three new treatments currently under investigation for limited use are bone marrow transplantation, immunotherapy, and monoclonal antibody therapy.

Bone marrow transplantation

Explain that this treatment replaces diseased bone marrow with healthy bone marrow and thus may enable the patient to manufacture normal blood cells. Usually, the healthy bone marrow is donated by the cancer patient's twin or another sibling. If this isn't possible, the doctor has two alternatives: he can transplant a donor's bone marrow that closely matches the patient's. Or, he can remove the patient's own bone marrow, treat it with antileukemic antibodies, and freeze it. After the treated bone marrow thaws, the doctor will reinfuse it into the patient.

To prepare the patient for bone marrow transplantation, reinforce the doctor's explanation of the procedure and answer any questions. Tell the patient that he'll first receive chemotherapy, radiation therapy, or both, to kill any residual cancer cells. He may also receive antibiotics to reduce the number of organisms normally present in the bowel. Then he'll be placed in reverse isolation, and the donated or treated bone marrow will be infused through a central venous (Hickman) catheter. Inform the patient that the bone marrow should be engrafted within 2 to 4 weeks. In the meantime, he'll be especially vulnerable to infection. As a result, all persons entering the patient's room will need to wear sterile gowns, masks, gloves, and shoe covers to prevent introducing germs into his environment.

Immunotherapy

Immunotherapy introduces antigens and other substances into the patient's body in an attempt to stimulate the immune system to recognize and attack cancer cells. Explain to the patient that immunotherapy is used in combination with other treatments, such as radiation therapy.

To prepare the patient for immunotherapy, inform him how it will be administered—by mouth, inhalation, or injection into the veins, skin, or tumor. Note that he may receive antihistamines and acetaminophen before immunotherapy. Teach him to watch for and report mild erythema and induration at the treatment site, pruritus, fever, chills, malaise, and anaphylaxis.

UNPROVEN TREATMENTS: HAZARDOUS TO YOUR PATIENT'S HEALTH

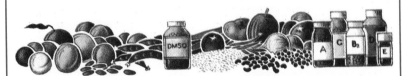

Fear of the prescribed therapy or feelings of despair as cancer progresses may make a cancer patient consider undergoing treatments that haven't gained medical acceptance—or that have received outright disapproval. When a patient chooses such a treatment, he risks delaying needed prescribed therapy and may also suffer damaging side effects.

How can you help your patient make an informed decision? First, listen to his concerns about his disorder and its prescribed therapy. If he mentions that he's considering an unproven treatment, be sure to point out what we know—and what we don't know—about it.

These are some of the most common unproven treatments for cancer.

LAETRILE

Also known as amygdalin, laetrile is derived from such foods as apricots, peaches, plums, almonds, cloves, and lima beans. Two theories exist concerning laetrile's actions against cancer cells. These postulate that:
• cancer cells contain an enzyme that releases cyanide from laetrile, and this kills the cancer cells.
• cancer is a vitamin deficiency, and laetrile is the missing vitamin B_{17}.

Extensive testing shows that laetrile is not effective as a cancer treatment. Also, it can cause cyanide toxicity, hypotension, vomiting, and motor disturbances. But its myth endures and it remains popular.

DIMETHYL SULFOXIDE (DMSO)

Widely used as an industrial solvent and a veterinary pharmacologic agent, DMSO is believed, but not proven, to reduce pain, increase the therapeutic benefits of chemotherapy, and decrease its side effects. But the only FDA-approved use of DMSO is for bladder instillation in interstitial cystitis.

MACROBIOTIC DIET

This diet is based on the Eastern philosophy of keeping a proper balance between one's self and the environment. Its supporters believe that cancer is related to an increased intake of so-called yin or yang foods. A macrobiotic diet usually includes cereals, vegetables, and beans, with limited fluids.

Besides having no proven effect as cancer therapy, a macrobiotic diet can cause decreased levels of essential vitamins, iron deficiency, and anemia.

VITAMIN THERAPY

Vitamins A and C are popular because they're widely available and thought to be generally beneficial and nontoxic. When taken in large doses, though, vitamin A *is* toxic—it causes vomiting, fatigue, and abdominal discomfort. And large doses of vitamin C can cause nausea and diarrhea. But because the body's need for vitamin C increases with stress and wound healing and in response to certain drugs used in cancer treatment, patients with cancer may benefit from eating more vitamin C–rich foods or from taking dietary supplements. Vitamin C also aids immune system function, and it may help the body fight infection.

Warn about muscle aches and fatigue if the patient receives interferon.

Monoclonal antibody therapy

Explain how monoclonal antibodies can help detect and treat cancer: when radioactive tracers are attached to monoclonal antibodies that are specific for selected cancer cells, they can accurately locate areas of that cancer in the body. And when used with chemotherapy, these antibodies can destroy cancer cells while leaving normal ones alone. Inform the patient that the use of monoclonal antibodies is still considered experimental.

To prepare a patient for monoclonal antibody therapy, reinforce the doctor's explanation of the procedure. Then check your hospital's protocol for administering the therapy. Explain how therapy will be given—for example, by injection into the veins, lymph nodes, or muscles. Describe the side effects the patient should watch for and report, including fever and chills. Also encourage him to discuss how he feels about the treatment. More than likely, he's already tried aggressive cancer treatment with conventional therapies. As a result, he may view monoclonal antibody therapy as his last hope for a cure.

Pain Control

Not all cancer patients experience pain, but those who do may find it difficult to manage. By teaching the patient what causes pain and how to relieve or reduce it, you can help him control it more effectively.

Identify causes of cancer pain

Explain that pain results from the growing cancer's intrusion on normal tissues; it doesn't radiate from the cancer itself, as many people erroneously believe. Pain may also result from diagnostic tests associated with cancer,

such as bone marrow biopsy, and from cancer treatments. Point out that the patient's emotional state can profoundly influence his perception of pain. Fear and anxiety about his body image, financial problems, and the future can exaggerate the frequency and intensity of pain.

How to relieve cancer pain

Discuss how pain can sometimes be relieved by removing the tumor or decreasing its size through surgery, chemotherapy, or radiation therapy. Pain can also be treated directly with medication and other techniques, such as distraction, relaxation, guided imagery, and cutaneous stimulation. (For more information, see Chapter 19.) When these conservative measures fail, you may need to teach the patient about neurosurgical techniques to relieve pain. (See "Surgery" in Chapter 9.)

Advise the patient to use nonprescription drugs judiciously to control mild pain. If he's receiving chemotherapy, inform him of any potentially harmful interactions (see *Special Alert: Chemotherapeutic Drug Interactions*, page 569).

If the patient is discharged with a prescription for a narcotic analgesic to control moderate or severe pain, make sure he understands the dosage instructions. If appropriate, demonstrate how to deliver the medication with an infusion pump. Teach the patient how to manage side effects of narcotics, such as constipation and drowsiness. Tell him to notify the doctor if side effects are persistent or troublesome.

HOME CARE

A cancer patient may have physical care needs that continue after he leaves the hospital. In many cases, you'll need to teach him and his family how to perform special procedures, such as tracheostomy care, as well as basic care measures, such as oral hygiene. You'll also need to help the caregiver learn how to avoid or manage stress and burnout (see *Helping the Caregiver Recognize—and Avoid—Burnout*).

To ensure competent home care, your teaching must stress the importance of maintaining optimal health through good nutrition and hygiene. In this way, you can help the patient and his family avoid or manage common complications of cancer and its treatment, including protein-calorie malnutrition and infection.

When teaching about home care, emphasize the variety of support systems that are available. Make sure your patient and his family realize that they don't have to face cancer alone.

Preventing Protein-Calorie Malnutrition

Among patients with cancer, the most common complication is protein-calorie malnutrition, a condition marked by weight loss, muscle wasting, apathy, lethargy, and compromised cellular immunity. Untreated, it can lead to cachexia and death.

To help prevent protein-calorie malnutrition, teach the patient and his family how to achieve a well-balanced, high-calorie, protein-rich diet. Identify specific foods and products that help supply adequate nutrition. For example, tell the patient to enrich foods and drinks with glucose polymers, which add 32 calories per tablespoon yet don't affect food taste. Or recommend sipping high-calorie, protein-rich supplements between meals. If these supplements cause diarrhea, suggest

---

HELPING THE CAREGIVER RECOGNIZE—AND AVOID—BURNOUT

As a nurse, you know that caring for a cancer patient can be stressful sometimes. And eventually, this stress may cause burnout—a condition marked by listlessness, difficulty making decisions, guilt, irritability, anger, and emotional withdrawal from others.

After the patient returns home, the family member or friend who's chiefly responsible for his care is also vulnerable to stress and the risk of burnout. How can you help? Teach your patient's caregiver to recognize the warning signs of burnout—for example, an inability to get organized, sudden and inexplicable outbursts of tears, and a constant feeling of urgency. Also recommend the following techniques to minimize stress:

Hobbies provide useful diversion. Some hobbies, such as exercise and sports, also release tension.

Proper nutrition and adequate rest help maximize energy.

Progressive muscle relaxation promotes overall relaxation through conscious tensing and relaxing of various parts of the body.

Imagery involves creating a tranquil scene in the mind, then concentrating on what it feels like to be there.

Meditation, a brief, structured mental escape from everyday routine, aims to reduce blood pressure and oxygen requirements through calm, restful concentration.

Humor has tension-relieving effects, according to some specialists in stress management.

Prayer, of course, can be helpful in achieving peace of mind.

Setting priorities helps promote a sense of control over the many demands on the caregiver's time.

Delegating tasks to other family members or friends helps the caregiver conserve his physical and emotional resources.

CARING FOR YOUR
CENTRAL VENOUS CATHETER

Dear Patient:

To keep your central venous catheter trouble-free at home, you must flush the catheter and change the dressing regularly.

How to flush the catheter
Flush the catheter at least once a day to prevent blood clots from forming inside it.

1

First, gather this equipment: bottle of heparin lock flush solution, disposable syringe with needle, two povidone-iodine swabs, $4'' \times 4''$ gauze pads, and tape. Now, wash and dry your hands. Then, open the bottle of heparin lock flush solution and wipe the bottle top with a povidone-iodine swab. *Don't touch the top after you've cleaned it.*

2

Next, remove the needle guard, and pull back the syringe plunger. Then, insert the needle into the bottle top, and push down on the plunger. Turn the bottle upside down, as shown at the top of the next column, and pull back on the syringe plunger to fill the syringe with solution. Remove the needle from the bottle, and put the bottle aside.

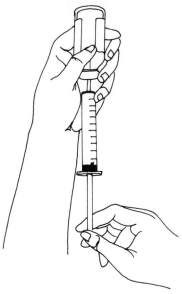

3

Remove and discard the gauze pad protecting the catheter cap. Using a clean povidone-iodine swab, wipe the top of the catheter cap. When the cap's dry, remove the catheter's clamp. Now, insert the needle into the cap.

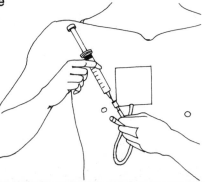

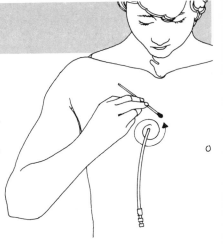

Push down on the plunger to inject the solution into the catheter. Replace the clamp after you withdraw the needle. Wrap the catheter cap in a sterile gauze pad and tape it on top of the dressing.

How to change the dressing

Change the dressing over the catheter every other day or whenever it becomes wet or dirty. When you change your dressing, carefully check the skin around the catheter. Call the doctor at once if you see any sign of infection—for example, redness, swelling, or pus. Also call him if you develop a fever or feel pain.

1

To change the dressing, first wash your hands and remove the soiled dressing. Wash your hands again. (If suggested by your doctor, you may want to put on sterile gloves to avoid possible contamination.)

Clean the skin around the catheter with an alcohol swab, beginning near the catheter and working outward in a circular motion, as shown at the top of the next column. Repeat the procedure, using a povidone-iodine swab.

2

Squeeze some povidone-iodine ointment onto a sterile gauze pad, and place the pad over the catheter exit site. Cover it with a dry sterile gauze pad.

3

Apply an adhesive bandage over both gauze pads, so that the bandage edges stick to your skin. For extra security, tape the bandage edges to your skin, as shown here.

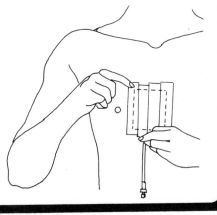

578

HOME CARE

TIPS TO STIMULATE APPETITE

Dear Patient:

Your loss of appetite is a common side effect of cancer and its treatment (chemotherapy and radiation therapy). Try the following tips to stimulate your appetite.

Make mealtime more enjoyable
• Create a pleasant dining atmosphere. Accompany meals with music, soft lights, a brightly colored table setting, or whatever makes you feel good while eating. If permitted, have a glass of wine or beer with your meal to increase your appetite.
• Arrange food attractively on the plate. Add a garnish, such as parsley or a slice of lemon, to make the food appealing.
• Share meals with your family or friends. Or try watching television or reading while you eat.
• Eat frequent, small meals instead of three large meals.
• Keep nutritious snacks on hand—nuts, fruit, and cheese, for example—and eat whenever you feel hungry.

Be creative with your cooking
• Vary your diet and try new recipes. Experiment with spices and seasonings to make food more flavorful.
• If you can tolerate dairy prod-

ucts, add margarine or butter to foods to improve flavor. Also try mixing canned cream soups with milk rather than water, and adding cream sauce or melted cheese to vegetables.
• Drink milk shakes, eggnog, or prepared liquid supplements between meals. You may want to enrich beverages with eggs, honey, or powdered milk.

Overcome obstacles to eating
• Take a walk or exercise moderately before meals to help build your appetite.
• If nausea discourages you from eating, try to curb it by eating low-fat meals. Avoid overly sweet or spicy foods. Eat dry foods, such as toast or crackers, when you get up in the morning.
• Minimize mouth soreness or dryness by avoiding foods that are very salty, highly spiced, or hot. Instead, eat cold foods— such as ice cream, frozen yogurt, milk shakes, or cold soups. Ice chips, flavored ice pops, hard candies, lemon slices, and dill pickles help keep your mouth moist.
• If you live alone, consider contacting "Meals On Wheels" or a similar community program when you don't feel like cooking.

diluting them with more water or cutting back on the amount.

Teach the patient and his family tips to combat anorexia, nausea, and vomiting—common side effects of chemotherapy and radiation therapy that may diminish the patient's desire to eat (see *Tips to Stimulate Appetite*). Also teach them how to cope with other problems, such as mouth dryness and mouth ulcers (see *How to Control Side Effects of Chemotherapy and Radiation Therapy*, pages 570 and 571).

Occasionally, enteral or parenteral nutrition may be necessary to maintain adequate nutrition. (For more information about enteral nutrition, see *How to Give an Intermittent Feeding* in Chapter 9.) If appropriate, teach the patient and his family how to administer parenteral nutrition through a central venous (Hickman) catheter. Stress measures to prevent infection at the catheter insertion site (see *Caring for Your Central Venous Catheter*, pages 576 and 577). Advise them to check the tubing frequently for kinks or loose connections. Instruct them to check the infusion rate every 30 minutes to prevent overly rapid infusion. Also teach them how to monitor the patient's daily weight and intake and output, and how to test his urine for glucose and acetone levels. Tell them to watch for and report such signs and symptoms as dyspnea, edema, distended neck veins, decreased urine output, chest pain or pressure, unusual weight gain, or a change in the patient's mental status.

Preventing Infection

Teaching the patient how to maintain optimal health through adequate rest and a high-calorie, protein-rich diet is the first step toward preventing infection. You'll also need to warn him about exposure to contagious illness. Stress how preserving skin integrity and performing frequent pulmonary hygiene can protect him from infection. Instruct the patient to notify the doctor if he develops signs and symptoms that may indicate infection, including fever, skin rash, persistent bleeding, dyspnea, or unusual pain. (For more information about patient teaching to prevent infection, see Chapter 17.)

Securing Support Services

After the patient is discharged, you may remain on call to teach and offer him support, especially if you were his primary nurse in the hospital. Depending on his needs, however, you may also need to refer him to a private-duty or visiting nurse. Securing the services of a private-duty or visiting nurse allows the family to participate in the patient's care without feeling totally burdened by the responsibility.

Also inform the patient and his family of the various community support services available to help them cope with cancer. For example, the American Cancer Society may be able to arrange for transportation to and from the hospital or treatment center.

When all curative medical therapies are discontinued and the patient is receiving only palliative treatment, you may refer him for hospice care. This can be delivered in the home, in an extended-care facility, or in a combination of the two. Its goal is to give the dying patient and his family as much control over his care as possible. When discussing hospice care, explain that the hospice nurse will teach the patient and his family how to care for the patient's physical needs and will prepare them emotionally to cope with his approaching death. For example, they'll be taught how to give injections and how to give a bed bath. After the patient dies, the hospice nurse will help the family through the grieving period.

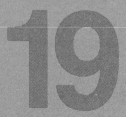

Comfort and Support

Comfort and Support

Introduction

Providing comfort and support. Day in and day out, we routinely carry out this key nursing responsibility. We seem to instinctively recognize that comfort and support are part of every patient's basic needs and rights. But what do these words actually mean?

To begin, *comfort* refers to physical and psychological well-being and entails relative freedom from pain and other unpleasant sensations. *Support* refers to use of resources—health care, social service, family, and other—to promote comfort. It includes, of course, emotional sustenance.

In the past, patients relied on their families—and, to some extent, on their nurses—for emotional support. And they relied almost exclusively on nurses and doctors for their physical comfort. But today, with increasing numbers of early hospital discharges and a growing public awareness of health issues, patients and their families are assuming a more active role.

You're in a position to promote this increasingly active role by teaching patients and families how to prevent or control discomfort and cope with the psychological stress dealt by physical changes. Teaching them about pain assessment and normal reactions to serious illness, changes in self-image, and death can give them a greater feeling of control and reduce their anxiety.

A personal experience
Because pain, altered body image, loss of a body part, and impending death are all highly personal experiences, your teaching will be most effective if you gain the patient's full participation.

Keep in mind that family members share the burden and can also help ease it. Teaching them assessment and intervention techniques will help them better support the self-sufficient patient or care more effectively for the bedridden or incapacitated patient.

If your patient's in pain, you'll need to teach him the difference between acute and chronic pain and specify the interventions that provide the best relief.

Comfort is equally personal. Your teaching about basic measures, such as good hygiene, adequate sleep, and appropriate exercise, will characteristically help the patient function as well as possible.

Mobilizing support
Whether your patient's coping with pain, body-image changes, or terminal illness, your teaching must prepare him and his family for a difficult adjustment. This will include encouraging them to draw on every possible support system to develop effective coping strategies.

COMFORT

Teaching about Basic Needs

To the debilitated and bedridden patient, comfort can mean something as simple as a daily bath and clean sheets. To the intubated patient, it can mean a mouth swab to relieve dryness. To the patient with terminal cancer, it can mean relief from unrelenting pain.

Regardless of his illness, your patient needs to understand the importance of certain basic needs: good hygiene, intact skin, adequate sleep, and appropriate exercise. Although these needs may seem unimportant—or even impossible to meet—to someone who's severely ill or in pain, explain that attending to them can actually improve health by promoting comfort, improving mood and self-esteem, stimulating circulation, improving muscle tone, preventing skin breakdown, and reducing the risk of infection.

We all know what makes us comfortable, and most patients will do as much of their own care as possible. But with a patient who is bedridden or in acute pain, you'll need to teach the family how to help him perform daily care or how to do it for him.

Promoting hygiene
Explain that hygiene is the most basic comfort measure. It includes bathing; hair, nail, and mouth care; and wearing comfortable, clean clothing. Stress the importance of a daily bath or shower. If the patient can't bathe himself or needs help, show the family how to bathe him in bed or in a chair. Teach them how to change the bed linens without getting the patient up.

Urge the patient to comb or brush his hair daily and to wash it as needed. Encourage women to set or style their hair as they did before they became ill. If the patient's bedridden, teach the family how to give a shampoo in bed, or help them find a beautician or barber who makes home visits.

Tell the patient to keep his fingernails and toenails trimmed and clean. If he's a diabetic or has poor peripheral circulation, warn him not to trim his own toenails; they should be trimmed by a podiatrist.

Emphasize the importance of mouth care. If the patient can provide his own care, urge him to brush after meals and to rinse and floss as necessary. If he's unconscious or debilitated, teach the family how to provide mouth care to prevent infection: After washing their hands, they should wrap a piece of gauze around a tongue blade and use it to wipe saliva and residue from the patient's mouth, teeth, and tongue. Then they should dip the gauze in salt water, mouthwash, or diluted hydrogen peroxide and wipe again. They should wipe a third time with plain water or, if possible, ask the patient to rinse with plain water. Next, they should apply lip moisturizer if the patient's lips are dry, and finish by washing their hands again. Warn the family not to insert fingers into the patient's mouth if he's unconscious or confused—he might bite. Also show them how to turn the patient's head to the side to prevent fluid aspiration.

Tell the patient or his family to change the patient's pajamas daily or more often if needed. Pajamas should be loose and comfortable to avoid causing skin irritation and breakdown.

Maintaining skin integrity
Explain to the patient and his family that skin breakdown poses a major risk for patients who are bedridden, not fully ambulatory, or unable to move body parts. Point out that decubitus ulcers can be prevented by regular position changes and good skin care.

DO'S AND DON'TS FOR BETTER SLEEP

Dear Patient:

If you're having trouble sleeping, follow these tips to help you fall asleep and have a restful night.

Do:

- If possible, exercise regularly during the day so you'll be physically tired at bedtime.
- Establish a bedtime routine. Performing the same activities in the same order can put you in the mood for sleep.
- Engage in relaxing activities, such as reading a novel or listening to soothing music, just before bedtime.
- Take a warm (not hot) bath before bedtime to relax your mind and your muscles. Or you can practice relaxation techniques an hour or two before going to bed.
- If your doctor prescribes a pain reliever, take it 30 minutes before you go to bed. That way, you're not as likely to be awakened by pain.
- Try to promote your overall comfort by using clean, wrinkle-free bedding and wearing comfortable sleepwear.
- Unless your doctor advises against it, drink a glass of warm milk or a glass of wine, brandy, or beer before bedtime.

Don't:

- Go to bed with worries. When possible, try to work them out well before bedtime. Even if you don't resolve your problems, just getting them out in the open can keep you from lying awake. However, if you can't share your problems with another person, do yourself a favor and try to put them out of your mind until the morning.
- Engage in strenuous physical activities just before you go to bed.
- Eat a large meal or drink a caffeinated beverage, such as coffee, tea, or cola, before bedtime. Also avoid drinking a large amount of alcohol before bedtime.
- Engage in mentally taxing activities, such as studying for an examination or balancing your checkbook, just before bedtime.
- Take naps during the day— they might interfere with your nighttime sleep needs. If you must take a nap, do so as early in the day as possible.
- Take diuretic medications just before bedtime, so you don't interrupt your sleep to go to the bathroom.

Aiding sleep

Tell the patient and his family that getting enough sleep promotes a feeling of relaxation, energy, and well-being and refreshes and renews the body and mind. Review the factors that influence sleep: age (the elderly usually sleep less than the young), emotions (anxiety and depression can cause insomnia or hypersomnia), illness (this can disrupt normal sleep cycles), and pain (this can prevent restful sleep, especially if the patient must be awakened to take medication).

Tell the patient and his family that they'll need to work together to ensure that the patient gets adequate sleep. For example, they should plan activities around the patient's sleep cycles and try not to awaken him for medications unless absolutely necessary.

If sleep continues to be a problem, give your patient suggestions to promote sleep (see *Do's and Don'ts for Better Sleep*, page 583). If these suggestions don't help, recommend that he ask his doctor about ordering a sedative. Caution him, though, not to rely on sedatives, since they can actually interfere with sleep patterns when used regularly. Also suggest that he ask his doctor about reviewing the timing and dosage of any prescribed analgesics to see if they might be contributing to insomnia.

Encouraging exercise and ambulation

Inform the patient and his family that exercise within the patient's limitations promotes his overall health, comfort, and well-being. Tell them that the doctor will prescribe an exercise program and set goals, and that the physical therapist will plan and initiate the program. Help the patient and his family understand the program, perform the exercises properly, and evaluate their effectiveness. (See *Performing Active Range-of-Motion Exercises*, pages 586 to 587.)

Explain that a therapeutic exercise program is indicated when a patient loses natural movement in a body part (as with a cerebrovascular accident) or when he stops moving a body part because of discomfort (as with arthritis). Review the objectives of the program: maintaining and increasing range of motion and function, and increasing muscle strength, endurance, coordination, and flexibility.

If the patient can't actively contract his muscles, you'll need to teach his family how to perform *passive* exercises to prevent contractures. If he can move some or all parts of his body but needs assistance, teach him and his family *active assistance* exercises to maintain and increase range of motion and function. If he can move without assistance, teach him *active* exercises. If he can perform active exercises easily, teach him mechanical or manual *resistance* exercises to maintain and increase range of motion, flexibility, and strength.

Depending on your patient's illness and abilities, he'll be ready to start walking again once he's built up his strength and flexibility with exercise. Tell him that a safe, consistent ambulation program helps prevent complications of immobility and also helps promote well-being and self-confidence.

First, teach the patient the importance of maintaining correct posture and body alignment. Tell him that using proper body mechanics will help him avoid injury and muscle strain, perform activities of daily living, and start walking again. Then describe exactly what the program involves, what is expected of the patient and family members, and what limitations, if any, will be placed on the patient. Also tell them to assemble any supportive or assistive devices.

Caution the patient not to overestimate his capabilities, reminding him that moderation is the key. Point out that he may feel dizzy if he stands up too quickly, especially if he's been bedridden for a prolonged period. Be sure to reinforce safety measures, such as

PROMOTING GOOD BODY MECHANICS

Although few people pay attention to how they sit, stand, or move about, use of good body mechanics is essential to prevent musculoskeletal injury and fatigue. That's why you'll need to demonstrate to the patient how to sit, stand, walk, recline, and lift and carry objects correctly, as described below.

How to sit
Sit with your back straight against the chair back, with your thighs supported by the chair seat as far as the curve of your knee. When you must sit for a long time, choose a firm, erect chair and change your position frequently.

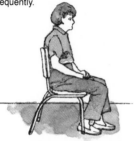

How to lie down and get up
Sleep on a firm mattress to keep your body aligned. The mattress should support all parts of your body equally—a sagging mattress can cause backaches.

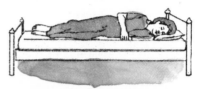

When rising, swing your legs off the edge of the bed, then push with both arms to assume a sitting position. Never "throw" yourself from a lying to a sitting position or leap out of bed.

How to stand
Stand erect with your head high and your chin pointed slightly downward. Move your chest out slightly and your shoulders back. Tuck in your pelvis and tighten your abdominal muscles to maintain good back posture. Keep your knees straight but relaxed, and your feet slightly apart, with your toes pointed straight ahead.

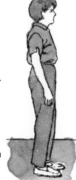

How to lift and carry objects
To lift an object, stand with your feet apart for a wide base of support. Bend at the knees while keeping your back straight. That way, your strong leg muscles, not your weaker back mus-

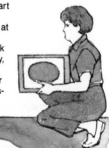

cles, will do most of the work. Avoid sudden twisting motions when lifting. Push—don't pull—objects that you can't lift.
To carry an object, hold it in front of you at waist level, as close to your body as possible.

How to walk
Walk with your body aligned the way it is when you're standing. Keep your feet parallel and close together. Push forward with your back foot, in an even, rhythmic stride, heel first, then the outside part of the sole, and then the forefoot. Swing your arms easily as you walk.

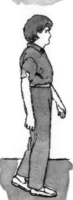

PERFORMING ACTIVE RANGE-OF-MOTION EXERCISES

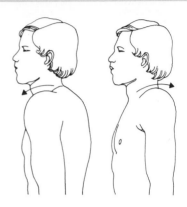

Dear Patient:

Do these active range-of-motion exercises to increase your muscle strength and make your joints move more easily.

Neck exercise
Slowly move your head as far back as possible. Then move it to the right toward your shoulder.

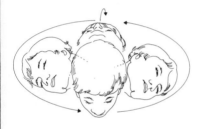

Next, lower your chin toward your chest as far as it will go. Then move your head toward your left shoulder and finally back to its normal upright position. Reverse the exercise and move your head in a circle, from left to right.

Shoulder exercise
Raise your shoulders, as if you were going to shrug. Next, move them forward in a circular motion, as shown at the top of the next column. Then move them backward in a circular motion.

Hip and knee exercise
Lie on your back with one leg bent and your foot flat on the bed or floor. Now bend your other leg and slowly bring the knee as far toward your chest as you can without discomfort. Then straighten this leg slowly while you lower it. Repeat the exercise with your other leg.

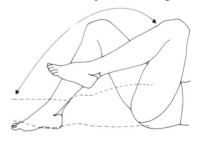

Elbow exercise
Extend your arm straight down to your side, palm up. Slowly reach back and touch your shoulder with your fingertips.

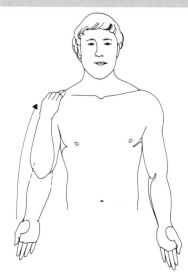

Then slowly straighten your arm again. Repeat with your other arm.

Wrist and hand exercise

Extend your arms, palms down and fingers straight. Keeping your palms flat, slowly raise your fingers and point them back toward you.

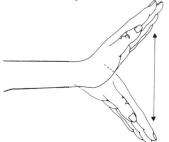

Then slowly lower your fingers and point them as far downward as you comfortably can.

Ankle and foot exercise

Lift one foot up and point it away from you. Make a circle with it, first right and then left. Next, point the foot back toward you. Make a circle with it again, first right and then left. Repeat with your other foot.

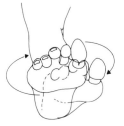

Tips for safety and success

• To get the most out of these exercises, do them daily.
• Repeat each exercise three to five times or as your doctor directs.
• Move slowly and gently so you don't injure yourself. If any exercise is painful, stop doing it. Ask your doctor whether you should discontinue that exercise.
• Remember, you don't have to do your exercises in a single session: you can space them out over the course of a day.

use of correct body mechanics and transfer techniques.

Instruct the patient and his family to keep a record of ambulation progress: distances, responses to increased activity, and so on. This helps them set goals or, if setbacks occur, begin the program again.

Teaching about Pain Control

Pain may result from physical injury, from tissue damage, from life-threatening conditions such as malignancies, or from non-life-threatening conditions such as osteoarthritis or migraine headaches. Pain may be acute, chronic, or both.

Regardless of the type of pain, explain to the patient and his family that quick, complete relief may not be possible. Then help them set realistic goals, such as improved pain relief; greater comfort, activity, and productivity; and less dependence on medication and the health care team.

Pain self-assessment
Teach the patient to do an accurate pain assessment. He'll need to learn about the nature and source of his pain and how to describe clearly the pain site, intensity, duration, and pattern. He and his family will also need to know how to evaluate the effectiveness of various pain control methods.

• *Identifying triggers.* Discuss pain's physical characteristics to explain how *internal* changes can trigger pain. To do an accurate and complete self-assessment, the patient must become attuned to his body's signals. First, advise him to become aware of his body when he's not in pain. Teach him to do a head-to-toe assessment for signs of freedom from tension, spontaneity and range of motion, and strength and duration of movement. Then teach him

how to keep a daily pain diary, identifying and recording the physical and emotional changes that accompany pain, so that he can recognize premonitory symptoms early enough to achieve more effective relief.

Once the patient can describe his pain and recognize its onset, show him and his family how to assess their environment for *external* contributing factors. Certain noises, foods, types of light, amounts of sleep, times of day, and even certain people can trigger a pain episode.

Next, you'll teach the patient and his family about pain control methods, including heat and cold, massage, relaxation breathing, and drug therapy. Tell them which types of pain respond best to which methods, and explain that a combination of methods usually works best. Suggest that they practice these techniques daily, if possible, when the patient's in minimal pain.

Heat therapy
Tell the patient and his family that heat controls pain in several ways. It promotes muscle relaxation and sedation, which reduce tension. It increases blood flow to injured areas, which helps restore proper nutrition and eliminate waste products from muscle and other tissues. It decreases the receptivity of sensory nerve fibers, which breaks the pain-spasm-pain cycle. And it softens exudate and increases suppuration in congested, inflamed, or infected areas, which localizes the infection and the painful area.

Suggest heat therapy to the patient with chronic pain, bruises, or muscle spasms. Warn him, though, not to use heat during the first 24 hours after an acute injury (when vasoconstriction is needed to reduce edema), during any acute inflammatory condition, or with undiagnosed pain of more than a few hours' duration. To prevent burns, tell the patient with circulatory or sensory impairment to apply heat cautiously.

Explain that heat may be moist or dry. Moist heat penetrates the skin more deeply, so most patients prefer it. Dry heat doesn't penetrate as deeply, so it may be applied at higher temperatures. When teaching about heat therapy, choose from the following commonly used methods.

• *Baths or showers.* Warm to hot baths or showers are simple, convenient, inexpensive ways to relax the body. A whirlpool further enhances the heat's effect by its massaging action. Suggest this technique if your patient has a sprain, muscle spasms, joint aches or stiffness, hemorrhoids, cystitis, or an episiotomy incision.

Instruct the patient to make the bath or shower water a comfortable temperature—105° to 110° F. (40.6° to 43.3° C.). Advise checking the water with a bath thermometer, so he'll know how the correct temperature feels. Since multiple short baths or showers are more beneficial than one long soak, suggest that he take four 15-minute baths or showers a day, if possible, and that he try to take one in the morning to relieve stiffness.

Depending on the patient's physical limitations, teach him how to safely enter and exit the tub or shower. Warn him that he might feel light-headed or weak from the vasodilation caused by warm water.

• *Hot water bottles.* Inexpensive and readily available, rubber hot water bottles stay hot for up to 30 minutes. Suggest this technique for deep muscle or ligament pain.

Tell the patient to fill the bottle two-thirds full of water heated to 115° to 130° F. (46.1° to 54.4° C.). He should place the filled bottle on a flat surface to remove residual air, then insert the stopper and check for leaks. Next, he should cover the bottle with a towel.

Since the bottle may be too heavy to feel comfortable on painful areas, advise the patient to lean the painful area against it, if possible. He should check for extreme redness and remove or reposition the bottle and wrap another towel around it if he notices this.

• *Heating pads.* Usually covered in plastic, with flannel cases, heating pads contain a web of wires that convert electrical current into heat. Pads conform easily to body contours. Also, they're lighter in weight and more comfortable than hydrocollator packs (see below) on painful areas and easier to use on extremities. Suggest this technique for muscle aches, low back pain, or menstrual cramps.

Instruct the patient to check the pad and its cord for defects before use. Then he should plug it in and adjust the temperature setting to a comfortable level. Warn the patient not to increase the temperature after he's used the pad for a while, because he'll be less sensitive to heat and might burn himself. Also caution him not to crush or fold the pad, since this can cause a malfunction or overheating; not to attach the cover with pins, since this can puncture the pad; and not to use the pad near water, since this can cause electrocution.

• *Hydrocollator packs.* These reusable, nonelectric, canvas-covered packs contain silicate gel. When they're placed in hot water (in a pot on the stove, for example), the gel becomes flexible and absorbs water. Packs come in various shapes and sizes and can be rolled to conform to body contours. They retain heat for 20 to 30 minutes. If your patient has musculoskeletal pain or pain in deep structures (such as the abdomen), suggest this method.

Instruct the patient to wrap the heated pack in a soft cloth or towel before application to provide insulation and prevent burns. Then he should assess the pain site to determine the safest, most beneficial placement. Because packs are heavy, they can cause discomfort if placed directly over a painful area; they can also slide off. So suggest that he rest the painful area on or against the pack.

Caution the patient not to use the pack for more than 30 minutes at a time to prevent skin maceration. Instruct him to check his skin for extreme redness at least every 5 minutes and to remove the pack immediately if he notices this. He may want to reposition it or add another protective cover.

If the patient will use the pack frequently, advise him to store it in water to prevent the gel from drying out and to shorten preparation time. If he won't be using it often, he can wrap it in plastic while it's still moist and store it in the refrigerator or freezer.

• *Aquamatic K pads.* These tubular rubber pads circulate distilled water at a constant temperature, as prescribed (usually 105° F., or 40.6° C.). A key locks in the temperature setting. The pads deliver dry heat and can also be laid over moist heat applications to sustain their warmth. Suggest this technique for muscle aches and low back pain.

Tell the patient to fill the control unit two-thirds full with distilled water, to check for leaks, and to clear the tubing of tangles and air (which interfere with heat conduction). He should tighten the cap, then loosen it a quarter turn to allow for heat expansion. After placing the pad in a pillowcase and securing it with tape, the patient may plug the unit in and turn it on. The pad warms in 2 minutes.

Caution the patient not to use tap water in the pad, since it leaves mineral deposits. He should also check the cord for defects before plugging it in and avoid using pins to secure the case, since they can puncture the pad.

• *Heat lamps.* A gooseneck lamp with an appropriate-watt bulb, placed a safe distance from a painful area, can provide radiant heat without weight or direct contact with the skin. Suggest this technique to relieve local discomfort, such as soft-tissue excoriation.

Tell the patient to cleanse the painful area, to drape the surrounding skin to prevent burns, and to lie or sit comfortably. If he's to use a 25-watt bulb, he should place it approximately 1' from his skin, a 40- or 50-watt bulb about 18″ to 20″ away, and a larger bulb about 24″ to 30″ away. Treatment should last from 15 to 30 minutes.

Caution the patient to check the area frequently for extreme redness and to stop the treatment if this occurs or if the heat feels excessive. Suggest setting a kitchen timer for the correct number of minutes, in case he falls asleep.

Cold therapy

Tell the patient and his family that cold controls pain by several means. It decreases edema and inflammation, which lowers tissue metabolism, bacterial activity in infection, lymph production, histamine release, and capillary permeability. It acts as a muscle relaxant and analgesic, which decreases nerve conduction velocity and peripheral sensory organ activity, thus breaking the pain-spasm-pain cycle. And it numbs the treated area, which deadens the pain sensation. Suggest cold therapy for acute pain, such as muscle sprains, and for chronic conditions, such as low back pain or osteoarthritis.

Explain to the patient that cold therapy produces vasoconstriction, decreases blood flow, and lowers heat exchange within the tissues, allowing deeper penetration than heat. Tell him that this treatment might feel uncomfortable at first because it increases muscle viscosity, thereby increasing stiffness. But exercising after treatment, before the analgesic effect wears off, can eliminate this problem.

When teaching about cold therapy, provide information about the following commonly used methods.

• *Moist cold compresses.* A towel or washcloth soaked in ice water can be used to relieve pain and inflammation in small body parts. This technique is ideal for eye injuries, tooth extractions, and sinus congestion.

Instruct the patient to wash his hands, to put the compress in a basin containing ice and a small amount of water, then to wring it out and apply it to the painful area. Its temperature should be 59° F. (15° C.). He should change the compress frequently since it absorbs body heat. Tell him to continue the treatment for 15 to 20 minutes and to repeat it every 2 to 3 hours.

• *Ice massage.* Rubbing ice on a painful area is a simple, safe technique that provides relief from acute or chronic pain for up to several hours.

Depending on the size of the painful area, recommend forming ice in an ice cube tray, plastic bowl, or styrofoam cup (using a popsicle stick handle). Instruct the patient to massage the area lightly and smoothly with circular or back-and-forth movements for 5 to 10 minutes. He'll experience four stages of sensation—coldness, burning, itching, and numbness. To obtain pain relief for 1 hour or longer, the patient should massage the area until it feels numb.

• *Cold packs, ice caps, and ice collars.* Consisting of a cloth, canvas, or rubber bag filled with chipped ice (which is easier to mold to the affected area than ice cubes), these devices are effective for many conditions, including bruises, cuts, sprains, postoperative orthopedic discomfort, muscle spasms, and arthritis.

Depending on the area being treated, suggest to the patient different inexpensive ways to make cold packs. For example, he can fill a rubber glove with ice and apply it to a swollen lip or painful I.M. injection site. Or he can moisten 4″ x 4″ gauze pads, freeze them in a plastic bag, and mold them to his nose, finger, knee, or ankle.

If the patient's using a commercial cold pack, instruct him to fill it two-thirds full with ice, to remove any air, to replace the cover to absorb condensation, then to fasten it with tape. Tell him that a 20- to 30-minute application, reapplied after 1 hour or several times a day, is usually effective. Instruct him to observe his skin for redness, discoloration, blanching, or mottling, indicating tissue damage, and to stop the treatment if these occur.

If he's using another commercial cold pack, such as a chemical cold pack, a cold hydrocollator pack, or an aquamatic K pad, tell him to follow the manufacturer's instructions and to use the same precautions as for all cold packs.

He can achieve deeper penetration by placing these cold packs over two layers of dampened towels.

Relaxation therapy

One of the best things you can do for your patient is to show him how to use relaxation techniques to reduce pain and the stress and fatigue that accompany it. Since family members can be especially helpful and supportive, include them in your teaching.

Tell the patient and his family that a stressful condition like pain increases heart rate, respirations, blood pressure, and muscle tension—all of which intensify pain. Relaxation can reverse this process and relieve pain and anxiety. Because the techniques require concentration, the patient won't be able to focus on his pain while he's performing them.

Explain that a wide range of relaxation techniques are effective for pain, especially chronic pain. But stress that relaxation doesn't preclude using other pain relief methods, such as analgesics, and that success with relaxation techniques doesn't mean that the pain was imagined or exaggerated.

Whether simple to learn, such as relaxation breathing, or more complicated, such as self-hypnosis, all relaxation techniques are virtually risk-free and require no special equipment or assistance once the patient's learned them. What's best, they let the patient participate actively in his care.

After you've reviewed relaxation techniques with the patient and his family, teach how to perform them. Then let the patient choose those he's most comfortable with. Many patients combine techniques and find that different types of pain require use of different techniques. Encourage your patient to experiment until he finds the techniques that suit him best.

Advise the patient to practice relaxation techniques at least 20 minutes a day. Since his goal is to *prevent* pain, he should use relaxation techniques not only during episodes of pain, but also before and after them, to extend his control over the experience.

For each technique, the patient should first select a quiet, comfortable environment. He should assume a relaxed position, sitting or lying down. (In fact, learning to relax in different positions will allow him to use these techniques anytime, anyplace.) He should choose a sound, word, or phrase to repeat silently or aloud, or an object to stare at.

If your patient has distracting thoughts while learning the techniques, tell him not to worry—most people have trouble concentrating at first, especially if they're in pain during the teaching session. Also caution him not to expect immediate results. He may even be *more* aware of his pain at first, but with practice the pain should decrease, replaced by the relaxation response: a slowdown of heart rate and other bodily processes accompanied by pleasant sensations, such as warmth, heaviness, lightness, or tingling.

• **Emergency techniques.** Occasionally, a patient's in so much pain that learning's nearly impossible. Or his pain may arise too suddenly to be relieved by practiced techniques. When this occurs, teach these two exercises:

☐ Tell him to relax his lower jaw, as if he were starting to yawn, and to rest his tongue on the bottom of his mouth. Then suggest that he breathe slowly and rhythmically through his mouth: inhaling, exhaling, then resting.

☐ Instruct him to close his eyes and imagine a star about 1″ from the tip of his nose. Then tell him to focus on the star and breathe deeply and slowly four times through his mouth.

• **Relaxation breathing.** Explain to the patient that in this technique, he breathes slowly and deeply until he relaxes. (See *Learning Relaxation Techniques,* pages 594 to 595.) Like all relaxation techniques, this one's effective for chronic pain. It also helps during painful procedures, between medication doses, and for episodes of acute pain. Caution wearers of con-

ventional contact lenses that they should remove lenses to prevent a corneal abrasion in case they fall asleep.

• **Progressive muscle relaxation (PMR).** Explain to the patient that in this technique, he systematically tenses and relaxes separate muscle groups. By learning to distinguish between muscle tension and muscle relaxation, he can consciously relax his muscles to reduce pain. Tell him that this technique is effective for acute or chronic pain, during painful procedures, or between medication doses.

Describe PMR as a three-step procedure: focusing on the muscles to be relaxed, tensing them, and gradually letting the tension go until he feels his muscles "unwind." Begin teaching the technique by having the patient focus on the muscles in his dominant hand. Then have him tense his forearm muscles and make a fist. When his muscles are tense, tell him to note the sensation. After 5 to 7 seconds, signal him to release his fist and relax his muscles. Ask him to think about the difference in feeling between the relaxed and tense states. Then tell him to tense and relax each major muscle group in his body. To end the exercise, tell him to open his eyes, to stretch, and finally, to walk around until he feels alert.

Although the patient may initially need guidance, he'll need, with practice, only minimal cues from you or a family member to achieve muscle relaxation. His goal: to learn to relax the muscles in the painful area and in any other area, on cue, in any setting.

For best results, suggest that the patient combine PMR with relaxation breathing and imagery. Because some patients with facial pain, migraines, or tension headaches find tensing and relaxing certain muscles quite painful, advise them to practice relaxation breathing, imagery, or other techniques first. Then, once their muscle tension is relieved, they can try PMR again.

• **Autogenic training.** Explain that this helpful addition to relaxation breathing and PMR uses self-suggestions about the sensations the patient feels when he's relaxed. Tell him that while he's learning, you'll softly and slowly describe the sensations—such as warmth or limb heaviness—that accompany relaxation in each part of his body. Eventually, he'll be able to do this silently for himself.

Tell the patient that this relaxation technique is most effective with chronic pain and that it also helps relieve anxiety and stress. It can be incorporated into PMR as the patient systematically relaxes each muscle group. Or it can be used following PMR to deepen or call his attention to the sensation of relaxation.

Be sure to tell the family how important their participation is in this technique; they can coach the patient and use it themselves to manage stress.

Since the patient may feel sleepy after performing this technique, tell him to practice it in a comfortable position and in a place where he can nap.

● *Imagery.* Explain that this technique, which involves concentration and imagination, can be practiced along with breathing and PMR to produce relaxation and fight pain. It's effective for both acute and chronic pain and during painful procedures. And it's quick and easy to learn.

Because many people have misconceptions about imagery, explain that it doesn't require giving up control, but it does require the ability to follow directions, to respond to suggestions, and to concentrate and create mental images. It doesn't involve sleeping, although it can be used to promote sleep.

Have your patient prepare himself by first practicing another technique, such as relaxation breathing, in a comfortable, distraction-free setting.

Before starting the imagery session, have the patient decide how long it should last. Fifteen to twenty minutes is usually adequate, unless he's undergoing a painful procedure that lasts longer. Emphasize that the image he uses is unimportant, but his involvement is critical. The more involved he gets, the less he'll focus on his pain.

● *Distraction.* Explain to the patient that distraction focuses his attention on something other than the pain, such as television programs, movies, or books, especially humorous ones. This temporarily increases pain tolerance and sometimes temporarily reduces pain intensity. Unlike imagery, distraction draws on actual physical stimuli in the patient's environment. Mention that this technique is easy to learn because most people use it naturally, often without even realizing it. Also explain to family members that by helping the patient practice this technique, they can increase their interaction with him while promoting his comfort.

Tell the patient that distraction is useful for both acute and chronic pain, but that the specific approaches differ. For brief episodes of pain, suggest combining distraction with relaxation breathing, massage, and imagery. For chronic pain, suggest getting involved in more complex or productive activities, such as doing home repairs or creating something.

Before teaching your patient to use distraction, ask if he's ever used this technique successfully on his own. If so, find out what worked and use it again; if not, find out what his interests are and incorporate them into distraction strategies. Then tell him not to expect total pain relief, just lessened awareness of pain and for only a brief time. Caution him to avoid any stimulus related to his pain; for example, he shouldn't look at the painful body part or think about or watch a painful procedure. His chosen distraction should involve as many senses as possible, since this more effectively blocks pain. And as pain worsens, he should make the distraction more complex; however, if pain becomes acute, he should simplify the distraction to prevent frustration. Advise him that brief distraction techniques should always include relaxation breathing.

Next, work with the patient and his

LEARNING RELAXATION TECHNIQUES

Dear Patient:

Relaxation techniques can help you cope with stress or pain. Practice these simple techniques daily.

Relaxation breathing

1

Close your eyes. Inhale slowly and deeply through your nose as you count silently: "In, 2, 3, 4." Notice how your abdomen expands first, then your rib cage, and finally your upper chest.

2

Hold your breath to the count of 4, but don't strain.

3

Exhale slowly through your mouth as you count silently: "Out, 2, 3, 4, 5, 6, 7, 8." Pretend you're breathing out through a straw to lengthen exhalation. Let your shoulders drop slightly as your upper chest, rib cage, and abdomen gently deflate.

Repeat this exercise four or five times.

Imagery

1

Begin by focusing on your breathing. Spend a few minutes breathing slowly and smoothly as you did for relaxation breathing.

2

As you breathe, slowly count backwards from 5, sinking deeper and deeper into a state of relaxation. Say to yourself, "I feel deeply relaxed."

3

Next, conjure an image of a pleasant, relaxing place—for example, a warm, quiet beach or a tranquil, fragrant garden. (Return to this special place every time you use imagery.) "Experience" the place with all your senses—sight, hearing, taste, smell, and touch. Remain there for about 5 minutes.

4

Then, slowly let the image dissolve or fade from the center of your attention as you focus again on your breathing. When you feel ready, count slowly to 5 and open your eyes.

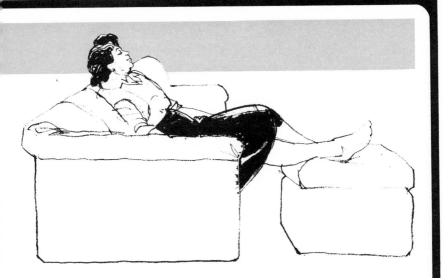

Autogenic training

To perform this technique, make yourself comfortable, close your eyes, and slowly repeat each of the following sentences to yourself:

1

"My feet feel heavy and relaxed. My ankles feel heavy and relaxed. My knees feel heavy and relaxed. My hips feel heavy and relaxed. My feet, ankles, knees, and hips all feel heavy and relaxed."

2

"My stomach and the center of my body feel heavy and relaxed."

3

"My hands feel heavy and relaxed. My arms feel heavy and relaxed. My shoulders feel heavy and relaxed. My hands, arms, and shoulders all feel heavy and relaxed."

4

"My neck feels heavy and relaxed. My jaw feels heavy and relaxed. My face feels heavy and relaxed. My forehead feels heavy and relaxed. My neck, jaw, face and forehead all feel heavy and relaxed."

5

"My whole body feels heavy and relaxed. My whole body feels very comfortable and relaxed." Repeat these last two sentences several times.

6

Remain relaxed for 2 to 5 minutes. When you feel ready, slowly open your eyes and remain relaxed for another 2 to 5 minutes.

family to develop creative, effective distraction techniques. For example, have the patient concentrate on a spot or object in the room while he or a family member massages the painful area (or a contralateral area) slowly and rhythmically. Or have him do rhythmic breathing (with or without massage and a concentration point), combining whatever rhythms he wishes (for example, slow, deep breaths; shallow breaths; or panting). Tell him to count "in, 1, 2; out, 1, 2, 3" or to say a short word on inhalation or exhalation, to increase the complexity of the distraction and provide a focus. His breaths per minute should stay under 60 and decrease as pain subsides. If he hyperventilates, tell him to breathe into a paper bag.

Point out to the patient other possibilities for distraction. He can sing, listen to music (using headphones works especially well), or tap his foot and massage to music, turning the volume up as pain worsens and down as pain subsides.

If a certain distraction doesn't work,

CLOSING THE GATE ON PAIN

What's the first thing you do when you stub a toe or bang an elbow? You rub the injured area to "make it better." In fact, this instinctive response can actually relieve pain by blocking its impulses before they can reach the brain. The gate control theory of pain, proposed by Melzack and Wall, explains how this works.

According to this theory, pain results from stimulation of small-diameter nerve fibers. These sensory (afferent) fibers penetrate the dorsal horn of the spinal cord and terminate within the spinal substantia gelatinosa. When sensory stimulation reaches a critical level, a so-called gate in the substantia gelatinosa opens, allowing transmission of the pain message to the brain.

In contrast, large-diameter sensory fibers function to inhibit pain transmission. Stimulation of these fast-conducting afferent fibers opposes the smaller fibers' input and causes the substantia gelatinosa gate to close, thus blocking pain transmission. In addition, descending (efferent) impulses along various tracts from the brain and brain stem can enhance or reduce pain transmission at the gate.

Unlike earlier pain theories, the gate control theory explains how external measures and cognitive strategies can affect pain transmission. For example, stimulation of large-diameter nerve fibers through massage, heat or cold application, or transcutaneous electrical nerve stimulation can override sensory input and block pain transmission at the gate. Cognitive strategies, such as distraction and relaxation breathing (which operate through the descending fibers), can also reduce pain by closing the gate.

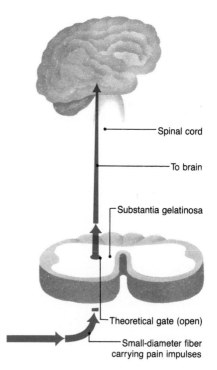

- Spinal cord
- To brain
- Substantia gelatinosa
- Theoretical gate (open)
- Small-diameter fiber carrying pain impulses

How we perceive pain
This illustration shows how pain impulses traveling along a small-diameter nerve fiber pass through an open gate in the substantia gelatinosa, then travel to the brain for interpretation.

encourage the patient to make it more or less complex or to explore new ideas with his family's help.

• *Massage.* Explain to the patient that this simple, instinctive response to pain provides both physical and mental comfort and can be used to relieve most types of acute or chronic pain, especially in the neck or back muscles. Given an accessible pain site, the patient may be able to perform it himself. Otherwise, he'll need to rely on a family member.

Describe how massage is believed to

Spinal cord

To brain

Large-diameter fiber carrying nonpain impulses

Substantia gelatinosa

Theoretical gate (closed)

Small-diameter fiber carrying pain impulses

What blocks pain transmission
Impulses carried by a large-diameter fiber can close the gate to small-fiber impulses, blocking pain transmission.

block pain transmission. (See *Closing the Gate on Pain.*) Explain that besides helping to alleviate pain, massage is an excellent way for the family to convey concern and become involved with the patient's care. It also offers an opportunity to observe for poor muscle tone, localized spasm or tension, and areas of poor circulation, pressure, or skin breakdown.

To make massage most effective, explain the importance of a soothing environment, comfortable massage surface, warm hands, and a lotion lubricant. Then teach the patient and family the various massage strokes that promote sedation, muscle relaxation or stimulation, and circulation. (See *How to Give a Back Massage,* page 598.)

Massage is safe for most patients, but caution family members to proceed with the strokes slowly, so the patient can adjust to them. Also warn against massaging calf muscles in a patient with thrombophlebitis, and point out that the obese or very muscular patient requires greater pressure to stimulate muscles.

• *Self-hypnosis.* Explain to the patient that self-hypnosis provides pain control through a heightened form of imagery that induces a state of intensely focused concentration. This concentration theoretically allows pain signals to be processed in the brain at an unconscious level and prevents the signals from penetrating to the consciousness.

Explain that self-hypnosis is effective for acute and chronic pain and can provide long-lasting pain relief. Since it's the object of much misunderstanding, reassure your patient that, although it will heighten his suggestibility to ideas, he'll still be in control of his behavior. In fact, self-hypnosis involves alertness, concentration, and individual control.

Inform your patient that self-hypnosis should be taught by a trained therapist. If appropriate, help him find a reputable therapist.

Once the patient's familiar with self-hypnosis, guide him in its use: Tell him to find a quiet room, to assume a com-

HOW TO GIVE A BACK MASSAGE

Dear Caregiver:

Before giving the person in your care a back massage, make sure your nails are trimmed and your hands are warm. Then follow these steps.

1

Position the person on his abdomen or side, with his back exposed. The room should be comfortably warm so he doesn't become chilled.

2

Apply a nonoily lotion to the person's skin to reduce friction. Warm the lotion first by placing the bottle in a bowl of warm water.

3

Using a circular thumb stroke, massage from the buttocks to the shoulders. Then, using a smooth stroke, return to the buttocks.

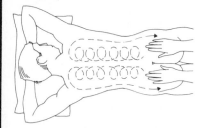

Be sure to keep your hands

parallel to the spine to avoid tickling the person.

4

Next, using your palm, stroke from the buttocks up to the shoulders, over the upper arms, and back to the buttocks. Use slightly less pressure on downward strokes.

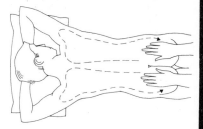

5

Using your thumb and forefinger, knead and stroke half the back and the upper arm, starting at the buttocks and moving toward the shoulder. Then knead and stroke the other half of the back, rhythmically alternating your hands.

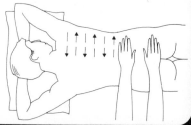

fortable position, and to loosen any tight clothing. Have him begin one of the relaxation breathing techniques. As his breathing slows and he becomes more relaxed, point out the physical signs of relaxation—heavy eyelids, decreased eye focus, limb heaviness, muscle relaxation, warmth, drowsiness, and tingling in the extremities. To deepen relaxation, tell him to count slowly backward.

Then tell the patient to focus on the positive image he selected ahead of time, such as a tranquil garden. The therapist will already have given him a posthypnotic suggestion about his power to induce relaxation, comfort, and analgesia. Now and throughout the procedure, you'll reinforce this ability.

Toward the end of the session, the patient can come out of hypnosis by imagining himself ascending a stairway or by counting forward. Afterward, tell him to relax with his eyes open and to gradually readjust to his environment.

Encourage the patient to adapt your suggestions to his own pain experience and to experiment until he finds the strategies that feel right for him. With practice, he'll be able to hypnotize himself within a few minutes.

• *Transcutaneous electrical nerve stimulation (TENS).* Explain that TENS is a noninvasive method of controlling pain. It consists of a battery-powered generator that delivers a mild electrical current through electrodes placed on the skin at or near the painful area. The current blocks transmission of pain impulses directly or by stimulating the release of endorphins.

The typical TENS user has chronic pain, such as low back pain, sciatica, or headaches. But the device is also effective in many acute musculoskeletal conditions: after knee, hip, or lower back surgery; for phantom limb pain, peripheral neuralgia, rheumatoid arthritis, or reflex sympathetic dystrophy; and for pain following cholecystectomy or thoracotomy—or for any postoperative pain in patients whose recovery could be complicated by narcotics.

Explain to the surgical patient that his TENS unit will be applied either in the operating room or immediately after he returns to his room. Reassure him that the current produces only a pleasant buzzing, tingling, vibrating, or massaging sensation and that the device is small enough to attach to his belt, so he can move about.

Teach the patient and his family how to use their unit. Advise them to try various electrode placements and to experiment with the device to find the most effective settings, but stress that an increase in intensity doesn't always provide relief; sometimes a decrease helps just as much. Inform the patient that to achieve effective pain relief, you'll need his input in adjusting these settings. For postoperative pain, he'll gradually decrease the duration and intensity of stimulation until he discontinues using the unit after 24 hours of nonuse. For chronic pain, he'll decrease duration and intensity until he finds an effective level of pain relief. Warn him to avoid using the unit for longer than 45 minutes; prolonged use may result in decreased effectiveness and skin irritation.

Emphasize to the patient and his family that they should become adept at making these adjustments, but warn them to change settings carefully, since the stimulator dials are quite sensitive. Once they find the desired setting, they should tape the dials in place.

If the patient will be going home with the TENS device, show him how to care for his surgical dressings, so he can check under the electrodes for dermatitis. Tell him that wound drainage is only a problem when excessive amounts disrupt electrode contact.

Also teach how to troubleshoot for problems if pain isn't relieved despite increased stimulation (loose electrodes and cable connections; weak battery; defective unit) or if a burn or shock results, especially with movement (buckling or loose electrodes, or elec-

TEACHING PATIENTS ABOUT DRUGS FOR PAIN

DRUG	ADVERSE REACTIONS	INTERACTIONS*
Narcotic adjuvants		
alprazolam (Xanax) **diazepam** (Valium) **lorazepam** (Ativan)	*Reportable:* confusion, depression *Other:* blurred vision, clumsiness, drowsiness, headache, nausea, vomiting, unusual weakness	• Tell the patient to avoid CNS depressants, such as antihistamines, and alcohol. • Inform him that nonalcoholic beverages and food don't influence the safety or effectiveness of these narcotic adjuvants.
amitriptyline (Elavil) **desipramine** (Norpramin) **doxepin** (Adapin, Sinequan) **imipramine** (Tofranil)	*Reportable:* blurred vision, confusion, severe constipation, irregular heartbeat, hypotension, unusually slow or fast pulse, shakiness, decreased urine output *Other:* mild constipation, dizziness, drowsiness, dry mouth, GI upset, headache, nausea, tiredness, weakness	• Tell the patient to avoid CNS depressants (such as antihistamines), products containing sympathomimetics (such as ephedrine), and alcohol. • Inform him that nonalcoholic beverages and food don't influence the safety or effectiveness of these narcotic adjuvants.
hydroxyzine (Vistaril)	*Reportable:* shakiness, trembling, rash *Other:* drowsiness, dry mouth	• Tell the patient to avoid CNS depressants, such as antihistamines, and alcohol. Inform him that nonalcoholic beverages and food don't influence the safety or effectiveness of hydroxyzine.
Narcotic analgesics		
codeine sulfate **hydromorphone** (Dilaudid) **methadone** (Dolophine) **morphine sulfate** **oxycodone** (Percocet, Percodan, Tylox) **propoxyphene** (Darvon)	*Reportable:* unusually slow breathing; confusion; unusually fast, slow, or pounding heartbeat *Other:* constipation, diaphoresis, dizziness, drowsiness, headache, unusual tiredness or weakness	• Tell the patient to avoid CNS depressants, such as antihistamines, and alcohol. • Inform him that nonalcoholic beverages and food don't influence the safety or effectiveness of this narcotic analgesic.

*Interactions include food, alcohol, and over-the-counter (OTC) drugs.

TEACHING POINTS

• Explain to the patient that the prescribed drug should reduce his anxiety, tension, and depression (especially if these symptoms are associated with chronic pain) by relaxing his muscles.
• Because drowsiness and incoordination occur during initial treatment, caution the pa-

tient to avoid activities requiring alertness at this time.
• Warn him not to discontinue the drug abruptly to avoid withdrawal symptoms.
• Remind him to also try other treatments for anxiety, depression, and pain, such as relaxation techniques.

• Explain to the patient that the prescribed drug should start reducing his depression, anxiety, and insomnia (especially if these symptoms are associated with chronic pain) within several days; however, its full effect won't be felt for several weeks.
• Because heavy sedation occurs during the first few days of treatment, tell the patient to check with the doctor about taking the entire dose at bedtime.
• Caution him to avoid activities requiring alertness during the first few days of treatment until heavy sedation subsides.
• Instruct the patient to take the drug with food if he experiences GI upset.

• Advise him to rise slowly from a sitting or lying position to minimize dizziness, lightheadedness, and fainting due to hypotension.
• Warn him not to discontinue the drug abruptly, as this can cause nausea, insomnia, muscle aches, and irritability.
• Discuss measures to prevent or relieve constipation, such as adding dietary fiber.
• Encourage the patient to rinse his mouth frequently and chew sugarless gum or suck on ice chips to relieve dry mouth.
• Caution the diabetic to monitor his blood glucose level closely, since this drug may raise or lower it.

• Explain to the patient that this drug should make his narcotic more effective in relieving pain and thus allow him to take a lower dose with fewer side effects. It should also promote comfort by relaxing his muscles and

decreasing tension, intestinal spasms, nausea, and vomiting.
• Suggest that he chew sugarless gum or suck on ice chips to relieve mouth and throat dryness.

• Explain to the patient that the prescribed drug should relieve moderate to severe pain and reduce anxiety.
• Explain that this drug is most effective when taken *before* pain becomes intense. Regularly scheduled doses often provide more consistent pain relief than doses ordered "as needed."
• Remind him to use this drug only for severe pain. When pain decreases, he should use a less potent pain reliever to avoid drug dependence and tolerance.

• Caution the patient to avoid activities requiring concentration, balance, and coordination, because narcotic analgesics can impair these functions.
• Advise him to rise slowly from a sitting or lying position to minimize dizziness, lightheadedness, and fainting due to lowered blood pressure.
• Discuss measures to prevent constipation, such as adding dietary fiber or fluids or increasing activity.

(continued)

**TEACHING PATIENTS ABOUT
DRUGS FOR PAIN** (continued)

DRUG	ADVERSE REACTIONS	INTERACTIONS*
Nonnarcotic analgesics		
acetaminophen (Tylenol)	*Reportable:* bloody urine, rash, signs of acute poisoning (chills, coma, delirium, diarrhea, excitation, fever, palpitations, psychological changes, seizures, sweating, vomiting, weakness), painful urination, yellowing of eyes and skin	• Tell the patient to avoid analgesics (including aspirin) and heavy alcohol consumption. • Inform him that nonalcoholic beverages and food don't influence the safety or effectiveness of acetaminophen.
aspirin (Bayer Aspirin, Ecotrin, St. Joseph's Aspirin for Children) **buffered aspirin** (Ascriptin, Bufferin) **choline and magnesium salicylates** (Trilisate) **magnesium salicylate** (Doan's Pills) **salsalate** (Disalcid)	*Reportable:* abdominal pain, bloody stools, bloody urine, unusually fast or deep breathing, chest tightness, confusion, severe diarrhea, severe drowsiness, uncontrollable flapping of hands, hallucinations, hearing loss, severe nausea, seizures, unusual sweating, unusual thirst, tinnitus, visual disturbances, vomiting (especially bloody or resembling coffee grounds), wheezing *Other:* heartburn, indigestion	• Tell the patient to avoid acetaminophen, antacids, other aspirin or salicylate products, cellulose-containing laxatives, and alcohol. • Inform him that nonalcoholic beverages and food don't influence the safety or effectiveness of aspirin or salicylates.
Nonsteroidal anti-inflammatory agents		
diflunisal (Dolobid) **ibuprofen** (Advil, Motrin, Nuprin) **indomethacin** (Indocin, Indocin SR) **meclofenamate** (Meclomen) **naproxen** (Anaprox, Naprosyn) **suprofen** (Suprol)	*Reportable:* unusual bleeding, bloody or tarry stools, bloody urine, blurred vision, rash, sore throat, swelling, decreased urine output, wheezing, yellowing of skin or eyes *Other:* diarrhea, dizziness, drowsiness, heartburn, indigestion, nausea, vomiting	• Tell the patient to avoid aspirin, acetaminophen, and alcohol. • Instruct him to take this drug on an empty stomach 1 hour before meals or 3 hours after meals for best absorption.
Sedative-hypnotics (benzodiazepine derivatives)		
flurazepam (Dalmane) **temazepam** (Restoril) **triazolam** (Halcion)	*Reportable:* confusion, depression *Other:* blurred vision, clumsiness, drowsiness, unusual weakness	• Tell the patient to avoid CNS depressants, such as antihistamines, and alcohol.

*Interactions include food, alcohol, and over-the-counter (OTC) drugs.

TEACHING POINTS

• Explain to the patient that this drug should relieve mild to moderate pain but will not reduce inflammation. When used in conjunction with a narcotic analgesic, acetaminophen can enhance pain relief and thus allow a lower narcotic dose with fewer side effects.
• Tell him that this drug takes effect 15 to 30 minutes after ingestion and provides relief for 3 to 5 hours.
• Advise against prolonged or excessive use of this drug, and urge the patient to see his doctor if pain, inflammation, or fever persists.
• If the patient has a bleeding or gastric disorder or is on anticoagulants, explain that this drug is an alternative to aspirin-containing analgesics.

• Explain to the patient that the prescribed drug should relieve mild to moderate pain (especially due to inflammation), reduce fever, and help prevent blood clots.
• Instruct him to take aspirin with food, milk, or a full glass of water to decrease stomach irritation. Inform him that enteric-coated aspirin (Ecotrin) avoids irritation by preventing drug breakdown in the stomach; commercially buffered aspirin (Bufferin) is only as effective in reducing irritation as food or milk.
• Advise against prolonged use of this drug.

If fever or pain persists, tell him to consult his doctor.
• If the patient requires large doses of aspirin to treat inflammation, tell him to maintain a regular dosage schedule to keep his blood levels constant. Emphasize that he must watch for early signs of overdose—tinnitus, dizziness, or impaired vision or hearing.
• Inform him that Trilisate causes less stomach irritation than aspirin and other salicylates and may also be taken less frequently.

• Explain to the patient that the prescribed drug should relieve mild to moderate pain. Note that it causes less stomach irritation than aspirin and doesn't interfere with blood clotting.
• However, suggest taking this drug with food, milk, or antacids if stomach irritation occurs.

• Caution him not to exceed the recommended dosage, since this increases the risk of adverse reactions. If his symptoms don't improve in a week, tell him to call the doctor.
• Tell him to use caution when performing activities that require alertness, since he may experience drowsiness and dizziness, especially during initial drug therapy.

• Explain to the patient that the prescribed drug should help him fall asleep. Note that it might not be effective for the first few nights, but that he should keep taking it anyway.
• Advise him to take this drug 1 to 2 hours before bedtime.

• Caution him not to perform any tasks requiring alertness after taking this drug.
• Instruct the female patient of child-bearing age to discontinue this drug immediately if she suspects that she's pregnant.

trodes placed less than their own width apart). Supply written instructions for the patient to refer to at home.

Warn the patient to watch for itching, skin irritation, and electrical burns resulting from some electrodes. If these occur, he should substitute hand cream or hydrocortisone cream for the conductive jelly, try another brand of jelly, change the type of adhesive tape or electrode, or vary electrode position. Also warn him never to immerse the unit in water and to turn off the unit during bathing to prevent electrical malfunction.

Drug therapy

Explain to your patient and his family that analgesics can modify pain perception without causing loss of consciousness. They're considered one of the most effective, reliable, and fast-acting pain control methods and can be combined with other techniques.

Although analgesics relieve all types of pain, point out that what works well for one patient may not work as well for another. Also point out that how a drug affects pain depends on the pain's severity, the drug used, the dosage, the route, the time of administration, and the patient's individual response. As with other types of pain control, finding the best combination is sometimes a matter of trial and error.

Inform the patient and his family that analgesics come in many forms—narcotics and their adjuvants (antidepressants and anxiolytics) and nonsteroidal anti-inflammatory drugs (see *Teaching Patients about Drugs for Pain*, pages 600 to 603). Then provide details about the patient's prescribed drugs. To break the pain cycle, emphasize that drugs must be taken on time or at the first prodromal symptom (as appropriate), *before* pain becomes severe. Explain peak effect time, and suggest that the patient schedule difficult tasks approximately ½ hour after taking his analgesic or that he try to perform these tasks when he feels the full drug effect. Also clarify your patient's drug order

by defining any directions, such as "p.r.n.," "b.i.d.," or "around-the-clock."

Teach your patient how to evaluate the effectiveness of his analgesic, and alert him to possible side effects. Tell him not to hesitate to call you or the doctor if his analgesic doesn't seem strong enough or effective for a long enough time, or if it seems to have stopped working altogether. If he's taking narcotics, reassure him that he won't become addicted if he takes them for a limited time. However, he should avoid their prolonged use for chronic pain unrelated to cancer.

Explain that analgesics are administered in several different ways—orally, I.M., I.V., or through special infusion systems. Patients on oral analgesics typically need little assistance or monitoring. However, patients receiving drugs I.M. or by infusion need help from family members. Even if the patient can take his own analgesics, be sure to include his family in your teaching.

• **Oral administration.** If your patient's taking his drugs orally, explain that this route has many advantages over other methods for long-term relief of chronic pain. Convenient and least expensive, it allows the patient maximum independence in controlling his pain. It also requires minimal learning: to interpret label directions, to follow the administration schedule correctly, and to recognize and report adverse effects.

Urge the patient to drink plenty of fluids with his analgesics. This prevents their lodging in his throat or esophagus, promotes dissolution, enhances drug passage into the small intestine, and increases absorption. Also remind him to follow the instructions on the medication label carefully, since some analgesics shouldn't be taken on an empty stomach or with antacids.

• **I.M. administration.** This route is usually ordered for patients who can't take food or liquids by mouth or who require analgesics that aren't as effective or well-absorbed when given orally.

If your patient's being discharged on I.M. analgesics, teach him and his family how to select injection sites and give the injections. (See *How to Give an Intramuscular Injection*, pages 606 to 609.) Explain how to assess for muscle, nerve, tissue, and bone damage. Tell him that after repeated injections, he may experience variable or decreased pain relief due to poor absorption, decreased muscle mass, lumps from previous injections, or variations in technique. Tell him to call the doctor immediately if any of these develop.

Because the patient may find the injections painful, give him this tip: puncture the skin quickly, inject slowly, and remove the needle quickly. Then apply ice to the site immediately.

• *I.V. administration.* This route is usually ordered for patients in severe acute or chronic pain or when the oral or I.M. route is unfeasible or ineffective. Explain to your patient and his family that I.V. administration provides immediate pain relief. Because the analgesic's administered directly into the bloodstream, relief is more rapid and the effective dose is often lower than with other methods, resulting in fewer side effects. However, the duration of action is usually shorter than with oral or I.M. administration.

If the patient's being discharged on I.V. analgesics, teach him and his family how to give the injections and monitor the equipment for proper function. Explain how to assess the degree of pain relief by noting the lowest effective dose and the duration of relief. Also inform them of possible side effects.

• *Continuous narcotic infusion (CNI).* This method delivers morphine or other narcotics continuously. It's usually ordered for patients with severe, chronic pain (for example, those with cancer) when regular I.V. therapy isn't possible or effective. Explain to your patient and his family that CNI provides stable analgesic levels for continuous pain control with few side ef-

fects. And it offers relief from the anxiety of waiting for analgesics to be administered or to take effect. Inform them that several boluses of analgesic may be required before an effective dose is established and that higher doses may still be needed later during increased pain. Once pain control has been established, the doctor will reduce the infusion rate to the lowest effective dose.

Because the patient on CNI can't be discharged until someone at home can monitor for side effects and care for the system, prepare family members for their responsibilities. Remind them that the dosage has been based on the patient's comfort level and tolerance of the analgesic without side effects, so they must never change it without checking with the doctor. Teach them how to assess the patient's comfort level by observing for signs of pain: restlessness, grimacing, guarding, and increased blood pressure and pulse. Teach the patient how to chart the effectiveness of the CNI through recordings in a pain diary. Also teach the family how to assess the patient's respiratory rate and level of alertness, especially during initial treatment and with dosage increases. Urge them to notify the doctor immediately if respiratory depression or any other adverse effects occur.

Since the family will need to purchase or rent an infusion system, supply the names of medical supply companies or home health care agencies specializing in I.V. therapy. After the equipment arrives, ensure that they know how to set it up and monitor it, and tell them about any specific precautions. For example, they mustn't immerse the system in water, expose the I.V. line to temperature extremes, or use the infusion pump around strong static electricity or electromagnetic fields. Then review with them the infusion process and other specifics for their type of CNI system.

Ambulatory infusion pumps attach to a specially designed harness or belt

HOW TO GIVE AN INTRAMUSCULAR INJECTION

Dear Patient:

To give yourself an intramuscular injection, follow these steps.

Selecting an injection site

First, choose from the sites illustrated here. The top and side of the thigh and the space just above the hip are most commonly used. If another person is giving you the injection, he may use the buttock sites or the upper arm. If possible, though, he should avoid using the upper arm, because the muscle there is small and very close to the brachial nerve.

If you'll be giving yourself a series of injections, rotate the sites. To reduce pain and improve drug absorption, don't use the same site twice in a row.

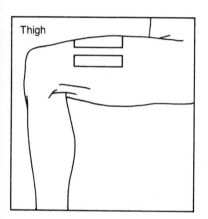

Thigh

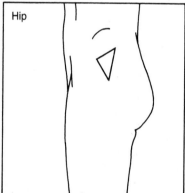

Hip

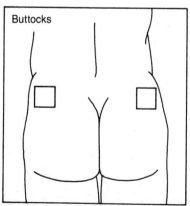

Buttocks

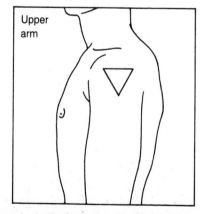

Upper arm

Giving the injection

1

Wash your hands and gather medication, alcohol swabs, syringe, and needle. Check the expiration date and make sure the medication's correct.

2

Remove the top of the medication bottle, and wipe the rubber stopper with an alcohol swab. Unwrap the syringe, and remove the needle shield.

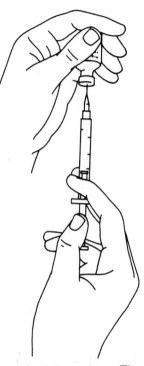

3

Pull back on the plunger of the syringe until you've drawn air into it in an amount equal to the medication you'll be injecting. Then inject this air into the bottle through the rubber stopper, without withdrawing the needle. This will prevent formation of a vacuum and will make withdrawing the medication easier.

the side of the syringe. Then withdraw the needle from the bottle.

4

Invert the medication bottle. With the needle positioned below the fluid level, draw the medication into the syringe by pulling back on the plunger, measuring the correct amount by checking the markings on

(continued)

HOW TO GIVE AN INTRAMUSCULAR INJECTION *(continued)*

5

Next, check for air bubbles. If you see any, hold the syringe with the needle pointing up, and tap the syringe lightly so the bubbles rise to its top. Then push the air out, and, if necessary, draw up more medication to obtain the correct amount.

Again hold the syringe with the needle pointing up, and pull back on the plunger just a little bit more. This will cause a tiny air bubble to form inside the syringe; when you inject the medication, this bubble will help clear the needle and keep the medication from seeping out of the injection site. Replace the needle shield.

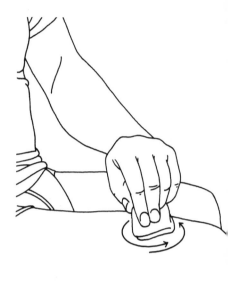

6

Check the injection site for any lumps or depressions in the skin. Then gently tap the site to stimulate nerve endings and minimize the initial pain of injection.

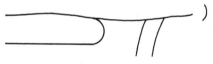

Let the skin dry for 5 to 10 seconds. If it's not dry, the injection might push some of the alcohol into the skin, causing a burning sensation.

7

Clean the site with an alcohol swab, beginning at the center and wiping outward in a circular pattern to move dirt particles away from the site.

8

Remove the needle shield. Now, with one hand, stretch the skin taut around the injection site. This makes inserting the needle easier and helps disperse the medication after the injection.

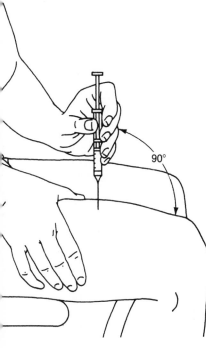

thing and start again. If no blood appears, inject the medication slowly, keeping the syringe and needle at a 90-degree angle. Never push the plunger forcefully.

10

When you've injected all the medication, press an alcohol swab over the needle and injection site, and withdraw the needle at the same angle as you inserted it.

Massage the site with the alcohol swab to help distribute the medication and promote its absorption.

11

To dispose of the used syringe and needle, first replace the shield on the needle. Then, holding the syringe, snap off the needle and shield. Put both in a covered shoe box, used only for disposal of needles and syringes. Keep the box in a safe place, out of a child's reach.

With your other hand, hold the syringe and needle at a 90-degree angle to the injection site and insert the needle with a quick thrust.

9

Holding the syringe firmly in place, pull back slightly on the plunger. If blood appears in the syringe, you've entered a blood vessel. Take the needle out and press an alcohol swab over the site. Then discard every-

and allow the patient to ambulate during treatment. They include a power pack, pump, disposable medication bag, and adjustable flow meter, and they provide a continuous infusion by the I.V. or subcutaneous route. Explain to the patient and his family that the doctor, pharmacist, or nurse will usually fill the medication delivery chamber, but that the rest will be up to them. Show them how to connect the pump to the I.V. tubing and prime the line, regulate the pump, connect the alarm system, and spot any mechanical problems. Be sure to describe the signs of infiltration. Also give the patient tips on how to perform activities while wearing the pump.

Implantable infusion pumps are surgically implanted systems that deliver a continuous infusion from a reservoir chamber to the vascular space. Typically, they're used for patients who require prolonged I.V. administration of medications when repeated venipuncture must be avoided and when vascular access is limited.

Implantable infusion ports are metal or plastic ports about 1″ in diameter that are placed under the skin of the patient's chest wall during surgery. The port will be attached to a silicone catheter inserted in a large artery or vein. Medication will be injected by a special needle into the port through the skin, either intermittently or by an I.V. line attached for continuous medication delivery.

Explain that this system is completely internal (only a small bump is visible), requires minimal care, rarely causes infection, and doesn't interfere with the patient's usual activities. Once the initial incision heals, the patient won't need a dressing, except during medication administration. Point out that medication delivery is usually started in the doctor's office or hospital outpatient clinic and that the patient returns home with the system attached to a small infusion pump. After that, heparinization to keep the line patent and to prevent clot formation is re-

quired only monthly and can be done in the doctor's office.

When appropriate, teach the patient and his family to access the infusion port for medication delivery, flushing, and heparinization. First, instruct them to wash their hands and put on sterile gloves. Then show them how to locate and stabilize the port by palpation and to cleanse the site with povidone-iodine. Next, demonstrate attaching a Huber (noncoring) needle to the appropriate syringe, extension, or I.V. tubing; inserting the syringe into the port; and applying a dressing to the site to protect needle placement during medication administration. Explain to them how to regulate, monitor, and discontinue the infusion, and how to perform a saline flush and heparinization.

Patient-controlled analgesia (PCA) systems allow the patient to regulate administration of his own pain medication. They consist of a computerized infusion device that piggybacks into the tubing for the I.V. or vascular access port. PCA systems are especially effective after surgery or major trauma, during sickle cell crisis, and with intractable cancer pain. The larger systems attach to I.V. poles; the new lightweight, portable models can be worn on a belt. PCA systems can be programmed to deliver narcotics three ways—at a continuous rate, at a continuous rate with intermittent boluses, or by bolus only—and specific systems may vary.

Explain to the patient that he'll press a button to administer a predetermined dose of narcotic (usually 0.5 to 1.5 mg of morphine sulfate) as needed for pain relief. Reassure him that the dose, refractory period, and maximum number of doses per hour are preprogrammed into the device by the doctor, so the patient can't accidentally overdose. Also explain that the device records how many times the patient attempts to obtain medication—information that helps determine the optimum dosage, the interval between doses, and the infusion rate.

Tell the patient and his family that the doctor will order the medication, dosage, concentration, and method of delivery. The pharmacist, doctor, or nurse will fill the detachable medication cassette under sterile conditions, and the medication cassette and programming instructions for medication delivery will be locked into the unit.

Then, working with their specific unit, teach the patient and his family how to attach the tubing to the pump, prime the pump, piggyback the tubing to the I.V. or vascular access port, and (if the pump is portable) secure the unit to the I.V. pole or patient pouch. They'll also need to know how to monitor the unit and I.V. line for correct function, how the alarm system works, and how to deal with characteristic mechanical problems.

SUPPORT

Every patient, regardless of his specific illness or treatment, needs emotional and physical support to help him cope with his condition, changes in body image, pain, or impending death. He—and his family—will be forced to draw on emotional reserves. But they'll also need all the help they can get from outside sources, such as friends, clergymen, health professionals, and support groups.

Although you can teach the patient and his family how to promote physical comfort, you can't teach them how to gain inner strength or how to give emotional support. But you *can* give them advice on dealing with illness, loss, and death. For example, you can tell them about the five stages of psychological coping that terminally ill patients or patients experiencing changes in body image or other types of loss often go

through. You can also reassure them that their ambivalent feelings are normal, even constructive.

Help the patient and his family learn to cope by stressing the importance of being honest and direct about their feelings. For the patient, this can mean coming to terms with his illness and opening the lines of communication with family and friends. For family members, this can mean working through their own feelings and becoming closer to the patient.

Family members should know that feelings of anxiety, guilt, and anger are normal responses for them. And the patient should know that feelings of uselessness, being a burden, losing control of physical or mental function, or being dependent on others represent normal reactions to chronic pain and disability, serious illness, or impending death. Often, though, the patient will be reluctant to voice these fears. So tell the family that they should ask open-ended questions to draw the patient out. These questions, which require more than a yes or no answer, allow the patient to express his feelings. A family member might ask, for example, "How does being in bed all the time make you feel?"

Emphasize that honesty can be hard for everyone involved. Family members and friends may feel uncomfortable at first, hearing the patient admit his feelings. And the patient will probably be quite sensitive to other people's reactions to his illness. So advise them all to be prepared for these eventualities and to try to be as understanding and compassionate as possible.

Explain that quiet time with the patient can be productive, too, and that families don't have to provide all the answers or always say "the right thing." Also urge them to express their feelings openly to each other, especially concerning role changes in the family. If they feel that outside help is needed, suggest support groups or recommend that they talk to a psychiatrist, family counselor, or clergyman.

Stress the importance of promoting the patient's sense of dignity and self-worth. Encourage the patient to retain some independence by doing everything he can within the limits of his condition. Urge him to be assertive about his need for privacy and "personal space." At the same time, encourage the family to include the patient in their activities, so he can lead as normal a life as possible. Tell them not to be afraid to say "no" to the patient; this encourages his independence and keeps him from assuming the "sick" role.

Also encourage the family to spend time away from the patient, and tell them that they needn't feel guilty for needing or doing this. Suggest that they ask another family member or friend to stay with the patient occasionally to ease their burden of responsibility.

Five Stages of Coping

Whether the patient's experiencing a loss related to his functional ability, body image, or impending death, he may go through various stages of coping—from denial to acceptance. Explain the stages of coping to him, stressing that what he's feeling is perfectly normal. Ask him how he's coped with loss or illness in the past, and encourage him to use these methods again if they were effective.

Stage 1: Denial
Explain that denial is a healthy defense mechanism when a patient first confronts loss. It acts as a buffer until he can develop long-term coping strategies.

Advise the family just to listen to the patient at this stage—he needs to express his feelings before he can progress to a more effective stage of coping. But caution them not to reinforce the

denial; instead, they should gradually present reality, as the patient gives clues that he's ready to accept it. Tell family members that they, too, can benefit from a sympathetic ear now.

Stage 2: Anger
Explain that, as denial begins to fail as a defense mechanism, anger often takes its place. At this stage, many patients try to control the situation by becoming demanding.

Advise the family to allow the patient maximum decision-making power in his care. Reinforce the importance of listening. Even though the patient might seem to be directing his anger at them, tell the family that he's simply responding to his own feelings of frustration and helplessness. And to cope with their own anger, suggest that family members talk honestly and openly together or with close friends to vent their frustrations.

Stage 3: Bargaining
Explain that at this stage, the patient attempts to postpone the loss or inevitable death, often by bargaining for time through promises to God (which may be kept secret). Again, impress on the family that the best approach is listening in a nonjudgmental manner. If the patient makes his bargains known to them but can't keep his promises, encourage the family to help alleviate his fears and guilt. And if family members find themselves engaged in similar bargaining, once again encourage them to confide in one another or in a close friend.

Stage 4: Depression
Explain that as the illness progresses, the patient becomes overwhelmed by the impact of the loss, and guilt and depression set in. Advise the family to do more talking at this stage—because the patient will be doing less. However, tell them to avoid trying to "cheer him up," since this only amplifies what's being lost or left behind.

Do urge them to allow the patient

time to be quiet and reflect. If he expresses guilt over leaving his family, unpaid debts, or uncompleted tasks, encourage the family to reassure him that things are under control by saying something like, "You've provided well for us. We'll really miss you, but we'll learn to manage." Also urge the family to be demonstrative and to touch the patient often. This can truly be more reassuring than words—for everyone involved.

Tell the patient and his family that, at this stage, they both need support from other family members, friends, and hospital staff. However, caution the family not to assume that the patient will automatically snap out of his depression—he might not. So teach them to evaluate its severity: Does the patient talk about suicide? Has he attempted it in the past? Has anyone else in the family ever been seriously depressed or suicidal? Does the patient have severe insomnia or anorexia? If so, suggest that they consult the doctor about ordering antidepressant medication and arranging psychological counseling.

If family members seem depressed, you might help them find a psychiatrist, family counselor, or support group. If they're churchgoers, encourage them to talk to their clergyman and attend services with the patient, if possible.

Stage 5: Acceptance

Explain that at this stage, the patient disengages himself from family, friends, and former life, often communicating less and becoming less involved with worldly events. Tell the family that he still requires support, but that he may want visitors limited to a few close friends and family. Also tell the patient that his family may need *his* support at this time, since they might not yet have arrived at the acceptance stage.

Abnormal grieving

Because everyone faces loss or death in his own way, "normal" behaviors vary.

However, some patients and family members react to grief in potentially harmful ways. Tell the family to watch carefully for these signs of abnormal coping in the patient: lack of emotional expression; reclusive behavior; severe depression; excessive feelings of guilt, bitterness, or self-reproach; or excessive activity with no apparent sense of loss. If they recognize any of these reactions, have them encourage the patient to vent his feelings and to consult a therapist.

Explain that the two most common abnormal reactions are delayed grieving and prolonged grieving. Grief that's delayed (sometimes for years) occurs when the patient or family member becomes trapped in the denial stage, refusing to recognize his own feelings at the time of the loss (usually to maintain morale and "spare" other people). This can postpone grieving (and final acceptance of loss) indefinitely, causing the person to express his grief at some later time.

With prolonged grieving, the patient or family member may also become trapped in the denial stage. Instead of delaying grief, though, he builds his life around it. In effect, he never "snaps back."

By focusing your teaching on the need to express feelings, to anticipate the personal impact of loss, and to work through the stages of grieving, you can guide the patient and his family to a healthy resolution of grief.

MAKING A DIFFERENCE

With issues of comfort and support, your careful, perceptive teaching can mean the difference between acquiescence and control for the patient, and between passivity and active involvement for his family.

20

Health Promotion

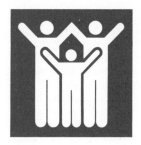

Health Promotion

Introduction

Research continues to provide mounting evidence that poor health practices contribute to a wide range of illnesses, a shortened life span, and spiraling health care costs. In contrast, good health practices have just the opposite effect: fewer illnesses, a longer life span, and lower health care costs. What's more, good health practices can benefit most people no matter at what stage of life they're begun. Of course, the earlier they're begun, the less they have to overcome. But, fortunately, later is better than never.

That's an important idea to remember, because poor health practices persist despite overwhelming evidence linking them to debilitating and even fatal illness. For example, we've known for over 20 years that smoking causes cancer and other serious illnesses. And we know that year after year far more people die from smoking-related lung disease than from car, plane, and train accidents combined. Despite this knowledge, millions still smoke.

However, on the positive side, even long-term smokers who quit may experience reversal of adverse cardiovascular and respiratory effects.

What is health promotion?

Quite simply, it's teaching good health practices and finding ways to help people correct their poor health practices. It's something that you'll do in a variety of settings—from your clinic, hospital, or patient's home to a community meeting, church social, or backyard barbecue.

But what specifically should you teach? Well, one good place to start is with the U.S. Surgeon General's 1976 report, which outlines our major health problems. This report divides the life cycle into five stages—infancy, childhood, adolescence, adulthood, and old age—and sets goals to promote health and reduce mortality for each stage.

You can use the Surgeon General's goals to direct your teaching. For example, to promote health in *infancy*, you'll need to stress the importance of prenatal care to help prevent low birth weight and certain birth defects. By educating parents about childbirth alternatives, you can also improve the chances of a safe delivery. Other topics that you'll need to cover include infant safety and nutrition.

Because accidents account for almost half of all fatalities in *childhood*, you'll need to emphasize such safety measures as consistent use of seat belts and precautions to prevent burns and poisoning. Your teaching must also stress nutrition to enhance growth and development, immunization against infectious diseases, and proper dental care.

To promote health in *adolescence*, you'll need to teach how to prevent motor vehicle accidents, drug and alcohol abuse, and suicide. You'll also need to provide information about contraception and proper care during pregnancy.

Some adolescent problems carry over into *adulthood*. However, the leading causes of death in this age-group are heart disease, cancer, and cerebrovascular accident (CVA). To promote health in adulthood, you'll need to cover such topics as how to quit smoking and how to perform self-examination of the breasts or testes.

To promote health in *old age*, you'll need to teach how to maintain independence through proper nutrition and exercise. You may also need to provide advice on coping with the effects of aging, such as hearing loss, and on preventing life-threatening infection.

HEALTH IN INFANCY

Providing Prenatal Instruction

How a woman cares for herself during pregnancy directly affects the health of her unborn infant. Two factors especially can jeopardize the infant's health: low birth weight (LBW) and birth defects. Any infant weighing less than 5½ lb (2.5 kg) at birth falls into this LBW category. Such infants are more likely to develop complications and less likely to survive them.

To promote the birth of a healthy infant, your teaching must stress the importance of early and ongoing prenatal care. Encourage a pregnant woman to schedule her first prenatal visit during the first trimester. After that, she should keep her appointments for follow-up visits, which are usually monthly through the 28th week of gestation, every 2 weeks between weeks 29 and 36, and then once a week until delivery.

During the first prenatal visit, you'll help obtain a thorough patient history and physical examination, including laboratory tests. When taking the history, be sure to ask about any genetic disorders in the patient's family and about any previous pregnancies. Next, obtain a baseline blood pressure reading, and measure the patient's height and weight. Explain laboratory tests, which may include VDRL, Pap smear, hemoglobin/hematocrit, urinalysis for glucose and protein, Rh factor and blood group, and rubella titer.

During the patient's subsequent prenatal visits, check her blood pressure and weight, and collect a urine specimen for analysis. Explain that the doctor will assess fetal well-being—usually by palpation and auscultation—and may recommend an amniocentesis, if indicated. However, focus most of your teaching efforts on prenatal nutrition and exercise and the adverse effects of cigarette smoking, alcohol, caffeine, and drugs on the fetus. Additionally, you'll want to teach her how to avoid exposure to certain infectious and toxic agents associated with birth defects. If the hospital in your area has childbirth education classes, suggest that the patient and her coach attend classes to prepare for labor and delivery and to learn about infant care.

Ensuring nutrition for two

Because the fetus relies on the mother for nourishment, poor nutrition during pregnancy can adversely affect intrauterine growth and development. Obstetricians once limited weight gain during pregnancy in the belief that smaller babies ensured easier—and thus, safer—deliveries. But now most recommend a weight gain of 25 to 30 lb during pregnancy.

This weight gain should not represent "empty calories" but a diet that's

EATING RIGHT: HELPING YOU HAVE A HEALTHY BABY

Dear Patient:

What you eat when you're pregnant affects both you and your unborn baby. That's why it's important to eat the right foods from the moment you learn you're pregnant. Just follow these nutrition tips.

Protein and calories

You need almost one and a half times the amount of protein now that you're pregnant. Choose from good protein sources, such as lean meat, milk, eggs, cheese, poultry, and fish.

You also need at least 1,800 calories per day and perhaps a lot more, depending on your height and weight. Ask your doctor or nurse-midwife for calorie requirements for a person your size. Generally, you should consume about 300 calories more per day than you usually do. When adding calories, choose from the following four groups: milk group (cheese, ice cream, and other milk products), meat group (meat, fish, poultry, eggs, cheese, or legumes), fruit and vegetable group (dark green or yellow vegetables, citrus fruit, or tomatoes), and bread and cereal group (whole grain bread or cereal, rice, or pasta).

Vitamins and minerals

Use only those supplements prescribed by your doctor or nurse-midwife. Don't take over-the-counter megavitamins since they might have an ill effect on your unborn baby.

Fiber and fluids

You need an adequate amount of fiber in your diet to help prevent constipation, which can cause hemorrhoids. Include whole grain breads and cereals, legumes, fruits, and vegetables. Add fiber to your diet gradually to avoid the possibility of diarrhea.

Remember to drink plenty of fluids, especially during the summer months and before, during, and after exercise. Unless your doctor directs otherwise, drink 4 to 6 glasses of water plus another 2 to 4 glasses of fluid each day.

Cautious consumption

Many health professionals advise steering clear or reducing consumption of "junk foods," dietetic products, caffeinated beverages like coffee and regular colas, and alcohol during pregnancy. Check with your doctor or nurse-midwife for instructions.

geared to the nutritional needs of the mother and her unborn child.

• **Caloric intake.** Advise the pregnant woman to increase her caloric intake by about 300 calories per day, depending on how rapidly she's gaining weight. Generally, she should be eating no fewer than 1,800 calories per day.

Make sure she understands the importance of selecting nutritious foods—and not "junk food"—to bolster her caloric intake. Also explain how the body metabolizes protein for energy if caloric intake is inadequate. This, in turn, robs the mother and fetus of protein for tissue growth.

• **Protein requirements.** Pregnancy increases a woman's protein requirement from 44 g of protein per day to 74 g per day. This extra protein supports increased maternal blood volume and tissue growth in the uterus, breasts, placenta, and fetus.

Because the American diet is high in protein, most expectant mothers are in no danger of protein deficiency. However, encourage the pregnant woman to eat high-quality protein of animal origin, such as plenty of meat, milk, eggs, cheese, poultry, and fish. If she's a vegetarian, teach her about protein alternatives, such as legumes, nuts, and meat analogues (soy).

• **Vitamin and mineral supplements.** Teach the pregnant woman that vitamins and minerals are intended to supplement, not replace, a well-balanced diet. Tell her to take prenatal vitamins and possibly an iron supplement, as directed by her obstetrician or nurse-midwife.

• **Salt restrictions.** Instruct her to limit her use of salt and to avoid high-sodium foods to prevent fluid retention.

• **Fiber.** To avoid constipation and hemorrhoids during pregnancy, teach the pregnant woman to add fiber—such as whole grain breads, high-fiber cereals, legumes, and fruits and vegetables—to her diet.

• **Fluid requirements.** Help her stay well hydrated during pregnancy by recommending that she drink at least 8 glasses of fluid each day, including 4 to 6 glasses of water.

Promoting fitness

The benefits of prenatal exercise are many. For example, it can reduce or eliminate back pain, stress, depression, fatigue, constipation, and calf cramps. However, warn the pregnant woman not to overdo it.

Instruct her to consult her doctor about an exercise program, especially if she is accustomed to a sedentary lifestyle; is obese or markedly underweight; has hypertension, anemia or other blood disorders, thyroid disease, diabetes, cardiac dysrhythmia or palpitations; or has a history of precipitous labor, intrauterine growth retardation, bleeding during pregnancy, or breech presentation in the last trimester. Under no circumstances should she exercise if she has ruptured membranes, premature labor, multiple gestation, an incompetent cervix, placenta previa, cardiac disease, or a history of three or more spontaneous abortions.

Warning about alcohol, caffeine, and drugs

Warn the expectant mother that alcohol consumption during pregnancy increases the risk of having an LBW infant or one with birth defects and/or mental retardation. Explain that researchers still don't know how many drinks per day during pregnancy is safe.

The stimulant caffeine can cause birth defects in animals when ingested in large quantities. While a link between caffeine and birth defects in humans hasn't been proven, encourage the pregnant woman to limit her intake of coffee, tea, soda, and chocolate.

Since many drugs cross the placenta to the fetus, also tell her not to take *any* medications, including aspirin, without her doctor's permission.

Discouraging smoking

One of the Surgeon General's warnings on cigarette packs reads "Smoking

EXERCISING SAFELY DURING PREGNANCY

Dear Patient:

Exercising during pregnancy helps you stay healthy and fit. But when you exercise, it's important not to take unnecessary risks that could harm you or your unborn baby. So, to exercise safely during your pregnancy, follow this list of do's and don'ts recommended by the American College of Obstetricians and Gynecologists:

Do:
• Exercise regularly rather than occasionally.
• Perform your exercises on surfaces that reduce shock and provide a sure footing.
• Warm up for 5 minutes before you exercise to stretch your muscles and raise your heart rate gradually. Cool down for 5 minutes, too.
• Measure your heart rate at times of peak activity. It should not exceed 140 beats per minute.
• Drink plenty of fluids before and after you exercise. Interrupt your activity, if necessary, to replenish fluids.
• Begin with mild exercise, if you normally exercise a little or not at all. Then gradually build up to more strenuous exercise.
• Stop any exercise right away

and consult your doctor if you develop any of these signs or symptoms: pain, bleeding, dizziness, faintness, shortness of breath, palpitations, or tachycardia (overly rapid heart rate).
• Increase your caloric intake to meet the extra energy demands of pregnancy—and of exercise.
• Plan your exercise program in collaboration with your doctor or nurse-midwife.

Don't:
• Exercise vigorously in hot, humid weather or when you have a fever.
• Perform strenuous exercise for more than 15 minutes.
• Engage in competitive sports.
• Bend deeply or greatly extend your joints.
• Participate in activities that require jumping, bouncing, jarring or jerky motion, or rapid changes in direction.
• Stand up abruptly after doing floor exercises.
• Exercise while lying on your back after the fourth month of pregnancy.
• Perform exercises that use the Valsalva maneuver.
• Exercise beyond your tolerance and comfort level.

causes lung cancer, heart disease, and emphysema, and may complicate pregnancy." And with good reason. Infants born to women who smoke weigh an average of 6 oz (170 g) less than infants born to women who don't smoke. Nicotine constricts blood vessels, which in turn decreases the oxygen level in the blood that reaches the fetus. Besides lowering an infant's birth weight, smoking during pregnancy increases the chance of spontaneous abortion or stillbirth. Pregnant women smoking one or more packs of cigarettes a day have a 50% greater risk of infant mortality.

Obviously, the less a pregnant woman smokes, the better. Many women are highly motivated to stop smoking, or at least to curb this habit, once they learn they're pregnant. Take this opportunity to encourage a woman to stop smoking for good.

Advising about rubella: Risk factor for birth defects

Exposure to rubella, or German measles, during pregnancy—especially in the first trimester—increases the risk of congenital abnormalities, such as blood dyscrasias, heart defects, hearing loss, and mental retardation. Most doctors recommend vaccination before pregnancy for women not previously exposed to rubella. If pregnancy occurs before vaccination, tell the woman to consult her doctor or nurse-midwife about serial testing for rubella antibody to detect infection.

Minimizing environmental hazards

Exposure to environmental radiation or chemicals, especially in the early weeks of pregnancy, poses a serious threat to fetal well-being. Instruct a woman to avoid X-rays, even dental X-rays, from the moment she suspects or knows that she's pregnant. Explain that high-dose radiation in utero increases the risk of fetal malformation and childhood leukemia and carcinomas. If a woman is accidentally exposed to radiation or chemicals during pregnancy, try to allay her fears and refer her to appropriate resources.

Exploring Choices in Childbirth

Parents today frequently choose to control the circumstances of their child's birth. For example, they may question the need for the routine administration of analgesics and anesthetics during labor instead of passively accepting it as part of a prescribed childbirth ritual. Or they may question the choice of a traditional hospital delivery room as the best delivery setting. When you're responsible for preparing a woman for labor and delivery, you'll need to explore childbirth options with her.

However, you'll first teach her how to detect—and correctly respond to—complications of pregnancy or labor and delivery. For example, if the woman is susceptible to toxemia, she should know how to recognize its early signs, such as rapid weight gain, headaches, or ankle or eyelid edema. And she should know to seek immediate medical attention if her membranes rupture early. To help her cope with complications during labor, explain the role of fetal monitoring. Also prepare her for the possibility of cesarean section.

The delivery

Because 20% of women experience some problem during labor (for example, hemorrhage, toxemia, or fetal anoxia), encourage a woman to select a delivery setting that's equipped to handle emergencies as well as provide the childbirth experience she desires. For example, birth centers are becoming increasingly popular. Usually located in the maternity unit of a hospital or operated by a childbirth association, a birth center offers a homelike environment with quick medical intervention available in an emergency.

Once a woman decides where she'd like to deliver, you'll need to help her prepare for the pain of childbirth. Most researchers agree that the less medication a mother receives during labor and delivery, the more responsive and healthy her baby will be. Encourage the woman to attend childbirth classes to learn how to control pain through breathing and relaxation techniques. But assure her that she can request an anesthetic during labor if pain becomes unbearable. Although not totally without risk, local and regional anesthetics are certainly preferable to a general anesthetic.

Providing Postpartum Instruction

After a woman delivers, your teaching will focus on postpartum nutrition and exercise as well as infant care, such as feeding and safety. For example, remind the mother and her partner to always use an infant car seat, beginning with the baby's trip home from the hospital.

Balancing nutrition and exercise

After delivery, many women think they can immediately resume their pre-pregnancy fitness program and start dieting to lose the weight gained during pregnancy. You'll need to stress the importance of *slowly* resuming exercise to avoid excessive fatigue. If a woman is breast-feeding, she should avoid dieting, which may interfere with her milk production as well as jeopardize her health.

Breast or bottle?

Because breast milk contains a unique balance of nutrients, it's considered the ideal food for infants. What's more, the maternal antibodies it contains help protect the infant against allergy and infection.

When a mother chooses to breast-feed, first explain the physiology of stimulating milk flow. Then teach her how to care for her breasts to prevent soreness and cracked nipples; how to position herself, place the infant at her breast, and stimulate him to suck; and how long to nurse on each breast. Also refer her to a local chapter of a support group, such as Nursing Mothers, for help with problem solving as she adjusts to breast-feeding. If a mother wishes to continue breast-feeding after returning to work, explain how to express breast milk and store it properly. Or, if she wishes to supplement her breast milk or opts not to breast-feed, teach her how to choose and prepare a commercial formula to ensure adequate nutrition. Also teach her the proper technique for bottle-feeding her infant.

Introducing solids

Inform parents that breast milk or formula (with appropriate vitamin and mineral supplements) is the only food their infant needs until he reaches age 3 to 6 months. Explain that introducing solid food too early can cause choking and food allergies and may predispose the infant to obesity.

When the infant's ready for solid food, teach parents to read commercial baby food labels for salt and sugar content. Also instruct them never to add salt or sugar to their infant's food.

To help parents learn what foods their infant likes or dislikes and to determine what foods may cause allergy, teach them to introduce foods in this order: rice cereal, then fruits and vegetables, and finally meats.

Dealing with special problems

Crib death, or sudden infant death syndrome (SIDS), is a chief cause of infant mortality, especially in those from 3 weeks to 7 months old. Typically, parents put the infant to bed and later find him dead, often with no indications of

EXERCISING AFTER CHILDBIRTH

Dear Patient:

After giving birth, you need to exercise regularly so that you can regain your strength, promote healing, and restore your figure. Use the exercises shown on these pages as a guide. Begin with the first exercise, and add a new one every day or so as you become stronger. Perform each exercise five times, twice a day, as your comfort and tolerance level allows. Or follow the special directions from your nurse, nurse-midwife, or doctor.

Note: Don't forget to perform your Kegel exercises at least 10 times, twice a day, as instructed by your nurse, to tighten your pelvic floor muscles.

1

Lie flat on your back, with your knees slightly bent. Breathe in deeply, so that your chest rises. Then slowly exhale through your mouth, and tightly pull in your abdominal muscles. Hold these muscles tight while counting to five; don't hold your breath. Now relax.

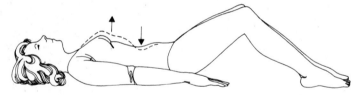

2

While lying in the same position, raise your head. As you do, try to keep the rest of your body still. Bring your head as close as possible to your chest; then slowly return to the starting position.

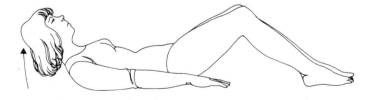

3

For this exercise, lie on your back with your legs apart and your knees slightly bent. Stretch your arms straight out from your shoulders. Then slowly raise them, until your hands meet directly above your chest. Without bending your elbows, lower your arms to the starting position.

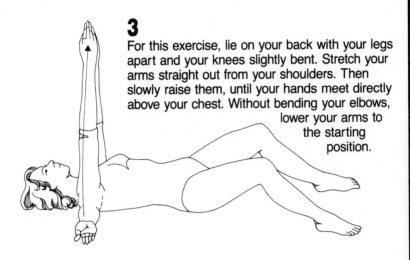

4

Next, lie flat on your back and straighten your legs. Raise your head and slightly bend one knee. Using your opposite hand, reach toward this knee, but don't touch it. Return to the starting position, and repeat this exercise with your other leg and hand.

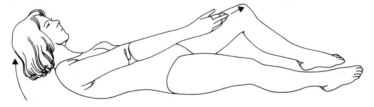

5

Lying on your back, bend one knee. Bring this knee toward your chin and the heel toward your buttock. Return to the starting position, and repeat the exercise with your other leg.

(continued)

EXERCISING AFTER CHILDBIRTH *(continued)*

6

Again lie flat on your back and keep your arms at your sides. Bend one knee toward your chin, and then straighten your leg until it's perpendicular to the floor. Lower this leg and repeat the exercise with your other leg.

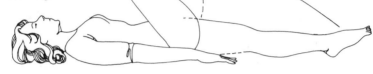

7

Now sit upright with your knees bent and your feet flat on the floor. Clasp your hands behind your head and lean back at about a 45-degree angle to the floor. Hold this position for several seconds; then sit upright again.

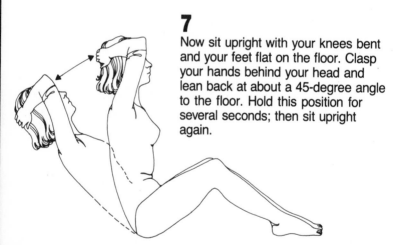

8

For the next exercise, lie flat, as you did in Exercise 6. This time, bend both knees toward your chin, and then straighten them until your legs are perpendicular to the floor. Then bend both knees back to your chin and lower your legs.

9

Now lie on your back with your knees bent and your feet flat on the floor, close to your buttocks. Keep your feet apart. Raise your buttocks slightly off the floor. As you raise your buttocks, tighten them and push your lower back down. Hold this position for several seconds; then return to the starting position.

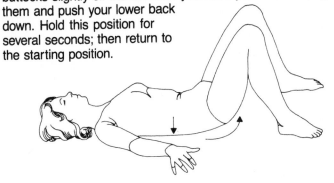

10

Repeat Exercise 9, this time raising your head and tightening your abdominal muscles as you lift your buttocks.

11

Finally, rest on your elbows and knees with your arms and legs perpendicular to your body. Hump your back upward (see arrow), tighten your buttocks, and draw in your abdomen. Then relax and take a deep breath.

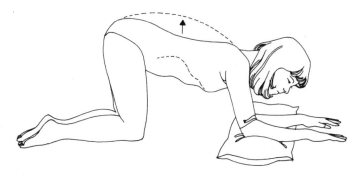

a struggle or distress of any kind. Even an autopsy doesn't reveal the cause of SIDS. Some infants may have had symptoms of a cold or another upper respiratory tract infection, but such symptoms are unusual. Although infants who die from SIDS often appear healthy, research suggests that many may have had undetected abnormalities, such as respiratory immaturity or dysfunction.

When an infant has a history of apneic periods, he's considered at risk for SIDS. You'll need to teach his parents about apnea monitoring. Also instruct them how to perform infant cardiopulmonary resuscitation. (Learning this skill is equally important for all parents. Why? Because suffocation from inhaling food or a small object is another common cause of infant mortality.)

When SIDS claims an infant, you'll need to focus on supporting the grief-stricken parents. Begin by reassuring them that they were not to blame. Provide basic information about SIDS and explain why an autopsy is necessary to confirm the diagnosis. Make sure the parents receive the autopsy report promptly. Then refer them to a local support group for SIDS.

HEALTH IN CHILDHOOD

Perhaps more than any other stage of life, childhood has a profound impact on health. During this period, an individual acquires many habits that may produce lifelong benefit—or harm. To promote healthy habits, you'll need to teach parents how to role-play with their child about significant issues, such as smoking. This open communication can prepare a child to confront the peer-group pressure that so often dominates adolescence.

Developing Sound Nutritional Habits

Usually, a child establishes his eating habits at an early age. Because poor eating habits can affect his growth and development, your teaching must stress the importance of sound nutrition during childhood. You'll also need to explain to parents how poor eating habits contribute to adult disease.

Begin by clearing up any misconceptions about eating habits. For example, tell parents that they shouldn't salt, butter, or sugar their child's food. Although they may prefer their food this way, these acquired tastes increase the child's risk of cardiovascular disease and dental caries.

Because a child needs protein and calcium for growth, parents were once encouraged to supply plenty of eggs, cheese, meat, whole milk, and ice cream in the diet. Research now shows that such a high-cholesterol, high-fat diet increases the risk of atherosclerosis. Therefore, urge parents to serve low-fat alternatives, such as skim milk, lean meat, poultry, and fish. Also suggest that they curb their child's consumption of nonnutritive snacks, such as candy and potato chips.

Teach parents to include a variety of foods in their child's diet to meet his vitamin needs. For example, milk, fish, liver, leafy green vegetables, and yellow fruits and vegetables supply vitamin A. Protein-rich foods, such as meat, and enriched breads and cereals supply the B-complex vitamins. Good sources of vitamin C include citrus fruits, tomatoes, raw cabbage, and green peppers. Fortified milk supplies vitamin D.

To help parents build good eating habits in their child, urge them to follow these tips:
• Serve food portioned out, instead of family style.
• Keep salt off the table.

- Never force a child to eat everything on his plate.
- If a child refuses to eat a certain food, try offering him an alternative from the same food group.
- Keep fresh raw vegetables, such as carrot sticks, ready for snacking.
- Praise a child for his healthy food choices.
- Recognize that a child will imitate his parents' eating habits. So try to avoid using salt, sugar, and butter on your own food, too.

Preventing Childhood Accidents

Each year, many children die or are injured as the result of automobile and recreational accidents, drownings, fires, and poisoning. Many of these deaths and injuries could have been prevented by observing proper safety measures. For example, a child can be taught how to float and swim or how to safely enjoy bicycles, swings, and other recreational equipment. Teaching parents about such safety measures ranks among your chief goals.

Encourage use of seat belts
More children die in automobile accidents than from any other single cause. That's why you'll need to stress the importance of *consistently* using a car seat for an infant or a young child and a seat belt for an older child. Tell parents that holding a child on their lap doesn't provide enough protection. Even at low driving speeds, the force of impact in a car crash can throw the child through the windshield or into the dashboard. Encourage parents to buckle up as an example for their child to follow.

Refer parents to the state department of transportation for guidance in selecting a car seat. The car seat should be crash-tested and should meet federal safety standards. It must also be suit-

SCHEDULE FOR CHILDHOOD IMMUNIZATIONS

Usually, childhood immunizations are given on a fixed schedule, as follows:

AGE	IMMUNIZATION
2 months	First dose: diphtheria/tetanus/pertussis (DPT) vaccine, polio vaccine
4 months	Second dose: DPT vaccine, polio vaccine
6 months	Third dose: DPT vaccine, polio vaccine
15 months	Measles, mumps, and rubella vaccine
18 months	DPT vaccine booster, polio vaccine booster
2 years	*Hemophilus influenzae B* vaccine
4 years	DPT vaccine booster, polio vaccine booster

Before immunization, ask the parent if the child receives corticosteroids or other drugs that depress the immune response, or if he's had a recent febrile illness. Obtain a history of allergies, especially to antibiotics, eggs, or feathers, and past reaction to immunization.

After immunization, tell the parents to watch for and report a severe reaction. Give them a record of their child's immunizations.

able for the child's age and size and be installed properly.

Warn against accidental poisoning
Thanks to the advent of lead-free paints and child-proof containers, fewer children die each year from accidental poisoning. However, poisoning still accounts for 5% of accidental deaths in children less than 5 years old. What can you do to improve this statistic? You can begin by teaching parents to

CHILDPROOFING YOUR HOME

Dear Parent:

As a parent, you know how quickly an active toddler can get into trouble. To protect your child, take these simple—but very important—precautions.

How to prevent burns
• Keep matches and lighters out of your child's reach.
• Don't let him play in the kitchen, unless he's in a playpen. You may trip over him or his toys, spilling hot food on him.
• Make sure electrical cords don't hang over counters, tables, or ironing boards. Your child may pull a hot toaster, iron, or Crockpot on himself.
• Don't let pot handles stick out over the edge of the stove. Your child may grab at them.

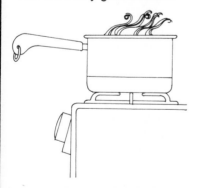

• Don't store candy or cookies on the stove or behind it—your child may try to climb on the stove to find them.

• Don't use tablecloths. A toddler may try to pull himself up by grabbing a tablecloth and pull everything on the table on top of him.

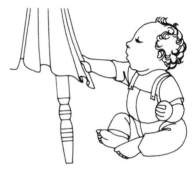

• Don't hold your child while drinking hot coffee or tea—or anything hot. If he bumps your arm, you may splash him with hot liquid.
• Don't leave your child alone in the bathtub—even for an instant. Remember, a child likes to turn knobs. He may turn on the hot-water faucet and burn himself. As an extra precaution, make sure your hot-water heater is set no higher than 130° F. (54.4° C.).
• Check labels on your child's clothing and bedding. Make sure all clothing and bedding are nonflammable.

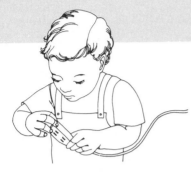

• Don't let him play with—or chew on—electrical cords, including extension cords.

• Be especially careful during holidays. Keep your child away from Christmas tree lights and cords. Don't allow him to play with fireworks or sparklers. And keep him away from flames, including candle flames, when he's dressed in a Halloween costume, especially a home-made costume.

How to prevent poisoning

• Teach your child that everything within reach is not good to eat. To prove the point, give him a taste of something bitter (such as vinegar) on the tip of your finger—but be sure to warn him that it *doesn't* taste good.

• Place poison identification stickers on all household poisons, such as cleaning solutions, polishes, weed spray, and bug killers. Lock them up, or store them on the top shelf of a closet or cabinet—out of reach. (Take care to store them away from food or eating utensils.) After using any poisonous product, *immediately* return it to a safe storage place.

Also keep cosmetics, such as nail polish, perfume, and hand cream, as well as all aerosol containers, out of your child's reach.

• Learn how to identify poisonous plants, and remove any you may find in your home or yard. Remember, many common houseplants, including dieffenbachias, are poisonous when eaten.

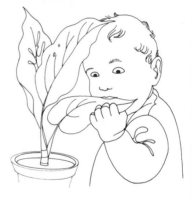

• If your child eats or drinks anything that may be poisonous, immediately call your local poison control center for help. Write the phone number on a label and tape it to the phone. Keep ipecac syrup handy in case the poison control center tells you to make your child vomit what he's swallowed.

place potentially poisonous products, such as household cleaners, bleaches, drugs, and pesticides, well out of the reach of children. Also warn them about lead poisoning, as appropriate. Typically, city children are at an increased risk for lead poisoning because they may ingest chipping lead-base paint from older buildings or inhale lead from automobile exhaust. Explain how lead poisoning damages the central nervous system, possibly leading to learning disabilities, mental retardation, or death. Recommend that parents strip any lead-base paint from walls, molding, and windowsills and then repaint these areas.

Forming Good Exercise Habits

While today's children appear healthy and are taller and heavier than previous generations, they often score poorly on tests of strength, endurance, and agility. Why? Because they're primed at an early age for a sedentary life-style. For example, instead of walking, they're often taxied by their parents to wherever they want to go. What's more, they frequently substitute an afternoon in front of the television for outdoor physical activity.

How can you help parents and children appreciate the benefits of exercise? First, teach them that exercise helps prevent constipation, stress, and obesity as well as delay degenerative and cardiovascular disease later in life. It also enhances good health by promoting strength, stamina, speed, agility, coordination, and balance.

Then encourage parents to support or initiate an exercise program that suits their child's abilities and interests. To improve cardiovascular fitness, recommend endurance exercises, such as swimming, cycling, running, jumping rope, walking, or hiking. Ideally,

the child should choose an exercise that he enjoys and in which he excels. Advise parents against unduly pressuring their child to win when he engages in competitive exercise. Also urge them to make exercise a family activity so that it becomes a healthy habit for the child. Remind them not to rely completely on school physical education programs to promote adequate exercise.

Learning to Deal with Stress

Even a very young child can experience stress, which may cause depression and jeopardize his psychological well-being. Stress also increases blood pressure and makes a child more susceptible to illness, such as streptococcal infection. To minimize these effects, your teaching must emphasize how to cope with stress effectively and, better yet, how to prevent it.

The most potentially stressful events in a child's life are divorce of his parents and illness or death in his family. Of course, he has no control over these events. However, he can choose to respond to them in either a healthy or a self-destructive way. Teach parents how to communicate with their child and to encourage him to turn to them for help when he's under stress. Also encourage parents to involve their child in school or community activities to help prevent stress.

To enhance a child's psychological well-being, suggest that parents devise projects and games that stimulate curiosity and creativity. Recommend that they limit the child's time for watching television and try to select educational shows. Also encourage parents to spend quality time with their child, especially if both work outside the home. Suggest that they spend the dinner hour with their child and regularly plan family activities.

HEALTH IN ADOLESCENCE

The adolescent years are often trying for both a teenager and his family. As he passes from childhood into adulthood, a teenager develops his own set of values and sense of identity, chiefly by testing and experimenting. Little by little, he withdraws from the family and asserts his independence. Typically, a teenager is motivated by a strong desire to belong to his peer group. He's also overly self-conscious about his appearance—largely a result of sexual maturation during adolescence.

These dramatic changes during adolescence can certainly affect a teenager's health. As a result, you'll need to teach about such varied health problems as poor nutrition, teenage pregnancy, and alcohol and drug abuse.

Meeting Growing Nutritional Demands

Because a teenager's body is growing so rapidly, he needs more calories than he did as a child. However, his diet should still be well balanced and varied. Recommend extra milk to supply needed calcium and protein for growth. When menstruation begins, suggest an iron supplement if adequate iron isn't provided by the diet.

Peer pressure makes food fads common among teenagers. Don't discourage a teenager from following such fads unless they jeopardize his health. Teach him about basic food groups to ensure a balanced diet and healthy weight. Most teenagers don't have a weight problem, but some are obese or suffer from anorexia nervosa.

Obesity

To help an obese teenager, first explore whether his weight problem results from inactivity, overeating, or both. Then try to encourage self-confidence so that he'll be motivated to lose weight. Stress that weight loss is crucial for good health and will also help him feel less ostracized by his peers. Refer him to a local weight-control program.

Anorexia nervosa

Sometimes an obese teenager or one who has a morbid fear of being fat develops a self-starvation disorder known as anorexia nervosa. Most common in teenage girls, this disorder may be life-threatening if untreated. Typically, the affected teenager is preoccupied with food but doesn't allow herself to eat even though she's emaciated. At the same time, she exercises compulsively. She may also demonstrate binge-eating, followed by spontaneous or self-induced vomiting or self-administration of laxatives. Because anorexia is a nutritional problem based on an emotional disturbance, it requires medical and psychiatric treatment. Refer the teenager and her family to Anorexia Nervosa and Associated Disorders (ANAD) for help in treating this disorder.

Preventing Teenage Suicide

Suicide, the third leading cause of death among teenagers, is usually accomplished by self-inflicted gunshot wounds, drug overdose, or carbon monoxide poisoning by automobile exhaust fumes. Most teenagers who successfully commit suicide have made previous attempts. What's more, a teenager will typically give warning signs of his intentions. Teach parents about such signs and advise them to seek counseling immediately if their teenager demonstrates these signs. Also suggest that parents keep guns and potentially lethal drugs properly secured.

Addressing Contraception and Teenage Pregnancy

Each year about half a million American teenagers give birth, commonly to an infant whose conception wasn't planned. Still other teenagers choose to have an abortion rather than carry an unwanted fetus. To help prevent an unwanted pregnancy, you'll need to provide basic information about how conception occurs and, most important, how it can be avoided.

Methods of contraception

If you're teaching a teenager about contraception, explain that the most effective form of birth control besides abstinence is the oral contraceptive. However, it can produce serious side effects, such as blood clots, CVA, and myocardial infarction (MI). These side effects, though, most commonly occur in women over age 35 or in those who are obese, who smoke more than 15 cigarettes a day, or who have hypertension, diabetes, or elevated serum lipid levels. Outline these risk factors, and encourage yearly gynecologic checkups.

Explain that the next most effective form of birth control is the intrauterine device. Somewhat less effective, but still satisfactory, are the diaphragm, the condom, and spermicides. Inform the teenager that using two of these forms of birth control at the same time improves effectiveness.

Teenage pregnancy

Teenage mothers are more likely than adult mothers to have premature or LBW infants and to develop toxemia. The mortality for their infants is also higher. One reason for this trend is that teenage mothers tend to delay seeking prenatal care and thus frequently don't realize the importance of proper nutrition during pregnancy.

You'll need to teach the pregnant teenager how her eating habits affect her unborn child. Explain that she needs extra calories—especially protein and calcium—to sustain her own growth spurts during adolescence as well as promote fetal growth. Emphasize that these calories should be supplied by a well-balanced, nutritious diet.

Curbing the Rise of Characteristic Adolescent Problems

Adolescence is a time of exploration and turmoil. Unfortunately, this combination too often leads to behavior that's dangerous to an adolescent and to others.

Motor vehicle accidents

Despite increased public awareness, alcohol-related motor vehicle accidents still rank as the leading cause of teenage deaths. Among other factors that contribute to these deaths are driving under the influence of marijuana or other drugs, driving too fast, and disregarding seat belts. Although driver education programs teach adolescents about safety, you too can promote sensible driving. For example, encourage a teenager to obey the speed limit, to always use a seat belt, and to wear a helmet when riding a motorcycle.

Alcohol and drug abuse

An estimated 3 million American youths between ages 14 and 17 are considered problem drinkers—that is, they become intoxicated at least once a month. Although teenagers drink less often than adults, they tend to drink larger quantities and thus are more apt to become intoxicated when they drink.

Teenagers today consume 30% more alcohol than they did 30 years ago. Not surprisingly, drug abuse is also on the rise. In fact, nearly 30% of youths between ages 12 and 17 have tried marijuana, with 10% of these smoking it every day. Among other substances that teenagers can abuse are amphetamines, cocaine, heroin, hallucinogens, and various illegally obtained prescription drugs.

As a nurse, you must educate both the teenager and his parents about the dangers of alcohol and drug abuse. Encourage parents to help their teenager cope with stress and develop enough self-confidence to say "no" despite peer pressure. When you discover that a teenager is abusing alcohol or drugs, refer him to a local Alcoholics Anonymous chapter, or suggest a rehabilitation center to help him overcome his dependence.

Smoking

Coinciding with the nationwide decline in the number of smokers, fewer teenagers smoke today than in previous years. In fact, smoking is becoming less socially acceptable, as laws passed to prohibit smoking in certain public areas confirm.

Why do some teenagers continue to smoke? Among other reasons, they may smoke to assert their independence, to act grown-up, or to imitate their friends. Also, teenagers are twice as likely to smoke if their parents smoke.

Take every opportunity to teach teenagers and their parents about the dangers of smoking. Explain how smoking shortens life expectancy and increases the risk of cardiovascular disease and lung cancer. When appropriate, refer the teenager to a community program to help him quit smoking.

Encouraging Exercise

The benefits of exercise during adolescence are many: it helps the teenager maintain a healthy weight, gives him an outlet for stress, and provides an opportunity to socialize with his peers. Because exercise isn't compatible with smoking and drug and alcohol use, it also tends to discourage him from practicing these unhealthy habits.

Encourage the teenager to take up an exercise—such as tennis or swimming—that he can continue as an adult. Or encourage him to continue a favored exercise that he began as a child. That way, it will more likely become a habit for him. Remind the teenager to increase his caloric intake to meet the extra energy demands of exercise. Also instruct the teenage girl to wear a properly fitting bra during exercise and the teenage boy to wear an athletic supporter.

Preventing accidents in team sports

Many teenagers participate in team sports, either at school or in the community. Although team sports teach important skills—such as working together to achieve a goal and sharing the spotlight—they can also increase the teenager's risk of physical injury and psychological stress.

To reduce the risk of physical injury, urge coaches and community sponsors to invest in and maintain proper equipment, such as helmets, mouthpieces, and shoulder pads. Also emphasize the importance of a clean and safe sports facility. Advise coaches to become certified in first aid so that they can respond promptly to any injury.

Before a teenager participates in a team sport, instruct him to have a complete physical examination. Then stress the importance of proper conditioning to promote better performance and to reduce the risk of injury. For example, to play football, a sport that requires strength, endurance, and agility, a teenager should perform a combination of aerobic and anaerobic exercises, such as running, calisthenics, and weight lifting. Remind him that conditioning also involves proper sleep and nutrition and rules out smoking and alcohol or drug use.

To minimize psychological stress, advise parents not to push a teenager to participate and excel in sports against his will. Teach them to support any interest in sports by encouraging the teenager to practice and to do the best he can. However, they should avoid placing him under stress to perform, to win, or to secure a spot on a specific team.

HEALTH IN ADULTHOOD

Adults in the prime of their lives—between ages 25 and 64—often fall victim to a number of health problems, such as heart disease, CVA, and cancer. Although genetic predisposition contributes to some of these problems, many are linked to specific unhealthy habits, such as overeating, smoking, and lack of exercise. Your teaching can help an adult recognize and correct these habits to help ensure a longer—and healthier—life.

Preventing Poor Nutrition

Once acquired, poor eating habits are especially difficult to change. To help an adult establish healthy eating habits, teach him to:
• include just enough calories each day to maintain a healthy weight
• limit saturated fats, cholesterol, salt, and sugar in his diet
• eat plenty of complex carbohydrates (whole grains, cereals, fruits, and vegetables)
• substitute more fish, poultry, and legumes (beans, peas, and peanuts) for red meat.

The link between diet and disease

Research shows that a strong correlation exists between diet and certain diseases, such as atherosclerosis, hypertension, and obesity. By teaching an adult how to modify his eating habits, you can help him reduce his risk of acquiring or aggravating such diseases.

• **Cardiovascular disease.** Encourage the adult to limit the amount of saturated fats and cholesterol in his diet. Increased serum cholesterol levels are clearly associated with atherosclerosis, which predisposes to MI and CVA. Stress that by modifying his diet an adult can retard, and possibly reverse, atherosclerosis.

To help prevent or control hypertension, instruct the adult to limit salt in his diet. For example, tell him to substitute herbs and other seasonings for salt when cooking and to avoid high-sodium prepared foods.

• **Cancer.** Research suggests that a high intake of animal protein or an inadequate intake of fiber may be associated with colon cancer. A high intake of saturated and unsaturated fats also may be linked to colon cancer as well as to ovarian and prostate cancer.

• **Obesity.** About 35% of adult women and 13% of adult men are considered obese. Besides being a social stigma, obesity is associated with a number of health problems, such as diabetes, gallbladder disease, and hypertension.

To help the obese adult, you'll need to stress the importance of *permanently* changing his eating habits. Otherwise, he's likely to become trapped in a cycle of losing and then regaining weight. Help him set realistic weight-loss goals and plan a dietary and exercise program to achieve these goals. Also refer him to a community support group, such as Weight Watchers.

Combating Inactivity

To promote cardiovascular fitness, an adult should exercise vigorously at least three times a week for 20 to 30 minutes. Unfortunately, most adults get little exercise at work or at home. Your teaching can help an adult understand the many benefits of a regular exercise program. Explain that exercise improves circulation and helps the heart and lungs function more efficiently. By helping the body metabolize carbohydrates and fats, exercise may reduce the risk of atherosclerosis. It can also make an adult feel more energetic, improve his ability to cope with stress, and help him get a good night's sleep. By burning calories and controlling appetite, exercise helps achieve and maintain a healthy body weight and increases muscle strength and stamina.

However, exercise can aggravate hidden or existing health problems and heighten the risk of injuries. So instruct the adult to consult his doctor before starting an exercise program if he:
• has diagnosed heart disease or a heart murmur, or has had an MI
• feels pain or pressure in the chest, left side of the neck, or left shoulder or arm during or after exercise
• feels faint or has dizzy spells
• experiences extreme breathlessness after mild exertion
• is hypertensive or hasn't had his blood pressure checked recently
• has bone or joint problems, such as arthritis
• is a male older than age 45 or a female older than age 50 who isn't used to vigorous exercise
• has a family history of coronary artery disease
• has any other medical condition, such as diabetes.

Refer the adult to the American Heart Association for brochures to teach him how to start an exercise program safely, what exercises he might enjoy, and how to avoid injuries.

Pointing Out Adult Safety Risks

In daily living, adults face a number of safety risks, such as toxic environmental agents, occupational hazards, and certain infectious diseases. Accidental injuries can also be potentially life-threatening or disabling. Some safety risks—like toxic waste disposal—are beyond the scope of individual action and require a community effort to affect them. Other risks can be minimized simply by following certain safety measures. For example, teach an adult to use a seat belt consistently, to read product warning labels, and to wear safety goggles when operating machinery. As always, encourage common sense to help prevent accidents. Also teach him precautions against infection, such as hand washing, and urge vaccination when appropriate.

Stress

Occasional stress during adulthood is normal and, in fact, helps an individual respond to his environment and improve his performance. However, chronic or overwhelming stress can tax his ability to cope, resulting in alcohol or drug abuse, depression or mental illness, hypertension, and GI upset.

Research shows that too many stressors occurring at once or consecutively can produce a cumulative effect that increases an individual's chances of becoming ill. Encourage the adult to plan stressors so that they're easier to manage. For example, suggest that a couple delay having a baby if they've just moved into a new home.

• *Coping skills.* Teach the adult specific skills to cope with stress, such as cognitive restructuring. This involves focusing on the positive side of events and downplaying the negative. For example, instead of viewing a traffic jam as a hardship and a waste of time, an individual can consider it an opportunity to relax and listen to music.

Point out that distractions, such as humor, reduce stress. Relaxation techniques can be of help, too. Suggest meditation, or teach the adult how to perform abdominal breathing. If he lives alone, you might recommend getting a pet. Research shows that petting a household cat or dog can significantly reduce blood pressure and stress.

However, one of the most important coping skills that you can teach an adult is time management. By managing his time effectively, he can gain a sense of control over his life. Begin by teaching an adult how to set priorities. Tell him to decide what is crucial to him, then to concentrate on that alone. Emphasize that he mustn't feel guilty when he can't accomplish everything. Also advise him to divide unpleasant tasks into small, manageable portions.

Smoking

Since the 1964 Surgeon General's report conclusively linked cigarette smoking to lung cancer, more than 30 million people have quit the habit. However, cigarette smoking remains the largest single cause of preventable illness and premature death. Smokers risk developing heart disease, CVA, chronic lung disease (such as emphysema), and cancer of the lung or other organs. In addition, smokers have a 70% greater chance of premature death than nonsmokers.

To encourage an adult to kick the habit, discuss these health hazards associated with smoking. Also point out the benefits of not smoking; for example, a nonsmoker can enjoy the taste of food more and isn't bothered by tobacco breath odor. Advise the smoker to ask his doctor about the use of nicotine resin complex gum to help him quit smoking. This prescription gum helps the smoker reduce blood levels of nicotine gradually, thereby minimizing withdrawal symptoms. Refer the smoker to the American Cancer Society for more information and support.

Teaching Early Signs of Illness

Part of your responsibility as a nurse is to teach adults about early signs of illness—especially cancer, MI, and

CVA. By doing so, you help ensure prompt treatment, which can be life-saving.

Signs of cancer

Teach the adult about the following types of cancer and their signs.

• **Breast cancer.** One out of 11 women develops breast cancer. What's more, it accounts for more cancer deaths in women than any other cancer. So you'll need to emphasize the importance of early detection through monthly breast self-examination and mammography. Explain that mammography can detect small lesions as well as cancer of the regional lymph nodes. The American Cancer Society recommends a baseline

INQUIRY

QUESTIONS PATIENTS ASK ABOUT P.M.S.

Why do I always feel this way before my menstrual period?

Although doctors aren't sure about the exact cause of premenstrual syndrome (PMS), they think it probably results from hormonal changes—chiefly involving progesterone and estrogen—during the menstrual cycle. Another hormone called prolactin may also contribute to PMS.

Do many other women also experience PMS?

Yes. In fact, up to 70% of women experience PMS. However, it affects each woman differently. Some women have only mild discomfort, while others have severe symptoms. For example, a woman may experience anxiety or panic attacks, depression, irritability, fatigue, food cravings, breast tenderness and swelling, bloating, swollen ankles or fingers, joint aches and pains, headaches, or even seizures.

How can I obtain relief from PMS?

Although your doctor may prescribe certain drugs or exercise to treat symptoms of PMS, you can help, too, by simply watching what you eat. Most important, you should try to steer clear of salt, caffeine, and sugar.

By reducing salt in your diet for 7 to 9 days before your period, you can help reduce water retention associated with uncomfortable bloating. This may also help to ease some of the aches and pains caused by water-swollen tissues pressing against nearby nerves.

Why reduce caffeine in your diet? Because caffeine can worsen the nervousness, irritability, and insomnia that you may already experience with PMS.

Hormonal changes in PMS also seem to affect your body's production of insulin, the hormone that causes your blood sugar level to drop. That's why most doctors recommend that you eliminate all sugars from your diet, including honey, molasses, brown sugar, candy, sweet desserts and snacks, and regular soft drinks. Your doctor may also suggest that you divide your daily caloric intake into three small meals and three between-meal snacks to avoid sudden drops in your blood sugar level.

One more point about what you eat. Because alcohol stimulates the release of insulin, it also can cause your blood sugar level to drop. So most doctors recommend that you avoid alcohol for two weeks before your period. But, if you're going to indulge, remember that you'll need only half your usual amount of alcohol to obtain the same effect. That's because PMS apparently makes you more susceptible to intoxication.

HOW TO EXAMINE YOUR BREASTS

Dear Patient:

Since 90% of breast cancers are discovered by patients themselves, it's important to learn and practice self-examination. You should examine your breasts once a month. If you've not yet reached menopause, the best time is immediately after your menstrual period. If you're past menopause, choose any convenient day.

Here's how to examine your breasts:

1

Undress to the waist, and stand or sit in front of a mirror, with your arms at your sides. Ob-serve your breasts for any change in their shape or size and any puckering or dimpling of the skin.

2

Raise your arms and press your hands together behind your head. Observe your breasts as you did before.

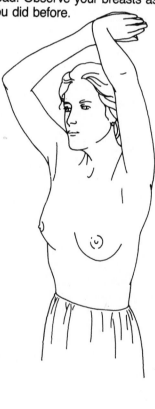

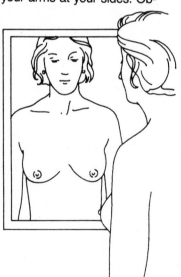

3

Press your palms firmly on your hips and observe your breasts again.

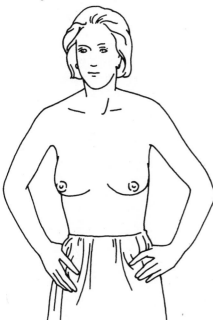

4

Now, lie flat on your back. This position flattens and spreads your breasts more evenly over the chest wall. Place a small pillow under your left shoulder, and put your left hand behind your head.

5

Examine your left breast with your right hand, using a circular motion and progressing clockwise, until you've examined every portion. You'll notice a

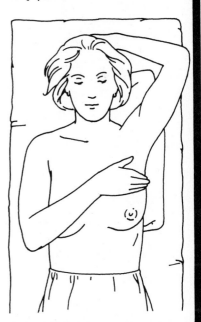

ridge of firm tissue in the lower curve of your breast; this is normal.

(continued)

HOW TO EXAMINE YOUR BREASTS *(continued)*

6

Check the area under your arm with your elbow slightly bent.

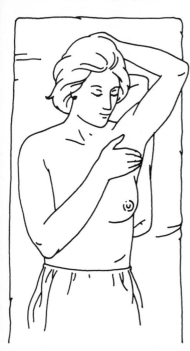

If you feel a small lump under your armpit that moves freely, don't be alarmed. This area contains your lymph glands, which may become swollen when you're sick. Check the size of the lump daily. Call the doctor if it doesn't go away in a few days or if it gets larger.

7

Gently squeeze your nipple between your thumb and fore-finger, and note any discharge.

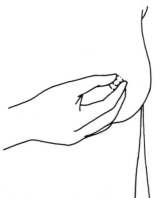

Repeat this examination on your right breast, using your left hand.

8

Finally, examine your breasts while in the shower or bath, lubricating your breasts with soap and water. Using the

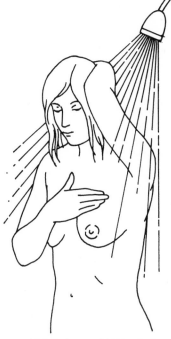

same circular, clockwise motion, gently inspect both breasts with your fingertips. After you've toweled dry, squeeze each nipple gently, and note any discharge.

9

If you feel a lump while examining your breasts, don't panic—most lumps aren't cancerous. First, note whether you can easily lift the skin covering it and whether the lump moves when you do so.

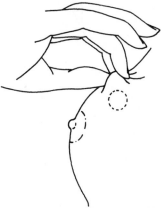

Next, notify your doctor. Be prepared to describe how the lump feels (hard or soft) and whether it moves easily under the skin.

Chances are, your doctor will want to examine the lump. Then he can advise you about what treatment (if any) you need.

Remember, although self-examination is important, it's not a substitute for examination by your doctor. Be sure to see your doctor annually or semiannually (if you're considered at special risk).

mammogram for women between ages 35 and 40. After that, a woman should have a routine mammogram as recommended.

• *Uterine cancer.* Thanks to the Pap smear and regular gynecologic checkups, deaths from uterine cancer have decreased by more than 70% over the past 40 years. The American Cancer Society recommends a Pap smear once every 3 years after a woman has had two negative tests performed 1 year apart. Explain that the Pap smear is especially effective in detecting cervical cancer. If a woman's at risk for endometrial cancer, though, her doctor may recommend an endometrial biopsy when she reaches menopause. Also instruct her to watch for warning signs of uterine cancer, such as unusual bleeding or discharge, and to notify her doctor if such signs develop.

• *Lung cancer.* Unfortunately, lung cancer is typically well advanced by the time it causes symptoms. As a result, focus your teaching on high-risk groups: smokers, especially if they've had the habit for more than 20 years, and adults exposed to asbestos or other industrial contaminants. Describe the warning signs of lung cancer, including a persistent cough, blood-streaked sputum, and chest pain.

• *Colorectal cancer.* Inform the adult that the American Cancer Society recommends these tests for early detection of colorectal cancer: a digital rectal examination performed annually after age 40; a fecal occult blood test performed annually after age 50; and a proctosigmoidoscopy performed every 3 to 5 years after age 50 following two negative annual examinations. Also teach him the warning signs of colorectal cancer: rectal bleeding, bloody stool, or a change in bowel habits.

• *Testicular cancer.* This uncommon cancer usually strikes men between ages 20 and 35. To emphasize the importance of monthly testicular self-examination, tell the adult male that 88% of such cancers have already spread by the time they're diagnosed.

Also teach him the warning signs of testicular cancer, such as a slight enlargement or a change in the consistency of the testes. A rapidly growing or hemorrhagic cancer may also cause sharp pain or discomfort, often described as "dragging" or "heaviness," in the testes.

• *Prostate cancer.* This cancer ranks as the second most common cancer in adult males (lung cancer is first). Describe the warning signs of prostate cancer, such as weak or interrupted urine flow, an inability to urinate or control urine flow, frequency (especially at night), blood-tinged urine, pain or burning on urination, and pain in the lower back, pelvis, or upper thighs. If the adult develops any of these signs or symptoms, instruct him to see his doctor to rule out other prostate problems.

Signs of MI

Teach the adult to seek medical help immediately if he experiences MI's cardinal symptom: persistent chest pain (often described as "heavy," "squeezing," or "crushing") that may radiate to the left side of the jaw or neck or to the left shoulder or arm. Mention that MI may also cause anxiety or a sense of impending doom, dizziness or fainting, sweating, nausea, and shortness of breath.

Signs of CVA

Describe these signs of CVA to the adult: sudden, temporary weakness or numbness of the face, arm, or leg on one side of the body; temporary loss of speech or inability to understand speech; temporary loss of vision or blurred vision, usually in one eye; unexplained dizziness, unsteadiness, or sudden falls. Explain that many severe CVAs are preceded by transient ischemic attacks. These attacks produce signs similar to a CVA and may occur days, weeks, or even months before a CVA. If the adult experiences any of these signs, have him notify his doctor promptly to help prevent death or severe disability.

HOW TO EXAMINE YOUR TESTICLES

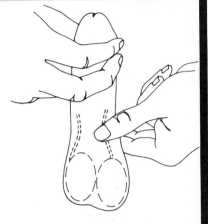

Dear Patient:

To help you detect abnormalities early, you should examine your testicles once a month. Eventually, you'll become familiar with them and will be able to recognize anything abnormal. Here's how to examine your testicles:

1

Remove your clothes and stand in front of a mirror. With one hand, lift your penis and check your scrotum (the sac containing your testicles) for any change in shape or size and for red, distended veins. Expect the scrotum's left side to hang slightly lower than the right.

2

Next, feel your testicles for lumps and masses. First, locate the cordlike structure at the back of your testicles. This is called the epididymis. Your spermatic cord extends upward from the epididymis.

3

Gently squeeze the spermatic cord above your right testicle between the thumb and first two fingers of your right hand. Then, using the thumb and first two fingers of your left hand,

examine the spermatic cord above your left testicle. Check for lumps and masses by squeezing along the entire length of the cords.

4

To examine your right testicle, place your right thumb on the front of the testicle and your index and middle fingers behind it. Gently press your thumb and fingers together; they should meet. Make sure you check your entire testicle. Then, use your left hand to examine your left testicle in the same manner. Your testicles should feel smooth, rubbery, and slightly tender, and you should be able to move them.

If you notice any lumps, masses, or changes, notify your doctor.

Preventing the Spread of Sexually Transmitted Disease

Each year, sexually transmitted disease (STD) strikes 10 million adults, most of them between ages 15 and 30. Although gonorrhea and syphilis are the best known types of STD, genital herpes and nonspecific urethritis (often caused by *Chlamydia*) also infect many adults. Because STD is often asymptomatic, it's difficult to detect and control. Unfortunately, thousands of infected women of childbearing age develop secondary pelvic inflammatory disease, which can cause sterility.

To help prevent and control STD, teach the adult that each type of STD is caused by a different organism. Note that he can have more than one STD at any given time. Remind him that reinfection is possible, too. Explain that condoms and some contraceptive creams and foams may protect against STD. Recommend limiting sexual contacts, avoiding infected partners, and urinating and cleansing the genitals right after intercourse. Urge an infected adult to inform sexual partners so they can seek treatment.

HEALTH IN OLD AGE

Today, more people live to old age than ever before. Fortunately, only 5% of the elderly need to be institutionalized; the rest can maintain their independence. However, 80% of the elderly suffer from at least one chronic health problem. Your teaching can help them cope with existing health problems as well as avoid new ones. What's more, it can improve their quality of life and help them continue as contributing members of society.

Emphasize that aging is a state of mind as well as of body. Urge the elderly person to continue as many activities as possible, depending on his mobility. Also help him explore new interests or hobbies. Recommend that he attend a hospital- or community-sponsored seminar on retirement. Such seminars usually cover topics like budgeting and health and fitness.

Perhaps the most powerful influence in old age is death. Besides contemplating his own mortality, an elderly person must often face the death of close friends or, most stressful of all, a spouse. By teaching him how to deal with grief, you can help the elderly person come to terms with such losses.

Ensuring Proper Nutrition

You'll need to suggest ways to help the elderly maintain good nutrition.

Caloric intake
Because metabolism slows with age, an elderly person requires fewer calories than before. However, metabolism still varies widely, so you'll need to help him adjust his caloric intake appropriately. For example, if he's moderately active, recommend 5% fewer calories for each decade between ages 40 and 59, 10% fewer calories between ages 60 and 69, and another 10% fewer after age 70.

Fiber and fluids
Encourage the elderly person to include adequate fiber in his diet. Fiber helps prevent constipation—a problem that the elderly are especially prone to because of reduced activity. It may also help prevent colon cancer, diverticulosis, and gallstones.

Because aging decreases the number

HOW TO SELECT—AND ENJOY— HEALTHFUL FOODS

Dear Patient:

A healthful diet means selecting the right foods to meet your body's needs. Here's how:

Selecting the right foods

Rely on the four basic food groups to ensure a healthful diet. The *fruit-vegetable* group includes all fruits and vegetables; the *bread-cereal* group, all grains and everything made from them, such as flour and pasta. The *meat* group includes beef and other meats, fish, poultry, and eggs; the *milk* group, milk and everything made from it, such as cheese, ice cream, and yogurt.

Each day, try to follow the 4-4-2-2 rule: 4 servings from the fruit-vegetable group, 4 servings from the bread-cereal group, 2 servings from the meat group, and 2 servings from the milk group.

Also remember these tips:
• To prevent or relieve constipation, make sure you're getting adequate fiber in your diet. That means eating a variety of fruits and vegetables as well as whole grain bread and foods like brown rice and barley.
• Watch your intake of cholesterol and saturated fats to lower your risk of heart disease. Eat more chicken and turkey (re-move the skin), rabbit, and fish rather than beef. And substitute low-fat or skimmed milk, cheeses like cottage cheese and ricotta, and yogurt for whole milk and its products. Just be sure not to neglect the milk group. Why? Because it provides calcium to help prevent your bones from becoming brittle.

Making mealtime more enjoyable

Once you've selected the right foods, follow these tips to make mealtime enjoyable:
• Since your taste buds become less sensitive as you grow older, you may need more seasonings to bring out the flavor in food. Try a variety of seasonings and herbs until you find what you like. However, avoid excessive use of salt, which can cause fluid retention and increase your risk of high blood pressure.
• If you live alone, try to eat with a friend. It's always more enjoyable to prepare a "sit-down" meal for two. You might even plan a picnic if the weather's nice.
• Buy a cookbook or take one out from the library, and plan some easy new meals.

of functional nephrons, instruct the elderly person to drink adequate fluids to promote excretion. Generally, he should drink 1 ml of water per calorie daily. Explain that he'll need to increase this amount if he's losing more water than usual, for example, with diarrhea, polyuria, use of diuretics, or excessive perspiration.

Vitamins and minerals

Because an elderly person requires fewer calories, he must be especially careful to eat healthy foods to get the vitamins and minerals he needs. Explain that calcium absorption decreases with age, increasing the risk for osteoporosis. To help prevent or delay osteoporosis, encourage the elderly person to increase his calcium intake, as recommended by his doctor. But instruct him not to take a calcium supplement without his doctor's approval. (For more information on its causes and treatment, see "Osteoporosis" in Chapter 10.)

Conveying the Benefits of Exercise

Encourage the elderly person to exercise for enjoyment and relaxation as well as to promote cardiovascular health. Explain how exercise can make him feel more energetic, help him cope with stress, and promote a good night's sleep. It also helps keep his joints limber and prevent backache.

Exercises most frequently recommended for the elderly include walking, swimming, bicycling, hiking, jogging, and yoga. When possible, suggest that he ask a friend to join him to make exercise more enjoyable.

Advise the elderly person to see his doctor before starting any exercise program. By performing an exercise stress test, the doctor can evaluate how well the person's heart responds to exercise.

Then, to promote safe exercise, encourage him to:
• begin his exercise program gradually over a period of weeks
• never exceed his tolerance level during exercise
• limber up gently and slowly
• be alert for muscle and joint pains as well as early warning signs of MI
• exercise on surfaces that reduce shock and provide a sure footing
• wear well-fitting support shoes
• drink plenty of fluids to replenish water lost through perspiration
• avoid vigorous exercise in hot, humid weather.

Coping with the Effects of Aging

Many elderly suffer from at least one chronic health problem—most commonly, arthritis, heart or respiratory disease, or impaired vision or hearing. Unfortunately, such problems often occur simultaneously in the elderly, taxing the individual's and his family's ability to cope. Your teaching can encourage an elderly person to perform self-care, when possible, and thereby maintain his independence. It can also guide his family in reallocating chores when disability forces the elderly person to relinquish his former role.

Minimizing the effects of immobility

If an elderly person has limited mobility, do all you can to link him with community services to avoid unnecessary institutionalization. For example, tell him about Meals On Wheels; transportation services to and from the doctor's office, church, or grocery store; homemaker services; and the role of visiting nurses and home health aides.

To help minimize immobility, stress the importance of exercise and a positive attitude. Also teach precautions against falls. For example, urge the elderly person to anchor throw rugs to the floor or to obtain throw rugs that have nonskid backing. Suggest installing grab rails in the bathtub to make getting in and out of the tub much easier—and safer. Applying nonslip strips or decals to the bottom of the tub also helps ensure good footing. Remember, the elderly are prone to fractures when they fall, and their healing time is also delayed.

Compensating for sensory loss

Aging commonly affects an individual's sense of taste, smell, hearing, and sight. That's why you'll need to teach the elderly person how to protect each of these senses and compensate for impaired function.

• *Taste and smell.* Research shows that taste buds diminish in number and sensitivity with age. Many elderly also have difficulty distinguishing odors. Because taste and smell contribute so much to food appreciation, an elderly person may develop poor eating habits. To stimulate his appetite, suggest how to arrange food attractively, and encourage him to vary his diet. If an elderly person has dentures, instruct him to see his doctor if he experiences pain when chewing; his dentures may need to be refitted.

• *Hearing.* Hearing loss is a widespread problem among the elderly. Unfortunately, they sometimes fall victim to fraud when buying hearing aids without guidance from trained medical personnel. If an elderly person suspects hearing loss, stress the importance of consulting an otolaryngologist or audiologist to determine its cause and proper treatment.

• *Sight.* To help an elderly person preserve his sight, stress the importance of routine eye checkups to detect glaucoma and to update his eyeglass prescription. Explain how a current prescription prevents eyestrain during reading and, even more important, promotes safety if he's driving. Encourage him to take advantage of free eye screening at a local health fair. Or suggest that he ask his family for eyeglasses as a Christmas or birthday present.

Preventing infection

Influenza and pneumonia are leading causes of death among the elderly, especially those weakened by chronic health problems. Just consider these statistics: pneumococcal pneumonia is responsible for more than 50,000 deaths a year. Compared to the rest of the population, the death rate is 2½ times higher for those between ages 65 and 74 and 10 times higher for those between ages 75 and 84.

Advise the elderly person to consult his doctor about vaccination against influenza and pneumococcal pneumonia, especially if he has chronic lung disease. Explain that chronic lung disease makes him less able to tolerate respiratory infection. Also remind him of other measures to prevent infection, such as hand washing.

A FINAL WORD

Whether you're addressing an elderly person or a young child, your health teaching can accomplish only so much. After all, it's up to the individual to modify his health habits. You can't force him to stop smoking or to use a seat belt consistently. But you can promote self-responsibility—the key to his willingness to follow your health teaching. To promote self-responsibility, recognize the individual's strengths, and praise his choice of healthy habits. Accept setbacks (for example, when he goes off his diet) without harsh criticism to avoid discouraging him.

Above all, be an example for him to follow by eliminating unhealthy habits from your own life.

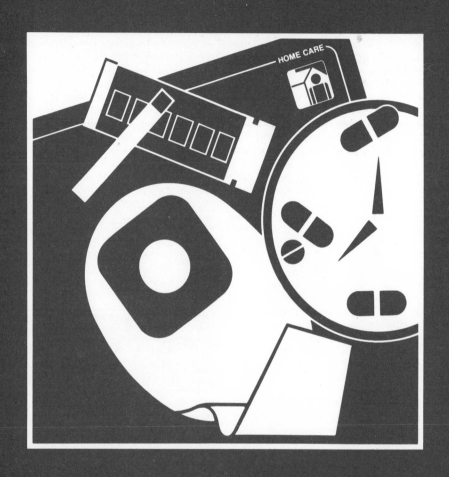

Appendices and Index

PATIENT TEACHING FOR SELECTED HEALTH PROBLEMS

This appendix supplements the main text of *Patient Teaching,* which provides comprehensive teaching considerations for hundreds of disorders, tests, and treatments. In contrast, the appendix summarizes key considerations for common disorders and symptoms that require limited, but significant, teaching as well as for uncommon ones that require extensive teaching.

For a minor health problem, such as a corn or a callus, your teaching will consist of sharing a few useful tips with your patient. But these tips can spell the difference between discomfort and relief and can prevent a minor nuisance from turning into a major problem. For a more serious problem, such as cystitis, your teaching will be more involved. You'll need to explain how successful home care—antibiotic therapy, ample fluids, and good hygiene—can eliminate the need for hospitalization. Finally, for a potentially life-threatening problem, such as anaphylaxis, you'll teach your patient when to seek medical help, while emphasizing measures to avoid such an emergency.

Acne vulgaris. An inflammation of the sebaceous glands, acne causes eruption of raised, red lesions on the skin.

Help the patient identify acne triggers—for example, certain foods or stress. Emphasize the importance of eating a well-balanced diet that provides adequate amounts of vitamins A, C, and E and the B-complex vitamins.

Help him develop an individualized skin care program: he should wash his skin frequently with a medicated soap or liquid cleanser, rinse thoroughly with warm water, and apply an astringent lotion. As needed, instruct him to apply antibacterial ointment and to use oil-free skin products. Advise him to shampoo his hair often, to keep his hair off his face. and not to squeeze or pick pimples or blackheads.

Discuss dosage instructions ,and side effects of prescribed medication. Tell a patient receiving tretinoin to apply the medication at least 30 minutes before washing his face and at least 1 hour before bedtime. Also instruct him to avoid sunlight or to use a sunscreen. Tell a patient receiving tetracycline to take the drug on an empty stomach and to avoid milk products.

Allergic rhinitis. A common immune reaction to inhaled allergens, allergic rhinitis can occur seasonally (hay fever) or year-round (perennial allergy). Common seasonal allergens include pollen and molds. Common perennial allergens include dust, cigarette smoke, and animal hair.

Describe the tests the doctor will perform to identify trigger allergens, and explain desensitization therapy. Teach the patient how to reduce environmental exposure to trigger allergens—for example, by using an air conditioner to filter pollens from the air. Also teach him how to use nasal sprays and to recognize side effects of antihistamines.

Anaphylaxis. This acute immune reaction occurs within seconds or minutes after exposure to an allergen. Common trigger allergens include vaccines, antibiotics (especially penicillin), insect venom, and certain foods.

Warn the patient at risk for anaphylaxis about the potential seriousness of this reaction. Also teach him what precautions to take. For example, if he's allergic to bee stings, tell him to avoid wearing dark clothing, especially black, which attracts bees. Advise him to carry an anaphylaxis kit whenever he goes outdoors. Make sure that he and his family know how to use the kit. Stress the importance of seeking emergency medical treatment if he experiences signs and symptoms of anaphylaxis. Also tell him to wear a Medic Alert bracelet.

Ankylosing spondylitis. Most common in males between ages 10 and 30, ankylosing spondylitis is characterized by bone and cartilage deterioration, primarily in the sacroiliac, apophyseal, and costovertebral joints. It can lead to fibrous tissue formation and, eventually, spinal fusion.

To relieve pain, instruct the patient to apply local heat, and teach family members how to massage the painful area. Discuss dosage instructions and possible side effects of prescribed anti-inflammatory medication.

To help maintain muscle strength and prevent deformity, teach the patient spine-extension exercises, chest-expanding exercises, and deep-breathing exercises. As needed, teach proper use and application of braces or splints.

To minimize deformity, advise the patient to avoid movements that stress his back, such as lifting heavy objects, slouching, or leaning over a desk. Advise against prolonged walking, standing, sitting, or driving. Also recommend sleeping in a prone position on a firm mattress.

Athlete's foot. Explain to the patient that athlete's foot results when excessive moisture, insufficient air circulation, or abrasion encourages fungus growth. If oozing lesions develop, instruct him to soak his feet every 4 hours with Domeboro or Bluboro powder solution. Show the patient how to separate his infected toes by using strips of soft cotton fabric rather than cotton balls. Tell him to wear only white cotton socks and to boil them after use.

To prevent recurrence, suggest that the patient use a skin toughener. Also tell him to wear sandals or shoes that "breathe," to keep his feet cool and dry, and to wash his feet daily.

B

Bell's palsy. A disease of the seventh cranial nerve, Bell's palsy produces unilateral facial weakness.

Teach the patient how to manage Bell's palsy and its treatment. To relieve pain, tell him to apply warm, moist compresses to the affected area. Also review dosage instructions for prescribed anti-inflammatory medication, and warn him about potential side effects. Instruct him to wear an eye patch when exposure to dust and wind is unavoidable. Advise him to eat soft foods and to chew on the unaffected side of his mouth. Teach him to exercise his facial muscles—initially, by massaging his face with a gentle upward motion; later, by grimacing—three times a day, for 15 minutes.

C

Carpal tunnel syndrome. A common, painful disorder of the hand and wrist, carpal tunnel syndrome results from compression of the median nerve at the wrist, within the carpal tunnel.

To relieve minor discomfort, tell the patient to take aspirin or acetaminophen. Then explain the recommended treatment—immobilization or surgery. If immobilization is ordered, teach him how to apply and remove the splint. Instruct him to watch for and report signs and symp-

toms of a poorly fitted splint, such as pain or cyanosis. When the splint is removed, have him perform gentle range-of-motion exercises with the affected hand. If surgery is ordered, teach him to exercise the hand and wrist in warm water after surgery. (Have him place a rubber glove over the dressing before immersing it in water.) Also show the patient how to apply a sling properly. Have him remove the sling several times a day and perform range-of-motion exercises for the shoulder and elbow.

Chalazion. Caused by inflammation of the meibomian gland, a chalazion is a hard, painless lump, usually pointed toward the conjunctival side of the eyelid.

Teach the patient to apply warm compresses to the affected eyelid four times a day, for 10 to 15 minutes. Also show him how to instill eye drops or ointment, as needed. After the chalazion heals, instruct him to wash his eyelids regularly with water and baby shampoo, applied with a cotton applicator. Have him apply warm compresses at the first sign of eyelid irritation to keep the gland lumen open.

Cleft lip and palate. A common congenital deformity, cleft lip and palate occurs when the palatine shelves fuse imperfectly with the front and sides of the face during the second month of gestation.

Before corrective surgery, show the parents how to hold the infant in a near-sitting position and direct the flow of formula to the side or back of his tongue. If the infant develops an ulcer on the underside of the nasal septum, teach the parents to feed him by directing the nipple to the side of his mouth. Instruct them to cleanse the ulcerated area with a cotton applicator dipped in half-strength hydrogen peroxide after each feeding. After surgery, teach the parents how to give enteral feedings until the infant's ability to suck returns.

Clubfoot. This congenital deformity is marked by a deformed talus and a shortened Achilles tendon. Typically, prompt treatment can correct clubfoot.

Teach parents how to care for their child's corrective cast and check circulation in the affected foot. Tell them to notify the doctor if the child develops signs of impaired circulation, such as numbness or cyanosis.

Emphasize the need for long-term orthopedic care to maintain correction. Urge parents to have the child perform prescribed exercises and wear corrective shoes and splints.

Cold injuries. Caused by overexposure to cold air or water, cold injuries may be localized (frostbite) or systemic (hypothermia). Untreated frostbite can lead to gangrene and may require amputation; severe hypothermia can be fatal.

For a patient with frostbite, explain the need for gradual rewarming of the affected area to avoid further tissue damage. Warn him not to rub the area until its temperature is restored.

For a patient with hypothermia, explain emergency treatment measures, such as the administration of warmed I.V. and nasogastric solutions and frequent monitoring.

To help prevent cold injuries, advise the patient to avoid alcohol and to eat a diet high in fats and carbohydrates before going outdoors in cold weather. Also advise him to wear mittens; windproof, multilayered clothing; and a hat or scarf when outdoors.

Conjunctivitis. Explain to the patient that inflammation of the conjunctiva, or conjunctivitis, may result from infection, allergy, or exposure to chemical irritants. Its telltale sign is eye redness, although discharge, tearing, pain, itching, and burning may also occur.

Teach the patient and his family how to use prescribed ointment or eye drops. To prevent spread of infection, instruct the patient to avoid rubbing the affected eye; to apply a clean, warm compress to the eye four times a day, for 10 to 15 minutes; and to wash his hands thoroughly before and after he touches the eye.

Constipation. Characterized by difficulty in passing stools or infrequent passage of hard stools, constipation is commonly caused by poor bowel habits, inadequate fluid and fiber intake, and lack of exercise. It's also associated with certain disorders and drugs and with laxative abuse.

To prevent or relieve constipation, instruct the patient to drink at least eight glasses of fluid a day and to eat high-fiber foods, such as grains, vegetables, and fruits. Also encourage him to exercise at least 1½ hours each week, if possible. Teach him how to schedule regular, unhurried bowel movements. Also warn that frequent use of laxatives may aggravate constipation. Tell him to notify the doctor if constipation lasts more than 2 weeks.

Corneal abrasion. The most common eye injury, corneal abrasion is a scratch on the surface of the cornea's epithelium. It usually results when a foreign body, such as dirt or metal, becomes embedded under the eyelid. It can also be caused by wearing contact lenses that are improperly lubricated or fitted, or by sleeping with hard or non-extended wear lenses in place.

Explain that most corneal abrasions heal in 24 to 48 hours if treated with antibiotics to prevent infection. Point out that untreated corneal abrasion can lead to ulceration and, possibly, permanent vision loss.

Teach the patient how to use prescribed eye drops or ointment and to apply an ophthalmic dressing and eye patch. Remind him to wash his hands before touching medication and sterile dressings. Prepare him for loss of depth perception when he's wearing the eye patch. If appropriate, tell him to check with his doctor before reinserting his contact lenses.

Corns and calluses. Corns and calluses are thickened pads of skin that develop in areas of constant pressure or friction. Both usually occur on the feet after wearing new or overly snug shoes, although calluses may also develop on the palms after doing manual work.

If the patient has a corn, teach him how to apply a salicylic acid plaster. After he removes the plaster, have him soak the affected area in water and remove the softened skin with a towel or pumice stone. Then have him apply a fresh plaster and repeat the procedure until the entire corn is removed. If the patient's corn has been excised or cauterized, show him how to change the dressing. Also instruct him to watch for and report signs of infection.

If the patient has a callus, teach him how to soften the horny layer of skin by applying emollients and keratolytic agents, as ordered. Have him soak the callus in warm water and smooth its surface with a pumice stone. Warn him never to cut the callus, and instruct him to watch for and report signs of infection.

Cor pulmonale. Cor pulmonale is defined as right ventricular hypertrophy resulting from a disorder of the lungs, pulmonary vessels, chest wall, or respiratory control center. Typically, it occurs in advanced disease.

To help the patient manage progressive dyspnea, teach him how to perform breathing exercises and use oxygen therapy at home. Instruct him to watch for and immediately report signs and symptoms of respiratory infection.

To prevent fluid retention, tell him to avoid drinking more than eight 8-oz glasses of fluid each day and to eat a low-sodium diet. Teach him how to monitor fluid balance by weighing himself at the same time each day, wearing the same type of clothing. Also teach him to measure his ankle girth and to check his skin for pitting, to assess peripheral edema. Tell him to notify the doctor immediately if his weight or peripheral edema increases.

Teach him how to check his radial pulse before taking digoxin. Have him notify the doctor if his pulse rate changes or if he develops signs and symptoms of digitalis toxicity.

To conserve energy, advise the patient to pace his activities and to rest frequently. Also recommend small, frequent meals to avoid fatigue during eating.

Cystic fibrosis. Marked by generalized dysfunction of the endocrine glands, cystic fibrosis is the most common fatal genetic disease affecting white children. Its clinical effects—including major aberrations in sweat gland, respiratory, and gastrointestinal function—may become apparent soon after birth or may take years to develop.

Discuss dietary management of cystic fibrosis with the child and his parents. Encourage the parents to keep the child's diet as normal as possible while limiting his intake of fat. To combat electrolyte loss through perspiration, instruct them to generously salt the child's food and to give him salt supplements during hot weather, as ordered. To offset pancreatic enzyme deficiency, tell them to include supplemental pancreatic enzymes with meals.

Teach the child and his parents how to maintain pulmonary hygiene through physical therapy, postural drainage, and breathing exercises. As needed, teach the parents to administer aerosol therapy and oxygen therapy at home. Warn them not to give the child over-the-counter antihistamines, which tend to dry mucous membranes. Also teach them to watch for and report symptoms of respiratory infection.

Cystitis. Common in women and catheterized patients, this inflammation of the urinary bladder results from bacterial infection. Untreated or severe cystitis may lead to pyelonephritis.

Teach the patient how to obtain a clean-catch urine specimen for culture and sensitivity analysis, if needed. To relieve dysuria, recommend sitz baths, aspirin, and application of heat to the perineum. Encourage the patient to drink at least 10 glasses of fluid per day to flush bacteria from the bladder.

To prevent recurrence of cystitis, instruct the patient to void immediately after intercourse, to empty the bladder completely during urination, and to always wipe the perineum from front to back. Teach a catheterized patient to maintain a closed drainage system and to change the urinary drainage bag once a month or whenever sediment accumulates. Stress the importance of completing the prescribed antibiotic therapy to help prevent reactivation of infection. Have the patient notify the doctor if fever, chills, or flank pain occurs.

D

Diarrhea. Characterized by unusually frequent and loose bowel movements, diarrhea is commonly caused by nervousness, intestinal infection, or ingestion of caffeine or contaminated, spicy, or high-fiber foods. Severe diarrhea may require medical intervention.

As ordered, recommend antidiarrheal agents, such as Kaopectate. Instruct the patient to drink plenty of fluids but to avoid milk and solid foods until diarrhea stops; then have him gradually add soft foods to his diet. Tell him to notify the doctor if diarrhea lasts more than 24 hours, contains blood, or occurs intermittently for an extended period.

E

Eczema. A noncontagious skin inflammation, eczema results from hypersensitivity to dust, perfumes, certain foods, or clothing made from animal products. Its characteristic thick, crusty skin lesions tend to flare up in response to ex-

tremes in temperature and humidity.

To help prevent such flare-ups, teach the patient to avoid known allergens and extremes in temperature or humidity. Also instruct him to take prescribed antihistamines, as ordered. Teach him strategies for coping with emotional stress, which may aggravate eczema.

Help the patient develop an individualized skin care plan. Advise him to limit bathing when eczema is severe and to use over-the-counter cleansers and shampoos formulated for persons with eczema. After bathing, tell him to lubricate his skin with a medicated cream or ointment. Instruct him to keep his fingernails short to avoid excoriation and secondary infection. Show the patient how to apply compresses of Domeboro or Bluboro solution to oozing skin lesions. If indicated, also show him how to apply hydrocortisone cream and nonocclusive dressings.

Epicondylitis. Any activity that requires a forceful grasp, wrist extension against resistance, or frequent rotation of the forearm can lead to epicondylitis, also known as tennis elbow. This painful inflammation involves the forearm extensor supinator tendon fibers where they attach to the lateral humeral epicondyle.

Teach the patient how to apply a splint to the affected forearm. Have him exercise every 2 to 4 hours while wearing the splint: he should stretch his arm and flex his wrist to the maximum, then press the back of his hand against a wall until he can feel a pull in his forearm, and hold this position for 1 minute. Tell him to remove the splint daily and gently move the arm to prevent stiffness and contracture. Review dosage instructions for prescribed anti-inflammatory medication, and warn the patient of potential side effects.

To prevent epicondylitis, advise the patient to warm up for 15 to 20 minutes before engaging in sports activity. Urge him to wear an elastic support or splint during any activity that stresses the forearm or elbow.

F

Fever. An abnormal elevation of body temperature, fever results from an imbalance between heat production and heat loss. Among its many causes are infection, severe trauma, and drug-related side effect. A fever's most important features are its duration and grade. Grade is labeled as low (oral temperature of 99° to 100.4° F. [37.2° to 38° C.]), moderate (100.5° to 104° F. [38.1° to 40° C.]), or high (above 104° F.).

Teach the patient (or his parents, if the patient's a child) how to take a temperature correctly. (See *How to Take a Temperature Correctly*, pages 654 and 655.) Instruct an adult patient to notify the doctor if fever rises above 104° F. or lasts longer than 24 hours. Instruct the parents of a pediatric patient to notify

654

HOW TO TAKE A TEMPERATURE CORRECTLY

Dear Patient:

Fever usually means that the body is fighting an infection or some other illness. You'll probably use a mercury thermometer or a digital thermometer to find out if you or a family member has a fever. You can take a temperature orally, rectally, or under the arm. A normal oral temperature is 97° to 99.5° F. (36.1° to 37.5° C.). Rectal temperature is generally 1 F. degree higher; underarm temperature, 1 to 2 F. degrees lower.

Using a mercury thermometer
Before using a mercury thermometer, wipe it with an alcohol-soaked gauze pad and rinse it off.

1

With your thumb and forefinger, grasp the thermometer at the end opposite the bulb. Then quickly snap your wrist to shake down the mercury.

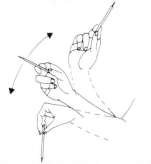

2

Next, hold the thermometer at eye level in good light and rotate it slowly until the mercury line becomes visible. Check for a reading of 95° F. (35° C.) or less. Now you're ready to take a temperature.

3

To take an oral temperature, place the bulb of the thermometer under the tongue, as far back as possible.

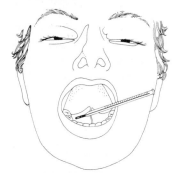

Leave the thermometer in place for 4 to 5 minutes to register the correct temperature. Then remove the thermometer and read it at eye level.

To take another person's rectal temperature, first dip the bulb end of the *rectal* thermometer in petrolatum (Vaseline). Then position the person on his side, with the top leg bent. Position an infant on his stomach.

Gently insert the thermometer into the rectum—about ½″ for an infant, 1″ for a child, or 1½″ for an adult.

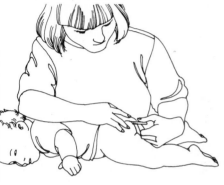

Hold the thermometer in place for 3 minutes. Next, carefully remove it and wipe it with a tissue. Read the thermometer at eye level.

To take an axillary (underarm) temperature, put the bulb of the thermometer in one armpit, and fold the arm across the chest. Remove the thermometer after 10 minutes, and read it at eye level.

Using a digital thermometer

If you wish, you can use a digital thermometer instead of a mercury thermometer to take an oral temperature reading.

1
Remove the thermometer from its protective case.

2
Next, position the thermometer tip under the tongue, as far back as possible. Leave the thermometer in place for at least 45 seconds.

3
Remove the thermometer and read the numbers on display. This is the temperature. Then clean the thermometer as the manufacturer instructs and replace it in its protective case.

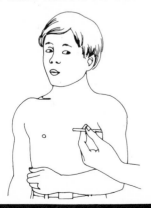

the doctor if the child's temperature rises above 101° F. (38.3° C.).

To reduce low- or moderate-grade fever, recommend that the patient take aspirin or acetaminophen, as directed. Also suggest that he lie in front of a fan or sponge his face, arms, and legs with lukewarm water and allow them to air dry. Tell the patient to rest during a fever episode and to drink eight or more glasses of water per day to prevent dehydration. Advise him to keep room temperature around 70° F. (21.1° C.).

Foreign body in the ear. Children sometimes put small objects—such as beans, beads, and bits of paper or cotton—into their ears. Insects can also find their way into the ears of children and adults alike.

If the patient has an insect in his ear, instruct him (or his parents, if he's a child) to kill the insect by instilling 70% isopropyl alcohol or a few drops of mineral oil into the ear canal. To remove other objects, instruct the patient or his parents to notify the doctor. Caution against using water to flush beans or paper from the ear canal: water may cause the object to swell, making removal more difficult. And, to prevent infection, tell the patient to avoid getting water in the ear for at least 24 hours after the object is removed. Instruct the patient or his parents to notify the doctor if fever, pain, erythema, or ear drainage occurs. Also teach them how to instill eardrops, if ordered.

G

Gastrointestinal reflux. In gastrointestinal (GI) reflux, gastric or duodenal contents flow upward past the lower esophageal sphincter into the esophagus.

Teach a patient who's predisposed to GI reflux tips to prevent it. For example, instruct him to avoid actions that increase intraabdominal pressure—such as bending, exercising vigorously, and wearing tight clothing—or that reduce sphincter control—such as smoking or ingesting alcohol, whole milk, tomatoes, or chocolate. Advise him to eat small, frequent meals and to sit upright for at least 2 hours after eating.

Gout. In this metabolic disease, urate deposits are responsible for painful, arthritic joints.

To relieve discomfort during an acute episode, teach the patient to apply hot or cold compresses to the affected joints four times per day, for 15 to 20 minutes. Also advise him to rest in bed with the affected joints elevated. Recommend aspirin or acetaminophen, if needed.

Explain specific treatment measures—for example, joint aspiration or intraarticular corticosteroid injection—if ordered. For chronic gout, stress the importance of taking the prescribed medication and returning to the hospital for

blood tests to measure uric acid levels. To avoid increasing urate levels, caution a patient taking probenecid or sulfinpyrazone to avoid aspirin or other salicylates. Also instruct him to avoid high-purine foods and drinks, such as anchovies, liver, sardines, kidneys, sweetbreads, lentils, and alcoholic beverages—especially beer and wine.

H

Heat injuries. Resulting from environmental conditions or internal problems that impair heat dissipation, heat injuries fall into three categories: heat cramps, heat exhaustion, and heat stroke.

Explain treatments to lower temperature—for example, an ice bath, application of ice packs, or administration of a cold I.V. solution.

To prevent heat injuries, instruct the patient to take these precautions in hot weather: wear lightweight, loose-fitting clothing; cover his head; rest frequently; and drink plenty of fluids. Advise the patient who is obese, elderly, or taking drugs that impair heat regulation—such as phenothiazines—to avoid overheating.

Hemorrhoids. This common problem results from conditions that increase pressure in the veins of the lower rectum and anus—for example, pregnancy, constipation, and prolonged sitting.

Tell the patient with hemorrhoids to use only white, unscented toilet paper and to clean the perianal area with soap and water after each bowel movement. To relieve pain and inflammation, instruct him to sit in a hot bath three to five times per day, for 10 to 20 minutes. Teach him how to instill rectal suppositories or ointment, and advise him to rest until discomfort subsides. Discuss strategies for preventing constipation, if needed. Tell the patient to notify the doctor if he develops sudden rectal pain or a large, firm lump near the anus—possible signs of thrombosed external hemorrhoids.

I J K

Infected skin laceration. Because the infection risk is so great, most skin lacerations—especially those with irregular edges or partially avulsed tissue—are considered contaminated injuries.

As ordered, explain the need for tetanus prophylaxis and the dosage instructions for prescribed antibiotics. Teach the patient how to change his dressing and irrigate the wound, if needed; however, stress that he should leave the wound undisturbed at all other times. Advise him to relieve pain by taking aspirin or acetaminophen and to reduce swelling by elevating the affected area. Tell him to watch for and report signs of worsening infection.

Infectious mononucleosis. Caused by a virus in the herpes group, this acute infection primarily affects young adults and children. It's characterized by fever, sore throat, cervical lymphadenopathy, and generalized weakness.

Tell the patient to drink plenty of water and fruit juice, especially while he has a fever. To relieve discomfort, tell him to take aspirin or acetaminophen, as ordered. Instruct the patient to gargle with saline solution to relieve sore throat. Stress that bed rest, especially in the acute phase, is essential to his recovery. Advise him not to return to his daily routine until he has fully recovered—which may take a month or longer.

Ingrown toenail (onychocryptosis). An ingrown toenail results when the free edge of a toenail penetrates and becomes embedded in soft tissue layers. To relieve discomfort, have the patient soak the affected foot in a warm solution of Epsom salts four times a day, for 15 to 20 minutes. Tell him to notify his doctor if pain persists. If the toenail is surgically removed, show him how to change his dressing, and tell him to watch for and report signs of infection. Advise the patient to wear loose-fitting shoes, to keep his feet clean and dry, and to trim his nails straight across the top of the toe to prevent recurrence.

Insect sting. The venom an insect injects by stinging its victim produces a local inflammatory reaction or, in sensitive individuals, anaphylaxis.

Instruct the patient to remove the stinger (if present) by scraping it with a fingernail, since pulling it out would release more toxins. Advise him to apply an ice compress to reduce spread of the toxin, decrease swelling, and relieve pain. Calamine lotion or hydrocortisone cream may reduce itching. Tell him to call the doctor immediately if he develops hives or has difficulty breathing. (See "Anaphylaxis," page 650.)

L

Laryngotracheobronchitis (croup). A severe inflammation of the upper airway, laryngotracheobronchitis (LTB) can lead to life-threatening airway obstruction in children. Usually, though, it can be managed successfully at home.

Teach parents to use a cool-mist humidifier at the first sign of LTB. If LTB progresses, advise them to carry the child into the bathroom, to shut the door, and to turn on the hot water in the shower. Usually, breathing the warm, moist air provides quick relief. However, if it doesn't, instruct the parents to notify the doctor immediately.

After an LTB episode, instruct the parents to monitor the child's temperature for fever. Tell them to give the child acetaminophen and sponge baths to reduce fever, and plenty of fluids to prevent dehydration. Also tell them to keep the child as quiet as possible. To relieve sore throat, recommend soothing fruit sherbet or popsicles. Caution them not to give the child milk products or beverages if he is producing heavy mucus or has trouble swallowing.

M

Ménière's disease. A dysfunction of the labyrinthine system, Ménière's disease produces attacks of severe vertigo, hearing loss, and tinnitus. It's believed to stem from autonomic nervous system dysfunction that temporarily constricts blood vessels supplying the inner ear.

To minimize vertigo during an attack, advise the patient to avoid reading and exposure to glaring lights. Warn him to avoid sudden position changes and tasks that vertigo makes hazardous.

Discuss dosage instructions and potential side effects of prescribed medication. If the patient experiences drowsiness, caution him against driving or operating machinery while taking medication.

Motion sickness. In motion sickness, the patient experiences loss of equilibrium with nausea and vomiting in response to irregular or rhythmic movements or the sensation of motion. To prevent or minimize motion sickness, tell him to avoid eating or drinking for at least 4 hours before traveling. Inform him that lying down, closing his eyes, and trying to sleep while traveling may relieve his symptoms. As ordered, teach the patient how to use antiemetics, such as dimenhydrinate.

Muscle cramp. A muscle cramp is a painful, sustained muscle contraction that commonly results from fatigue, poor circulation, exposure to cold, calcium or vitamin B_1 deficiency, or sodium or potassium loss.

To relieve a muscle cramp, have the patient stretch the affected muscle. For example, to relieve a muscle cramp in the calf, tell him to straighten the knee and pull the foot upward or to stand up and point the toe toward the ceiling. Suggest massaging the affected muscle and applying a warm compress. After the cause is identified, teach the patient how to prevent muscle cramps—for example, by replacing fluids and electrolytes lost during strenuous activity or by taking calcium or vitamin B_1 supplements to correct deficiency.

Muscular dystrophy. Muscular dystrophy (MD) is actually a group of congenital disorders characterized by progressive skeletal muscle wasting without neural or sensory deficits. However, these wasted muscles tend to enlarge because of connective tissue and fat deposits, giving an erroneous impression of muscle strength.

Teach the patient and his family how to apply

and use orthopedic devices, if ordered. Also teach the patient proper techniques for coughing, deep breathing, and diaphragmatic breathing. Stress that performing prescribed exercises will help maintain mobility. To prevent constipation associated with muscle weakness, advise the patient to drink 8 to 10 glasses of fluid per day and to eat high-fiber foods.

N

Neurogenic arthropathy. Caused by sensory nerve impairment, neurogenic arthropathy is a progressive degenerative disease of peripheral and axial joints.

To control joint pain, tell the patient to take aspirin or acetaminophen and to apply warm compresses to the affected joints four times a day, for 15 to 20 minutes. As ordered, teach him how to immobilize the affected joint, apply and remove braces or splints, and walk with crutches. Also teach him to pace daily activities, to rest often, to avoid physically stressful actions, and to take safety precautions, such as removing throw rugs from the floor. Advise him to report persistent joint pain, swelling, or instability to his doctor.

O

Obesity. Defined as a body weight more than 20% above the ideal weight, obesity results from excessive caloric intake in relation to energy expenditure. Rarely, obesity is associated with hormonal disturbances; most commonly, it's caused by overeating.

Discuss the patient's prescribed diet—usually, a well-balanced, low-calorie diet that eliminates foods high in fat and sugar. Caution him to check with the doctor before using over-the-counter appetite suppressants. Also help him develop an individualized exercise program, and stress the importance of increasing physical activity to burn calories. Emphasize that he must *permanently* change his eating and exercise habits to maintain the proper weight.

Occupational lung disease. Fibrotic lung damage may result from chronic exposure to environmental pollutants, such as silica (silicosis), asbestos (asbestosis), beryllium (berylliosis), or coal dust (coal worker's pneumoconiosis).

To help loosen secretions, advise the patient to increase his fluid intake and to use a humidifier. Also teach him and his family how to administer chest physical therapy and, if needed, oxygen therapy at home.

To help prevent infection, teach the patient to avoid crowds and persons with colds or flu. Also advise him to receive influenza and pneumococcal vaccines.

Tell the patient to pace his activities and to rest frequently to conserve his energy. How-ever, encourage regular exercise to increase his tolerance.

Otitis externa. Also known as swimmer's ear, otitis externa is an inflammation of the external ear canal and auricle. It may result from swimming in contaminated water, exposure to dust and other irritants, using earphones, and cleaning the ear canal with objects that cause irritation or introduce microorganisms.

Teach the patient how to clean and care for the infected ear. Show him how to clean the ear without damaging delicate tissue and how to apply heat to the periaural region. Also teach him how to instill eardrops properly—by pulling the pinna up and back for an adult or down and back for a child.

To prevent future bouts of otitis externa, tell the patient to keep shower water out of his ears with lamb's wool earplugs coated with petrolatum (Vaseline), to use earplugs when swimming, and to instill 2 to 3 drops of 3% boric acid solution in 70% alcohol in each ear before and after swimming. Caution him against cleaning the ears with cotton swabs, bobby pins, or foreign objects.

P Q R

Paget's disease of the bone. In this progressive metabolic bone disease, abnormal bone resorption and formation lead to painful deformities and susceptibility to pathologic fractures.

Outline drug therapy for the patient, and warn him about potential side effects and interactions. To relieve pain, recommend analgesics such as aspirin and acetaminophen. Show the patient how to administer calcitonin I.M., if ordered. Have him notify the doctor if he develops nausea, vomiting, fever, facial flushing, itchy hands, or pain and redness at the injection site. Tell a patient receiving etidronate to take the drug with fruit juice 2 hours before or after meals and to notify the doctor if he develops stomach cramps, diarrhea, or increasing pain. Tell a patient receiving plicamycin to notify the doctor if he develops easy bruising, bleeding, and fever. Stress the importance of returning for follow-up blood studies.

As needed, teach the patient how to use assistive devices and perform prescribed exercises. Also teach him to observe good body mechanics and safety measures, such as removing throw rugs and clutter from the floor. Suggest that he use a firm mattress or a bed board to minimize spinal deformities.

Pediculosis (lice). Pediculosis is caused by parasitic forms of lice, which lay their eggs (nits) in body hairs or clothing fibers. After the nits hatch, the lice must feed on human blood. A louse bite injects a toxin into the skin that produces mild irritation and a purpuric spot.

If the patient has head lice, instruct him to

apply 30 ml of undiluted lindane (Kwell) shampoo to the hair, work it into a lather, rinse thoroughly after 5 minutes, and dry. To remove nits, tell him to comb his hair with a fine-toothed comb dipped in vinegar; to remove crusts, tell him to wash his hair with ordinary shampoo.

To remove body lice, tell the patient to bathe in warm soapy water, to apply a thin layer of prescribed ointment to the affected area, and to wash off the ointment after 8 to 12 hours. Instruct him to remove lice from clothing by washing or dry-cleaning the items and storing them for at least 30 days. Tell him to disinfect bed linens and pillows after treatment by washing them in hot water.

Poison ivy, sumac, and oak. In a sensitive individual, physical contact with poison ivy, sumac, or oak produces a red, papular, pruritic skin rash, which darkens as the allergic reaction intensifies.

Inform the patient that the rash usually reaches its peak within 5 days after exposure and gradually resolves within 7 to 14 days. To treat severe itching and burning, teach the patient to apply compresses soaked in cold water or Burow's solution four times a day, for 20 minutes. If a large area of skin is affected, recommend bathing in Domeboro or Bluboro solution. Tell the patient to apply a thin layer of steroid cream or calamine lotion after soaking or bathing and to wash his hands thoroughly after touching the affected area.

To prevent skin exposure, tell the patient to wear protective clothing (long pants and sleeves, closed shoes) when walking in areas where poison oak, sumac, or ivy grows. If skin exposure occurs, advise him to wash as soon as possible with cold water and bar laundry soap. Warn against burning poison oak, sumac, or ivy. Inhaling smoke from bonfires made with these vines may cause serious respiratory tract inflammation.

Psoriasis. Characterized by recurrent flare-ups, psoriasis produces erythematous papules covered with telltale silvery scales. Tell the patient that no cure exists for psoriasis, but assure him that flare-ups can usually be controlled with therapy. Also explain that psoriasis is not contagious.

Help the patient develop an individualized skin care program: advise him to bathe in tar-based over-the-counter preparations to relieve itching and to wash his hair with a medicated shampoo. Recommend baby oil or petrolatum to soften scales. Tell him to apply a thin layer of steroid cream or ointment several times a day. Have him rub the cream well into his skin. Also teach him to apply an occlusive dressing after cream application, or recommend covering the skin with plastic wrap, plastic gloves, or a vinyl exercise suit. Describe potential effects of steroid cream, such as acne. If he's using anthralin concurrently with steroid cream, tell

him to apply it with downward strokes to avoid rubbing it into the follicles. Advise him to stay out of the sun on the day of anthralin therapy and to wear sunglasses if he goes outdoors the day after therapy. Inform him of potential side effects, such as burning, itching, and nausea.

S

Sarcoidosis. This chronic granulomatous disease typically produces lymphadenopathy, pulmonary infiltration, and skeletal, liver, eye, or skin lesions. Its cause is unknown.

Focus your teaching on helping the patient cope with the diverse effects of sarcoidosis. Instruct him to take analgesics, as ordered, to relieve arthralgia. Advise him to eat a nutritious, high-calorie diet and to drink plenty of fluids. If appropriate, recommend limiting his calcium intake to correct hypercalcemia. Tell him to notify the doctor immediately if he experiences shortness of breath, chest tightness or pain, extreme or progressive muscle weakness, or decreased visual acuity.

Reinforce the doctor's explanation of steroid therapy, and teach the patient how to minimize its side effects. For example, because steroids increase appetite, recommend a diet that's high in protein and carbohydrates but low in fat, to prevent obesity. Also advise him to decrease his salt intake to avoid fluid retention. Stress the importance of returning to the hospital for blood tests to monitor steroid therapy. Also warn him not to discontinue or change the steroid dosage without checking with his doctor.

Scabies. This skin infection results from infestation with the itch mite and is predisposed by overcrowding and poor hygiene—conditions that can make it endemic. Typically, scabies causes itching that intensifies at night. It's marked by erythematous nodules that usually become excoriated.

Teach the patient how to treat scabies and prevent reinfection. Instruct him to bathe thoroughly with soap and warm water and to apply a thin layer of the prescribed cream or lotion from the neck down over his entire body. Tell him to allow 15 minutes between applying the lotion and dressing, and to wait 24 hours before bathing again. Stress that all contaminated clothing and linens must be washed in hot water or dry-cleaned. Explain that itching may continue for several weeks after effective treatment. If needed, hydrocortisone cream can be used to relieve itching.

Scleroderma. Progressive systemic scleroderma is characterized by fibrotic, degenerative, and occasionally inflammatory changes in the skin, blood vessels, synovium, skeletal muscles, and internal organs. This diffuse connective tissue disease affects women more than men, especially between ages 30 and 50. Its cause is unknown.

Explain the disease process and the recommended treatment—for example, chemotherapy, steroid or antibiotic therapy, esophageal dilation, dialysis, or physical therapy for joint stiffness. Stress the importance of returning to the hospital for laboratory tests to monitor immunosuppressive therapy. Also advise the patient to report any abnormal bruising or nonhealing abrasions immediately. To lessen hand and foot debilitation, have her wear warm socks and gloves and avoid exposure to cold. Caution her to avoid burns and cuts, to minimize digital ulceration, and to treat any local infections immediately. Advise her to use skin-softening lotions, soaps, and bath oils to prevent skin dryness. To minimize dysphagia, tell her to eat small, frequent meals; to chew food slowly; and to drink liquids with meals. After meals, she should take an antacid and sit upright for 30 to 45 minutes to prevent heartburn. Recommend using extra pillows or raising the head of the bed to prevent nocturnal esophageal reflux.

Scoliosis. Scoliosis is a lateral curvature of the spine found in the thoracic, lumbar, or thoracolumbar spinal segment.

Explain the recommended treatment: generally, curvature less than 25 degrees is treated with special exercises to strengthen torso muscles and prevent progression. Curvature between 25 and 60 degrees requires a spinal brace as well as exercise. Curvature greater than 60 degrees requires corrective surgery.

As indicated, teach the patient how to perform prescribed exercises, including sit-up pelvic tilts, hyperextension of the spine, and breathing exercises. If the patient requires a spinal brace, make sure he knows how to apply and care for it properly. Advise him to remove the brace during prescribed exercises. To prevent skin breakdown, tell him to keep his skin clean and dry, to wear a snug T-shirt under the brace, and to avoid use of skin lotions, ointments, and powder. Advise him to gradually increase his activity while wearing the brace but to avoid strenuous sports. If the patient requires corrective surgery, teach his family how to care for him while he recuperates. Also teach cast care, if needed.

Severe combined immunodeficiency disease. In this genetic disorder, both T cell and B cell immunity are either completely absent or severely deficient, leading to extreme susceptibility to infection and a shortened life span. Only males are affected, and most die from infection during the first year of life.

Although nursing care is primarily supportive, you'll also need to teach parents how to care for their infant at home. Instruct them to watch for and report signs and symptoms of infection, and teach them how to set up and maintain sterile isolation. Explain that the child will require a stimulating atmosphere in order to promote growth and development.

Stye. A localized, purulent staphylococcal infection, a stye can occur externally (in the glands of Zeis or Moll's glands) or internally (in the meibomian gland).

To alleviate pain and to facilitate drainage, instruct the patient to apply warm compresses over the stye four times a day, for 10 to 15 minutes. Have him wash his hands thoroughly after each application. To prevent spreading infection, have him discard or launder the compress cloths separately and avoid sharing face and hand towels with other family members. Teach the patient how to instill eye drops or ointment. Also warn him not to squeeze the affected eye.

Sunburn. Most people become sunburned while trying to acquire suntans. Explain to the patient that exposure to the sun's ultraviolet rays damages skin cells and that extensive exposure can eventually lead to skin cancer.

To relieve sunburn pain, tell the patient to apply an anesthetic ointment or cool compresses of witch hazel, diluted Burow's solution, or baking soda and water several times a day, for 15 minutes. Recommend aspirin or acetaminophen if pain persists.

To prevent future sunburn, advise the patient to stay out of the sun between 10 a.m. and 2 p.m. and to avoid surfaces that reflect ultraviolet rays. Recommend a sunscreen with the proper sun protection factor for his skin type.

T

Tendinitis and bursitis. Inflammation of a tendon (tendinitis) or bursa (bursitis) can result from trauma, postural misalignment, or various musculoskeletal disorders.

Review dosage instructions for prescribed anti-inflammatory agents, and warn the patient of potential side effects or interactions. For example, tell him to notify the doctor immediately if he develops gastrointestinal distress.

Explain that resting the joint by immobilization also helps relieve pain. For example, to support the arm and shoulder, teach the patient and his family how to apply a triangular sling. Instruct him to replace the sling with a splint at night.

To maintain joint mobility and prevent muscle atrophy, teach him how to perform prescribed exercises. However, advise against excessive exercise or physical work that stresses the painful joint.

Tooth avulsion. In many cases, an avulsed tooth can be successfully reimplanted if its root hasn't been severely damaged. To help ensure successful reimplantation, tell the patient (or his parents, if he's a child) to place the avulsed tooth in a cup of cold milk and then see the dentist as soon as possible. To reduce bleeding, instruct him to apply gauze over the gum and apply pressure.

U

Urticaria. Urticaria is a skin eruption characterized by transient wheals with well-defined erythematous margins and pale centers. It's produced by the local release of histamine or other vasoactive substances as part of a hypersensitivity reaction—most commonly, to certain drugs, foods, or insect bites or to cold or sun exposure. Angioedema is characterized by the acute eruption of wheals involving the mucous membranes and, occasionally, the arms, legs, or genitalia. It can be life-threatening if it involves the throat.

Describe the testing procedure to identify allergens, and explain desensitization therapy. Also teach the patient how to recognize and avoid trigger allergens. Tell him to notify the doctor immediately if he develops angioedema or if his throat begins to itch.

If appropriate, instruct the patient to apply corticosteroid creams. Also discuss dosage instructions and side effects of antihistamines.

V

Vitiligo. Caused by loss of pigment cells, vitiligo produces stark white skin patches that are usually bilaterally symmetrical with sharp borders. Although the cause of vitiligo is unknown, genetics and stress seem to be contributing factors.

Instruct the patient to use repigmentation medications as ordered: systemic psoralens should be taken 2 hours before sun exposure; topical solutions, 30 to 60 minutes before exposure. Warn the patient to use a sunscreen to protect both affected and unaffected skin. If sunburn occurs, advise the patient to temporarily discontinue repigmentation therapy.

Vocal cord paralysis. Vocal cord paralysis results from disease of or injury to the superior or recurrent laryngeal nerve. Depending on the cause, paralysis may be unilateral or bilateral and may produce vocal weakness or airway obstruction.

If the patient has unilateral paralysis, explain the procedure for injecting Teflon into the paralyzed cord, under direct laryngoscopy. Emphasize that this will improve his voice but won't return it to normal.

If the patient has bilateral paralysis, reinforce the doctor's explanation of the recommended treatment—tracheostomy or arytenoidectomy. If he'll be undergoing tracheostomy, describe the procedure and mention that it will be performed under a local anesthestic. Reassure the patient that he'll be able to talk after surgery by covering the lumen of his tracheostomy. Teach him how to suction, clean, and change the tracheostomy tube. If he'll be undergoing arytenoidectomy, describe the procedure and explain that he'll require a temporary tracheostomy until swelling subsides.

Vomiting. Defined as the forceful expulsion of stomach contents through the mouth, vomiting can be triggered by emotional upset, overeating, excessive alcohol intake, minor food poisoning, or viral gastroenteritis. It's also associated with more serious disorders, such as bowel obstruction, appendicitis, and head injury.

Tell the patient to take small, frequent sips of fluid, such as water or flat ginger ale. Advise him not to eat solid food until vomiting subsides. After vomiting subsides for 4 hours, have him eat plain toast or crackers; he can resume his regular diet after 24 hours. Tell the patient to notify his doctor if vomiting persists for more than 24 hours, is bloody or excessive, or is accompanied by other symptoms, such as fever or severe abdominal pain.

Vulvovaginitis. Vulvovaginitis is an inflammation of the vulva and vagina. Acute vulvovaginitis results from bacterial, fungal, or viral infection or from parasitic infestation. Chronic vulvovaginitis is associated with debilitating diseases, decreased estrogen levels, and poor personal hygiene.

Teach the patient how to administer prescribed vaginal suppositories or ointment. Tell her to lie down for at least 30 minutes after administration, to promote absorption. Suggest that she use a sanitary pad to avoid staining her underpants. To relieve pruritus, tell her to apply cool compresses or to take warm sitz baths. To avoid irritating the perineal area, have her wash with mild soap and use white, unscented toilet paper. Urge her to wear all-cotton underpants and to avoid clothing that traps moisture in the genital area, such as tight-fitting pants and panty hose.

W X Y Z

Wiskott-Aldrich syndrome. In this genetic disorder, inadequate cell-mediated or humoral immunity decreases resistance to infection and malignancy and causes thrombocytopenia with severe bleeding. Wiskott-Aldrich syndrome results from an X-linked recessive trait that occurs only in males, most of whom die by age 4.

Explain the disease process to the parents, including its impact on the child's life-style. Teach them to watch for and report signs of bleeding, such as easy bruising, painful swollen joints, and tenderness in the trunk area. Instruct them to have the child avoid contact sports and to encourage less traumatic activities, such as swimming.

To prevent infection, teach the parents to carefully cleanse any wounds. Also stress the importance of meticulous mouth and skin care, good nutrition, and adequate hydration. Advise against exposing the child to crowds or to persons with active infections. Teach the parents to watch for and report signs of infection, such as fever.

SOURCES OF INFORMATION AND SUPPORT

Al-Anon Family Group Headquarters
1372 Broadway, New York, N.Y. 10018,
(212) 302-7240

Alzheimer's Disease and Related Disorders Association
70 E. Lake St., Suite 600, Chicago, Ill. 60601-5997, (800) 621-0379

American Allergy Association
P.O. Box 7273, Menlo Park, Calif. 94026,
(415) 322-1663

American Anorexia/Bulimia Association
133 Cedar Lane, Teaneck, N.J. 07666,
(201) 837-1800

American Cancer Society (ACS)
90 Park Ave., New York, N.Y. 10016,
(212) 599-8200

American Diabetes Association
National Service Center, 1600 Duke St., Alexandria, Va. 22314, (800) 232-3472

American Heart Association
7320 Greenville Ave., Dallas, Tex. 75231,
(214) 750-5300

American Kidney Fund
7315 Wisconsin Ave., Suite 203E, Bethesda, Md. 20814-3266, (800) 638-8299

American Lung Association
1740 Broadway, New York, N.Y. 10019,
(212) 315-8700

American Parkinson Disease Association
116 John St., Suite 417, New York, N.Y. 10038,
(800) 223-2732

American Reye's Syndrome Association
701 S. Logan, Suite 203, Denver, Colo. 80209,
(303) 777-2592

The Amyotrophic Lateral Sclerosis Association
15300 Ventura Blvd., Suite 315, Sherman Oaks, Calif. 91403, (818) 990-2151

Arthritis Foundation
1314 Spring St. N.W., Atlanta, Ga. 30309,
(404) 872-7100

Cystic Fibrosis Foundation
6000 Executive Blvd., Suite 510, Rockville, Md. 20852, (800) 344-4823

Endometriosis Association
P.O. Box 92187, Milwaukee, Wis. 53202,
(414) 962-8972

Epilepsy Foundation of America
4351 Garden City Dr., Landover, Md. 20785,
(301) 459-3700

Gay Men's Health Crisis (AIDS)
P.O. Box 274, 132 W. 24th St., New York, N.Y. 10011, (212) 807-6655

Guillain-Barré Syndrome Support Group
P.O. Box 262, Wynnewood, Pa. 19096,
(215) 649-7837 or (215) 896-6372

Herpes Resource Center
P.O. Box 100, Palo Alto, Calif. 94306,
(415) 328-7710

Leukemia Society of America
733 Third Ave., New York, N.Y. 10017,
(212) 573-8484

Lupus Foundation of America, Inc.
P.O. Box 12897, St. Louis, Mo. 63141; Missouri residents: (314) 872-9036; Out-of-state residents: (800) 558-0121

March of Dimes Birth Defects Foundation
1275 Mamaroneck Ave., White Plains, N.Y. 10605, (914) 428-7100

Medic Alert Foundation International
2323 Colorado Ave., Turlock, Calif. 95381-1009,
(209) 668-3333

Mended Hearts (Cardiac Surgery)
7320 Greenville Ave., Dallas, Tex. 75231,
(214) 750-5442

Muscular Dystrophy Association
810 Seventh Ave., New York, N.Y. 10019,
(212) 586-0808

Myasthenia Gravis Foundation
7-11 S. Broadway, Suite 304, White Plains, N.Y.
10601, (914) 328-1717

**National Association of Anorexia Nervosa
and Associated Disorders (ANAD)**
P.O. Box 7, Highland Park, Ill. 60035,
(312) 831-3438

National Association of Sickle Cell Disease
4221 Wilshire Blvd., Suite 360, Los Angeles,
Calif. 90010, (213) 936-7205

**National Easter Seal Society (Crippled Chil-
dren and Adults)**
2023 Ogden Ave., Chicago, Ill. 60612,
(312) 243-8400

National Hemophilia Foundation
110 Green St., Room 406, New York, N.Y.
10012, (212) 219-8180

National Kidney Foundation
Two Park Ave., New York, N.Y. 10016,
(212) 889-2210

National Leukemia Association
Roosevelt Field, Lower Concourse, Garden
City, N.Y. 11530, (516) 741-1190

National Lupus Erythematosus Foundation
5430 Van Nuys Blvd., Suite 206, Van Nuys,
Calif. 91401, (818) 885-8747

**National Maternal and Child Health Clearing-
house**
38th and R Sts. N.W., Washington, D.C. 20057,
(202) 652-8410

National Multiple Sclerosis Society
205 E. 42nd St., New York, N.Y. 10017,
(212) 986-3240

**The National Neurofibromatosis Foundation,
Inc.**
141 Fifth Ave., Suite 7-S, New York, N.Y.
10010, (212) 460-8980

National Parkinson Foundation
1501 N.W. Ninth Ave., Miami, Fla. 33136; Flor-
ida residents: (800) 433-7022; Out-of-state residents: (800) 327-4545

National Reye's Syndrome Foundation
426 N. Lewis, Bryan, Ohio 43506,
(419) 636-2679

**National Sudden Infant Death Syndrome
Clearinghouse**
8201 Greensboro Dr., McLean, Va. 22102,
(703) 821-8955

**National Sudden Infant Death Syndrome
Foundation**
Two Metro Plaza, Suite 205, 8240 Professional
Place, Landover, Md. 20785, (800) 221-SIDS

Premenstrual Syndrome Action
P.O. Box 16292, Irvine, Calif. 92713,
(714) 752-6355

Reach to Recovery
90 Park Ave., New York, N.Y. 10016,
(212) 599-8200

Resolve, Inc. (Infertility)
P.O. Box 474, Belmont, Mass. 02178,
(617) 484-2424

Scleroderma International Foundation
704 Gardner Center Rd., New Castle, Pa.
16101, (412) 652-3109

Smokenders
214 S. 42nd St., Philadelphia, Pa. 19104,
(215) 386-1403

Stroke Club International
805 12th St., Galveston, Tex. 77550,
(409) 762-1022

United Cerebral Palsy Association, Inc.
66 E. 34th St., New York, N.Y. 10016,
(212) 481-6300

United Ostomy Association, Inc.
2001 W. Beverly Blvd., Los Angeles, Calif.
90057, (213) 413-5510

VD National Hotline
260 Sherican Ave., Palo Alto, Calif. 94306; California residents: (800) 982-5833; Out-of-state
residents: (800) 227-8922

REFERENCES AND ACKNOWLEDGMENTS

Advice for the Patient, vol. II. Rockville, Md.: United States Pharmacopeial Convention, Inc., 1985.

The American Medical Association. *Straight-Talk No-Nonsense Guide to Back Care.* New York: Random House, 1984.

Barber, Triphy C., and Langfitt, Dot E. *Teaching the Medical-Surgical Patient: Diagnostics and Procedures.* Bowie, Md.: Robert J. Brady Co., 1983.

Beam, Ida Marlene. "Alzheimer's Disease: Helping Families Survive," *American Journal of Nursing* 84(2):229-32, February 1984.

Bell, W.C., et al. *Home Care and Rehabilitation in Respiratory Medicine.* Philadelphia: J.B. Lippincott Co., 1984.

Bennett, R.L., and Griffin, W.D. "Patient Controlled Analgesia," *Contemporary Surgery* 22(4):75-89, April 1983.

Bethea, Doris C. *Introductory Maternity Nursing,* 4th ed. Philadelphia: J.B. Lippincott Co., 1984.

Bille, D.A. *Practical Approaches to Patient Teaching.* Boston: Little, Brown & Co., 1981.

Boos, M.L. "A Program of Home Traction for Congenital Dislocation of the Hip," *Orthopaedic Nursing* 1(2):11-16, March/April 1982.

Brodoff, A. "Optimizing Care for the AIDS Patient," *Patient Care* 18(2):125-31, January 30, 1984.

Cancer Chemotherapy Handbook. Association of Pediatric Nurses, 1985.

Cardiovascular Disorders. Nurse's Clinical Library. Springhouse, Pa.: Springhouse Corp., 1984.

DeWys, W. "Management of Cancer Cachexia," *Seminars in Oncology* 12(4):461-65, December 1985.

Diagnostics, 2nd ed. Nurse's Reference Library. Springhouse, Pa.: Springhouse Corp., 1986.

Diseases, 2nd ed. Nurse's Reference Library. Springhouse, Pa.: Springhouse Corp., 1986.

Dodson, Margaret E. *The Management of Post-Operative Pain.* Baltimore: Edward Arnold, 1986.

Dodd, M.J., and Mood, D.W. "Chemotherapy: Helping Patients to Know the Drugs They Are Receiving and Their Possible Side Effects," *Cancer Nursing.* 4(4):311-18, August 1981.

D'Onofrio, C.N. "Evaluating Patient Education: Purposes, Politics, and a Proposal for Practitioners," in *Patient Education, An Inquiry into the State of the Art.* Edited by Squyres, W.D. New York: Springer Publishing Co., 1980.

Drug Information for the Health Care Provider, 5th ed. Rockville, Md.: United States Pharmacopeial Convention, Inc., 1985.

Ellenberg, M., and Rifkin, Harold, eds. *Diabetes Mellitus: Theory and Practice,* 3rd ed. New Hyde Park, N.Y.: Medical Examination Pub. Co., 1983.

Endocrine Disorders. Nurse's Clinical Library. Springhouse, Pa.: Springhouse Corp., 1984.

Falvo, Donna R. *Effective Patient Education: A Guide to Increased Compliance.* Rockville, Md.: Aspen Systems Corp., 1984.

Fithian, J. *Understanding the Child with a Chronic Illness in the Classroom.* Phoenix, Ariz.: Onyx Press, 1984.

Garrett, Elise. "Parkinsonism: Forgotten Considerations in Medical Treatment and Nursing Care," *Journal of Neurosurgical Nursing* 14(1):13-18, February 1982.

Gill, Frances M. "Treatment of Sickle Cell Disease," in *Conn's Current Therapy.* Edited by Rakel, R. Philadelphia: W.B. Saunders Co., 1984.

Guzzetta, Cathie E., et al. *Cardiovascular Nursing: Body Mind Tapestry.* St. Louis, Mo.: C.V. Mosby Co., 1984.

Hershman, J. *Endocrine Pathophysiology: A Patient-Oriented Approach,* 2nd ed. Philadelphia: Lea & Febiger, 1982.

Jensen, M., and Bobak, I. *Maternity and Gynecologic Care: The Nurse and the Family.* St. Louis, Mo.: C.V. Mosby Co., 1985.

Joseph, K., et al. "Home Traction in the Management of Congenital Dislocation of the Hip," *Clinical Orthopaedics and Related Research* 165:83-90, 1982.

Kaufman, Joseph J. *Current Urologic Therapy.* Philadelphia: W.B. Saunders Co., 1986.

Kernaghan, Salvinija. "Preadmission Preoperative Teaching: A Promising Option," *Promoting Health* 6(2):6-8, March/April 1985.

Kess, Rachelle. "Suddenly in Crisis: Unpredictable Myasthenia," *American Journal of Nursing* 84(8):994-98, August 1984.

Larson, Elaine. *Clinical Microbiology and Infection Control.* Boston: Blackwell Scientific Publications, 1984.

Mandell, G.G., et al., eds. *Principles and Practices of Infectious Diseases.* New York: John Wiley & Sons, 1985.

McCorkle, R., and Germino, B. "What Nurses Need to Know About Home Care," *Oncology Nursing Forum* 11(6):63-69, November/December 1984.

Medication Teaching Manual: A Guide for Patient Counselling. Bethesda, Md.: American Society of Hospital Pharmacists, 1983.

Mulley, D.A. "Harnessing Babies' Dysplastic Hips," *American Journal of Nursing* 84(8):1006-8, August 1984.

Neoplastic Disorders. Nurse's Clinical Library. Springhouse, Pa.: Springhouse Corp. 1985.

Newell, Frank W. *Ophthalmology: Principles and Concepts.* St. Louis, Mo.: C.V. Mosby Co., 1982.

Notelovitz, M., and Ware, M. *Stand Tall! The Informed Woman's Guide to Preventing Osteoporosis.* Gainesville, Fla.: Triad Publishing Co., 1982.

Nursing87 Drug Handbook. Springhouse, Pa.: Springhouse Corp., 1987.

Oski, Frank, and McMillan, Julia. "Iron in Infant Nutrition," in *Textbook of Pediatric Nutrition.* Edited by Robert Suskind. New York: Raven Press Pubs., 1981.

Parker, Susan. *Pediatric Care: A Guide for Patient Education.* Norwalk, Conn.: Appleton-Century-Crofts, 1983.

Pellino, T. "Chymopapain: Alternatives to Laminectomy for Herniated Lumbar Discs," *Orthopaedic Nursing* 2(2):14-21, 1983.

Petton, S. "Easing the Complications of Chemotherapy: A Matter of Little Victories," *Nursing84* 14(2):58-64, February 1984.

Rankin, Sally H., and Duffy, Karen. *Patient Education: Issues, Principles, and Guidelines.* Philadelphia: J.B. Lippincott Co., 1983.

Regan, Patricia, ed. *Massachusetts General Hospital Teaching Guide for Patients with Neurologic Disorders.* Reston, Va.: Reston Publishing Co., 1984.

Reich, Paul R. *Hematology: Physiopathologic Basis for Clinical Practice,* 2nd ed. Boston: Little, Brown & Co., 1984.

Respiratory Disorders. Nurse's Clinical Library. Springhouse, Pa.: Springhouse Corp., 1984.

Ridder, Marie. "Nursing Update on Alzheimer's Disease," *Journal of Neurological Nursing* 17(3):190-200, June 1985.

Ruzicki, D.A. "Evaluation: It's What You Do with What You've Got That Counts," *Promoting Health* (9-10):6-9, September/October 1985.

Sadler, Diane. *Nursing for Cardiovascular Health.* Norwalk, Conn.: Appleton-Century-Crofts, 1984.

Sergi-Swinehart, P. "Hospice Home Care: How to Get Patients Home and Help Them Stay There," *Seminars in Oncology,* 12(4):461-65, December 1985.

Sheard, C.M. "How Effective is Our Advice to Diabetics? A Preliminary Evaluation," *Human Nutrition: Applied Nutrition* 38(2):138-41, April 1984.

Shipes, E. "Effective Patient Teaching," in *Principles of Ostomy Care.* Edited by Broadwell, D., and Jackson, B. St. Louis, Mo.: C.V. Mosby Co., 1982.

Signs & Symptoms. Nurse's Reference Library. Springhouse, Pa.: Springhouse Corp., 1986.

Silvers, I.J., et al. "Assessing Physician/Patient Perceptions in Rheumatoid Arthritis: A Vital Component in Patient Education," *Arthritis and Rheumatism* 28(3):300-7, March 1985.

Smith, Dorothy L. *Medication Guide for Patient Counseling,* 2nd ed. Philadelphia: Lea & Febiger, 1981.

Snyder, Mariah, ed. *A Guide to Neurological and Neurosurgical Nursing.* New York: John Wiley & Sons, 1983.

Spivak, Jerry L., ed. *Fundamentals of Clinical Hematology,* 2nd ed. Philadelphia: Harper & Row Publishers, 1984.

Vaughn, Daniel, and Asbury, Taylor. *General Ophthalmology,* 10th ed. Los Altos, Calif.: Lange Medical Pubns., 1983.

Veenker, C.H. "Evaluating Health Practice and Understanding," *Health Education* 16(2):80-82, February 1985.

Walsh, P.C., et al. *Campbell's Urology.* Philadelphia: W.B. Saunders Co., 1986.

Wintrobe, Maxwell M., et al., eds. *Clinical Hematology,* 8th ed. Philadelphia: Lea & Febiger, 1981.

Woldum, Karyl, et al. *Patient Education: Foundations of Practice.* Rockville, Md.: Aspen Systems Corp., 1985.

Acknowledgments

p. 13: "Saving Time for Teaching" adapted from Gerri George, RN, MSN, "If Patient Teaching Tries Your Patience, Try This Plan," *Nursing82* 12(5):50, May 1982.

pp. 140-141: Chart reprinted with permission of Marlene Ruiz, Director, Inservice and Patient Education, Kaiser Foundation Hospital, San Diego.

p. 355: Illustration adapted from an original drawing by David E. Cook.

Index

A

Abdominal breathing, 178i
Abdominal ultrasonography, 143t
ABG. See Arterial blood gas analysis.
Ability to learn, assessment of, **37-43**
Abnormal grieving, 613
Abrasion, corneal, 652
Abscess, due to premature cessation of therapy, 512
Acceptance, as stage of coping, 613
Accident prevention
in Alzheimer's disease, 258
motor vehicle, 633
in team sports, 634
Accidental poisoning, in children, 627, 629i, 630
Acebutolol, 158-159t
Acetaminophen, 602-603t
Acetazolamide, 384-385t, 492, 502-503t
Acetohexamide, 434-435t
Acid perfusion test, 233t
Acne vulgaris, 650
Acquired immune deficiency syndrome, **466-470**
as complication of hemophilia treatment, 443
transmission of, 468-470
ACS. See American Cancer Society.
Active assistance exercises, 584
Active exercises, 584
range-of-motion, 586-587i
Acute angle-closure glaucoma, 489, 490i, 491, 492-493
Acute renal failure, **352-356**
phases of, 352-353
Acyclovir, 532-533t
Adaptation
assessment of, 28-29i
stages of, 28-29
Addison's disease, 402
Admission procedure, as teaching opportunity, **83**
Adolescence, health promotion during, **631-634**
Adolescent cancer patient, special problems of, 545i
Adolescent suicide, **631-632**
warning signs, 632

Adrenal crisis
as complication of adrenocortical insufficiency, 402, 404-405i
prevention, 406
Adrenergics, 502-503t
Adrenocortical insufficiency, **402-407**
Adulthood, health promotion during, **634-644**
Adult learner, development of, 12
Affective learning domain, 14, 16t, 17
learning goals in, 47, 48t
Age, as risk factor in CAD, 114-115t
Aging, effects of, coping with, **646-647**
AIDS. See Acquired immune deficiency syndrome.
Airborne transmission of infection, 508-509
Albuterol, 202-203t
Alcohol
avoidance of, during pregnancy, 618
and smoking, as cancer risk factors, 544-545
Alcohol abuse, in adolescence, 633
Alcoholism, as cause of cirrhosis, 208
Alimentary hypoglycemia, 424-425
Allergens, 167
Allergic rhinitis, 650
Allopurinol, 348-349t
Alpha-adrenergic blockers, 382-383t
Alprazolam, 600-601t
Alzheimer's disease, **256-258**
guidelines for caring for person with, 258
Alzheimer's Disease and Related Disorders Association, 662
Amantadine, 306-307t, 532-533t
Ambenonium, 306-307t
Ambulation, 584, 588
Ambulatory electrocardiography, 143t
Ambulatory infusion pump, for continuous narcotics infusion, 605, 610
Ambulatory monitoring, 143t

American Allergy Association, 662
American Anorexia/Bulimia Association, 662
American Cancer Society, 662
American Diabetes Association, 662
American Heart Association, 662
American Kidney Fund, 662
American Lung Association, 662
American Parkinson Disease Association, 662
American Reye's Syndrome Association, 662
Amiloride, 162-163t
Aminocaproic acid, 460-461t
Aminopenicillins, 534-535t
Aminophylline, 202-203t
Amiodarone, 150-151t
Amitriptyline, 600-601t
Amniocentesis, 393t
Amoxicillin, 534-535t
Ampicillin, 534-535t
Amputation, 341
wrapping stump after, 342-343i
Amygdalin, 573
Amyotrophic lateral sclerosis, **259-264**
Amyotrophic Lateral Sclerosis Association, 662
Analgesics, 474, 600-601t, 602-603t
Anaphylaxis, 650
as transfusion reaction, 447
Androgens, 458-459
Anecdotal notes, as evaluation technique, 78
Anemia
iron deficiency, **448-449**
sickle cell, **449-454**
Anger
as barrier to learning, 26
as stage of coping, 612
Angina, 112-113
Angiography, 143-144t
Anisotropine, 382-383t
Ankle exercises, 287i
Ankylosing spondylitis, 650-651
Anorexia nervosa, 631
Antacids, 244-245t
Antegrade pyelography, 372t
Antepartal external fetal monitoring, 393t
Anterior cerebral artery syndrome, 267i

Boldface page numbers indicate major entries; i refers to an illustration, t to a table.

C

Boldface page numbers indicate major entries; i refers to an illustration, t to a table.

Boldface page numbers indicate major entries; i refers to an illustration, t to a table.

Boldface page numbers indicate major entries; i refers to an illustration, t to a table.

Boldface page numbers indicate major entries; i refers to an illustration, t to a table.

Boldface page numbers indicate major entries; i refers to an illustration, t to a table.

Boldface page numbers indicate major entries; i refers to an illustration, t to a table.